MW01009132

Essentials of Youth Fitness

Avery D. Faigenbaum, EdD

Rhodri S. Lloyd, PhD

Jon L. Oliver, PhD

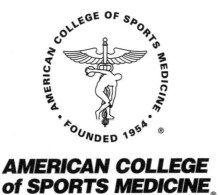

**AMERICAN COLLEGE
of SPORTS MEDICINE**®

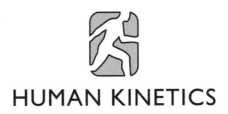

HUMAN KINETICS

Library of Congress Cataloging-in-Publication Data

Names: Faigenbaum, Avery D., 1961- author. | Lloyd, Rhodri S., author. |
 Oliver, Jon L., author. | American College of Sports Medicine, author.
Title: Essentials of youth fitness / Avery Faigenbaum, EdD, Rhodri Lloyd,
 PhD, Jon Oliver, PhD, and American College of Sports Medicine.
Description: Champaign, IL : Human Kinetics, [2020] | Includes
 bibliographical references and index.
Identifiers: LCCN 2019010081 (print) | LCCN 2019011398 (ebook) | ISBN
 9781492591078 (epub) | ISBN 9781492591061 (PDF) | ISBN 9781492525790
 (print)
Subjects: LCSH: Physical fitness for youth. | Exercise for youth.
Classification: LCC RJ133 (ebook) | LCC RJ133 .F345 2020 (print) | DDC
 613.7/042--dc23
LC record available at https://lccn.loc.gov/2019010081

ISBN: 978-1-4925-2579-0 (print)

Copyright © 2020 by Avery Faigenbaum, Rhodri S. Lloyd, Jon L. Oliver, and American College of Sports Medicine

Human Kinetics supports copyright. Copyright fuels scientific and artistic endeavor, encourages authors to create new works, and promotes free speech. Thank you for buying an authorized edition of this work and for complying with copyright laws by not reproducing, scanning, or distributing any part of it in any form without written permission from the publisher. You are supporting authors and allowing Human Kinetics to continue to publish works that increase the knowledge, enhance the performance, and improve the lives of people all over the world.

Care has been taken to confirm the accuracy of the information present and to describe generally accepted practices. However, the authors, editors, and publisher are not responsible for errors or omissions or for any consequences from application of the information in this publication and make no warranty, expressed or implied, with respect to the currency, completeness, or accuracy of the contents of the publication. Application of this information in a particular situation remains the professional responsibility of the practitioner; the clinical treatments described and recommended may not be considered absolute and universal recommendations. The authors, editors, and publisher have exerted every effort to ensure that drug selection and dosage set forth in this text are in accordance with the current recommendations and practice at the time of publication. However, in view of ongoing research, changes in government regulations, and the constant flow of information relating to drug therapy and drug reactions, the reader is urged to check the package insert for each drug for any change in indications and dosage and for added warnings and precautions. This is particularly important when the recommended agent is a new or infrequently employed drug. Some drugs and medical devices presented in this publication have Food and Drug Administration (FDA) clearance for limited use in restricted research settings. It is the responsibility of the health care provider to ascertain the FDA status of each drug or device planned for use in their clinical practice.

For more information concerning the American College of Sports Medicine certification and suggested preparatory materials, call (800) 486-5643 or visit the American College of Sports Medicine website at www.acsm.org.

The web addresses cited in this text were current as of May 2019, unless otherwise noted.

Senior Acquisitions Editors: Amy N. Tocco and Michelle Maloney; **Developmental Editor:** Laura Pulliam; **Managing Editors:** Shawn Donnelly and Julia R. Smith; **Copyeditor:** Tom Tiller; **Indexer:** Nan N. Badgett; **Permissions Manager:** Martha Gullo; **Senior Graphic Designer:** Joe Buck; **Cover Designer:** Keri Evans; **Cover Design Associate:** Susan Rothermel Allen; **Photographs (cover and interior):** Daniel Erman/© Human Kinetics, unless otherwise noted; **Photo Asset Manager:** Laura Fitch; **Photo Production Coordinator:** Amy M. Rose; **Photo Production Manager:** Jason Allen; **Senior Art Manager:** Kelly Hendren; **Illustrations:** © Human Kinetics, unless otherwise noted; **Printer:** Sheridan Books; **ACSM Publications Committee Chair:** Jeffrey A. Potteiger, PhD, FACSM; **ACSM Chief Content Officer:** Katie Feltman; **ACSM Development Editor:** Angie Chastain

Printed in the United States of America

10 9 8 7 6 5 4 3 2 1

The paper in this book is certified under a sustainable forestry program.

Human Kinetics
P.O. Box 5076
Champaign, IL 61825-5076
Website: www.HumanKinetics.com

In the United States, email info@hkusa.com or call 800-747-4457.
In Canada, email info@hkcanada.com.
In the United Kingdom/Europe, email hk@hkeurope.com.

For information about Human Kinetics' coverage in other areas of the world,
please visit our website: **www.HumanKinetics.com**

E6740

Tell us what you think!
Human Kinetics would love to hear what we
can do to improve the customer experience.
Use this QR code to take our brief survey.

We dedicate this book to all parents, coaches, teachers, professionals, and volunteers who work to keep children healthy, fit, and strong. You provide youth with the opportunity to experience the many benefits offered by sport and exercise, thus helping them to develop skills that will last a lifetime. This book was written for you and for aspiring youth fitness specialists. In it, we hope you find ideas that positively influence your practice and help inspire the children with whom you work.

CONTENTS

PREFACE

In pediatric exercise science, as in many disciplines, it is essential for scientists and practitioners to exchange knowledge and cooperate. This approach enables us to help youth of all ages and abilities to participate in evidence-based training programs. Too often, however, scientific research and practical teaching, or coaching, are viewed as separate and even opposing entities. We firmly believe that science and practice can, and should, interact synergistically to maximize the exercise experience for all youth. The desire to blend up-to-date scientific theory with real-world application has shaped this textbook at each step of the process, from the initial conceptual design right through to the final product, which we believe will stand alone in the field of pediatric exercise science due to its ability to blend science with practice.

The book will also provide great value to students (both undergraduate and postgraduate), teachers and professors, coaches, and health care providers. We hope that it will be found not only in university libraries but also in the training facilities used by youth fitness instructors, strength and conditioning coaches, and athletic trainers, as well as the clinical settings of physiotherapists and sport physicians.

Essentials of Youth Fitness is organized in a way that takes you on a journey of learning and discovery. Part I introduces you to the fundamental concepts of pediatric exercise science by covering pediatric physiology, growth and maturation, long-term athletic development, and pedagogical strategies for youth fitness specialists. These early chapters provide you with grounding principles that will help you develop a robust understanding of the topics covered in the rest of the book.

Part II begins with chapters on assessing youth fitness and conducting a warm-up, then moves into a series of chapters devoted to the development of various fitness components, including motor skills, strength and power, speed and agility, and aerobic and anaerobic fitness. This part of the book closes with a chapter on integrative program design, which focuses on the science and art of designing training programs. Throughout the chapters included in part II, you will be given insights into how the development of fitness can be influenced by interactions between growth, maturation, and training; you will also be shown how to design training sessions to meet the needs of young people with varying abilities.

Part III presents a collection of chapters covering key modern-day topics in pediatric exercise science. Population-specific chapters focus on young athletes participating in organized sport, overweight and obese youth, and individuals diagnosed with certain clinical conditions. The final chapter addresses the important topic of nutritional approaches for youth populations.

Throughout *Essentials of Youth Fitness*, a number of key features are included to enhance your learning experience. For instance, each chapter sets out clear chapter objectives, which you can refer back to in order to check for understanding. In addition, boxes titled "Do You Know?" provide bits of information in much the same way that a succinct message might be shared on a social media platform. Each chapter also includes teaching tips to help contextualize important themes or highlight key messages, as well as a list of key terms (bolded in the text) to stimulate reflective discussion. In part II, some chapters include sample training programs with accompanying exercise photos.

Although it is possible to simply pick up this book and read individual chapters, the best way to use the text is to read the chapters in sequence while making full use of the learning aids. This approach not only provides you with information that is immediately useful but also allows the book to serve as a seminal resource that you can refer back to in order to facilitate your ongoing prescription and delivery of exercise to all youth.

ACKNOWLEDGMENTS

It has been said that you can see farther if you stand on the shoulders of giants. This metaphor captures our appreciation and admiration for the pioneers in pediatric exercise science, sports medicine, and youth fitness who have led us to where we are today. While it is not possible to recognize every pediatric researcher, clinician, or practitioner who has influenced our thinking, careers, and lives, we specifically recognize Neil Armstrong, John Cronin, William Kraemer, Lyle Micheli, Greg Myer, Tom Rowland, Wayne Westcott, and Craig Williams.

We thank the American College of Sports Medicine for entrusting us with the opportunity to coauthor this book. It has been an honor and a privilege, and we are grateful for the unwavering support provided by Angie Chastain and Katie Feltman over the past five years. Thanks are also due to Karin Pfeiffer, PhD, FACSM, at Michigan State University for insightful feedback on the book. In addition, we owe a huge debt of gratitude to the staff at Human Kinetics, especially Michelle Maloney and Laura Pulliam, for their guidance, direction, and editorial prowess. Many people at Human Kinetics supported our vision for this book and worked hard to coordinate the final production. We also thank Daniel Erman, Sylvia Moeskops, Tom Mathews, and the models for their outstanding work during the photo shoot.

We acknowledge the many colleagues, students, and children with whom we have crossed paths. You have influenced our careers and provided ongoing support and inspiration for our work in pediatric exercise science. We are humbled by the opportunity to write this book, and we extend our deepest gratitude to each of you.

Finally, we acknowledge those who have helped and endured the most as we have made this journey: our loved ones. Taking on the formidable challenge of writing this text was hugely rewarding but often all consuming. Our loved ones offered unconditional support and understanding throughout the process, and we would not have made it through without them.

To Tamara, for your unwavering love and support.

   Avery D. Faigenbaum

To my immediate family—in particular, Mum, Dad, and Rhys—for your unconditional support. To my beautiful wife, Rhia, for your encouragement, understanding, love, and friendship. To our two amazing children, Ava and Oliver, for being my constant source of inspiration.

   Rhodri S. Lloyd

To Melissa, Isla, and Ivy—for everything. *xxx*

   Jon L. Oliver

PART I
FUNDAMENTAL CONCEPTS

CHAPTER 1

Physical Activity and Children's Health

CHAPTER OBJECTIVES

- Discuss worldwide trends in youth physical inactivity
- Explain the long-term effects of physical inactivity on disease risk
- Identify the physical, mental, and cognitive benefits of physical activity for youth
- Introduce physical activity recommendations from infancy through adolescence
- Provide an overview of age-related strategies for activating youth
- Justify the role of the youth fitness specialist

KEY TERMS

athleticism (p. 15)

children (p. 4)

developmental milestone (p. 7)

exercise (p. 4)

exercise deficit disorder (p. 7)

fundamental movement skill (p. 13)

muscular fitness (p. 12)

ontogenetic (p. 4)

phylogenetic (p. 4)

physical activity (p. 4)

physical fitness (p. 13)

physical inactivity (p. 4)

physical literacy (p. 4)

primordial prevention (p. 10)

sedentary behaviors (p. 6)

self-efficacy (p. 4)

Introduction

The belief that daily **physical activity** is essential for health and well-being predates the historical writings of classical Greek philosophy and medicine. Although some early observers suggested that disease resulted from superstitious and mystical forces, physicians such as Hippocrates and Galen spoke of the health-related effects of **exercise** and the importance of establishing positive lifestyle habits. Thus, more than 2,000 years ago, these physicians and other notable healers recognized the salutary benefits of daily physical activity and the importance of prescribing the right "dose" of exercise to enhance health and well-being without overuse. Hippocrates in particular is credited with the famous statement, "If we could give every individual the right amount of nourishment and exercise, not too little and not too much, we would have found the safest way to health."

Although Hippocrates' early conviction focused on the importance of an exercise regimen for adults, current findings indicate that youth also benefit from this sage counsel. However, during the past decade, epidemiological reports and clinical observations indicate that some **children** and adolescents are not as active as they should be, whereas others experience overuse injuries and burnout due to overemphasis on intensive sport training at an early age (Aubert et al., 2018; Brenner & Council on Sports Medicine and Fitness, 2016; Collings et al., 2014; Corder et al., 2016; LaPrade et al., 2016; Tremblay et al., 2016). Fortunately, youth fitness specialists are becoming more aware of the importance of prescribing the right dose of physical activity during the growing years in order to optimize training adaptations while sparking an ongoing interest in free play, fitness activities, and youth sport. In fact, the need to encourage participation in physical activity as part of a healthy lifestyle is so compelling that the American College of Sports Medicine (ACSM) launched a program called Exercise Is Medicine to promote collaboration between health care providers and exercise professionals. This global health initiative is grounded in the belief that physical activity is critical to preventing and treating diseases and that exercise professionals play an essential role in educating the community about the benefits of physical activity across the lifespan (Sallis, Matuszak, et al., 2016).

In view of the consequences of **physical inactivity**— for global health and for the economic, environmental, and social dimensions of life—we need strategies for establishing healthy behaviors early on, before youth become resistant to targeted interventions. More specifically, we need developmentally appropriate programs in schools, recreation centers, and sport facilities to help school-age youth gain the skills, strength, and confidence they need in order to participate robustly in a variety of physical activities. Interventions that promote healthy living, improve physical fitness, and optimize athletic performance can be developed by youth fitness specialists who understand the essential principles of pediatric exercise science, teach effectively, and appreciate the developmental diversity of boys and girls.

Youth Fitness Specialists

The goal of pediatric exercise is not simply to engage in at least 60 minutes of moderate to vigorous physical activity daily but to enhance a child's competence and confidence for participating in a variety of games, activities, and sports with energy, vigor, and interest. Youth tend to be active in different ways and for different reasons than older populations, and their needs, abilities, and interests are often inconsistent with exercise programs and training philosophies designed for adults. Consequently, the essential principles of pediatric exercise science need to be balanced with pedagogical expertise to improve learning outcomes, optimize training adaptations, and enhance **physical literacy**. Youth who are physically literate value human movement and enjoy participating in active play, exercise, and sport activities. They are cognizant of the benefits of physical activity, competent and confident in a range of movement skills, and help others make healthy lifestyle choices. This confluence is where the art and science of youth exercise programming come into play, because the quantitative aspects of prescribing exercise must be balanced with the qualitative aspects of implementing programs (Faigenbaum & Rial, 2018; Pesce, Faigenbaum, Goudas, & Tomporowski, 2018).

Simply having played a college sport or being trained to work with older adults does not necessarily qualify an exercise professional to design, implement, and assess youth fitness programs for participants with diverse needs, goals, and abilities. To the contrary, for the safety and well-being of all participants, exercise professionals who want to work with youth—whether in schools, fitness centers, or sport programs—should design programs with an acute awareness of age-specific concepts, teaching strategies, and principles of developmental physiology. The most effective youth programs include education and training by youth fitness specialists who are skillful in teaching youth and who understand how adaptations from exercise programs are influenced both by **ontogenetic** factors (related to growth and development) and by **phylogenetic** differences (related to genetic endowment) (Rowland, 2005).

Youth fitness specialists who genuinely appreciate the physical and psychosocial uniqueness of younger populations are well positioned to foster **self-efficacy**

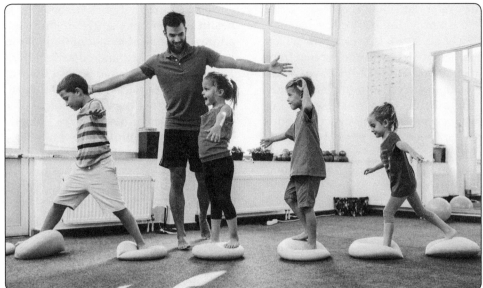

BraunS/E+/Getty Images

Youth fitness specialists should educate, motivate, and inspire all participants.

(confidence in one's ability to perform a specific task) and deliver youth exercise programs that are safe, effective, and enjoyable. Moreover, when practitioners model appropriate behaviors and develop a philosophy that is consistent with the physical and psychosocial uniqueness of youth, they are better prepared to teach positive lessons and spark lifelong interest in physical activity. By learning about the essentials of youth fitness, practitioners can best prepare themselves to help young people become the best they can be.

Physical Inactivity and Public Health

The term *physical inactivity* is used when an individual does not accumulate the recommended amount of regular physical activity. The American College of Sports Medicine (2018) recognizes physical inactivity as a modifiable risk factor for the prevention and control of noncommunicable diseases. Moreover, large-scale reports have confirmed that physical activity and chronic disease mortality are marked by a dose–response relationship (Arem et al., 2015; Yu, Yarnell, Sweetnam, & Murray, 2003; Zhao et al., 2014). In adult populations, it has been estimated that inactive living increases the relative risk of coronary artery disease, stroke, hypertension, and osteoporosis by 45 percent, 60 percent, 30 percent, and 59 percent, respectively (Booth & Lees, 2007). The public health burden and economic costs associated with physical inactivity have resulted in calls to increase population-level amounts of physical activity and to promote collaboration between health care providers and other professionals

in order to encourage active living (W. Kraus et al., 2015; B. Lee et al., 2017; Sallis, Matuszak, et al., 2016). It has also become clear that some physical activity is better than none and that we need a paradigm shift toward disease prevention and comprehensive care.

Years ago, the term *hypokinetic disease* was used to describe a condition resulting from insufficient movement and exercise (H. Kraus & Raab, 1961); the word *hypokinetic* literally means "less" (*hypo*) "movement" (*kinetic*). At that time, a lack of physical activity, particularly in a growing child, was recognized as a medical condition comparable to long-term vitamin deficiency. Accordingly, health care providers were taught to recognize the potential dangers of underexercise in order to prevent their wards from experiencing disease from "motion-deficiency" as much as from contagion or lack of vitamins (H. Kraus & Raab, 1961). Years later, Rowland (1990) emphasized the importance of diagnosing "exercise deficiency" early in life by directly questioning family members about their exercise habits, leisure activities, and sport involvement. Indeed, the lifestyle habits of parents should not be overlooked, because young children who receive greater parental support for physical activity are more than six times as likely to be highly active as they are to be inactive (Zecevic, Trembla, Lovsin, & Michel, 2010).

In view of the global effect of physical inactivity on health and well-being, some observers suggest that this issue should be described as a pandemic with far-reaching consequences (Kohl et al., 2012). Indeed, the proportion of youth worldwide who engage daily in at least 60 minutes of moderate to vigorous physical activity (MVPA) is troublingly low (Aubert et al., 2018;

Guthold, Cowan, Autenrieth, Kann, & Riley, 2010; Hallal et al., 2012; Kalman et al., 2015; Konstabel et al., 2014; Tremblay et al., 2016). In one report, which described physical activity levels of adolescents from 105 countries, only 20 percent of 13- to 15-year-olds engaged in the recommended 60 minutes of daily MVPA (Hallal et al., 2012). Even worse, emerging awareness of objectively measured MVPA in U.S. adolescents revealed that fewer than 9 percent meet current physical activity recommendations and that this low level persisted through the transition to adulthood (Li et al., 2016). Other researchers objectively assessed the physical activity levels of European children (2.0 to 10.9 years old) and reported that the percentage of children complying with current MVPA recommendations ranged from 2 percent in Cyprus to 15 percent in Sweden (Konstabel et al., 2014). In addition, the volume and intensity of after-school physical activities (e.g., dance, sport) also falls short of expectations because young people spend a large proportion of time in sedentary or light physical activities (Cain et al., 2015; Guagliano, Rosenkranz, & Kolt, 2013; Leek et al., 2010; Ridley, Zabeen, & Lunnay, 2018).

Given that school-age youth spend a large proportion of their waking hours being sedentary, we need to examine the associations between **sedentary behaviors** and health indicators (Colley et al., 2011; Matthews et al., 2008). The term *sedentary behavior* refers to any waking behavior characterized by an energy expenditure of less than or equal to 1.5 METS (metabolic equivalent units) while seated, reclining, or lying (United States Department of Health and Human Services, 2018). Examples of sedentary behavior include television viewing, computer use, and compulsive texting. Although different types of sedentary behavior may affect health differently, higher durations of sedentary behavior, particularly screen time, are generally associated with unfavorable health outcomes in youth (Carson et al., 2016). Current recommendations limit recreational screen time to no more than two hours per day, and additional health benefits are seen with lower screen time (Tremblay, Leblanc, et al., 2011). The American Academy of Pediatrics discourages the use of electronic media by children younger than two years; instead, it encourages unstructured, unplugged play, which is more valuable for the developing brain (Council on Communications and Media, 2016).

DO YOU KNOW?

Though all children must engage in some sedentary behavior throughout the day, scheduling sedentary behavior in shorter bouts may be associated with improved health outcomes.

Physical inactivity has become the biggest public health problem of the 21st century, and in order to address it we need to mount multidisciplinary efforts in advocacy, policy, and education (Kohl et al., 2012; I. Lee et al., 2012; United States Department of Health and Human Services, 2018). Yet physical inactivity has yet to garner the recognition of other risk factors for cardiovascular disease even though it contributes more to poor health than do high blood pressure or high blood glucose (Blair, 2009; W. Kraus et al., 2015; Fletcher, 2018). Fortunately, the incontrovertible effects exerted by childhood physical inactivity on lifelong pathological processes have at least encouraged some creative initiatives to disseminate practice-based evidence and enhance public awareness of the benefits of physical activity.

For example, physical activity report cards have been used in many countries to analyze global variations in physical activity among youth and to improve the grades in all countries (Aubert et al., 2018; Tremblay et al., 2016; Tremblay et al., 2014); an example is provided in figure 1.1. Researchers from 49 participating countries were encouraged to use the best available evidence to create a report card based on 10 common indicators: overall physical activity, organized sport and physical activity, active play, active transportation, sedentary behaviors, physical fitness, family and peers, school, community and environment, and government. The grading framework for physical activity ranged from a grade of A (≥87% of youth meeting recommendations) to a grade of F (<20% of youth meeting recommendations). In terms of overall physical activity, the average grade around the world was D (low/poor), and troubling trends were observed across countries with diverse socioeconomic, cultural, and geographical contexts (Aubert et al., 2018). These observations are consistent with findings from a 50-country comparison focused on the 20-meter shuttle run and involving over one million participants aged 9 to 17 years (Lang, Tremblay, Léger, Olds, & Tomkinson, 2018). Youth in Africa and Central and Northern Europe were among the best performers, and those from South America were among the worst. Collectively, these findings provide valuable information that can be used to alter the current trajectory of low physical activity and stimulate the cross-fertilization of ideas for improving the physical activity behaviors of children and adolescents worldwide.

DO YOU KNOW?

Screen time and work obligations in developed countries appear to be slowly replacing active play during free time.

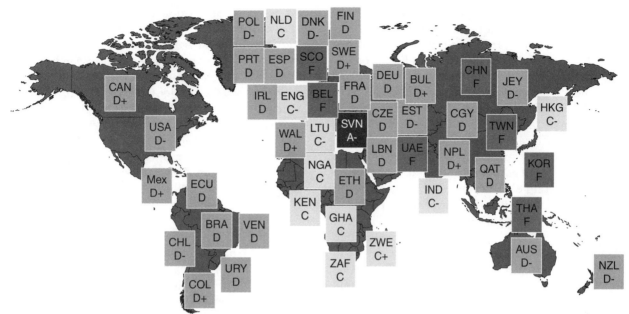

FIGURE 1.1 Grades for overall physical activity among children and adolescents.
Data from Aubert, Barnes, Abdeta, et al. (2018).

The effect of physical inactivity on lifelong patho-logical processes is so compelling that physical inactivity should be recognized as a disease in its own right. In fact, the term **exercise deficit disorder** (EDD) has been introduced to convey a fresh view of this condition, which is characterized by low levels of MVPA that are inconsistent with public health recom-mendations and long-term well-being (Faigenbaum & Myer, 2012; Myer et al., 2013; Stracciolini, Myer, & Faigenbaum, 2013). The construct of EDD is unique because there are no clinical markers or laboratory tests for identifying an inactive child or teenager with poor movement skills. Moreover, there are no medications to treat this condition, and it is unlikely that an inactive child will simply "outgrow" EDD without structured intervention. Therefore, youth who do not meet the current recommendation of at least 60 minutes of MVPA per day (i.e., 420 min per wk) should receive a developmentally appropriate exercise plan with ongoing support to participate in active play, exercise, and sport activities.

The use of the word *exercise* in *exercise deficit disor-der* does not suggest that free play is inconsequential; rather, it emphasizes the premise that youth should participate daily in a variety of physical activities that are safe, meaningful, and enjoyable. The construct of EDD can be used to educate youth about the link between exercise and health, to inform parents about positive lifestyle choices, and to identify barriers (both real and perceived) to sustainable collabora-tion between health care providers and youth fitness specialists. Currently, health agencies and health care providers have been urged to advance universal health through key actions that include screening for physical inactivity, counseling about physical activity, and investing in comprehensive policies to promote physical activity (Kohl et al., 2012; W. Kraus et al., 2015; Sallis, Matuszak, et al., 2016). Concerted efforts are needed to promote physical activity and reduce time spent in sedentary behaviors in order to improve health indicators in youth.

DO YOU KNOW?

Physical inactivity is now the fourth-leading risk factor for global mortality.

The importance of screening all youth for physi-cal inactivity early in life should not be overlooked in the health care setting (Myer et al., 2013; Walker, Stracciolini, Faigenbaum, & Myer, 2018; World Health Organization, 2018). Even though inactive infants and toddlers may reach **developmental milestones**, such as taking the first step or kicking a ball at the desired age, they may not be accumulating the desired amount of physical activity daily. In most pediatric clinics, however, health screening relates mainly to vision, hearing, and body mass index and is typically void of any meaningful assessment of physical activity. This failure constitutes a missed opportunity to assess current physical activity habits, provide anticipatory guidance, and promote regular participation in age-ap-propriate activities that are consistent with individual needs, goals, and abilities.

In contrast, screening for a condition such as EDD encourages early detection, promotes intervention, and helps identify youth who may need additional guidance related to motor skill development and fitness conditioning. Along these lines, Healthy People 2020 contains leading health indicators with the overarching goal of attaining high quality lives free of preventable disease, disability, injury, and premature death (United States Department of Health and Human Services, 2016). Notably, Healthy People 2020 objective PA-11.2 aims to increase the number of child and adult patients who receive counseling about exercise in primary health care settings (United States Department of Health and Human Services, 2016). Daily physical activity and other healthy behaviors can also be promoted through policy strategies and medical training designed to achieve competence in lifestyle counseling (Hivert et al., 2016; Thornton et al., 2016). Healthy People 2030 will build upon lessons learned over the past four decades and continue to promote healthy behaviors across the lifespan. Figure 1.2 provides a theoretical algorithm for assessing physical activity and identifying youth at risk for EDD.

Although most parents believe their children are physically active on a daily basis, research observations indicate that adults tend to overestimate their children's MVPA (Corder, Crespo, van Sluijs, Lopez, & Elder, 2012; Corder et al., 2010). Throughout childhood and adolescence, daily MVPA appears to decline with age, with an observable drop starting during primary school, at about seven or eight years of age (Nyberg, 2009; Tudor-Locke, 2010; Farooq, 2018; Schwarzfischer et al., 2019). In addition, girls have been reported to be less active than boys during childhood and adolescence (Francis, Morrissey, Letuchy, Levy, & Janz, 2013; Metcalf, Hosking, Jeffery, Henley, & Wilkin, 2015), and youth with physical disabilities or mobility limitations are even less physically active than their typically developing peers, which can negatively affect their functional independence and quality of life (Bloemen et al., 2015; Sit et al., 2017; Wilson, Haegele, & Zhu, 2016).

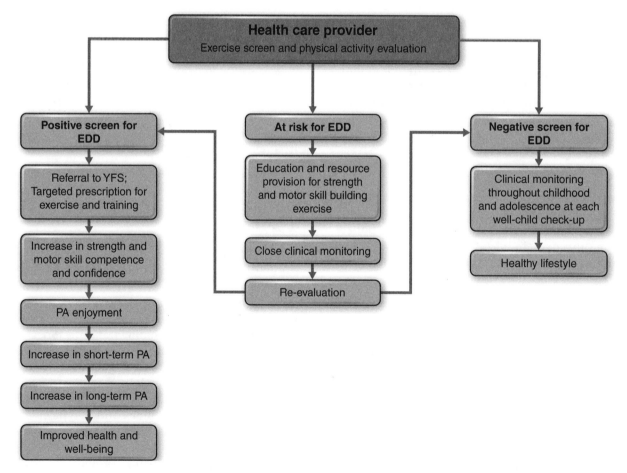

FIGURE 1.2   Theoretical algorithm for assessing physical activity and identifying youth at risk for excercise deficit disorder (EDD). YFS=youth fitness specialist. PA=physical activity.

Adapted by permission from A. Stracciolini, G. Myer, and A. Faigenbaum, "Exercise Deficit Disorder in Youth: Are We Ready to Make the Diagnosis?" *The Physician and Sports Medicine* 41, no. 1 (2013): 94-101.

Disease Prevention Starts Early

Physical inactivity increases the risk of many chronic conditions; moreover, if current trends continue, the health-related consequences of physical inactivity will likely place an unprecedented burden on youth, their families, and our health care systems. The decline in physical activity tends to emerge early in life, and targeted interventions are needed to promote healthy lifestyle choices during the growing years in order to minimize health risks later in life. By the time students reach high school, many already have a low prevalence of ideal behaviors related to cardiovascular health (Fyfe-Johnson et al., 2018; Shay et al., 2013). In addition, we are now seeing risk factors for cardiovascular disease (e.g., hypertension, dyslipidemia, elevated fasting plasma glucose) both in youth who are overweight or obese and in youth of normal weight (May, Kuklina, & Yoon, 2012; Steinberger et al., 2016).

In order to combat the pandemic of physical inactivity and prevent the inevitable cascade of adverse health outcomes, as well as the associated health care costs, we need to begin developmentally appropriate interventions and treatment strategies early in life. Support for early intervention is provided by the landmark Pathobiological Determinants of Atherosclerosis in Youth (PDAY) study, which found strong relationships between risk factors and the severity and extent of atherosclerosis (measured after death) in 15- to 34-year-olds who died accidentally of external causes (Strong et al., 1999). Specifically, the report found a striking increase in severity and extent of disease as the number of risk factors increased; it also found that the absence of risk factors was associated with a virtual absence of advanced atherosclerotic lesions. In other words, establishing healthy habits early in life may prevent the development of risk factors and the progression of pathological processes; therefore, we must work to reduce, if not eliminate, poor lifestyle choices during the formative years of life (Daniels, Hassink, & Committee on Nutrition, 2015; Steinberger et al., 2016; Tanrikulu, Agirbasli, & Berenson, 2017).

This view is supported by observations from the Cardiovascular Risk in Young Finns Study (Laitinen et al., 2012) and the Special Turku Coronary Risk Factor Intervention Project for Children (Pahkala et al., 2013). Both of these projects showed that the number of ideal cardiovascular health behaviors present during childhood and adolescence predicted cardiometabolic health in adulthood. In adolescents who participated in the Special Turku Coronary Risk Factor Intervention Project, ideal cardiovascular health during the teenage years was inversely associated with aortic intima-media thickness and directly associated with elasticity (Pahkala et al., 2013). Aortic intima-media thickness is an important atherosclerotic risk marker and is measured by assessing the thickness of the innermost layers of the walls of the vessel with ultrasound images. Collectively, these findings indicate that the prevalence of obesity, hypertension, and dyslipidemia will likely get worse unless positive health behaviors are established early in life and sustained throughout adolescence and adulthood.

The rise in physical inactivity and obesity early in life is accompanied by a disturbing prevalence of metabolic syndrome, type 2 diabetes, and cardiovascular complications among youth (Bjerregaard et al., 2018; Cote et al., 2015; Kallio et al., 2018). The progression to established type 2 diabetes from an impaired glucose tolerance state seems to occur more rapidly in youth than in adults, and the likelihood that these trends will continue is both real and alarming (Centers for Disease Control and Prevention, 2011; Kehler et al., 2014; Ligthart et al., 2016). One dire projection suggests that the steady rise in life expectancy during the past two centuries may soon come to an end due to the rapid rise in obesity and unhealthy lifestyle behaviors (McCrindle, 2015; Olshansky et al., 2005).

Teaching Tip

FIRST THOUSAND DAYS

The first thousand days of life are recognized as a critical period for optimal nutrition and improved health outcomes (Black et al., 2013). We also need to make concerted efforts to establish habitual physical activity behaviors early in life. Infants who spend too much time in front of a television or in a stroller may experience a delay in motor development. In contrast, playful behaviors—such as crawling, reaching, and "tummy time"—can help infants grow and develop. Therefore, parents and caregivers should limit screen time, dedicate periods of time throughout the day to interactive movement behaviors (Tremblay et al., 2017), and establish healthy eating patterns early in life.

DO YOU KNOW?

Having a television in a child's bedroom is associated with an increased risk of weight gain.

Current trends toward physical inactivity and unhealthy lifestyle behaviors among youth appear to be caused at least in part by a lack of healthy environments (for living, learning, and playing) that support disease prevention, as well as a lack of sustained interventions such as early screening for inactivity. In order to reverse the negative trajectory of physical inactivity and reduce chronic disease, we need to stop considering physically inactive children to be "healthy," regardless of whether they are of normal weight or overweight. Moreover, because the development of chronic disease conditions begins during childhood, interventions that promote health-enhancing behaviors must also begin early in life (Berenson, 2011; Juonala et al., 2010; Tanrikulu et al., 2017). Focusing interventions only on children who are obese, or on adolescents with hypertension, will likely foster a symptom-reactive treatment strategy that is ineffective in the long term.

Whereas primary prevention is designed to treat disease risk factors and prevent disease, **primordial prevention** involves preventing the risk factors themselves (Weintraub et al., 2011). This approach requires broad changes in school curriculums and health policies to minimize the presence of social and environmental conditions that increase the risk of disease. The general concept calls for creating an environment in which healthy behaviors are the norm. Remember, physical activity is a learned behavior that is influenced by a child's family, friends, and environment. Consequently, children who grow up in an environment that provides

insufficient opportunities to participate in a variety of physical activities may not develop the motor skill repertoire and confidence to be physically active later in life. In this situation, the eventual decline in physical activity typically begins to emerge during childhood, and this decline can exert a troubling effect on inactive youth who tend to opt out of fitness activities and sports as their confidence and competence decrease (Belcher et al., 2010; Dishman, McIver, Dowda, & Pate, 2018; Nyberg, Nordenfelt, Ekelund, & Marcus, 2009).

This view is supported by researchers who found that participation in MVPA and vigorous physical activity (VPA) for at least 55 minutes per day was associated with lower odds of obesity, independent of sedentary behavior, in a large multinational sample of children (age 9 to 11 years) from 12 countries (Katzmarzyk et al., 2015). Others observed that 5-year-old boys and girls in the highest quartile of accelerometry-measured MVPA had a lower fat mass at ages 8 and 11 than did 5-year-old children in the lowest quartile of MVPA (Janz et al., 2009). Even among 3- to 5-year-old preschoolers, those with better motor skill proficiency tend to engage more frequently in more advanced physical activities than do children with poor motor skills (O'Neill et al., 2014). These findings support current physical activity recommendations and highlight the importance of making skill-building physical activities a habitual part of every child's life.

Children who do not engage in daily MVPA and do not develop a prerequisite level of motor skill performance early in life may later be unable to break through a hypothesized "proficiency barrier" that prevents them from participating in a variety of physical activities with energy and enthusiasm (Seefeldt, 1980). Although the concept of such a barrier was put forth some four decades ago, the contention that children,

Teaching Tip

FAMILY FITNESS PORTRAIT

Typical vital signs include heart rate, breathing rate, blood pressure, and body temperature. In some medical centers, health care providers also obtain a vital sign for physical activity by asking adult patients about their weekly physical activity habits (Sallis, Baggish, Franklin, & Whitehead, 2016). Similarly, health care providers and youth fitness specialists should paint a family fitness portrait for children by asking them and their parents about their daily physical activity habits. We can shed light on families' activities and their intensity levels by asking follow-up questions about the amount of time spent participating in outdoor games, recreational sports, and fitness activities that require breathing hard. Physical activity should be encouraged from birth, and youth who are not accumulating the recommended amount of daily physical activity should be identified and treated before they become resistant to targeted interventions later in life. If we identify inactive youth and provide their parents with specific recommendations for achieving physical activity goals, we can encourage positive change that is supported within the family structure.

adolescents, and young adults with low motor skill competence are unlikely to achieve desirable levels of MVPA remains relevant today (De Meester et al., 2018; Myer, Faigenbaum, Ford, et al., 2011; Stodden, True, Langendorfer, & Gao, 2013). The concept is particularly relevant for children and adolescents with intellectual or physical disabilities, who should be provided with ample opportunities in school, at sport clubs, and in the community to gain confidence and competence in their physical abilities (Bloemen et al., 2015; Shields, King, Corbett, & Imms, 2014).

Decline and disinterest in physical activity begin even earlier in youth who perceive physical activity to be boring, discomforting, or simply not fun. As illustrated in figure 1.3, children who do not develop adequate levels of muscular fitness and movement skill early in life are less likely to engage in the desired amount of MVPA and more likely to experience disease risk factors and negative health outcomes later in life. Incremental lifetime medical costs are substantially higher for obese children than for children of normal weight, and they will likely increase further unless cost-effective strategies are targeted at preventing excessive weight gain and reducing the prevalence of obesity (Finkelstein, Graham, & Malhotra, 2014; Hollingworth et al., 2012). On a larger scale, direct health care costs, productivity losses, and disability-adjusted life years attributable to physical inactivity contribute to the growing economic burden of this global pandemic (Ding et al., 2016; B. Lee et al., 2017).

Effective, sustainable treatments for childhood obesity are challenging to formulate, costly to implement, and often associated with poor clinical outcomes; therefore, school- and community-based initiatives should be prioritized in order to establish and reinforce healthy behaviors, keep children physically active,

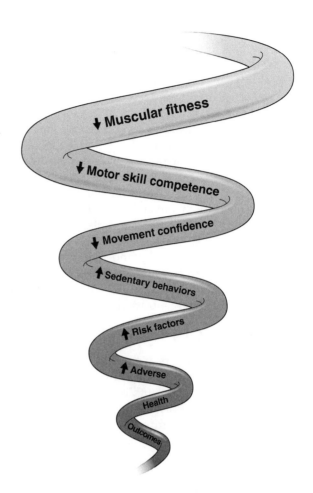

FIGURE 1.3 Downward spiral of adverse health consequences resulting from physical inactivity.

Adapted by permission from A.D. Faigenbaum, R.S. Lloyd, and G.D. Myer, "Youth Resistance Training: Past Practices, New Perspectives, and Future Directions," *Pediatric Exercise Science* 25, no. 4 (2013): 591-604.

Teaching Tip

RIGHT FROM THE START

Although all youth can benefit from developmentally appropriate exercise interventions, childhood in particular provides a unique opportunity to develop and reinforce desired movement patterns due to the high degree of neuromuscular plasticity that characterizes this developmental period (Myer et al., 2015). As compared with adolescents, most children are less self-conscious about making mistakes and therefore tend to be more willing to try new activities. In contrast, older youth with poor motor skills are less likely to be willing to display their low motor competence in front of family members and peers. Fortunately, youth fitness specialists who know how to teach and sensibly progress a variety of games and activities in a supportive environment can create positive learning experiences that give all participants an opportunity to establish proper movement patterns, gain confidence in their physical abilities, and develop healthy behaviors right from the start.

and help them maintain a healthy weight (Institute of Medicine, 2015). Some observers have argued that the absence of a sound strategy for promoting and sustaining physical activity for youth is tantamount to mass child neglect (Weiler, Allardyce, Whyte, & Stamatakis, 2014). Such comparisons highlight the critical need to address this public health crisis and reverse the negative trajectory of physical inactivity and the resulting medical conditions. The undeniable effect of physical inactivity on lifelong pathological processes demands that we expand school programs, active environments, and pediatric research initiatives to develop new diagnostic tools, implement treatment plans, strengthen policy frameworks, and escalate advocacy in order to increase physical activity and reduce sedentary behaviors in youth (Institute of Medicine, 2015; United States Department of Health and Human Services, 2012; World Health Organization, 2018).

Benefits of Physical Activity

Much of what we understand about the stimulus of exercise has been gained from research on adults. Yet we need only watch youth on a playground, in a gymnasium, or on a sport field to find support for the premise that both structured physical activity (e.g., sport, physical education) and unstructured physical activity (e.g., recess, outdoor play) provide children and adolescents with benefits for health and fitness. These observations are supported by research investigations and public health reports that highlight the potential physical, psychosocial, and cognitive benefits of physical activity for school-age youth (Bangsbo et al., 2016; Donnelly et al., 2016; Poitras et al., 2016). Regular participation in developmentally appropriate physical activities is associated with positive physiological adaptations, healthy social interactions, improved academic performance, and meaningful learning experiences that are essential for normal growth and development. More specifically, table 1.1 outlines potential physical, psychosocial, and cognitive benefits

associated with youth physical activity (Bangsbo et al., 2016; Donnelly et al., 2016; Poitras et al., 2016).

Youth fitness specialists possess the necessary information to justify physical activity programs for children and adolescents because of the numerous benefits that have been documented through research (Ortega, Ruiz, Castillo, & Sjostrom, 2008; World Health Organization, 2010). Perhaps equally important, children who are physically active early in life tend to be more active later in life (de Souza et al., 2014; Telama et al., 2014). Children begin to assimilate health-related behaviors at a young age, and early exposure to active play, ball games, and various outdoor activities can help shape their attitudes and values related to physical activity. With this reality in mind, we should consider it *abnormal* for children to remain inactive throughout the day, merely watching television, surfing the web, and texting on smartphones. Youth fitness specialists who teach meaningful content and provide opportunities for all participants to be creative in a supportive environment will likely exert the greatest positive effect on students' lifelong health, fitness, and well-being.

DO YOU KNOW?

All patterns of physical activity—whether sporadic, in bouts, or continuous—improve health indicators in both children and adolescents.

Young people enjoy participating in games, exercises, and activities that are engaging, challenging, and fun. In addition to improving aerobic performance and **muscular fitness** (e.g., muscular strength, muscular power, local muscular endurance) beyond naturally occurring adaptations, regular MVPA can improve markers of cardiovascular and metabolic health. Youth who engage regularly in MVPA tend to have lower adiposity, improved blood lipids, better insulin sensitivity, enhanced endothelial function, and higher bone mineral content and density (Garcia-Hermoso, 2019;

TABLE 1.1   POTENTIAL BENEFITS OF YOUTH PHYSICAL ACTIVITY

Physical	Psychosocial	Cognitive
Enhanced health-related fitness Enhanced skill-related fitness Enhanced musculoskeletal strength Improved body composition Enhanced blood vessel function Improved glucose metabolism Improved blood lipids Improved sleep quality Reduced risk of activity- and sport-related injuries	Improved mental health Improved self-esteem Promotion of positive social interactions Decrease in depressive symptoms Stimulation of feelings of well-being	Enhanced concentration Improved classroom behavior Improved academic performance

Gutin & Owens, 2011; Ortega et al., 2008; Rowland, 2007). In contrast, inactive children exhibit significantly higher clustered cardiometabolic risk scores and lower cardiorespiratory fitness (Boddy et al., 2014).

As youth gain confidence and competence in their **fundamental movement skills**, they are more likely to reinforce desirable movement patterns, engage in different types of physical activity, and realize the health benefits associated with a physically active lifestyle (Cattuzzo et al., 2016; Lubans, Morgan, Cliff, & Barnett, 2010; Utesch, Bardid, Büsch, & Strauss, 2019). Fundamental movement skills are basic movement patterns that are commonly categorized as involving locomotion (e.g., running, jumping), object control (e.g., catching, throwing), or stability (balance and rotation). When children participate regularly in exercise interventions that improve motor skill performance and enhance muscular fitness, they become better prepared for the demands of more advanced exercise programs while reducing the risk of activity- and sport-related injuries (Lauersen, Bertelsen, & Andersen, 2014; Morgan et al., 2013; Sugimoto, Myer, Barber Foss, & Hewett, 2015). When designing programs for children and adolescents, youth fitness specialists also need to be cognizant of individual differences in fitness abilities, because youth with low habitual levels of physical activity are at increased risk for injury during recreational and sport activities (Bloemers et al., 2012; Nauta, Martin-Diener, Martin, van Mechelen, & Verhagen, 2014). Therefore, we need to be careful when prescribing the intensity, volume, and frequency of youth exercise programs and advance them sensibly over time.

Regular participation in MVPA may improve mental health in children and adolescents by decreasing or preventing depressive symptoms (Brown, Pearson, Braithwaite, Brown, & Biddle, 2013; McMahon et al., 2017). Participation in physical activities that are developmentally appropriate and engaging may also stimulate feelings of well-being, improve self-esteem, and promote high-quality sleep at night (Biddle & Asare, 2011; Ekstedt, Nyberg, Ingre, Ekblom, & Marcu, 2013; Galland & Mitchell, 2010). Although more studies are needed to identify the mechanisms that mediate the relationship between physical activity and mental health in school-age youth, it appears that both physiological mechanisms (e.g., hormonal responses) and psychological factors (e.g., positive social interactions) may play a role (Eime, Young, Harvey, Charity, & Payne, 2013; Martikainen et al., 2013). If physical activity programs for youth are nonthreatening and taught by qualified youth fitness specialists, then participants have the opportunity to gain confidence and competence in their physical abilities while making friends, learning something new,

and having fun. However, excessive physical activity with a focus on winning can exert a negative effect on mental health indicators; in some cases, it can even be considered a form of abuse (Hallal, Victora, Azevedo, & Wells, 2006; Oliver & Lloyd, 2014).

Emerging evidence indicates that physically challenging and mentally engaging activities can exert a positive effect on cognitive function and brain health in children and adolescents (Donnelly et al., 2016; Hillman & Biggan, 2017; Lubans et al., 2016). MVPA has been found to improve academic performance by enhancing concentration, focusing attention, and improving classroom behavior (Centers for Disease Control and Prevention, 2010; Donnelly et al., 2016; Ericsson & Karlsson, 2012; Howie & Pate, 2012). Evidence from a nine-month after-school intervention demonstrated a causal effect of physical activity on improvements in cognitive performance and brain function in children, and this finding supports the notion of enhancing brain health through structured MVPA consisting of aerobically demanding exercises and skill-based games (Hillman et al., 2014). We still need to understand more about which specific characteristics of the physical activity stimulus promote changes in brain function and cognition. In the meantime, however, we should remember the importance of multifaceted exercise training that combines aerobic, motor, and muscular training to improve the structure and function of the developing brain (Esteban-Cornejo et al., 2019).

DO YOU KNOW?

Even a single bout of MVPA can have a positive effect on brain function in school-age youth.

Developmental Fitness

Markers of health and fitness change throughout childhood and adolescence. Although children follow the same general trajectory over developmental time, daily physical activity can alter the development of motor skills and the improvement of physical capacity. Figure 1.4 illustrates the possible outcomes of exercise training in school-age youth. The dashed line represents expected gains in physical fitness as a result of growth, development, and periodic bouts of physical activity (e.g., active transportation, free play). For example, a 14-year-old girl will generally jump higher and run faster than an 8-year-old girl, even without structured training.

Further gains in **physical fitness** that might be made through fitness training are illustrated by the bold line. Physical fitness is a state of well-being that enables an individual to perform daily physical activities with energy, vigor, and enjoyment (Malina,

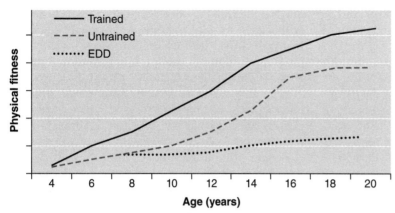

FIGURE 1.4   Possible outcomes of exercise training in youth.

Bouchard, & Bar-Or, 2004). At any age, a child or adolescent who participates in a structured fitness program (e.g., gymnastics, martial arts, fitness conditioning) will gain a performance advantage over age-matched peers who are untrained, and that advantage will be even greater for children who build a strong foundation early in life.

In contrast, the dotted line shows what might happen if a child suffers from EDD and does not participate in adequate MVPA. Likely outcomes include suboptimal gains in physical fitness and a worsening of health markers over time. Without intervention, the divergence in performance between youth with EDD and trained youth will likely widen over developmental time. From a practical perspective, children need to learn how to move with confidence and competence early in life. At the same time, youth fitness specialists need to be aware that for inactive children some physical activity is better than none.

It is a misconception that children innately know how to throw, catch, kick, and jump with proper technique. However, when school-age youth participate in developmentally appropriate physical activities, whether structured or unstructured, they gain opportunities to develop fundamental movement skills that serve as the building blocks for an active lifestyle. Without meaningful instruction, directed movement practice, and a sensible progression of age-appropriate activities, physically inactive children are unlikely to develop the necessary competence and confidence in their physical abilities to be motorically proficient adults.

Longitudinal research has found that proficiency in fundamental movement skills early in life predicts physical activity later in life (Barnett, Van Beurden, Morgan, Brooks, & Beard, 2008; de Souza et al., 2014; Henrique et al., 2018; Lopes, Rodriques, Maia, & Malina, 2011; Utesch, Bardid, Büsch, & Strauss, 2019). Even young children (five to six years of age) with high levels of motor proficiency have been found to engage in more physical activity than their peers with lower motor proficiency (Kambas et al., 2012). Not only do children with higher motor competence possess higher levels of physical fitness, but also they participate more often in sport than do less able children (de Souza et al., 2014; Fransen et al., 2014). These observations highlight the importance of ongoing participation in a variety of skill-building physical activities early in life.

The low level of physical fitness among modern-day youth is fueled at least in part by techno-

Teaching Tip

KEEP EDUCATION PHYSICAL

Although most children and adolescents spend a substantial part of their day in school, it is nearly impossible for all students to accumulate the recommended amount of MVPA through physical education and other school-based strategies that involve physical activity. In addition, in a growing number of school districts, the quality and quantity of physical education have been reduced—and the number of nonspecialists delivering physical education has been increased—due to political and economic pressures to improve standardized test scores. Consequently, we need to make concerted efforts to educate parents, school administrators, and government officials about the critical importance of physical education that is taught by physical education teachers. To reiterate, students who are physically literate and enhance their physical fitness are more likely to learn better in the classroom, engage regularly in physical activity, and support a healthy school environment (National Association for Sport and Physical Education & American Heart Association, 2016; ParticipACTION, 2018; Society of Health and Physical Educators, 2014).

logical advances. Along with declines in aerobic fitness among children and adolescents (Craig, Shields, Leblanc, & Tremblay, 2012), it is common to see lower levels of muscular fitness and motor skill (Cohen et al., 2011; Hardy, Barnett, Espinel, & Okely, 2013; Runhaar et al., 2010). Unless these trends are addressed through age-appropriate interventions targeting exercise deficits early in life, they will likely continue, and the gap between youth with low and high levels of physical fitness will widen across developmental time. Although unstructured physical activities, such as free play, make important contributions to a child's physical growth and psychosocial development, we must emphasize the enduring influence of structured exercise programs in which all participants have an opportunity to learn meaningful content in a supportive environment. Important considerations in such interventions include developing motor skills, enhancing muscle strength, fostering new social networks, and promoting healthy behaviors. Such programming can be provided through sport centers, community programs, and school-based physical education taught by qualified professionals. These approaches have the potential to provide participants with the strength, skills, and abilities they need in order to participate in a variety of lifetime activities with energy and interest.

Structured programs that are purposely designed to enhance the **athleticism** of children and adolescents beginning early in life provide a logical and evidence-based approach to their long-term physical development (Faigenbaum, Lloyd, MacDonald, & Myer, 2016; Granacher et al., 2016; Lloyd & Oliver, 2012). The concept of athleticism addresses the ability to move competently, confidently, and consistently in a variety of settings with speed, style, and precision. Because athleticism is grounded in both skill- and health-related components of physical fitness (see figure 1.5), the concept of athleticism is applicable to inactive youth as well as to aspiring young athletes. An inactive 8-year-old who develops increased athleticism will be better prepared to play outside with friends and to participate actively in physical education classes and recreational fitness opportunities. Similarly, a 14-year-old basketball player who balances sport training with conditioning will be a better player with a broader base of athletic abilities.

Thus children and adolescents need to participate in a range of physical activities that enhance both health- and skill-related components of physical fitness. Instead of prolonged periods of moderate-in-

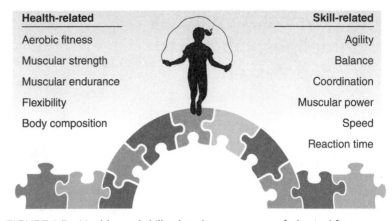

FIGURE 1.5   Health- and skill-related components of physical fitness.

tensity aerobic exercise—which may be less appealing for some youth—exercise programs for children and adolescents should (as tolerated) integrate various types of physical activities with intermittent bouts of vigorous-intensity exercise (Faigenbaum et al., 2011; Myer, Faigenbaum, Chu, et al., 2011). This type of exercise helps young people master fundamental movement skills, improve movement mechanics, and gain confidence in their physical abilities. It may also offer additional value for health and fitness because vigorous-intensity bouts of physical activity are associated with greater improvements in cardiorespiratory fitness, cardiometabolic health, and body composition than less intense bouts of physical activity in school-age youth (Aadland et al., 2018; Hamer & Stamatakis, 2018; Laguna, Ruiz, Lara, & Aznar, 2013).

Given the high degree of neuroplasticity during preadolescence, the earlier we ingrain the concept of athleticism and related lifestyle behaviors (e.g., proper nutrition, adequate sleep), the greater the benefit will be for lifelong health and well-being. Children who enhance their athleticism will gain the needed confidence and competence in their physical abilities to enable later learning of more complex movements and sport skills. In fact, the dynamic and reinforcing relationships between the health- and skill-related components of physical fitness and the outcomes of athleticism are consistent with the existence of a positive feedback loop. As illustrated in figure 1.6, youth who enhance both health- and skill-related components of fitness are more likely to participate in moderate and vigorous bouts of physical activity (e.g., free play, fitness activities, sport). As their athleticism improves, they are motivated by physical, psychosocial, and cognitive rewards to participate in outdoor activities, fitness programs, and sport activities—all of which continue to reinforce desired muscle actions and health behaviors.

Physical Activity Guidelines: Infancy to Adolescence

Youngsters who learn how to engage in different types of physical activity and who enjoy playing age-related games are more likely to sustain this desired behavior. Consequently, a primary goal of youth physical activity is to help participants become aware of the intrinsic value, as well as the sheer pleasure, of physical activity so that they become active adults. Indeed, high levels of enjoyment have been found to be associated with higher levels of MVPA and lower levels of sedentary behavior in youth (Bai, Allums-Featherston, Saint-Maurice, Welk, & Candelaria, 2018). We should begin promoting and encouraging movement exploration and skill development during infancy in order to establish healthy habits and lay a strong foundation for later participation in age-appropriate games and free play. The earlier that youngsters are exposed to daily movement and active play, the more likely they are to develop healthy habits and avoid unhealthy weight gain (Institute of Medicine, 2011; National Association for Sport and Physical Education, 2009; Utesch, Bardid, Büsch, & Strauss, 2019).

Infants (birth to one year old) should be provided with opportunities throughout the day to explore their indoor and outdoor environments while engaging in

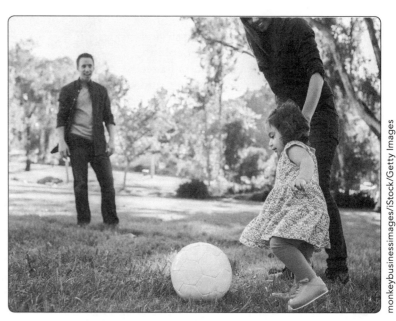

Active parents tend to have more active kids.

interactive play under adult supervision (Tremblay et al., 2017). Even during infancy, excess subcutaneous fat can delay motor development, which may lead to reduced levels of age-appropriate exploration and physical activity (Kanazawa et al., 2014; Slining, Adair, Goldman, Borja, & Bentley, 2010). Consequently, caregivers need to understand the importance of daily physical activity very early in life. For infants younger than six months of age, "tummy time" (time spent in the prone position) can help strengthen the upper back

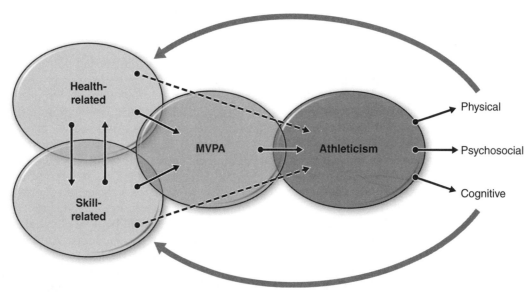

FIGURE 1.6 Conceptual framework illustrating interrelationships of health- and skill-related components of physical fitness, MVPA, and athleticism in youth.

and neck muscles, thus enabling infants to support their head as they crawl, roll, reach, grasp, and stand. Both structured activities (e.g., baby games such as pat-a-cake and peekaboo) and unstructured activities (e.g., playing with textured balls and squeeze toys) can support the development of fundamental movement skills and awaken an infant's senses (National Association for Sport and Physical Education, 2009). Adults can use verbal and nonverbal expressions to encourage infants to explore their environment while facilitating the development of movement skills.

Fundamental movement skills—such as running, jumping, throwing, kicking, and striking—begin to develop during the first few years of life (roughly, years one through three). As proficiency in these skills begins to emerge, new opportunities become available to participate in playground games and other recreational activities. Sedentary time should be minimized for toddlers (except during sleep!), and they should be given ample opportunities throughout the day to learn and practice fundamental movement skills. Guidelines suggest that toddlers should engage in at least 30 minutes of structured physical activity and at least 60 minutes of unstructured physical activity on a daily basis (National Association for Sport and Physical Education, 2009) or be physically active for at least 180 minutes spread throughout the day (Australian Government Department of Health, n.d.; Canadian Society for Exercise Physiology, 2012; Department of Health Social Services and Public Safety, 2011). Appropriate activities for toddlers include chase games, movement with active follow-along songs, playground activities, and playing with large balls and inflatable toys.

Youth fitness specialists should counsel parents about appropriate strategies for increasing children's physical activity and reducing sedentary behavior throughout the day. When toddlers are exposed regularly to various movement experiences that encourage peer play, foster creativity, and promote the development of motor skills and muscular fitness, they are more likely to maintain their interest in physical activity. Young children should be guided away from long periods of sedentary behavior, such as excessive television watching. In addition, parents and caregivers should use strollers for toddlers and preschoolers only when necessary and should avoid withholding physical activity as a punishment. Providing daily opportunities for light, moderate, and vigorous bouts of physical activity marks an important first step toward establishing healthy patterns and preventing excess weight gain during this early period (Institute of Medicine, 2011).

DO YOU KNOW?

Youth who spend more time outdoors are more likely to engage in adequate MVPA.

Although most preschoolers (three to five years old) enjoy participating in simple games and outdoor activities, prevalence reports indicate that most do not meet physical activity guidelines (Pate et al., 2015; Spittaels et al., 2012). Although an individual's developmental status, skill level, and personal interests are important considerations, preschoolers should generally be encouraged to participate in a variety of movement skills and activities during this developmental stage. Parents and caregivers should provide preschoolers with opportunities throughout the day to learn and practice basic movement skills while offering instruction and positive reinforcement (De Bock, Genser, Raat, Fischer, & Renz-Polster, 2013; Pate et al., 2016). Preschoolers should be physically active for at least 180 minutes throughout the day (Australian Government Department of Health, n.d.; Department of Health Social Services and Public Safety, 2011) or accumulate

Teaching Tip

FUNDAMENTAL FITNESS

Although time spent in MVPA provides a measure of the outright quality of physical education or youth sport practice, youth fitness programs should also provide opportunities for all participants to make friends while learning FUNdamental movement skills that are enjoyable, engaging, and developmentally appropriate (Bukowsky, Faigenbaum, & Myer, 2014). Youth fitness specialists should help participants understand what they are doing, why they are doing it, and how it can contribute to their health, fitness, and performance. Effective strategies are needed to teach participants game tactics and sport skills in an environment that is physically stimulating, mentally engaging, and generally enjoyable. The time has come to expand our conceptual thinking about youth physical activity and implement a more complex model that is designed to identify and treat inactive youth with well-designed interventions before they proceed too far down the path of chronic disease (Faigenbaum, Rial Rebullido, & MacDonald, 2018).

TABLE 1.2 PHYSICAL ACTIVITY (PA) GUIDELINES FOR YOUNG CHILDREN BY AGE AND COUNTRY

Age (yr)	Australia	Canada	United Kingdom	United States
Infant (≤1)	Playful activities and push-and-pull games with balls and soft toys	Daily activity, particularly interactive floor-based play	Play that encourages infants to use their muscles and develop motor skills	Varied bouts of play that promote skill development and movement exploration
Toddler (1-3)	≥180 minutes throughout the day (games, movement to music, active toys, dance)	≥180 minutes throughout the day to develop movement skills	≥180 minutes throughout the day (energetic play, chasing games, minimal sedentary time)	≥30 minutes of structured PA and ≥60 minutes of unstructured PA throughout the day
Preschooler (3-5)	≥180 minutes throughout the day (games, movement to music, active toys, dance)	≥180 minutes at any intensity (variety of activities in different settings)	≥180 minutes throughout the day (energetic play, chasing games, minimal sedentary time)	≥60 minutes of structured PA and ≥60 minutes of unstructured PA throughout the day

Data from Australian Government Department of Health (n.d.); O'Donovan, Blazevich, Boreham, et al. (2010); Tremblay, LeBlanc, Janssen, et al. (2011); United States Department of Health and Human Services (2008); World Health Organization (2010); and Poitras, Gray, Borghese, et al. (2016).

at least 60 minutes of structured physical activity and at least 60 minutes of unstructured physical activity each day (National Association for Sport and Physical Education, 2009).

If preschoolers gain confidence and competence in their ability to perform basic movement skills, they will be better prepared to perform more complex movement tasks when they begin school. For example, activities such as dancing to music, aquatic movements, tumbling exercises, and child-initiated experiences on playground equipment can enhance a preschooler's repertoire of movement skills and promote social interaction with peers and parents. Although the specific design of an activity program should depend on a participant's health history and movement competence, general physical activity recommendations can be made for infants, toddlers, and preschoolers (see table 1.2).

Throughout childhood and adolescence (6 to 17 years old), young people should be encouraged to participate in *at least* 60 minutes of MVPA daily as part of play, games, sports, transportation, recreation, physical education, or planned exercise. Notwithstanding the potential value of replacing sedentary activities (e.g., television viewing) with less intense physical activities (e.g., playing a musical instrument), physical activity for children and adolescents should include moderate to vigorous bouts of aerobic exercise (e.g., bicycling, swimming, dancing) and muscle- and bone-strengthening activities (e.g., playground games, resistance training) that enhance the structure and function of the cardiorespiratory and musculoskeletal systems.

Summary

Daily physical activity in the context of family, school, and community programs can provide young people with physical, psychosocial, and cognitive benefits. Yet despite these potential returns, physical activity levels among youth fall short of expectations, and the decline in physical activity appears to emerge early in life. Thus we are faced with an urgent need to raise awareness about the importance of daily physical activity and invest in health promotion policies and practices that provide equal access to activity-friendly environments for children and adolescents. Without initiatives that focus on disease prevention and health promotion early in life, new health care concerns will continue to emerge as youth engage in unhealthy behaviors, learn bad habits, and suffer sport-related maladies including overuse injuries.

Regular participation in a variety of physical activities that enhance both health- and skill-related components of physical fitness is a critical component of disease prevention and health promotion. Improved communication between health care providers and youth fitness specialists will facilitate the development of sustainable interventions that are consistent with the needs, abilities, and interests of all youth. If exercise is medicine, then the dose needs to be properly prescribed and advanced, as well as consistent with the needs, abilities, and interests of younger populations. Youth fitness specialists who are well versed in pediatric exercise science and skilled at teaching youth are well positioned to foster sustainable programming that enhances physical fitness and promotes healthy lifestyle choices.

CHAPTER 2

Principles of Pediatric Exercise Science

CHAPTER OBJECTIVES

- Understand the fundamental concepts of pediatric exercise science
- Describe how biological and physiological systems develop during childhood and adolescence
- Analyze how developmental physiology interacts with acute and chronic responses to exercise
- Recognize that children are not miniature adults and therefore require developmentally appropriate exercise interventions

KEY TERMS

adenosine triphosphate (ATP) (p. 38)

anabolic (p. 27)

autonomic nervous system (p. 21)

cardiopulmonary system (p. 36)

cardiovascular system (p. 36)

catabolic (p. 27)

creatine kinase (p. 39)

endochondral ossification (p. 29)

endocrine system (p. 24)

growth plate (p. 29)

lactate dehydrogenase (p. 39)

minute ventilation (p. 37)

muscle hyperplasia (p. 33)

muscle hypertrophy (p. 33)

osteogenesis (p. 29)

osteoporosis (p. 29)

overtraining (p. 21)

pediatric exercise science (p. 20)

peripheral nervous system (PNS) (p. 21)

phosphofructokinase (p. 39)

puberty (p. 25)

somatic nervous system (p. 21)

stretch–shortening cycle (p. 23)

vulnerable population (p. 20)

Introduction

Our knowledge and understanding of how children and adolescents respond to physical activity must be grounded not in myths and misconceptions but in evidence. Well-grounded knowledge, in turn, should influence policy and practice, thus helping youth fitness specialists to design exercise programs that are developmentally appropriate. In determining how to engage youth in physical activity and stimulate positive adaptations, we can turn to decades of pediatric exercise research confirming that children are not miniature adults (Bailey, 2012). **Pediatric exercise science** applies scientific principles and inquiry to exercise by children and adolescents. Youth form a unique population—separate from older populations—due to the biological processes of growth and maturation and their influences on both acute and chronic responses to exercise. Whereas adults have reached a fully mature and relatively stable state, children and adolescents experience constant change while evolving physically, psychologically, socially, biochemically, and physiologically (Rowland & Saltin, 2008). This constant state of change, extending from childhood to adulthood, affects the structure, function, and capacity that determine the markers of exercise or physical performance (e.g., endurance, strength, speed, balance, agility). Thus pediatric exercise science aims to understand how these complex processes of growth and maturation affect performance and influence responses to exercise in youth.

Research in pediatric exercise science requires clinicians and scientists to work with what is considered a **vulnerable population**—in this case, children and adolescents. As a result, they must take extra care in determining research design and collecting data. They must ensure that their research poses no unnecessary risk to participants and that they have put in place robust safeguards. Williams and colleagues (2011) suggest that the welfare of young research participants depends both on any personal benefit they may gain from participating and on the risks of doing so. The authors continue that most of this research falls into the category of "minimal risk with no direct benefit to the participant" and is ethical if the research procedures are no different from those a child might experience in everyday life. As a result, protocols such as X-rays, blood sampling, and maximal exercise testing may be considered ethical. More complete guidelines are available on issues of ethics, recruitment, participant welfare and safeguarding, and conduct of research staff involved in pediatric exercise research (Williams et al., 2011).

The discipline of pediatric exercise science hinges on studying the interaction of development and physical activity. As youth develop, natural growth and maturational processes make them larger; alter their body proportions; change their body composition; and refine the biological, physiological, and neural mechanisms that contribute to their physical functioning. As a result of these developmental changes, fitness and physiological capacities generally improve throughout childhood and adolescence, provided that a child lives a healthy lifestyle. This natural development is nonlinear and includes periods of little change interspersed with periods of rapid change. This pattern can be observed at the whole-body level (e.g., changes in size), the systems level (e.g., changes in circulating

Teaching Tip

"CONTEMPORARY" ISSUES IN PEDIATRIC EXERCISE SCIENCE

Pediatric Exercise Science was the first international journal dedicated to understanding exercise in children and adolescents. In the inaugural issue, published in 1989, editor Tom Rowland identified the following key issues that were considered contemporary at that time:

- Worldwide concern about physical activity levels in youths
- Low levels of fitness and the implications for future health
- Effects of intensive training on youth athletes
- Effectiveness of exercise as a therapy for youth with chronic disease

In the ensuing 30 years, the accumulation of research has extended our understanding of how youth develop and respond to exercise. However, the same issues identified by Rowland in 1989 remain contemporary today; in fact, they are arguably now more relevant than ever. As research in pediatric exercise science continues to grow, the resulting scientific knowledge needs to be widely translated into policy and practice in order to promote the positive development of all youth.

hormones), and the cellular level (e.g., changes in metabolism). It is also reflected in changes in physical fitness (e.g., endurance, speed, strength, power).

DO YOU KNOW?

Half of the sport-related injuries that occur among youth result from overuse (Difiori et al., 2014).

As shown in chapter 1, physical activity and training during the growing years can positively influence physical fitness and well-being. For instance, resistance training has been shown not only to increase strength in children and adolescents (Behringer et al., 2010) but also to translate into improved motor abilities, such as running, jumping, and throwing (Behringer et al., 2011). We must also recognize, however, that development can be influenced negatively by inappropriate exercise. **Overtraining**, for instance, is associated with increased injury risk and negative physiological, psychological, and sociological consequences (Difiori et al., 2014; Matos et al., 2011). It can be attributed partly to the fact that some youth sport systems expose young athletes to adult training volumes and ignore the fact that youth athletic development is built on a constantly changing base of normal growth and development (Bergeron et al., 2015). As a result, young athletes require lower training volumes and plenty of time for recovery and natural growth processes (American Academy of Pediatrics, 2000; Brenner, 2016).

Developmental Physiology

Tasks such as walking, running, jumping, twisting, throwing, and kicking may seem relatively simple, but all physical activity requires the integrated response of multiple physiological systems to produce coordinated movements. Specifically, the central and peripheral nervous systems must stimulate muscles to contract, the muscle–tendon system must generate and transmit mechanical forces, and the metabolic system must provide the energy required to produce a contraction. Simultaneously, the cardiopulmonary and cardiovascular systems must transport oxygenated blood to working muscles in order to allow continued movement and support metabolic recovery. At the same time, hormones help regulate respiratory, cardiac, and metabolic responses during exercise and stimulate growth and repair afterward. All of these physiological systems develop throughout childhood and adolescence, and those developments affect the body's acute and chronic responses to exercise. Therefore, we need to understand this process of development and its implications for exercise among youth.

Central and Somatic Nervous Systems

The nervous system consists of the brain, the brain stem, the spinal cord, the sensory organs, and the nerves that connect these organs with the rest of the body, thereby allowing us to control both voluntary and involuntary actions. The central nervous system (CNS) consists of the brain (including the brain stem) and the spinal cord. The CNS is connected to the limbs and organs by the **peripheral nervous system** (PNS), which allows neural signals to reach the extremities and enables feedback to be relayed to the CNS. The PNS, in turn, consists of the **somatic nervous system** and the **autonomic nervous system**. The somatic nervous system controls voluntary activation of skeletal muscle and mediates involuntary reflexes; more specifically, efferent nerves stimulate muscle contraction, and afferent nerves provide sensory feedback from the periphery to the CNS. The autonomic nervous system, in contrast, regulates the internal organs, blood vessels, and glands and controls respiratory and cardiovascular responses to exercise. This system is further divided into the sympathetic and parasympathetic

Teaching Tip

CHILDREN ARE NOT MINIATURE ADULTS

Children are not merely smaller than adults; to the contrary, they are physically and psychosocially less mature. In addition, whereas adults tend to participate in a narrow range of physical activities that require specialized skills, children need to develop a variety of movement skills by taking part in a wide range of activities. Moreover, whereas adults may exercise continuously for prolonged periods of time, children tend to engage in short bouts of vigorous and spontaneous exercise interspersed with rest as needed. Children and adults may also differ in both their acute physiological responses to exercise and their long-term adaptations to training. Consequently, children should not be trained like miniature adults. Instead, youth fitness specialists should consider the unique developmental needs of children and adolescents when designing and implementing exercise programs.

systems, the first of which mobilizes the body for action (e.g., fight-or-flight response) and the latter of which is responsible for energy conservation and resting functions.

Development of the Neural System

The neural system experiences rapid growth during the early years of life. Figure 2.1 shows the growth of the neural system as compared with that of the reproductive system. The figure clearly shows that both systems exhibit nonlinear development but with different timing. The rapid postnatal growth of the neural system means that about 95 percent of the total adult size of the central nervous system and related structures is achieved by age seven, followed by small steady gains to complete the process (Malina et al., 2004).

Although figure 2.1 shows a smooth developmental growth curve for the nervous system, the maturation process is more complex for the component parts, particularly within the brain. Total brain volume reaches 95 percent of maximum size by 6 years of age, peaks around 11.5 years in females and 14.5 years in males, and then diminishes slightly in size by adulthood (Lenroot & Giedd, 2006). Even more specifically, white matter, which consists primarily of myelinated nerve axons, increases continually throughout childhood and adolescence. Myelination allows rapid conduction of signals and is essential for correct and efficient functioning of nerves. In contrast, gray matter—which consists primarily of nerve cell bodies, dendrites, and synapses—displays an inverted U trend of increasing density before puberty and decreasing density after puberty. Moreover, the timing of gray matter development itself varies across brain regions. Gray matter associated with the control of movement peaks at 7.5

years old in girls and 10 years old in boys (Lenroot & Giedd, 2006). That development is followed by pruning, wherein rarely used synapses are selectively removed and remaining nerves are myelinated to become more adept at transmitting information (Johnson et al., 2009).

The combined effects of neuromaturation can be summarized as synaptic overproduction, pruning of rarely used connections, and myelination of retained nerves—the timing of which is specific to each region of the brain. Parts of the brain that control more basic functions have been shown to mature earlier than areas that control complex functions (Gogtay et al., 2004). This sequence means that motor and sensory functions mature first, though refined control of motor coordination takes longer. Given the early maturation of motor control and the observable effect of environment on both pruning and enhancement of brain function, we must regularly expose youth to a wide variety of physical stimuli in order to promote their neural development during the first two decades of life.

DO YOU KNOW?

Physical inactivity weakens the architecture of the developing brain.

Some of the later-developing areas of the brain are associated with more complex functions of cognition and emotion, and these areas may not fully mature until the third decade of life (Johnson et al., 2009). The delayed development of more complex functions has been associated with adolescents' relative lack of judgment and greater inclination to take risks; late-developing functions have also been associated with goal setting and one's ability to respond to the environment (Johnson et al., 2009). This pattern may

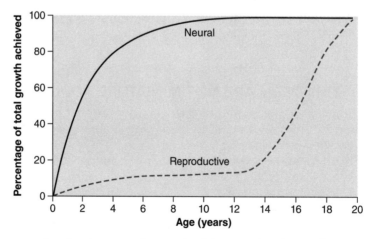

FIGURE 2.1   Scammon's curve showing the systemic growth of the neural and reproductive systems.

Adapted from Scammon (1930).

hold implications for whether one chooses to engage in daily physical activity or how well one responds to challenging situations in sporting environments.

Because it is difficult to directly monitor the autonomic nervous system, development has been examined through indirect markers of sympathetic and parasympathetic activity. Sympathetic-mediated responses of heart rate, blood pressure, and blood flow do not appear to differ between children and adults (Rowland, 2005). Sympathetic activity stimulates the release of norepinephrine, a hormone that acts as a neurotransmitter. Resting levels of norepinephrine have been shown to increase with pubertal stage in boys (related to testosterone) but not in girls (Weise et al., 2002). This finding suggests that sexual maturation influences development of the sympathetic nervous system in boys. Both sympathetic and parasympathetic activity influence the regulation of the heart, causing variability in the beat-to-beat interval, which can be measured as heart rate variability. At rest, children have been shown to have greater high-frequency variability and a lower ratio of low-frequency to high-frequency variability than adults, reflecting greater parasympathetic activity (Ohuchi et al., 2000). Thus the evidence suggests that parasympathetic activity is greater and sympathetic activity lower in children than in adults.

Acute Response of the Neural System to Exercise

In terms of acute response, the neural control of exercise can differ between children, adolescents, and adults. Children may be less able than adults to recruit motor units and may do so in a manner that is less coordinated and less efficient. The evidence, however, can be conflicting. For instance, Blimkie (1989) reported lower motor-unit activation in boys than in men (78 percent versus 95 percent) during knee extension exercise but no between-group differences in elbow flexion. The size principle dictates that motor units are recruited in ascending order of size; consequently, lower activation levels in untrained children are thought to reflect an inability to fully recruit larger type II motor units (Dotan et al., 2012). This notion holds implications for the ability of untrained youth to generate high levels of force and power and also for the metabolic consequences of high-intensity exercise. An activation deficit would limit the recruitment of type II motor units, which in turn would reduce force production and reliance on anaerobic energy.

As children develop and practice learned movements, they become more coordinated, which can be observed in their ability to execute increasingly complex skills. At the muscle level, we can also observe development of recruitment patterns. For example, let us consider co-contraction of agonist–antagonist muscles, which can help provide joint stability but also increases the energy cost of exercise and reduces force output. It has been shown that during running, co-contraction in the lower limbs decreases with age in childhood and adolescence, meaning that younger children are less economical due to greater activation of antagonist muscles (Frost et al., 2002).

During activities such as running, jumping, and throwing, muscles contract in a coordinated sequence known as the **stretch–shortening cycle**. In rebounding activities, muscles are preactivated before ground contact in order to help tolerate impact loads, and stretch reflexes provide excitatory bursts of activity to help produce rapid and forceful movements. Both preactivation and stretch-reflex activity during rebounding exercise have been shown to develop with maturation (Lloyd et al., 2012; Oliver & Smith, 2010). This finding suggests that the neural strategies that prepare muscles for impact and provide feedback in activities such as running and jumping develop toward a more excitatory response as a child moves toward adulthood. Similarly, the rate of rise of muscle activation (i.e., the speed at which activation increases) during explosive actions is known to be lower in children than in adults and is related to a reduced rate of force development (Dotan et al., 2012; Waugh et al., 2013). These differences can hold implications for speed, agility, and explosiveness and may even influence economy.

DO YOU KNOW?

As children mature, the CNS develops a less inhibitory and more excitatory response to exercise.

In theory, the increase in sympathetic nervous activity that comes with maturity should promote a faster physiological response to a stimulus. However, research is equivocal when examining the response of heart rate, blood pressure, and blood flow to exercise in children and adults (Rowland, 2005). The norepinephrine response to maximal exercise has been shown not to differ between boys and men, and the lack of a difference has been attributed to high variability in individual responses (Lehmann et al., 1981; Rowland at el., 1996). Conversely, greater high-frequency heart rate variability at rest has been correlated with a faster decline in heart rate after exercise in children than in adults (Ohuchi et al., 2000). This finding supports the notion that greater parasympathetic activity in children modulates a quicker recovery of heart rate after exercise than is the case in adults.

Chronic Response of the Neural System to Exercise

Direct evidence is sparse in regard to chronic adaptation of the nervous system to training in youth. Even so, training programs intended to increase strength, speed, and power are often designed to promote neural adaptation. In children and adolescents, a large body of evidence does show that strength, speed, and power all respond positively to training (Behm et al., 2017; Behringer et al., 2011; Lloyd et al., 2014; Moran et al., 2017; Rumpf et al., 2012), thus providing indirect evidence of neural adaptation. This is particularly true in prepubertal children, in whom circulating androgens may limit any size or structural adaptations contributing to performance gains. Mitchell and colleagues (2011) directly measured muscle activation in groups of power- and endurance-trained boys of ages 7 to 12 with varied training histories. The results showed that gymnasts achieved a higher rate of muscle activation than did endurance-trained children, who in turn achieved greater activation rates than minimally active nonathletes. These findings suggest that in prepubertal and early-pubertal boys, the neural system is capable of adapting to chronic power training, especially in explosive sports such as gymnastics. In addition, Ozmun and colleagues (1994) provided direct evidence of chronic neural adaptation in prepubertal boys and girls; in particular, arm strength increased by 23 percent and muscle activation amplitude increased by 17 percent following an eight-week strength training intervention.

Limited research has examined chronic adaptations in the autonomic nervous system in response to exercise. Mandigout and colleagues (2002) reported that 13 weeks of endurance training increased some measures of parasympathetic activity in prepubertal children, which would support the observation that increased fitness improves recovery rates. Research has also shown that exposing prepubertal children to 20 minutes of moderate physical activity five times per week can improve both sympathetic and parasympathetic activity (Nagai et al., 2004). Nagai and colleagues (2003) found that obese children had lower autonomic nervous system activity than did non-obese sedentary individuals and that the magnitude of depression in sympathetic and parasympathetic activity related to the duration of obesity. In a follow-up study, Nagai and Moritani (2004) revealed an interaction between autonomic nervous system function, physical activity, and body fat. Children who were lean and active had the greatest autonomic activity, and children who were obese and inactive had the lowest. Children who were obese and active had autonomic function similar to that of children who were lean and inactive. In another study, four months of physical activity improved the parasympathetic activity of 7- to 11-year-olds who were obese, but this positive adaptation was lost with four months of detraining (Gutin et al., 2000). Thus, regular physical activity improves autonomic function in lean and obese children, but the stimulus of exercise must be maintained in order to ensure that adaptations are not lost.

Endocrine System

The **endocrine system** is a collection of glands that produce hormones to regulate the body's growth, metabolism, sexual development, and functioning. Pediatric exercise science is particularly interested in the development of the sex and growth hormones, which exert a profound effect on body size, composition, and function, as well as the development of physical fitness. As shown earlier, in figure 2.1, the development of the reproductive system follows a different time course than the central nervous system. Whereas the CNS experiences rapid growth in the first six to seven years of life, the reproductive system experiences very little growth until the onset of puberty, after which a cascade of events leads to rapid changes in body size and function. Puberty is accompanied

Teaching Tip

LEARN TO MOVE

In order to lead an active life, youth need to master a variety of life skills. As a point of reference, Hernandez (2012) found that third-grade children who could read were four times more likely to graduate than were children with poor reading skills. Similarly, failing to develop motor skills in early life can negatively affect one's lifelong development. For instance, low competence in movement skills in childhood is associated with lower levels of physical activity (Aaltonen et al., 2015; Lopes et al., 2011) and reduced cardiorespiratory fitness in adolescence (Barnett et al., 2008). The early years are critical for learning life skills, and youth fitness specialists should capitalize on the adaptability of the central nervous system to adapt to motor skill training during this time.

by alterations in the levels of circulating hormones, which affect increases in body size and changes in body composition, skeletal development, muscle–tendon architecture and function, cardiorespiratory function, metabolism, and cognitive development. In short, puberty and the development of the hormonal system are responsible for a myriad of physiological changes that influence physical fitness and both acute and chronic responses to exercise.

Development of Sex and Growth Hormones

Puberty is a period of transition between childhood and adulthood that takes place in several sequential steps controlled by complex neuroendocrine factors (Naughton et al., 2000). The development of reproductive function occurs in response to the presence of the sex hormones estrogen (in females) and testosterone (in males). These sex hormones initiate and control reproductive development but lead to very different outcomes in boys and girls. Changes in the circulating levels of sex hormones in the first 18 years of life are shown in figure 2.2. In the first decade of life, boys and girls have similarly low levels of both estradiol (the most active of the estrogen hormones) and testosterone. With the onset of puberty, divergent responses appear in boys and girls in the levels of estradiol and testosterone, and this divergence contributes to differences in physical fitness that become increasingly apparent during the pubertal years. For instance, increased

testosterone provides a physical performance advantage for males, since testosterone stimulates relatively greater increases in muscle mass, cardiac size, and red blood cell volume.

Figure 2.2 shows the development of sex hormones relative to puberty. Childhood here is the prepubertal state, adolescence is the period from the onset to the end of puberty, and the cessation of puberty signifies the attainment of adulthood. The timing of pubertal onset can differ by as much as five years between individuals (Malina et al., 2004); therefore, chronological age should not be used to conclude that puberty has begun. During childhood, prepubertal estradiol levels are slightly higher in girls than in boys. With the onset of puberty, estradiol increases rapidly in females, in whom it stimulates ovulation, reproductive maturation, and breast development while also promoting increased body fat. Childhood testosterone levels are very low in both boys and girls. During adolescence, girls experience a minimal increase in testosterone, whereas boys experience at least a 20-fold increase in the circulating level of testosterone by the time adulthood is reached (Malina et al., 2004). In males, increased testosterone promotes sexual development, which can be observed in increased penis and testicular size, appearance of pubic and facial hair, and deepening of the voice. Increased testosterone also promotes increases in muscle mass and linear growth, which is why males at full maturity are on average taller than females and carry more muscle tissue.

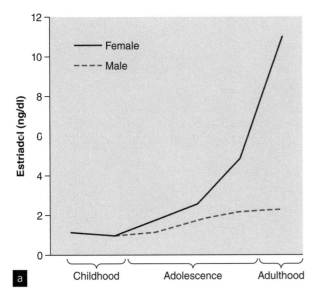

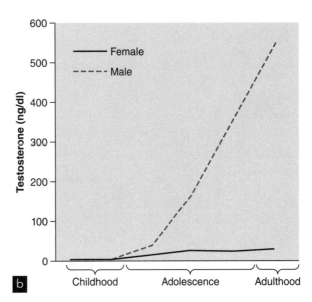

FIGURE 2.2 Blood concentrations of (a) estradiol and (b) testosterone in childhood, in adolescence (the period of puberty), and at attainment of adulthood.

Adapted by permission from R.M. Malina, C. Bouchard, and O. Bar-Or, *Growth, Maturation, and Physical Activity*, 2nd ed. (Champaign, IL: Human Kinetics, 2004), 414. Data from Esoterix Inc.

DO YOU KNOW?

Testosterone levels in males are maintained from the end of adolescence into the third and fourth decades of life.

Activation of the hypothalamic–pituitary–gonadal axis stimulates progressive secretion of sex hormones during puberty (Naughton et al., 2000). An established hypothesis supposes that a critical level of body fat is needed to stimulate the onset of puberty, which provides a link between reproductive function, maturation, exercise, and nutrition. The role played by body fat in the initiation of puberty can be supported by the observations that prepubertal girls accumulate more body fat than boys do and begin puberty earlier (Rowland, 2005), that girls with a negative energy balance (whether from high levels of physical activity, low levels of energy consumption, or both) experience delayed onset of puberty and the menstrual cycle, and that obesity is associated with earlier onset of puberty (Kaplowitz et al., 2001). These observations suggest that we need to consider both diet and physical activity in order to promote healthy development and maturation.

Puberty is associated with a period of rapid growth in stature, and this growth is mediated by the synergistic interaction of sex and growth hormones. Concentrations of growth hormones rise slightly during childhood, increase further in puberty (peaking at the time of the adolescent growth spurt), and then decline (see figure 2.3). Growth hormone is released in pulses throughout the day, and the magnitude of these pulses (rather than their frequency) is elevated during puberty. This increase in growth hormone relates to the adolescent growth spurt, wherein the rate of height increase follows a similar trend to that of growth hormone concentration. Growth hormone promotes tissue growth both through direct biological effects on tissue and through effects mediated by the hormone known as insulin-like growth factor 1, or IGF-1 (Malina et al., 2004). IGF-1, which is produced in the liver and other tissues in response to stimulation by growth hormone, helps to regulate skeletal development and protein synthesis, among other things.

During puberty, the entire endocrine system is radically altered. Sex hormones control the development of the reproductive system and stimulate and interact with growth hormones to promote growth, tissue synthesis, and functional changes. Whereas sex hormones remain at peak values into adulthood, growth hormone and IGF-1 both peak in puberty and then decline throughout the remainder of adolescence. Changes in circulating growth hormone can be observed indirectly in the rapid increase in stature that is typical of adolescence (figure 2.3). Circulating levels of sex and growth hormones exert a profound effect on physical fitness and influence both acute and chronic adaptations to exercise in children and adolescents.

Acute Response of Sex and Growth Hormones to Exercise

Endocrine development influences hormone-mediated increases in muscle–tendon size and characteristics, cardiac size, blood volume, respiratory capacity, and energy metabolism—all of which affect a child's ability to exercise. Both children and adolescents may display an acute hormonal response to exercise, although the magnitude of the response may be greater in those

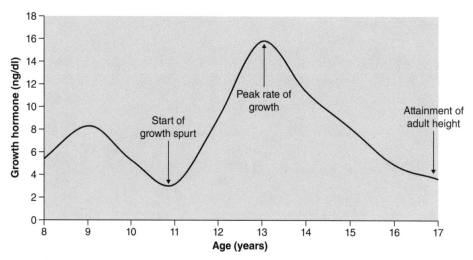

FIGURE 2.3 Mean 24-hour plasma concentrations of growth hormones in boys of advancing chronological age. Changes in circulating growth hormone are associated with the growth spurt and rapid increase in stature that occurs during the adolescent years.

Adapted from Martha, Rogol, Veldhuis, et al. (1989).

with advanced maturity. For instance, Viru and colleagues (1998) reported that after a bout of moderate-intensity exercise, estradiol increased by 27 percent in girls just entering puberty but by 43 percent of those at an advanced stage of puberty. Similarly, Marin and colleagues (1994) reported that growth hormone increased in response to a treadmill test in boys and girls and that the magnitude of the response related to pubertal status (but with no sex differences in the response at any given pubertal stage).

It has been suggested that the acute growth-hormone response to exercise is mediated by both circulating testosterone and intensity of exercise and that increased exercise intensity is a particularly potent stimulant at all stages of maturation (Jurimae & Jurimae, 2008). Whereas some authors have suggested a limited acute response of testosterone to exercise in boys (Pomerants, et al., 2006; Vingren et al., 2010), Di Luigi et al. (2006) showed that 90 minutes of soccer training stimulated an increase in testosterone in boys and that the magnitude of the response related to maturity and resting testosterone levels. It has also been suggested that in order to experience an acute testosterone response to exercise, a child must have accumulated some level of training history (Jurimae & Jurimae, 2008). Eliakim and colleagues (2009) reported that elite volleyball players aged 13 to 18 years significantly increased both testosterone and growth hormone following one hour of volleyball practice; no differences appeared between girls and boys in the magnitude of the **anabolic** response to training. It has also been shown that submaximal exercise can acutely increase testosterone levels in mid- to late pubertal girls but not in prepubertal girls (Viru et al., 1998), and Nemet and colleagues (2009) reported that a cross country training session substantially increased growth hormone in adolescent girls.

Relevant findings were also reported by Eliakim and colleagues (2014) in a review of their previous work. Specifically, they found that growth hormone responds to acute bouts of sport practice in adolescents and that this response does not seem to differ between males and females or between team and individual sports. The authors did find that the response was blunted in water polo, and they speculated that water, or water temperature, inhibits the release of growth hormone. In addition, although growth hormone appeared responsive to many types of sport training, IGF-1 did not increase in any circumstance. This lack of response was potentially attributable to real-life sport practices simply being insufficiently intense to cause an increase.

In a comprehensive review of children's hormonal responses to resistance training, Falk and Eliakim (2014) noted some equivocal results with regard to changes in testosterone, growth hormone, IGF-1, and cortisol. The balance of evidence suggests that youth can experience acute changes in anabolic and **catabolic** hormones following resistance training. Our understanding is limited, however, by the fact that most of the relevant studies have been conducted with adolescent boys; that is, few studies have addressed immature boys, and none have addressed girls.

Although more research is needed in order to fully understand the acute effects of exercise on hormone secretion in youth, evidence does suggest that exercise plays a role. It can cause an acute hormonal response in children and adolescents, though the magnitude of the response may depend on maturity. Hormonal response to physical activity is likely also affected by exercise mode and intensity, training history, and lifestyle (e.g., nutrition, sleep).

Chronic Response of Sex and Growth Hormones to Exercise

In pre- and early pubertal children, resting levels of testosterone and growth hormone have been shown to differ between those who participate in different sports (Tsolakis et al., 2003). This finding suggests that relatively immature children experience chronic adaptation of the hormonal system that is specific to the demands of the activity in which they participate. In both children and adults, prolonged endurance activity has been associated with a reduction in circulating testosterone, and resistance training has been associated with an increase in circulating testosterone (Tsolakis et al., 2003; Jurimae & Jurimae, 2008). Tsolakis and colleagues (2003) exposed a group of sedentary pre- and early pubertal boys aged 11 to 13 years old to a two-month exercise intervention. Their findings showed that, following the intervention period, circulating testosterone increased by a trivial amount in the control group (+0.5 nmol/L), by a small amount in a group undertaking aerobic training (+1.52 nmol/L), and by a large amount in a group undertaking resistance training (+6.06 nmol/L).

Figure 2.4 shows findings from another study involving changes in testosterone in prepubertal and pubertal boys in response to a two-month resistance training intervention followed by a detraining period (Tsolakis et al., 2000). The training, performed three times per week, consisted of six upper-body exercises with three sets of 10-repetition-maximum, one minute of rest between sets, and three minutes of rest between exercises. Both prepubertal and pubertal groups showed a similar absolute increase in testosterone, which was maintained over a two-month detraining period. The difference in baseline testosterone suggests

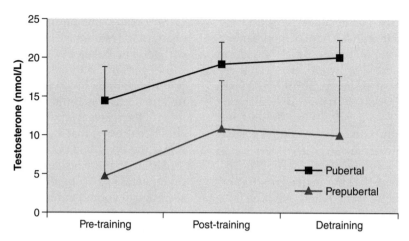

FIGURE 2.4 Changes in resting testosterone in prepubertal and pubertal boys following a two-month, upper-body resistance training program and a subsequent two-month detraining period.

Data from Tsolakis, Messinis, Stergiolas, and Dessypris (2000).

that prepubertal boys experience a greater relative increase in testosterone than do pubertal boys (124 percent versus 32 percent) but that the latter retain an advantage of higher absolute testosterone after training.

More generally, however, the evidence is equivocal regarding chronic hormonal changes following resistance training in children and adolescents. Falk and Eliakim (2014) concluded that available evidence demonstrates that children are more likely to experience increases in testosterone than adolescents following resistance training, whereas for other hormones a change is unlikely or the available data are insufficient. Research has indicated that adolescent female runners increase their testosterone, both at rest and in response to a bout of exercise, following a seven-week period of training (Kraemer et al., 2001). The increase may be explained at least in part by the fact that the training

included high-intensity interval sessions rather than just prolonged endurance exercise.

The anabolic effects of testosterone have often been examined in conjunction with cortisol, which suppresses the immune system and exerts a catabolic effect on bone and muscle tissue. Summarizing the available evidence, Jurimae and Jurimae (2008) concluded that resting levels of cortisol are not influenced by training during sexual maturation. Consequently, testosterone appears sensitive to favorable chronic adaptations in response to exercise in youth without an associated negative increase in cortisol. However, individual responses are likely to vary substantially and will be influenced by a variety of factors, including maturation, exercise intensity, and training history.

A prolonged negative energy balance, caused by a mismatch between energy expenditure and intake, can lead to negative outcomes for growth, bone health, and

Teaching Tip

ENERGY DEFICIT AND HORMONES

Exercise and nutrition interact to influence growth hormone and IGF-1, and their secretion is regulated in part by energy balance. Youth who take on high training loads or who take in inadequate energy may enter a state of negative energy balance (expending more calories than they consume). In this scenario IGF-1 may decrease and physical growth may slow. If energy balance is restored, by either reducing the training load or increasing energy intake, IGF-1 and physical growth will recover. A prolonged energy deficit can lead to more serious consequences, particularly in girls, who may experience suppression of estrogen, delay or disruption of menstruation, and weakening of the bones. With these risks in mind, youth fitness specialists must ensure that young athletes avoid overtraining and undereating so that they can maintain healthy growth and development. To this end, we must help young people manage their training loads, allow for sufficient recovery and time away from sport, and promote a positive attitude toward eating.

reproductive development and function. Eliakim and colleagues (Eliakim, Brasel, Mohan, Barstow, Berman, & Cooper, 1996; Eliakim, Brasel, Mohan, Wong, & Cooper, 1998) found that when adolescent girls and boys completed five weeks of endurance training, IGF-1 was reduced. This finding was attributed to the possibility that the increased training load led to negative energy balance and a catabolic state. In female athletes, prolonged negative energy balance is associated with delayed menarche (the first menstrual cycle) as well as amenorrhea (disruption or cessation of the menstrual cycle) (Rowland, 2005). This association has been attributed to a "caloric drain" resulting from the combination of training stress and caloric inadequacy, which leads to the suppression of estrogen production and impairment of reproductive function (Rowland, 2005).

The observation that amenorrhea also occurs in malnourished nonathletes suggests that diet plays a particularly important role in the occurrence of this state. In one area of major concern, estrogen controls bone maturation in both males and females, and estrogen suppression reduces bone density. This concern is heightened by the fact that adult bone mineral density is largely established during childhood and adolescence (Bass, 2000).

Overall, then, evidence suggests that the hormonal system may experience both positive and negative adaptations in response to the cumulative effect of exercise and nutrition throughout maturation.

Skeletal System

The skeleton provides the framework to support body mass. It develops throughout childhood and adolescence and into later life, as bone is continually remodeled in response to the internal milieu and external loading. Speaking broadly, the skeletal system may be considered fully mature when adult stature is reached. Its maturity can also be assessed more directly through the use of radiographs to identify adult bone morphology and epiphyseal union (the point at which the **growth plate** between the end and the shaft of a bone is no longer distinguishable).

Although bone ceases to grow when the fully mature state is achieved, it is continually remodeled throughout life. The formation of bone, known as **osteogenesis**, begins during fetal development. At birth, the skeleton is formed primarily of cartilage, which, in most of the body, is remodeled into bone through the process of **endochondral ossification** (the skull relies on more rapid intramembranous ossification, or bone formation in the absence of cartilage). The hard substance of bone is provided by definitive bone cells known as osteocytes; in turn, these cells are formed by others, known as osteoblasts, that become entrapped on the bone surface. Bone cells are resorbed by osteoclasts, which release minerals back into circulation; this process occurs throughout growth in order to maintain the shape of individual bones.

Development of the Skeletal System

The process of endochondral bone formation is shown in figure 2.5. Initially, primary ossification occurs near the center of the shaft; a secondary center of ossification appears in the cartilage of the extremities of long bones. Ossification of the primary center forms the diaphysis (shaft), whereas bone that is ossified from the secondary center forms the epiphysis (end). The cartilage of the epiphysis is progressively ossified, leaving only a thin layer of cartilage—the epiphyseal plate, or growth plate—separating the epiphysis from the diaphysis (Gilsanz & Ratib, 2005). As long as the epiphyseal plate exists, the epiphysis and diaphysis will continue to grow. The growing end of the bone (located on the diaphysis side) is referred to as the metaphysis. Eventually, as the diaphysis and epiphysis become fused, the epiphyseal plate becomes ossified and growth ceases. Skeletal growth can vary in individual bones and around joints. In the lower limbs, the femur experiences more growth than does the tibia, and growth around the knee joint accounts for two-thirds of the increase in lower-limb length (Hume & Russell, 2014). Periods of rapid skeletal growth may be associated with increased risk of overuse injuries in youth (DiFiori et al., 2014).

Bone mass increases at the same rate in prepubertal girls and boys, but at the beginning of puberty bone mass increases faster in boys than in girls (Hemper, 2008). Maximal bone mass is achieved in the late teens or early twenties, and bone mass at the end of adolescence accounts for most of the variability in bone mass at older ages (Clark & Rogol, 1996). The National Osteoporosis Foundation suggests that the degree to which indicators of bone strength track from childhood to peak bone mass and beyond make it vitally important to optimize bone development in youth to help ensure lifelong skeletal health (Weaver et al., 2016). Consequently, we need to promote exercise and a healthy diet in childhood and adolescence in order to promote good bone health in adult life. In contrast, low bone-mineral density at the end of adolescence is associated with reduced bone health into adult life and, potentially, increased risk of fracture (Bass et al., 2000; Davies et al., 2005). Females are at greater risk of **osteoporosis** than men are, both because they are likely to accumulate lower levels of bone mineral density during adolescence and because they lose bone mass at a higher rate following menopause (Hemper, 2008).

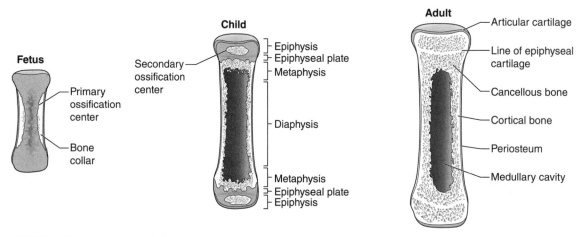

FIGURE 2.5   Endochondral formation of a long bone.

DO YOU KNOW?

Measures of bone health track strongly from childhood through adolescence and into adulthood.

Bone remodeling during growth is a function of hormonal factors and mechanical loading. Consequently, growth, maturation, and physical activity interact to promote bone development, and the process needs to be supported by a diet that provides sufficient energy and calcium. Normal bone maturation in both males and females is determined primarily by the hormone known as estrogen (Rowland, 2005). In addition, central hormonal factors maintain circulating calcium concentrations within a limited range (Hemper, 2008). Calcium is crucial for skeletal development; indeed, almost 99 percent of the body's calcium is deposited in the skeleton.

The primary role of estrogen in bone development is to suppress the activity of osteoclasts, thus inhibiting bone mineral resorption and allowing bone mass to accumulate during growth. Estrogen is required only in low levels to promote bone growth, which explains why it can mediate skeletal maturation in both boys and girls; higher levels, however, are associated with more rapid skeletal maturation (Cutler, 1997). Although prepubertal levels of estradiol are low for both sexes, they are still significantly higher for girls, and this difference has been suggested as a reason for the fact that girls experience faster skeletal maturation (Cutler, 1997).

Mechanical loading (through muscle actions or impact with the ground) can stimulate a stress adaptation response in bone. If the stress is large enough, it promotes calcium accumulation within the bone, as osteoclasts remove damaged structures and osteoblasts repair them (Burger & Klein-Nulend, 1999). If the mechanical stress is too low, it provides insufficient stimulus for remodeling. If it is too high, bone removal outstrips bone repair, which leads to microfractures due to structural fatigue. Consequently, youth fitness specialists should consider each child's exercise history: Inactive children may respond to low-impact loading by improving bone mass, whereas more active children will need more mechanical load in order to promote skeletal response (Weaver et al., 2016).

Bone adaptation is influenced not only by hormonal development and mechanical stress but also by their interaction, which may in fact be particularly important. One longitudinal study found that more than 35 percent of bone mineral content was laid down in the four years encompassing puberty, and that the rate of accrual was particularly rapid in the two years following the growth spurt and the observation of peak height velocity (Bailey, 1997). These findings mean that gains in bone mineral density lag behind gains in bone length, which may in turn mean that bones are more susceptible to injury (e.g., fracture) during this time. Therefore, during this period of growth and development, it is critical that youth consume sufficient calcium and vitamin D to support their skeletal growth (Institute of Medicine, 2010). For more on nutrition, see chapter 16.

Acute and Chronic Response of the Skeletal System to Exercise

Studying the direct effects of acute exercise on bone is challenging as bone remodeling is a chronic process. As noted earlier, estrogen concentrations can be elevated in response to exercise in girls, and this increase may provide some benefit for bone remodeling. At the same time, skeletal development in youth is believed to be stimulated by mechanical stress, particularly the intensity of the forces acting on the bones rather

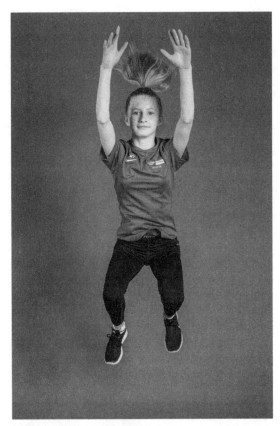

FIGURE 2.6 Jump-landing and rebound tasks can provide the type of mechanical loading needed to stimulate bone adaptation.

than the duration of exercise (Hemper, 2008). An acute mechanical stimulus can be provided through weight-bearing and weight-loading activities, which, if varied and repeated over time, elicit a positive chronic adaptation of increased bone density (see figure 2.6).

Habitual physical activity exerts a positive influence on bone health in youth. Bailey and colleagues (1999) monitored adolescents longitudinally for a six-year period and found that, respectively, physically active boys and girls accrued 9 percent and 17 percent more bone mineral content than did their inactive peers. Large differences have also been found in side-to-side bone mass and bone mineral density in the arms of young players of racket sports once the adolescent growth spurt is reached (Haapasalo et al., 1998). Moreover, the greatest differences were observed in those who started playing when they were prepubertal (Kannus et al., 1995).

In a similar finding, the training age of prepubertal female gymnasts has been shown to influence the magnitude of positive increases in bone mineral density, and increased bone mass appeared to last well into adulthood following retirement from the sport (Bass et al., 1998). In addition, greater bone mineral density has been reported in 17-year-old Junior Olympics weightlifters than in either age-matched controls or adults, and as much as 65 percent of the variance was explained by strength (Conroy et al., 1993). In contrast, bone mineral density in young swimmers has been found to develop at a rate similar to that of sedentary youth and slower than that of youth involved in weight-bearing sports; moreover, the difference increased with advancing age (Gomez-Burton et al., 2016). Collectively, this evidence indicates that habitual, weight-bearing physical activity and resistance training promote the development of bone health in children and adolescents.

Table 2.1 provides a review of interventions that have examined the benefits of training on bone mineral content and bone density in youth ranging from 7 to 16 years old. All of the studies compare participants' gains in measures of bone health following an intervention period with any gains observed in a control group. The use of a control group is a particularly important aspect of experimental design with this population because markers of bone health in youth are expected to increase even without intervention due to natural growth and maturation processes. Therefore, researchers must distinguish whether any observed

Teaching Tip

PHYSICAL ACTIVITY AND BONE

According to Turner (1998), bone cells become less responsive to routine mechanical loading and appear to react best to exercise characterized by high dynamic loads with an unexpected and irregular pattern and relatively short duration. These requirements can be largely fulfilled by providing children with regular opportunities for outdoor play, varied fitness activities, and participation in recreational sport. Children tend to take part in dynamic short-burst activities that typically involve jumping, skipping, dodging, hopping, and bounding—all of which can positively affect bone development. Providing youth with opportunities to engage in a wide variety of weight-bearing activities during the growing years will help to optimize their gains in bone health.

TABLE 2.1   SKELETAL LOADING INTERVENTION STUDIES IN YOUTH

Reference	Age (yr)	Sex	Duration and frequency*	Intervention	Findings**
Fuchs et al. (2001)	7.5	M & F	7 mo, 3×10	Progression of drop jumps to reach 100 jumps per session from a 61 cm (24 in.) box	Gains in spine and hip BMC
Valdimarsson et al. (2006)	7.7	F	12 mo, 5×40	Ball games, running, and jumping	Gains in spine BMC, BMD, and bone width
McKay et al. (2000)	8.9	M & F	8 mo, 3×10-30	10 tuck jumps three times per week and jumping activities included in physical education classes	Gains in femur BMD
Morris et al. (1997)	9.5	F	10 mo, 3×30	Mixed exercise including aerobics, team games, dance, and resistance training	Gains in total-body, spine, and femur BMD and BMC
Bradney et al. (1998)	10.0	M	8 mo, 3×30	Mixed exercise including aerobics, team games, dance, gymnastics, and resistance training	Gains in total-body, spine, and leg BMD
McKay et al. (2005)	10.1	M & F	8 mo, 5×3	10 countermovement jumps at the start of each school day	Gains in femur BMC
MacKelvie et al. (2001)	10.1 and 10.5	F	7 mo, 3×10	Circuit of various jumping activities	10.1 yr (prepubertal): no gains in total-body, spine, or femur BMD or BMC 10.5 yr (early pubertal): gains in spine and femur BMD and BMC
MacKelvie, McKay, et al. (2002)	10.3	M	7 mo, 3×10	Circuit of various jumping activities	Gains in total-body BMC but no gains in boys of high body mass index (BMI)
Yu et al. (2005)	10.4	M & F	1.5 mo, 3×75	Strength training with aerobic and agility training	Gains in whole-body BMC
Heinonen et al. (2000)	11.0 and 13.7	F	9 mo, 2×20	Jumps from floor and from a 30 cm (12 in.) box	11.0 yr: gains in spine and femur BMC 13.7 yr: no gains in spine or femur BMC
Weeks et al. (2008)	13.8	M & F	8 mo, 2×10	Various jumping activities	Girls: gains in neck BMC and spine BMD Boys: gains in whole-body BMC
Witzke & Snow (2000)	14.6	F	9 mo, 3×30-45	Resistance training (weighted vests) and plyometric exercises	No gains in total-body, spine, or femur BMC
Álvarez-San Emeterio et al. (2011)	14.7	M & F	24 mo, 3× (not given)	Strength training and alpine skiing	Gains in spine BMD
Blimkie et al. (1996)	16.2	F	6.5 mo, 3× (not given)	Resistance training, four sets of 10-12 reps, 13 exercises	No gains in total-body or lumbar-spine BMD or BMC

*Duration and frequency are shown as program duration in months (mo) and number of sessions per week × session duration in minutes.

**Gains are expressed relative to a control group. BMC indicates bone mineral content, and BMD indicates bone mineral density.

change is due to an imposed intervention or simply reflects normal developmental progress.

The research is almost unanimous in finding that various exercise interventions improve bone health in girls and boys aged 11 years or under—in other words, in participants who can be considered prepubertal or early pubertal. In two studies that included older, adolescent females, interventions did not improve markers of bone health above the improvement experienced by control groups. Accordingly, it has been suggested that during the very early stages of puberty, bone may be particularly responsive to weight-bearing activities and safely executed high-impact exercises in a range of fitness activities and youth sports (MacKelvie, Khan, et al., 2002). In contrast, older, more mature children who have accumulated more exercise experience may require a greater progression toward unfamiliar exercises and mechanical loading patterns in order to promote continued bone adaptation beyond the level provided by growth and maturation alone. Given the implications of this research, youth fitness specialists should be aware of the different types of exercise that can help promote bone health. For example, the Bounce at the Bell intervention studied by McKay and colleagues (2005) showed that as little as three minutes of jumping at the start of each school day improved bone mineral content in the femur of 10-year-old children.

Muscle–Tendon System

The muscle–tendon system enables the production of mechanical work during exercise. Specifically, when skeletal muscle receives a neural stimulus of sufficient strength, it contracts and produces force, which is then transmitted through the tendon to generate tension and movement. Both muscle mass and tendon size increase substantially due to growth and maturation throughout childhood and adolescence, and these gains underpin the large improvements in fitness that can be observed in active youth during these periods. Growth and maturation also lead to qualitative structural changes in muscles and tendons that positively influence their ability to generate and transmit force. These positive adaptations can be further enhanced through exercise and training in youth.

Development of the Muscle–Tendon System

The total number of muscle fibers is determined largely by genetics (De Ste Croix, 2008), and the increases in muscle size that occur during childhood result from **muscle hypertrophy** (which increases protein content and fiber size) rather than from **muscle hyperplasia** (which increases the number of muscle fibers) (Yan et al., 2013). During prepuberty, muscle mass increases linearly with age, and boys experience slightly greater gains than girls do. With the onset of puberty, increases in IGF-1 and growth hormone promote protein synthesis in both boys and girls, but the additional anabolic effect of increased testosterone means that boys experience much greater gains in muscle mass during puberty than girls do. From age 5 to 17 years, relative muscle mass increases from 42 percent to 54 percent of body weight in boys but only from 40 percent to 42 percent in girls (Malina et al., 2004). For girls, the relative contribution of muscle mass peaks at 46 percent around 13 years of age, then decreases as absolute muscle mass is maintained but increasing fat mass adds additional body weight (Malina et al., 2004). Maturation also brings changes in the distribution of muscle mass around the body. At birth, about 40 percent of muscle mass is located in the lower extremities, and this proportion increases to about 55 percent at sexual maturity in both boys and girls (De Ste Croix, 2008).

DO YOU KNOW?

In a fetus, skeletal muscle development is primarily achieved by muscle hyperplasia and affected dramatically by maternal nutrition (Yan et al., 2013).

One primary determinant of muscle strength is muscle cross-sectional area, which is determined by the number and size of fibers in parallel. For instance, figure 2.7 shows changes in cross-sectional area in upper-arm muscle from age 1 to age 18 years. Differences in muscle cross-sectional area between the sexes largely explain the differences in absolute strength that are consistently observed between males and females following the onset of puberty. Given the large influence exerted on muscle size by growth and maturation, the cross-sectional area of muscles around the elbow increases by about 200 percent in boys and 70 percent in girls between the ages of 9 and 24 years (Deighan et al., 2006). By adulthood, muscle cross-sectional area in the limbs is about 30 percent to 40 percent greater in males than in females (Miller et al., 1993).

Increases in muscle volume result from changes in both muscle cross-sectional area and muscle length. Linear growth of the skeletal system has been proposed as providing the stimulus for continued increases in muscle length during childhood and adolescence, as bone growth increases tension on the muscle and provides the stimulus to adapt muscle length (Round et al., 1999). This model is consistent with the observation that bone growth precedes

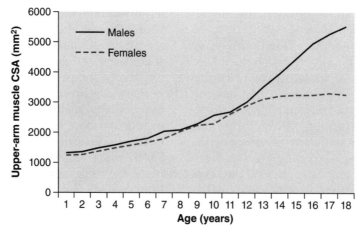

FIGURE 2.7   Changes in upper-arm muscle cross-sectional area (CSA) from 1 to 18 years old (*n* = 5467).
Data from Frisancho (1981).

increased muscle length, as well as the implication of temporarily increased muscle tension in growth- and sport-related conditions such as Osgood-Schlatter disease.

Increases in strength above increases in muscle cross-sectional area during childhood and adolescence suggest qualitative changes in muscle structure and function. Muscle is typically considered in terms of slow- and fast-twitch fibers; the former are also referred to as type I fibers, and the latter are further classified as type IIA and type IIB fibers. Each fiber type is distinguished by certain characteristics in terms of size and function, which are summarized in table 2.2. As implied in the table, having a high percentage of slow-twitch fibers is beneficial for endurance exercise, whereas having a high percentage of fast-twitch fibers is beneficial for high-intensity and explosive activities. Some debate exists as to whether fiber type changes with maturation. Malina and colleagues (2004) concluded that the distribution of the different fiber types appears to be stable from about one year of age and that little difference appears in distribution

of muscle fiber types in children and adolescents. In contrast, Armstrong and Fawkner (2008) suggest a consistent age-related decline in the percentage of type I fibers from childhood to early adulthood.

The angle at which muscle fibers meet tendon is referred to as the pennation angle. Greater pennation reduces the efficiency of force transmission, but this reduction is more than compensated for by the fact that pennation increases the number of fibers in parallel, thus increasing the functional cross-sectional area. As a result, pennation ultimately allows for greater force production. Whether pennation angle increases with growth and maturation remains unclear. Binzoni and colleagues (2001) reported that pennation of the gastrocnemius increases until the adolescent growth spurt, then stabilizes. In contrast, O'Brien and colleagues (2010a) found no difference in pennation of the quadriceps muscles when comparing nine-year-old boys and girls with adults, and it may be that any changes with maturation are specific to each muscle.

In comparison with muscles, tendons have greater capacity for energy storage and higher recoil speed

TABLE 2.2   BASIC CHARACTERISTICS OF SLOW-TWITCH (TYPE I) AND FAST-TWITCH (TYPE IIA AND TYPE IIB) SKELETAL MUSCLE FIBERS

	Type I	Type IIA	Type IIB
Size	Small	Large	Very large
Contraction speed	Slow	Fast	Very fast
Force production	Low	High	Very high
Aerobic capacity	High	Medium	Low
Anaerobic capacity	Low	High	Very high
Fatigue resistance	High	Low	Very low

and force (Blavezich et al., 2013). Tendons usually extend into the muscle as aponeuroses; to produce mechanical work, muscles must transmit forces through the aponeuroses and tendons to create force across a joint. Development of tendon properties during childhood and adolescence has been examined in limited research. In a mixed sample of males and females, cross-sectional area in the Achilles tendon doubled from childhood (five to seven years old) to adulthood (Waugh et al., 2012). When each sex was analyzed separately, the increases were found to be considerably larger in males than in females (O'Brien et al., 2010b), which is similar to differences found in the development of muscle cross-sectional area.

With maturation, tendon length increases more in males than in females, due to the increased skeletal growth and longer limb lengths attained by males. In addition, both Waugh and colleagues (2012) and O'Brien and colleagues (2010b) report greater mechanical tendon stiffness in adults than in children, which suggests that maturation involves microstructural adaptation of the tendon. It has been proposed that tendon adaptation, like bone adaptation, is stimulated by maturation and mechanical loading—in this case, most likely in the properties of the tendon's collagen matrix (O'Brien et al., 2010b, Waugh et al., 2012).

Acute Response of the Muscle–Tendon System to Exercise

The nearly identical growth curves of muscle mass and strength confirm the relationships between muscle size, strength, sex, age, and maturation (Rowland, 2005). Due to differences in muscle size, absolute force production is generally lower in females than in males; it is also generally lower in immature children than in more mature children, although this difference is less obvious in girls than in boys. The question of whether force production increases relative to body size with growth and maturation remains under debate. Increased relative force production with maturation is supported by increased performance of tasks requiring body mass to be moved, such as jumping. These relative changes in acute function represent changes in the interaction of the neural system and the muscle–tendon system.

When a muscle is activated by the nervous system, a time lag occurs before the muscle generates force, and this electromechanical delay has been shown to be longer in younger girls than in older ones (De Ste Croix et al., 2014). The larger electromechanical delay in younger, more immature children is related to lower tendon stiffness and slower rate of force development, which indicates less effective transfer of muscle forces (Waugh et al., 2013). Increasing muscle–tendon stiff-

ness from childhood to adulthood also correlates with increased stretch-reflex response (Grosset et al., 2007). Consequently, changes in the muscle–tendon properties with maturation facilitate a more excitatory feedback response from the neural system, which should benefit performance in activities such as sprinting, jumping, and throwing.

The ability to produce a greater peak rate of force development with advancing maturity can also be attributed to the fact that the ability to produce peak force increases (due largely to increased muscle mass), whereas contraction times do not change; therefore, with growth, more force is developed over the same contraction time (Grosset et al., 2005). This change can provide a benefit in physical activities. In sprinting, for instance, although adolescents do not increase stride frequency with development, their increased force production during ground contact produces a longer stride, thus increasing their sprinting speed (Meyers et al., 2015).

Chronic Response of the Muscle–Tendon System to Exercise

The notion that children can increase muscle size with training may appear to be supported by anecdotal evidence—in particular, observations of body size and shape in children involved in intensive training programs in sports such as gymnastics and rugby. However, there is only a limited amount of direct evidence to support training-induced increases in muscle size in children and adolescents. In a review of 22 training studies in prepubertal and early pubertal youth, Malina (2006) concluded that resistance training programs exerted no influence on body mass and only limited influence on body composition, thus suggesting an absence of hypertrophy. However, the training programs lasted only 8 to 12 weeks and were not specifically designed to induce muscular hypertrophy, which requires muscular and metabolic stress.

In another study, Granacher and colleagues (2011) concluded that high-intensity resistance training was unable to affect muscle size in prepubertal children. However, hypertrophy would be unlikely to result in any case from the program's 10-week duration and three- to four-minute rest between sets. Alternatively, Fukunaga and colleagues (1992) reported that 12 weeks of resistance training increased muscle cross-sectional area in both boys and girls as compared with controls. The increase positively correlated with skeletal age and amounted to about 50 percent of that observed in adults. Although the limited existing body of research might suggest that hypertrophy is not achievable during prepuberty or early puberty, we must be cautious about drawing conclusions, due to the limitations of existing research. Debate also remains open about whether muscle hypertrophy is a desirable chronic training goal in prepubertal children. Finally, though it is generally accepted that training-induced hypertrophy can be achieved following the onset of puberty, this hypothesis has been examined in only a limited amount of research.

Only a few studies have examined chronic training adaptations in the tendon or qualitative muscle factors found in children and adolescents. In one study, resistance training was found to exert no influence on the contractile properties of muscle in prepubescent boys; specifically, no changes were found in contraction or relaxation times (Ramsay et al., 1990). This finding is consistent with the earlier observation that contraction times do not change from childhood to adulthood, which suggests that contraction times are relatively fixed. Achilles tendon stiffness, on the other hand, has been found to increase in prepubertal children following 10 weeks of resistance training that consisted of calf-raise exercises (Waugh et al., 2014). In addition, a study in young men (18.8 years old) revealed that plyometric training increased Achilles tendon stiffness without any concomitant increase in cross-sectional area (Foure et al., 2010). Thus it may be speculated that chronic training adaptations can be achieved in the tendon in children and adolescents; to confirm this speculation, however, further evidence is needed.

Cardiopulmonary System

Sustained physical activity depends on a well-developed **cardiopulmonary system**. This system consists of the heart and lungs, whereas the **cardiovascular system** consists of the heart and blood vessels. Together the cardiopulmonary and cardiovascular systems transport oxygen, blood, nutrients, and other needed compounds throughout the body. During exercise, oxygen is needed by the working muscles to enable aerobic metabolism, and blood is also needed to help regulate muscle temperature and pH, supply energy substrates, transport hormones, and remove waste products.

Development of the Cardiopulmonary System

Cardiopulmonary function is driven by a 20-fold increase in heart size from birth to adulthood (Rowland, 1996). Resting and maximal heart rates decrease for both boys and girls throughout childhood and adolescence, whereas stroke volume increases 10-fold from birth to late childhood (4 to 40 mL) and 15-fold from birth to adulthood (Stratton & Oliver, 2014). Increasing stroke volume means that maximal cardiac output

also increases throughout childhood and adolescence.

The increase in heart size is closely associated with increased body size, as heart mass is related to body surface area during childhood and adolescence. Expressing cardiac output and stroke volume in relation to body surface area provides relative measures known as cardiac output index and stroke volume index. These measures have been shown to remain stable with growth, thus indicating no maturational influence (though females have values that are about 10 percent lower than those of males) (Rowland, 2008). In fact, when cardiovascular variables are scaled appropriately to body size, no quantitative or qualitative maturation-related differences appear in terms of peak cardiac index, stroke index, exercise factor, ventricular systolic or diastolic function, cardiovascular drift, patterns of stroke volume, or alterations in heart chamber size (Rowland, 2008). However, blood composition does change during puberty. In particular, hematocrit increases from 30 percent in infancy to 40 percent or even 45 percent in adult males and to 38 percent or even 42 percent in adult females; in addition, hemoglobin increases from 10 grams per deciliter in childhood to 14 in adult females and 16 in adult males (Stratton & Oliver, 2014).

As with the heart, the lungs experience rapid growth from birth to adulthood. Lung mass increases from 65 grams (2.3 oz) to 1.3 kilograms (2.9 lb), the number of alveoli increases from about 20 to about 300 million, and the number of breaths at rest decreases from about 25 per minute to about 15 (Stratton & Oliver, 2014; Fawkner, 2008). The growth of lung volume follows the general pattern of the growth of body size; therefore, peak lung growth occurs around the time of the adolescent growth spurt. Lung capacity is closely related to the cube of height, and it increases from about 2 liters at a body height of 1.2 meters (3 ft 11 in.) to 6 liters at a height of 1.8 meters (5 ft 11 in.) (Fawkner, 2008). A similar relationship is observed with alveoli surface area. Growth in the diameter of the airways means that airway resistance decreases from childhood to adulthood even as compliance of the lungs increases, all of which influences breathing patterns both at rest and during exercise. The changes in lung volume, structure, and breathing frequency enable maximal minute ventilation during exercise to increase from 50 liters per minute at five years of age to 100 liters per minute at adulthood.

DO YOU KNOW?

With growth, cardiac output increases in proportion to body surface area, and lung volume increases in proportion to height.

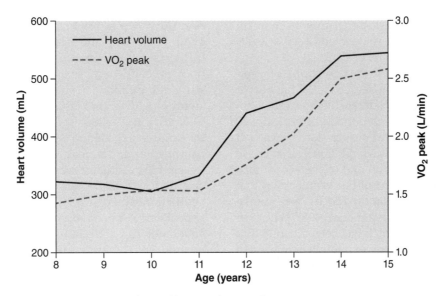

FIGURE 2.8 Increases in peak oxygen uptake and heart volume in boys.
Adapted from Hollman, Bouchard, and Herkenrath (1967).

Functionally, development of the cardiopulmonary and cardiovascular systems is often examined in terms of peak oxygen uptake ($\dot{V}O_2$peak), which is the maximal rate at which oxygen can be delivered to and used by exercising muscles. $\dot{V}O_2$peak more than doubles from 1.2 to 2.7 liters per minute in boys between the ages of 6 and 12; values for females are about 0.2 liters per minute lower than those of males (Rowland, 2005). Boys then experience an accelerated increase in $\dot{V}O_2$peak during puberty due to the anabolic influence of testosterone in increasing muscle mass and heart size, whereas in girls the absolute values plateau. Figure 2.8 shows that the age-related increase in $\dot{V}O_2$peak in boys tracks with increases in heart volume. This parallel is not surprising given that $\dot{V}O_2$peak is determined primarily by maximal cardiac output.

Acute Response of the Cardiopulmonary System to Exercise

Although the underlying mechanism remains unclear, it is well known that maximal heart rate decreases with age. This reduction means that in vigorous activity the maximal heart rate of younger children is higher than that of older children or adults. Nonetheless, though individual variation is still apparent, a reasonably valid equation for predicting HRmax in both children and adolescents has been suggested in the predictive equation of 208–(0.7 × age) (Mahon et al., 2010). Moreover, when appropriately accounting for the influence of size, it has been concluded that the qualitative and quantitative features of the cardiovascular response to an acute bout of progressive exercise are similar in children and adults (Rowland, 2008). For instance, the pattern of the stroke volume response to exercise is similar in children and adults (Nottin et al., 2004). In addition, both children and adults have been shown to have an "exercise factor" of about six liters; this factor quantifies the increase in cardiac output that is required in order to increase oxygen consumption by one liter per minute (Rowland, 2005).

DO YOU KNOW?

Heart rates over 200 beats per minute are normal and expected when healthy children participate in active play, fitness training, or sport.

Children and adults may differ in the pattern of change in breathing frequency and tidal volume (the amount of air expired in each breath) in response to an acute bout of exercise. The product of breathing frequency and tidal volume is **minute ventilation**. During incremental exercise in adults, minute ventilation increases, initially due to a rise in tidal volume, but there's only limited change in breathing frequency; at higher intensities, however, tidal volume plateaus and breathing frequency increases, but the opposite response has been reported in children (Fawkner, 2008). As background for this finding, note that during exercise the arterial partial pressure of carbon dioxide increases, and the level that stimulates increased ventilation, known as the set point, has been shown to be lower in children than in adults (Rowland, 2005). Consequently, children experience greater ventilatory drive during an acute bout of exercise and use greater minute ventilation to expire a given amount of carbon dioxide. It has been suggested that this mechanism allows children to better regulate blood acidity levels during intense exercise (Ratel et al., 2002).

Ventilation kinetics involve the time course of respiratory dynamics at the onset of exercise. At the start of constant-load exercise of moderate intensity, the time constant for change in oxygen uptake is typically 20 to 40 seconds in adults, and steady state is reached in about three minutes (Rowland, 2005). If exercise is prolonged, then ventilation and oxygen consumption gradually drift upward. It has been shown that children have faster ventilation and oxygen uptake kinetics than do adults (Cooper et al., 1987; Welsman et al., 2001), the latter of which has been attributed to both faster delivery and faster extraction of oxygen in children (Leclair et al., 2013). These findings mean that in response to a bout of submaximal exercise, children increase their oxygen consumption and reach steady state more quickly than adults do.

Chronic Response of the Cardiopulmonary System to Exercise

As compared with untrained children, those who are trained as cyclists have exhibited higher peak oxygen uptake and greater resting and exercise cardiac dimensions and stroke index but similar patterns of stroke volume response to exercise and no differences in maximal heart rate, cardiac contractility, or arteriovenous oxygen difference (Nottin et al., 2002; Rowland et al., 2002). When 10- and 11-year-old children were exposed to 13 weeks of training (three times per week for one hour at an intensity of more than 80 percent HRmax), the gains observed in peak oxygen uptake in both boys and girls were attributable entirely to increases in maximal stroke volume and not to changes in maximal heart rate, cardiac contractility, or arteriovenous difference (Obert et al., 2003). Similar findings were reported previously by Eriksson and Koch (1973). In contrast with adults, increased stroke volume in children following endurance training is associated with increased left ventricular cavity dimensions without concomitant increases in wall thickness (Obert et al., 2003). When prepubertal children experienced morphological adaptations in the heart following three months of exercise training, those adaptations were lost within two months of detraining (Obert et al., 2001).

Examination of swimmers suggests that this mode of exercise promotes pulmonary adaptation. In particular, trained swimmers exhibit increased lung function and larger lung volume relative to height than do nonswimmers, and the difference is more marked in older children (Andrew et al., 1972; Zinman & Gaultier, 1986). In contrast, it has been shown that prepubertal and postpubertal youth who partake in land-based training do not experience any pulmonary adapta-tion (Eriksson & Koch, 1973; Hamilton & Andrew, 1976). Therefore, land-based training may exert less influence on pulmonary function than swim training does, probably because land-based training does not stress the pulmonary system to the same degree as swimming (Fawkner, 2008).

Nourry and colleagues (2005) found that prepubertal children exposed to eight weeks of high-intensity running training increased lung volume and function, lowered the ventilatory response to submaximal exercise, and increased peak oxygen uptake and minute ventilation. Thus the high-intensity basis of the study appears to have been sufficient to promote pulmonary adaptation in children. Increased minute ventilation in children following training results from increases in tidal volume (not breathing frequency) and is correlated with increased peak oxygen uptake (Nourry et al., 2005; Rowland & Boyajian, 1995).

DO YOU KNOW?

Swimming improves lung function and cardiopulmonary fitness in youth with asthma (Beggs, 2013).

Metabolic System

As children grow and mature, they become able to perform more work during exercise. This improved physical function is supported by the development and interaction of the various physiological systems. One crucial aspect in this process is the ability to derive metabolic energy in order to produce mechanical work. The metabolic requirements of physical activity relate to exercise intensity, and the ability to continue exercising or to work at higher intensities is dictated by the ability to resist fatigue. The ability of the metabolic system to provide energy is a potential limiting factor in exercise and performance, and it is clear that some metabolic capacities develop from childhood into adulthood. These changes in exercise metabolism interact with other developmental processes, such as altered motor unit recruitment strategies (e.g., co-contraction and activation deficits), to contribute to differences between children and adults in the ability to perform work and resist fatigue.

Development of the Metabolic System

Adenosine triphosphate (ATP) is the high-energy phosphate that is broken down to allow the contractile elements of skeletal muscle to produce mechanical work. Muscle ATP levels increase rapidly in the first year of life (Malina et al., 2004), and available data suggest that after two years of age ATP stores are the same in children and adults (Rowlands, 2005). What may differ between children and adults is the ability to resynthesize ATP in order to allow exercise to continue at a desired rate, as well as the ability to tolerate the fatiguing effects of some metabolic by-products. ATP stores are rapidly resynthesized through the use of high-energy phosphocreatine (PCr) by what is known as the ATP-PC system. In terms of providing energy for work, this system is high in power, low in capacity, and limited by the availability of PCr. Muscle biopsies on a small sample of boys have shown that muscle PCr stores increase from 11 years old to reach adult values by 15 years old (Eriksson & Saltin, 1974). The ATP-PC reaction is catalyzed by an enzyme, **creatine kinase**, that is active to a similar level in both children and adults (Berg et al., 1986).

The functional capacity of the glycolytic pathway is greater in adults than in children (Rowland, 2005). Although glycogen storage and availability becomes a limiting factor in prolonged exercise, it is unlikely to limit exercise performance for youth in most scenarios. Muscle glycogen concentrations have been shown to increase by more than 50 percent in boys from 11 to 15 years of age and to reach adult levels by the end of that period (Eriksson & Saltin, 1974). Table 2.3 summarizes levels of stored metabolic substrates in boys aged 11 to 15 years.

The end product of glycolysis is pyruvate. At lower exercise intensities, pyruvate enters what is known as the Krebs cycle and is metabolized aerobically. In contrast, at higher exercise intensities, the capacity to metabolize pyruvate aerobically is exceeded, and pyruvate is converted to lactate. This conversion is catalyzed by the enzyme **lactate dehydrogenase** (LDH). Haralambie (1982) showed that the activity of LDH and of **phosphofructokinase** (PFK)—a key regulatory enzyme of glycolytic activity shown to increase in concentration during childhood (Malina et al., 2004)—did not differ between adolescents (boys and girls) and adults (men and women). In a younger age range, of 6- to 13-year-olds, Berg and colleagues (1986) reported a 143 percent increase in LDH activity. Therefore, based on the limited available evidence, it has been suggested that prepubertal children have lower glycolytic enzyme activity than do adults (Rowland, 2005).

The ratio of glycolytic to oxidative anaerobic enzyme activity has been reported to be 59 percent higher in 17-year-olds than in 6-year-olds, reflecting a more anaerobic profile with more advanced maturity (Armstrong & Fawkner, 2008). Though it is difficult to study the influence of hormones on energy metabolism, the balance of evidence suggests that glycolytic activity in children may be reduced by a lower sympathetic and excitatory hormonal response (Armstrong & Fawkner, 2008). As a result, children are less reliant on glycolysis and convert less pyruvate to lactate (more pyruvate is oxidized) as compared with adults. Accordingly, children have been reported to be more reliant than adults on fat oxidization when working at a given relative or absolute intensity. For instance, Timmons and colleagues (2003) reported that 9-year-old boys used 73 percent more lipids and 23 percent less carbohydrate then men did during the second half of a 60-minute cycle. More generally, Stephens and colleagues (2006) examined substrate usage in males of varying maturation and concluded that fully mature fuel use occurs sometime between mid and late puberty.

It has been suggested that children are "metabolic nonspecialists" (Bar-Or & Rowland, 2004). In practice, this notion suggests that a child could often excel in both sprint and endurance events, whereas for adults the best sprinter would not be the best endurance athlete (Ratel & Williams, 2008). This observation has been attributed to the development of metabolic properties with maturation, including the shift to a more anaerobic profile. Ratel and Williams (2008) state that the notion of children as metabolic nonspecialists has been accepted as an established fact that is rarely challenged.

Although the literature does support changing metabolic profiles as children mature, we lack studies that examine the integrative metabolic response to exercise. For instance, metabolic response is influenced by fiber type distribution within muscle. As noted earlier, debate continues about whether fiber type distribution changes with age and maturation. Certainly, such a change is suggested by some research. Lexell

TABLE 2.3   RESTING VALUES* OF SKELETAL MUSCLE ATP, PCr, AND GLYCOGEN IN BOYS AGED 11 TO 15 YEARS

Group (age in yr)	ATP	PCr	Glycogen
11.6	4	15	55
12.6	5	20	70
13.5	5	17	70
15.5	5	24	85

*All values are given in terms of millimoles per kilogram wet weight.

Data from Eriksson (1980).

and colleagues (1992) reported that the distribution of type I fibers decreased from 65 percent at 5 years old to 50 percent at 20 years old. Type I fibers have greater mitochondrial density, which would increase reliance on aerobic metabolism and therefore support the belief that children are more predisposed toward that type of metabolism. As children mature, they develop anaerobic capabilities at a faster rate than aerobic capabilities (Ratel & Williams, 2008).

Acute Response of the Metabolic System to Exercise

The breakdown of ATP and phosphocreatine during exercise occurs at the same rate in children and adults (Berg et al., 1986; Malina et al., 2004). However, the lower glycolytic enzyme activity in children means reduced reliance on glycolysis during exercise and reduced conversion of pyruvate to lactate. Coupled with children's lower muscle mass, this difference means that the muscle and blood lactate observed in children in response to a bout of high-intensity exercise is considerably lower than that observed in adults. The lower accumulation of lactate is linked to an attenuated lowering of muscle pH in children in response to high-intensity exercise. Given that lower muscle pH (reflecting cellular acidosis) is associated with fatigue, the blunted lowering response in children may partly explain their ability to resist fatigue during all-out intense efforts of exercise. Direct examination of muscle following exercise confirms that children and adolescents experience lower levels of acidosis than do adults (Kuno et al., 1995; Zanconato et al., 1993).

Although children and adults can both fully deplete phosphocreatine during intense exercise, debate exists as to whether children are able to resynthesize these stores at a faster rate during recovery. Taylor and colleagues (1997) reported that resynthesis kinetics in 6- to 12-year-old boys are about twice as fast as those in adults (12 versus 27 seconds to recover half of phosphocreatine stores). In contrast, Barker and colleagues (2008) reported no differences when comparing 9-year-old boys with adults. In another study, examining the ages of 11 to 16 years, the decrease in glycogen stores during exercise was three times lower in the younger children (Eriksson & Saltin, 1974).

Given their reduced reliance on glycolysis and anaerobic metabolism, children have a relatively greater reliance on aerobic metabolism, particularly on lipid oxidization, at any exercise intensity. This response may help to preserve the lower muscle-glycogen stores in children, which is supported by the observation that the blood glucose response to prolonged submaximal exercise does not change with age or maturation (Boisseau & Delamarche, 2000). In children, in response to prolonged exercise, lower glycogen stores and glycolytic rate are compensated for by increased fat metabolism, which allows children to maintain adequate levels of blood glucose. Figure 2.9 provides a complete summary of acute physiological responses to a bout of exercise in children as compared with adults.

Chronic Response of the Metabolic System to Exercise

The experimental difficulty inherent in measuring metabolic properties means that only limited research has examined changes in these properties following training interventions in youth. In addition, the research that is available must be interpreted with caution due to the absence of control groups to account for changes that could be attributed to growth and maturation. In a landmark study, Eriksson and colleagues (1973) exposed 8- to 13-year-old boys to a four-month training intervention about which little detail was provided. The authors reported that resting values of ATP increased by about 12 percent, phosphocreatine by 39 percent, and muscle glycogen by 32 percent. No posttraining change occurred in ATP or PCr depletion rate during exercise, but increased glycolytic rates were observed, along with a 56 percent increase in muscle lactate accumulation.

Teaching Tip

FATIGUE AND RECOVERY DURING INTENSE EXERCISE

Children may experience less metabolic stress than adults in a single bout of all-out exercise; they may also fatigue less and recover more quickly in repeated intense bouts. For instance, Ratel and colleagues (2004) reported that during a 10-repetition set of 10-second cycle sprints separated by 15 seconds of recovery, peak power was reduced by only 18 percent in 11-year-old boys but by 43 percent in men. At the same time, the increase in blood lactate was 2.5 times greater in adults. Improved recovery rates in children have been associated with faster phosphocreatine resynthesis, increased oxidative capacity, better acid–base regulation, faster cardiopulmonary readjustment, and lower production and faster removal of metabolic by-products (Armstrong & Fawkner, 2008).

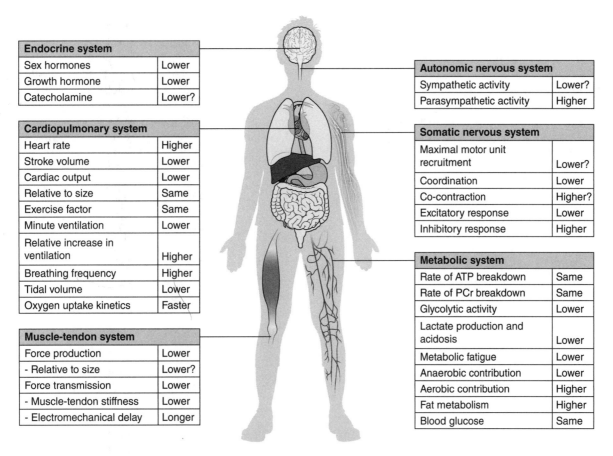

Endocrine system

Sex hormones	Lower
Growth hormone	Lower
Catecholamine	Lower?

Cardiopulmonary system

Heart rate	Higher
Stroke volume	Lower
Cardiac output	Lower
Relative to size	Same
Exercise factor	Same
Minute ventilation	Lower
Relative increase in ventilation	Higher
Breathing frequency	Higher
Tidal volume	Lower
Oxygen uptake kinetics	Faster

Muscle-tendon system

Force production	Lower
- Relative to size	Lower?
Force transmission	Lower
- Muscle-tendon stiffness	Lower
- Electromechanical delay	Longer

Autonomic nervous system

Sympathetic activity	Lower?
Parasympathetic activity	Higher

Somatic nervous system

Maximal motor unit recruitment	Lower?
Coordination	Lower
Co-contraction	Higher?
Excitatory response	Lower
Inhibitory response	Higher

Metabolic system

Rate of ATP breakdown	Same
Rate of PCr breakdown	Same
Glycolytic activity	Lower
Lactate production and acidosis	Lower
Metabolic fatigue	Lower
Anaerobic contribution	Lower
Aerobic contribution	Higher
Fat metabolism	Higher
Blood glucose	Same

FIGURE 2.9 Acute responses to exercise in children as compared with adults. The question marks indicate where there is either limited evidence available or conflicting evidence. "Exercise factor" is the increase in cardiac output that is needed to increase oxygen consumption by one liter per minute.

Fournier and colleagues (1982) reported that sprint training in adolescent boys increased PFK activity by 21 percent and that endurance training increased aerobic enzyme activity by 39 percent, although the values returned to baseline with detraining. Thus metabolic adaptations are specific to the demands of a training program, and any metabolic gains may be lost once training is ceased. Cadefau and colleagues (1990) noted substantial gains in glycogen content and glycolytic and aerobic enzyme activity after 16- to 18-year-old boys were exposed to power, sprint, and endurance training. From this limited collection of research it appears that both substrate storage and glycolytic and aerobic enzyme activity can positively adapt to training in children and adolescents.

Summary

Pediatric exercise science involves the application of scientific inquiry and principles as they relate to exercise in children and adolescents. Research has provided an evidence base that describes how children and adolescents respond and adapt to different types of exercise. Understanding both acute and chronic responses to exercise can help youth fitness specialists design exercise programs that are safe, effective, and developmentally appropriate. In any physical activity or sport, the outcome results from the interaction of the nervous, skeletal, muscle–tendon, hormonal, cardiorespiratory, and metabolic systems. These systems develop dynamically throughout childhood and adolescence, and one's current developmental state can exert a profound effect on both acute responses to a bout of exercise and chronic adaptations to exercise training. Children are not simply miniature adults; therefore, exercise programming should be consistent with their developmental needs and abilities—a concept that is revisited throughout Part II of this book.

Children and adults respond differently to an acute bout of exercise, and the differences can be applied to any exercise scenario. Consider a child running around a playground or an adolescent competing in a distance race. In both cases, the metabolic, hormonal, and cardiorespiratory systems may favor a more aerobic response than they would in an adult, but the nervous and muscle–tendon systems may not generate or transmit force as effectively as in an adult.

Throughout childhood and adolescence, all physiological systems appear sensitive to training, although the magnitude of chronic training adaptations may vary depending on maturity. Exercise-induced adaptations in the skeletal system may peak in prepuberty and early puberty. Similarly the central nervous system may adapt more quickly to training in younger children. These observations reinforce the importance of engaging youth in physical activity early in life. Although training-induced gains in fitness are likely to subside if the exercise stimulus is removed, the time course of detraining varies across physiological mechanisms. From a practical perspective, youth should be provided with daily opportunities to engage in various types of physical activity in the context of family, school, and community activities in order to promote long-lasting adaptations that enhance their health, fitness, and well-being.

CHAPTER 3

Growth, Maturation, and Physical Fitness

CHAPTER OBJECTIVES

- Define and distinguish between growth, chronological age, maturation, and the broader concept of development
- Explain the difference between skeletal, sexual, and somatic maturation
- Introduce a range of methods available for measuring growth and maturation
- Describe how growth and maturation influence the development of physical fitness

KEY TERMS

Introduction

The rapid physical development that marks childhood and adolescence is readily apparent: Basic skills should be quickly mastered—for instance, walking, running, and jumping. Substantial changes occur in body size, shape, and composition. And physical competence should improve markedly in tasks of strength, speed, and endurance. This rapid development is underpinned by interaction between genetics and environment, which promotes biological, physiological, and neurological adaptations that determine observable characteristics and, ultimately, physical fitness. Environmental factors such as nutrition and exercise exert profound influence on growth, development, and physical fitness.

During childhood and adolescence, growth and maturation represent the pathway to reaching adult size and maturity. This pathway to adulthood is influenced by considerable variability across individuals, which also influences physical fitness during childhood and adolescence. Typically, physical development is nonlinear, including periods of relatively little change interspersed with periods of rapid development in both growth and maturation. Even among individuals of the same chronological age, maturation can vary substantially, which raises issues when comparing or grouping **youth** based on chronological age. Consequently, we must understand the fundamentals of growth and maturation in order to appreciate the natural development of physical fitness and how this process may affect physical activity and selection for participation in youth sport.

Growth, Maturation, and Development

Chronological age is generally easy to measure and define. Debate continues, however, about the exact chronological ages used to distinguish periods of early life and about inconsistent definitions of the terms *growth, maturation,* and *development.* These terms are often used interchangeably, and *growth* and *maturation* may even be used synonymously, but this practice should be avoided because each refers to specific biological activities (Malina et al., 2004). Operational definitions are provided for these terms in the following subsections.

Chronological Age

Chronological age is a simple measure in which birth represents zero time and chronological age is the time point away from birth. Within the domain of growth and maturation, chronological age is used to identify specific stages of early life:

- Infancy—the first year of life
- Early childhood—the preschool years, or chronological age of 1.00 to 4.99 years
- Mid childhood—5.00 to 7.99 years
- Late childhood—8.00 years to the onset of **adolescence** (thus requiring identification of the onset of sexual maturation)

Adolescence is the transitional period from late childhood to the attainment of adulthood, including puberty and the progression from sexually immaturity to full sexual maturity. Consequently, late childhood and adolescence cannot be described by fixed chronological boundaries; however, the total period of **childhood** can be defined as the period from the first birthday to the onset of adolescence. In contrast, school and sport systems routinely categorize pupils and participants into chronological age groups, typically with one-year intervals. This approach is used, for example, when allocating children to a year group at school or an age-based tennis team. This method allows convenient grouping of individuals who might be viewed as occupying a similar developmental stage.

From a movement perspective, children of the same chronological age have had the same amount of time to learn and develop skills—provided, of course, that they have been exposed to the same experiences. Even on this basis, however, grouping children in one-year intervals can be problematic, because the oldest and youngest individuals in the group can differ in age by nearly 12 months. Of even more concern, chronological age categories may not adequately group individuals who are at similar developmental stages. This is particularly true during adolescence, when maturation can exert a profound effect on growth, body size, and development at different chronological ages across individuals. Figure 3.1 demonstrates the potentially large differences in maturation and body size across children of the same chronological age.

Growth

Growth can be defined as an increase in the size of the body or specific parts of the body (Malina et al., 2004). It is the most significant biological activity that occurs during the first two decades of life, from birth to full maturity. Physical growth can be considered the most important factor in the development of physical fitness, and rate of growth is largely responsible for differences in physical performance across individuals of similar age in pediatric populations (Rowland, 2005). These growth-related gains in physical performance are related to increases in stature and mass, particularly lean mass, as well as increases in organ size (e.g.,

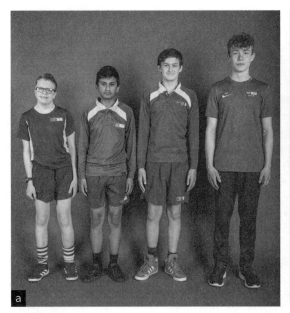 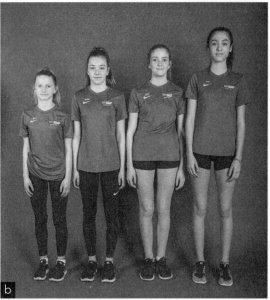

FIGURE 3.1 Children of the same chronological age (year group) but contrasting maturity and body size.

heart size). Three processes contribute to growth from conception through adulthood:

- Hyperplasia—increase in cell number
- Hypertrophy—increase in cell size
- Accretion—increase in intercellular substances

All three of these processes contribute to growth, but their predominance varies from conception to adulthood. Hyperplasia typically predominates in the prenatal period or shortly after birth, whereas hypertrophy accounts for the predominant, nonlinear growth process from childhood to adulthood.

Maturation

In the simplest terms, **maturation** can be defined as the process of becoming mature (Malina et al., 2004; Stratton & Oliver, 2014). One's level of maturity consists of one's current state, or how far along the pathway from immaturity to full maturity one has traveled at a given point in time. Maturation is a biological process that occurs in all tissues and affects both size and function. Consequently, maturity status is often quantified in terms of biological age, which provides a measure of how developed a biological system is on the continuum from immature to fully mature. However, specific biological processes can mature at different rates, which makes it difficult to define and measure maturity.

Typically, maturity and biological age are considered in three possible contexts:

- **Skeletal age** provides a rating of biological age based on the progress of the skeleton from cartilage to bone. Full skeletal maturity is identified as a fully ossified skeleton.

- **Sexual age** provides a rating of biological age based on secondary sexual characteristics, such as developments related to the breasts, genitalia, and pubic hair. Full sexual maturity is identified with fully functional reproductive capability.

- **Somatic age** provides a rating of biological age based on progress and rate of development toward full adult size and proportion. Full somatic maturity is identified as the achievement of final adult stature.

Some debate exists about how well the different measures of biological age relate to one another. Some researchers suggest a reasonable relationship (Tanner, 1990), whereas others suggest a relatively poor relationship (Malina et al., 2012). Therefore, we must exercise caution when comparing maturation markers.

The fact that somatic maturity can be based on the rate of change in body shape and size demonstrates the close association between growth and maturation. Both are dynamic and directional processes with the goal of achieving the adult state. However, the timing and tempo of progress toward the mature biological state can vary dramatically between individuals. In this context, *timing* refers to the occurrence of specific maturational events, and *tempo* refers to the rate at

Teaching Tip

THE UNFAIR ADVANTAGE OF SIZE

Children competing in chronological age groups can vary markedly in both maturation and size. Roy and colleagues (1989) showed that a group of small ice hockey players under age 13 were nearly a foot (30 cm) shorter, weighed only half as much, and had only half the strength of a group of large players in the same age category. Organizers in some sports (e.g., American football, rugby union in some countries) have tried to resolve this issue by setting minimum and maximum thresholds for body mass within age categories. In this approach, players who fall outside of the limits move up or down by one age grade in order to be more closely matched for body size.

which maturation progresses through the stages, from immaturity to full maturity. Although growth and development are influenced by environmental factors (e.g., nutrition, exercise), the timing and tempo of maturation are largely under genetic control.

DO YOU KNOW?

Timing of the growth spurt can vary by as much as six years between individuals.

Though adolescence is defined as the period from the end of late childhood until the attainment of adulthood, it can be difficult to identify with exactness due to the variable maturation of different biological processes and the variations that occur in timing, tempo, and termination of maturation. Therefore, in the interest of simplicity, the period of adolescence is sometimes described in terms of a broad range of chronological ages (e.g., World Health Organization, 2015). However, it is more appropriate to use measures of biological age, rather than chronological age. Indeed, adolescence is functionally represented by the period of sexual maturation, starting with initial changes in the neuroendocrine system, which precede observed changes in physical characteristics, and ending with a fully mature reproductive system.

Adolescence may be more easily identified from a structural perspective; in this view, it begins with the onset of the growth spurt and ends when full adult stature is attained. Consequently, identification of the onset of maturation provides the time point by which childhood and adolescence are separated.

Quantification of biological age allows identification of current maturity status. Specifically, it can be compared with references for developmental rates and chronological age in order to place an individual into one of three categories:

- *Early maturing*—biologically ahead of chronological age

- *Average maturing*—biologically on time with chronological age
- *Late maturing*—biologically behind chronological age

Development

Within the domain of growth and maturation, **development** can be defined as a broad conception of progress toward the adult state, which incorporates both biological and behavioral perspectives. Biologically, development is considered in qualitative terms with reference to the differentiation, specialization, and refinement of cells and the ways in which all of this relates to function. Differentiation occurs primarily in the prenatal period, and functional refinement takes place throughout childhood and adolescence. The behavioral context, on the other hand, reflects development toward adult behaviors. This dimension has been viewed as including the development of social, cognitive, and emotional competence, as well as psychomotor skills (Malina et al., 2004; Stratton & Oliver, 2014).

Cultural environment and social interaction play primary roles in the development and expression of physical, intellectual, social, and moral competencies. Though biological and behavioral development are somewhat independent, they are not mutually exclusive concepts. In particular, sexual maturation is triggered by changes in the endocrine system, which facilitate sexual and physical development, but it can also be associated with altered psychological function. For instance, increased testosterone in males during adolescence is associated with heightened levels of joyfulness but also increases in aggressive behavior and greater levels of depression and anxiety (Christiansen, 2001). As a result, adolescent males may begin to experience more exaggerated emotions, which can be observed in more extreme or variable moods. However, given the sparsity of existing research, more work is required to confirm the nature of any associa-

Teaching Tip

MATURATION OF BIOLOGICAL SYSTEMS

Maturation, the biological process of becoming fully mature, influences both size and function. Different biological processes mature at different rates, and maturity is typically considered in terms of skeletal, sexual, and somatic maturation. These dimensions, though somewhat interrelated, are not the same. Indeed, the timing and tempo of maturation can vary significantly between different biological systems—for instance, the skeletal system and the reproductive system. Various methods are available for quantifying biological age, which can be used to categorize youth as either early maturing, average maturing, or late maturing. This information can help explain differences in physical fitness among children and adolescents of similar chronological ages. Evaluating maturation can also inform exercise prescription, because both acute and chronic responses to physical activity can vary with maturity status.

tion between changes in testosterone with changes in mood and behavior during adolescence (Duke et al., 2014). In females, estrogen increases markedly during adolescence and alters the activity of serotonin, a cerebral neurotransmitter, which can negatively alter perception of pain and motivation to exercise.

Measuring Growth and Maturation

Growth and maturation play significant roles in determining one's physical performance capabilities (in addition, of course, behavioral development affects one's motivation to engage in physical activity). Therefore, accurately measuring growth and maturation provides us with information to inform our judgments when promoting the physical and psychosocial development of children and adolescents. Among other things, this information can be used to help us accurately interpret data related to fitness level, prescribe appropriate exercise, and enhance young people's engagement in physical activity.

Measuring Growth

Measurement of growth involves measuring body size, or the size of specific parts of the body, and tracking how size increases over time. The methods used to measure body size and proportions are referred to collectively as anthropometry, and they are extremely reliable if practiced by skilled assessors (Stratton & Oliver, 2014). Measurements are taken by using appropriate instruments for anatomical landmarks at certain reference points while the participant is placed in specific positions. To ensure reliable results, the assessor must be well practiced at taking measurements and must follow exactly the same procedures each time a measurement is taken. Overall body size is measured

most simply and commonly in terms of stature (height) and body mass (weight). Other measures include length, breadth, circumference, proportion (or ratio) between two measures, and body composition.

Body Size

Stature, or standing height, is a linear measurement of the distance from the floor to the vertex of the skull and is most commonly reported in feet and inches or in meters (or centimeters). Due to gravitational forces compressing the spine when upright, stature decreases slightly throughout the day. Therefore, in the interest of consistency, an individual's stature should be measured at a consistent time of day and by means of the same procedures each time. Ideally, body mass would be measured with the individual unclothed, but this approach is of course impractical, often unethical, and inconsistent with codes of conduct in schools and sport clubs. Alternatively, body mass can be measured with the subject in minimal clothing, such as shorts and T-shirt (no shoes).

To monitor a child's growth, we can plot stature and body mass on a growth chart. Such charts provide reference values for measures of body size with increasing chronological age. In addition, growth curves are provided in percentiles for the population. The 50th percentile indicates the average body size for boys or girls over the first two decades of life, and other percentiles show those who sit more toward the extremes of size. Population growth curves are shown in figures 3.2 and 3.3 for both stature and body mass for males and females, respectively.

Growth is monitored by plotting stature or body mass on the appropriate chart and plotting serial measurements over time. Data are assessed to determine where a child is placed relative to the reference population (i.e., in terms of percentiles) and whether this placement changes over time. In infancy and early

Teaching Tip

ESTROGEN EFFECT

The influence of rising estrogen on serotonin levels has been suggested as a contributing factor to the decline in physical activity and performance observed in females during the teenage years (Rowland, 2005). However, adolescent girls are responsive to training and can benefit from regular physical activity. Consequently, youth fitness specialists should seek to overcome the increased risk of disengagement from exercise in adolescent girls by providing continued motivation and encouragement to help them maintain interest in physical activity.

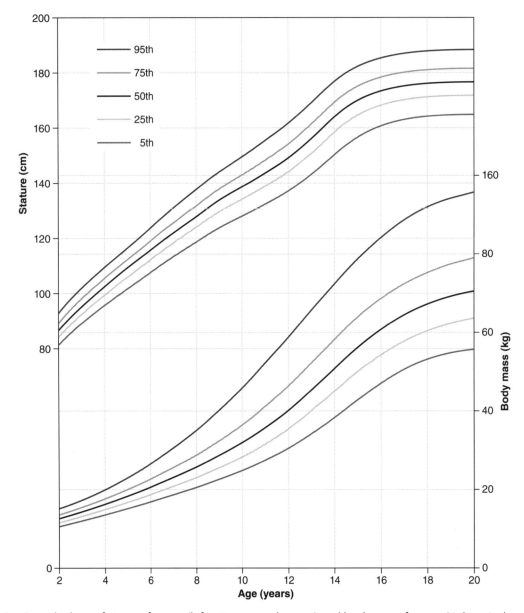

FIGURE 3.2   Growth chart of stature for age (left axis, upper data set) and body mass for age (right axis, lower data set) with percentiles for males aged 2 to 20 years old.

Data for American children from CDC National Center for Health Statistics, Percentile Data Files with LMS Values (https://www.cdc.gov/growthcharts/percentile_data_files.htm).

childhood, a child might be quite variable and move across percentiles while progressing toward the genetically predetermined size. After about four years of age, an individual's percentile is generally expected to track quite well from childhood to adulthood (Cole & Wright, 2011), especially for stature. Chart position may get disrupted, however, when the adolescent growth spurt occurs. This is the case because growth charts are based on chronological age and do not account for

variability in the age at which maturation takes place. To a large extent, growth of stature is determined genetically, whereas growth of mass is more susceptible to environmental influence, thus providing more potential for movement across percentiles over time.

DO YOU KNOW?

By age two years, children have achieved about half of their adult height.

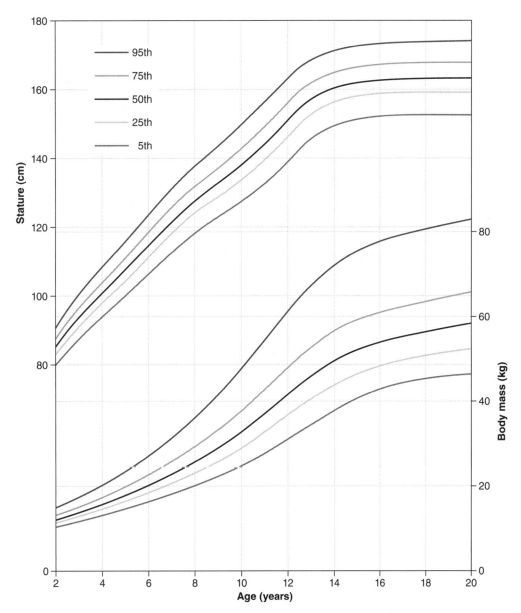

FIGURE 3.3 Growth chart of stature for age (left axis, upper data set) and body mass for age (right axis, lower data set) with percentiles for females aged 2 to 20 years old.

Data for American children from CDC National Center for Health Statistics, Percentile Data Files with LMS Values (https://www.cdc.gov/growthcharts/percentile_data_files.htm).

Body Mass Index and Body Composition

Comparing measures of both stature and mass can provide further insight into size and proportion. For example, a child who is at the 50th percentile for body mass but the 90th percentile for stature would be tall and lean. In contrast, an individual who has relatively large mass in proportion to height could either be stocky and muscular or carrying excess fat, the latter of which would be worthy of further investigation. The most common measure that combines stature and body mass to identify potential fatness is the **body mass index** (BMI), also referred to as the Quetelet Index:

$$\text{Body mass index} = \text{body mass (kg)} / \text{stature}^2 \text{ (m)}$$

Be cognizant of the fact that BMI is an indirect measure of fatness; it does not measure body composition directly. In addition, children and adolescents carry less weight for their height than do adults, and adolescents typically grow taller before adding additional mass. Consequently, adult criteria for BMI should not be applied to younger populations. Doing so would risk categorizing an overweight or obese child as having normal weight, thus missing an important opportunity to intervene in terms of lifestyle factors in order to prevent adult obesity. For instance, although a high BMI can be used to identify someone as being overweight or obese, a young athlete might have a high BMI due to large muscle mass relative to height; this situation might be observed, for instance, in American football or rugby union. Therefore, when a high BMI is identified, the finding should be followed up with further assessment in order to confirm whether excess fat mass is an issue. One simple way to supplement BMI when classifying body fatness is to use waist circumference (Cornier et al., 2011).

Patterns of change in body composition are similar for boys and girls in prepuberty but then diverge due to hormone-mediated developments associated with maturation. Specifically, increased testosterone in males promotes greater increases in muscle mass, whereas increased estrogen in females promotes increased fat mass.

Body composition can be measured directly by using underwater densitometry, air plethysmography, or dual-energy X-ray absorptiometry (DEXA). However, these methods are often infeasible due to practical limitations related to cost and required expertise. Therefore, body composition of youth is often measured indirectly in terms of skinfold thickness. Common sites of skinfold measurement include the triceps, biceps, subscapular, suprailiac, thigh, and calf areas, though normally only some of these sites are measured. Skinfolds involve the layer of subcutaneous adipose tissue, and the measurements are used in a predictive equation to estimate percentage body fat. A number of predictive equations are available, and the most appropriate should be chosen to reflect the characteristics (e.g., age, sex, ethnicity) of the person or population being measured (e.g., Cameron et al., 2004; Rodriguez et al., 2005; Slaughter et al., 1988).

Length, Breadth, Circumference, and Proportion

Most body dimensions follow a developmental profile similar to those of stature and body mass: rapid growth in infancy and early childhood, slower growth in mid childhood, accelerated growth during adolescence, and finally a slowing followed by termination when adult size is reached. However, the exact timing of growth spurts can differ between body segments. On the population level, measures of size and proportion are similar between immature boys and girls, and sex-specific differences become apparent with the onset of maturation. Because success in some sports depends partly on a specific body size or shape, body dimensions and proportions have been used to identify youth with the necessary profile to excel.

Other common measures of growth include leg length and sitting height, which are used to separate growth of the lower limbs and of the trunk. Sitting height is measured in the same way as stature but with the child sitting on a raised surface with the legs hanging freely. Figure 3.4 shows examples of measuring standing height and sitting height of a child. The latter provides a measure from the sitting surface to the top of the head, which can be subtracted from standing height to calculate leg length.

This information can also be used to calculate the ratio of sitting height to stature, or Cormic index, which in turn can be multiplied by 100 to express sitting height as a percentage of standing height. This result can be used to identify individuals with relatively short or long legs for their stature; for example, a higher ratio represents a relatively longer trunk and relatively shorter legs. Because growth spurts in the legs and trunk occur at slightly different times, this ratio can also be useful for estimating somatic maturity.

DO YOU KNOW?

The long bones of the limbs have an earlier growth spurt than do the short bones of the trunk.

Breadths are measured at specific anatomical landmarks and are used as indicators of skeletal robustness

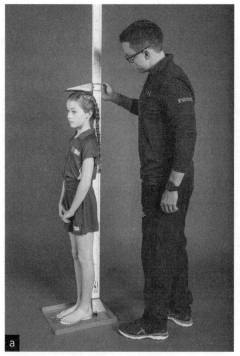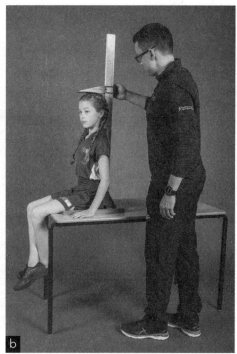

FIGURE 3.4 Measuring (a) standing height (stature) of a child and (b) sitting height of a child. Subtracting sitting height from standing height provides a measure of leg length.

(Malina et al., 2004). Common breadth measurements include the following:

- *Biacromial*—distance between the acromial processes of the left and right scapulae, providing a measure of shoulder broadness
- *Bicristal*—distance between the most lateral parts of the iliac crests of the pelvis, providing a measure of hip breadth
- *Biepicondylar*—distance between the epicondyles on either the femur or the humerus, providing a measure of knee and elbow breadth, respectively

The shoulders-to-hips proportion is similar for boys and girls during childhood but diverges with maturation. For females, the hips widen relatively more during adolescence; for boys, shoulder breadth increases relatively more.

Circumferences are sometimes used as indirect measures of muscularity. It is assumed that muscle is the primary determinant of a circumference, although other types of tissue (e.g., bone, fat) contribute as well. Limb circumferences are usually measured in either the limb's proximal portion (e.g., thigh) or its distal portion (e.g., calf), and measurements are typically taken at the portion's midpoint, where the circumference is greatest. Chest circumference, which may be

used as a measure of trunk muscularity, is measured at the middle of the sternum, with the arms by the sides, and following a normal exhalation.

Measures of Maturation

Maturation, which reflects an individual's biological progress toward the fully mature state, can be measured in terms of biological age. Biological systems mature at different rates, and biological age is most commonly measured as skeletal, sexual, or somatic age. Evaluating maturity is important because maturation influences physical performance, exercise and training prescription, training adaptation, and injury risk (Lloyd et al., 2014). Youth of similar chronological age are likely to vary considerably in biological age, and this variation needs to be considered when designing exercise programs or selecting youth for sport teams.

It is debatable whether there is a gold standard or criterion measure of maturity. However, skeletal maturity (rather than sexual or somatic maturity) is often considered to provide the best method of assessing biological age (Lloyd et al., 2014; Mirwald et al., 2002).

Skeletal Age

Maturation of the skeletal system involves long-term transition from prenatal cartilaginous structures to fully developed bones of the skeleton by adulthood. The characteristics of individual bones change in a uniform and irreversible manner, from initial ossification to achievement of a fully mature adult state, thus allowing skeletal age to be quantified (Malina, 2011). Assessment of skeletal age is based on radiographs of the hand–wrist skeleton, which includes the radius, ulna, carpals, metacarpals, and phalanges. Each radiograph is assessed against standard criteria to determine skeletal age. Consequently, clinical equipment is required, and only appropriately trained individuals (e.g., radiographers) are able to collect and analyze these data.

As the skeleton continually develops, skeletal age provides a measure of biological maturity throughout childhood and adolescence. Although X-rays and radiographs expose a child to some level of radiation, modern technology has reduced the amount to less than would be expected with daily background radiation (Malina, 2011); therefore, measuring skeletal age in this manner is considered safe and ethical. Skeletal maturity is commonly assessed by means of three methods that are all based on hand–wrist radiography but use different assessment criteria. A sample right hand–wrist radiograph of a 19-year-old male is shown in figure 3.5.

Greulich-Pyle Method

This method is based on reference radiographs collected from white American children of high socioeconomic status (Greulich & Pyle, 1959). It is also referred to as the atlas method because it involves comparing a hand–wrist radiograph against an atlas of reference plates depicting skeletal maturity from birth to adulthood. Skeletal age is determined by selecting the reference plate that most closely matches an individual's radiograph. This method is limited by the fact that it determines skeletal age based on matching to a single best reference plate of overall hand–wrist development; therefore, it does not consider variation in the rate of development of individual bones.

Tanner-Whitehouse Method (TW)

The first two versions of this method (TW1 and TW2) are based on data from a population of British children (Tanner et al., 1962, 1975), whereas the third version (TW3) is based on data from a wider sample of European, Argentinian, American, and Japanese youth (Tanner et al., 2001). In this method, either 13 or 20 bones are individually rated for maturity status against a series of statements and shapes (representing the maturity status of each bone). All scores are then summed and converted to a rating of skeletal age. This type of

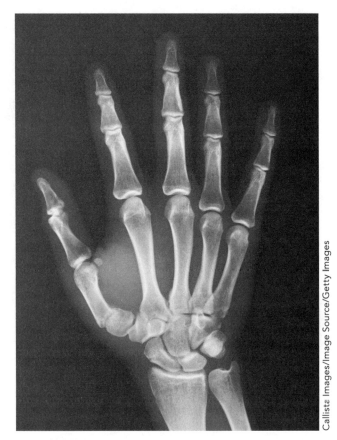

FIGURE 3.5 Sample right hand–wrist radiograph of a 19-year-old male.

Callista Images/Image Source/Getty Images

evaluation is a fairly complex and time-consuming process that requires a reasonable amount of subjective decision making (Lloyd et al., 2014).

Fels Method

This method is based on data from a middle-class U.S. population in Ohio (Roche et al., 1988). It involves grading bones of the hand–wrist according to age and sex, measuring ratios between the length and width of the epiphysis and metaphysis, and noting the presence and degree of ossification of the pisiform (a small sesamoid bone that makes up part of the hand–wrist joint) and the adductor sesamoid (a small bone in the thumb). Measurements are entered into a software package and weighted for sex and chronological age in order to calculate skeletal age and standard error of estimate. The degree of error is lower in immature individuals and increases with maturation.

The three methods for assessing skeletal age provide results that are correlated but not equivalent (Malina, 2011). For instance, Malina, Chamorro, Serratosa, and Morate (2007) reported that the TW3 and

Fels methods yielded significantly different skeletal ages in a population of elite youth soccer players. Therefore, the different methods should not be used interchangeably or compared directly. However, all of the methods do provide a measure of skeletal age in years, which can be compared against chronological age to provide a classification of maturity status. For instance, a child with a chronological age of 10 years but a skeletal age of 12 years is considered to be an early maturer because biological age is far ahead of chronological age. The difference between skeletal age and chronological age can be used to generate the following classifications:

- *Early maturing*—skeletal age older than chronological age by at least one year
- *Average maturing*—skeletal age within one year of chronological age
- *Late maturing*—skeletal age younger than chronological age by at least one year

The threshold of plus or minus one year of difference between skeletal age and chronological age approximates the standard deviation of skeletal age within a given chronological age in 10- to 17-year-olds (Malina, 2011). The approach of applying a standard deviation should mean that the majority of children (68 percent) are classified as *average maturing* and the remainder are evenly split between *early* and *late maturing*. Given the need for access to clinical equipment and expert assessors, it has been suggested that widespread use of skeletal age is likely only with the use of low-dose radiation scans (such as dual-energy X-ray absorptiometry) and automated computer analysis of images (Stratton & Oliver, 2014).

The Greulich-Pyle method has been applied to a large sample that included Asian, black, white, and Hispanic boys and girls (Zhang et al., 2009). The authors reported that bone age was significantly overestimated in Asian and Hispanic children of both sexes because those populations mature sooner. In another study, Cole et al (2015) used the TW3 method to compare skeletal maturity in white and black African boys and girls. The researchers found that black African boys matured seven months later than their white counterparts but that no such difference existed for girls. Given that skeletal maturation is influenced by multiple factors—including genetic differences, diet, and energy balance (Zhang et al., 2009)—it can be debated whether apparent ethnic differences in maturation actually result from nature or from nurture. In the study by Cole and colleagues (2015), the later maturation of black African boys was attributed to that population's lower socioeconomic status and exposure to more adverse environmental circumstances. Moreover, given that ethnicity seemingly did not influence skeletal maturation in girls, the study's findings supported an existing hypothesis that skeletal maturity is more sensitive to environmental factors in boys than in girls.

Sexual Age

Sexual age provides a measure of progress toward a fully functioning adult reproductive system. It can be used to classify children who are prepubertal (with puberty defined as the period of sexual maturation). However, the fact that prepubertal children are sexually immature does not mean that they form a homogeneous group; in fact, skeletal age can vary dramatically among prepubertal children of similar chronological age. This potential for variation highlights the notion that the timing and tempo of maturation can differ between biological systems.

Sexual age is assessed by observing and rating secondary sexual characteristics, most commonly pubic hair, breast, and genital development. Observations are compared against reference criteria, and each characteristic is rated into one of five categorical stages, referred to as stages of sexual maturation, usually according to Tanner's criteria (Tanner, 1962). Ordinarily, ratings can be made only through direct

Teaching Tip

SKELETAL AGE: GOLD-STANDARD MEASURE OF MATURATION?

Skeletal age is often viewed as the gold-standard measure of maturation. However, the need for specialized equipment and experienced assessors means that this method is inaccessible to many people. The assessment of skeletal age is also not without its limitations, which include exposure of the child to radiation (albeit low-level), disagreement between different methods for calculating skeletal age, and reference samples that lack ethnic diversity. Youth fitness specialists should be aware of these limitations and apply caution if using skeletal age. Where skeletal measurements are not practical, youth fitness specialists should appreciate that maturity can also be estimated through more accessible and noninvasive methods, such as assessment of somatic maturation.

observations in a clinical setting by a trained practitioner (i.e., pediatric clinician). This approach was used by Sun and colleagues (2002) to compare the effect of race on the timing of sexual maturation in 4,000 Mexican-American and non-Hispanic white and black boys and girls. The authors reported that black American boys and girls both started sexual maturation earlier than their white and Mexican-American peers but that the time taken to reach full maturity was the same across all groups. These findings highlight ethnic differences in the timing but not the tempo of sexual maturation, and of course these differences carry implications in terms of changes in body size and physical fitness.

Assessment of secondary sex characteristics has been a popular method of assessing and describing maturation in pediatric research. However, it has limited applicability outside of clinical settings because of the necessary invasion of personal privacy. In fact, some researchers consider assessment of sexual maturation to be unethical because the process may be unpleasant for a child or adolescent and because other, less invasive methods exist. Self-assessment techniques have been developed that allow children to self-rate by using a mirror to compare their own sexual characteristics with reference drawings or photographs (Duke et al., 1980; Schlossberger et al., 1992). However, the accuracy of self-assessment may be insufficiently valid; indeed, when using this method,

boys tend to overestimate and girls to underestimate their sexual development (Rasmussen et al., 2015).

Brief descriptions of the secondary sexual characteristics used in Tanner's criteria are shown in table 3.1; other sources provide full descriptions and images of the criteria (e.g., Malina et al., 2004; Tanner, 1962). Stages 1 and 5 refer to the prepubertal and adult state, respectively, and the adolescent period is assigned to stages 2, 3, and 4. This staging limits the system to describing maturation in terms of a categorical system with relatively few classifications available. For instance, the categorical format does not differentiate between a child at the start of a given stage and a child at the end of that stage, even though substantial variation may occur between these points. In addition, this approach is most useful when comparing children of the same chronological age. The subjective process of making assessments is likely responsible for the reported low levels of reliability and validity when comparing ratings across physicians and between physicians and self-assessments (Faria et al., 2013; Hergenroeder et al., 1999). Due to a combination of these factors, the utility of Tanner's criteria for rating sexual maturation in school and youth sport settings has been questioned (Lloyd et al., 2014; Malina et al., 2004).

For females, maturity status can also be classified in terms of age at menarche (no equivalent measure exists for males). **Menarche** is the first menstrual cycle, and all females can be classified as either pre- or

TABLE 3.1   SECONDARY SEXUAL CHARACTERISTICS ACCORDING TO TANNER'S CRITERIA

Stage*	Description
P1	Prepubertal state, pubic hair absent
P2	Minimal growth of sparse, slightly colored, straight or slightly curled hair
P3	Pubic hair sparse but considerably darker, coarser, and more curled than in P2
P4	Pubic hair now adult in type but covering less area
P5	Pubic hair adult in type and quantity, spreading to inner surface of thighs
B1	Prepubertal state, breast development absent
B2	Areola elevated and larger than in childhood
B3	Further enlargement of breast and areola without separation in contour
B4	Nipple and areola projecting from breast to form a mound
B5	Breast now adult, areola markedly colored, only nipple projecting
G1	Prepubertal state, genitals as in early childhood
G2	Scrotum and testes enlarged but minimal change in penis
G3	Penis longer but little change in thickness, scrotum now hanging below base of penis
G4	Penis, scrotum, and testes further enlarged; end of penis conical; scrotum darker
G5	Penis, scrotum, and testes marked by adult size and shape

*Stages of maturity: P = puberty, B = breast, and G = male genitalia.

Adapted from Malina, Bouchard, and Bar-Or (2004), pp. 285-289.

postmenarcheal. However, due to the temporal delay between the onset of puberty and that of menarche, a premenarcheal state does not necessarily indicate a prepubertal state—a fact that limits the usefulness of this approach for assessing sexual maturation.

On average, menarche occurs at 13 years of age, and a threshold of plus or minus one year around this age is used to identify females as either early, average, or late maturing. Due to ethnic variation in the age of menarche, population-specific norms should not be applied. Age at menarche is typically measured retrospectively by asking an individual to recall the age at which menarche occurred. The ability to accurately recall that age diminishes with more time elapsed since the event, and by two years postmenarche less than half of females accurately recall the time at which it occurred (Koo & Rohan, 1997). As for any effect of menarche on physical performance, analysis across a range of measures has found no consistent trend to peak before, at, or after menarche (Malina et al., 2004).

Another noninvasive option for assessing maturity is the pubertal development scale (PDS; Petersen et al., 1988). In this approach, children are asked five questions—three general questions (relating to growth of height, appearance of body hair, and appearance of the skin and acne) and two sex-specific questions. Boys are asked about facial hair and deepening of the voice, and girls are asked about breast growth and menarche. Each response is scored on a scale of 1 to 4, where 1 = not yet started, 2 = barely started, 3 = definitely started, and 4 = seems complete (menarche is scored as either a 1 or a 4). The pubertal development score is calculated by totaling the scores for three questions (for boys, questions about body hair, voice, and facial hair; for girls, questions about body hair, breast growth, and menarche). Scoring is interpreted as follows: 3 = prepubertal, 4 or 5 = early pubertal, 6 through 8 = mid pubertal, 9 through 11 = late pubertal, and 12 = postpubertal.

The PDS has been shown to be reliable and valid (Petersen et al., 1988) and to distinguish between different populations (Robertson et al., 1992). It has also been found to exhibit moderate agreement with ratings of sexual maturation based on Tanner's criteria and has been suggested as a better alternative for use in school-based settings due to it being less invasive (Bond et al., 2006). However, it is subject to the pitfall of missing data when children either do not answer a question or indicate that they "don't know." In fact, in a study by Carskadon and Acebo (1993), one-third to one-half of boys and girls were missing data for at least one item.

Somatic Age

Somatic age provides a measure of progress toward attainment of adult body size. In this approach, measures of body size and proportion are taken to provide indirect markers of maturation rather than direct measures of biological process. Body size and shape both change as part of skeletal and sexual maturation. For instance, the onset of sexual maturation, along with marked changes in the endocrine system, promotes rapid skeletal maturation, which can be observed indirectly in a rapid increase in stature, otherwise known as "the adolescent growth spurt." Consequently, monitoring changes in body size and proportion can allow us to describe maturation and help identify important events, such as onset of adolescence and attainment of adulthood.

Because of the association of events in sexual and skeletal maturation and the growth spurt, somatic age is typically identified from longitudinal measurements of stature. Here, instead of plotting cumulative stature (as was presented earlier, in figures 3.2 and 3.3), measurements are used to calculate the rate of growth in stature in centimeters per year, thus providing a measure of height velocity. **Peak height velocity** (PHV) is the maximal rate of growth in stature during the adolescent period, and age at PHV is most often used to describe somatic maturity.

Figure 3.6 shows examples of growth rate curves for stature and thus depicts the nonlinear nature of maturation. The curves show a slowing of growth in late childhood, then a sudden upturn in growth rate, which eventually peaks before slowing and stopping. This pattern of change can be used to identify the

Teaching Tip

GROWTH RATE AND SOMATIC MATURATION

Measuring body size can enable us to describe growth. Taking longitudinal measurements of body size can enable us to describe rate of growth, or growth velocity, which can be used to assess maturation indirectly. The process of assessing somatic maturity is noninvasive and inexpensive and requires only limited equipment, thus making it a readily accessible method for evaluating maturation. A rapid increase in standing height signals the start of the growth spurt and is used to help identify the onset of adolescence. Peak height velocity, or the rate of growth at its fastest, is used along with age at PHV as a landmark of adolescence. Cessation of growth in stature indicates a fully mature state.

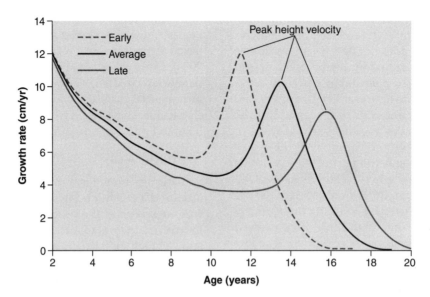

FIGURE 3.6 Examples of height velocity curves for early-, average-, and late-maturing males reaching the same final adult stature.

Based on hypothetical data.

onset of adolescence (i.e., onset of the growth spurt), peak height velocity (maximal rate of growth), and adulthood (cessation of growth). It has been suggested that longitudinal measurements of body size should be taken at intervals of three months or longer to allow detection of worthwhile changes in size and calculation of growth rates (Stratton & Oliver, 2014). Intervals of six months are often used and may be preferable.

PHV typically occurs around age 12 years in girls and age 14 years in boys (Mirwald et al., 2002; Malina et al., 2004). In other words, as compared with girls, boys experience two more years of preadolescent growth, as well as a higher peak in growth rate. These differences explain why males are, on average, 5 inches (13 cm) taller than females once adulthood is reached. Age at PHV also varies with ethnicity. After reviewing available data for various samples of North American, Japanese, and European children, Malina and colleagues (2004) concluded that in most instances PHV occurred between 11.6 and 12.1 years of age in girls and between 13.8 and 14.1 years in boys. Among notable exceptions, earlier maturation was observed in black American girls (10.8 years) and in Japanese boys and girls (about 12.5 and 11.0 years, respectively). Thus, even though Japanese children and adolescents are on average shorter than their age-matched peers in Europe and the United States, they are advanced in maturity (Malina et al., 2004).

For both girls and boys, the standard deviation for the mean age at PHV is about plus or minus one year (Malina et al., 2002; Sherar et al., 2005). This variability is used to categorize maturity. Specifically, reaching PHV within one year of the mean population age at PHV constitutes average maturing, reaching it more than a year before the population mean constitutes early maturing, and reaching it more than a year after the population mean constitutes late maturing. Figure 3.6 shows hypothetical data for early-, average-, and late-maturing boys who achieve their PHV at the ages of 11.5, 13.5, and 15.8 years old, respectively. Although the timing and magnitude of PHV differs between the three boys, they all ultimately attain the same adult stature—they just do so at different ages (about 16.5, 18.6, and 20 years, respectively). Thus the early-maturing boy gains an initial size advantage that is beneficial in many sports, but the average- and late-maturing boys eventually catch up.

Although PHV is the most common measure of somatic maturity, other indicators of size can also be monitored. These indicators typically demonstrate a growth curve similar in shape to that of height velocity, but the timing can vary. Longitudinal monitoring of body mass allows identification of **peak weight velocity** (PWV), which occurs after PHV. This pattern can be observed in an adolescent who first grows tall and lanky, then "fills out" by gaining additional body mass. Boys typically achieve PWV within six months of achieving PHV, adding mass at a peak rate of 20 to 22 pounds (9-10 kg) per year. The gap between PHV and PWV may be longer in girls, ranging from a few

Teaching Tip

PEAK HEIGHT VELOCITY (PHV)

The age at which PHV occurs can vary from 11 to 16 years old in boys and 10 to 15 years old in girls. On average, at PHV, stature increases at a rate of about 4 inches (10 cm) per year in boys and about 3 inches (8 cm) per year in girls. At the individual level, however, peak rate of growth can range from about 2.4 to 5.1 inches (6-13 cm) per year in boys and about 2 to 4.3 inches (5-11 cm) per year in girls. Thus, considerable individual variation exists in both the timing and the magnitude of the adolescent growth spurt. With longitudinal monitoring, PHV cannot be identified until after the event, when rate of growth falls below the level of the peak. The age at which PHV occurs can be estimated using predictive equations based on measures of body size and age (e.g., Mirwald et al., 2002). However, these equations tend to be valid only around the period of PHV.

months up to a year; when experiencing PWV, girls add mass at a rate of about 15 to 20 pounds (7-9 kg) per year (Malina et al., 2004). The composition of the mass added during adolescence also varies between the sexes; in particular, lean mass increases at peak rates of about 11 and 20 pounds (5 and 9 kg) per year in girls and boys, respectively. These differences in the growth of lean mass are largely responsible for the considerable divergence in physical performance capabilities that become increasingly apparent throughout adolescence.

DO YOU KNOW?

Children "stretch out" before they "fill out"; that is, they grow taller before adding more muscle mass.

Growth rates for stature represent a total measure of increases in both the lower and the upper parts of

the body. However, different body segments experience differential timing of growth spurts, and these differences can be useful in identifying somatic maturity. Specifically, the longer bones of the limbs experience an earlier growth spurt than do the shorter bones of the trunk. Consequently, the ratio of leg length to sitting height changes during adolescence; an increasing ratio suggests that an individual is pre-PHV, whereas a decreasing ratio suggests that an individual is post-PHV.

Figure 3.7 shows the changing proportion between leg length and sitting height during adolescence. The ratio increases prior to PHV, as the legs grow faster than the trunk, but the opposite holds true after PHV. The need for longitudinal data to use in calculating growth rates constitutes a limitation of monitoring somatic maturity; moreover, peak rates cannot be identified until after they have occurred. When long-term serial measurements are not available, short-term longitudinal monitoring of the ratio of leg length to

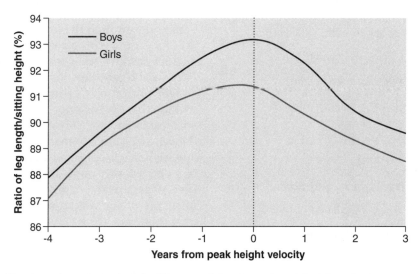

FIGURE 3.7   Ratio of leg length to sitting height (%) around the time of peak height velocity.

Data from Mirwald, Baxter-Jones, Bailey, and Beunen (2002).

sitting height may help identify whether an individual is pre- or post-PHV.

Prediction of Somatic Maturity

In some circumstances, youth fitness specialists do not have access to serial measures of body size and therefore cannot calculate growth rates or use them to identify important maturational events. This lack has led researchers to develop methods by which maturation can be estimated from somatic measures taken at a single point in time. Mirwald and colleagues (2002) developed equations to estimate somatic maturity based on data gathered from a sample of Canadian and Belgian children. The predictive equations were based on the differential timing of peak rates of growth in stature, mass, leg length, and sitting height; the interaction between leg length and sitting height plays a particularly important role in the estimation.

The equations provide a measure, known as the maturity offset, that estimates the number of years by which the individual is either before or after PHV. For instance, a value of −2.0 indicates a child estimated to be 2 years prior to experiencing PHV. The maturity offset can be subtracted from chronological age to give age at PHV, which in turn can be used (per the method described with longitudinal monitoring) to categorize individuals as either early, average, or late maturing. For example, a boy with a chronological age of 12 years and an estimated maturity offset of −2 years is predicted to have an age at PHV of 14 years, thus categorizing him as average maturing.

Here are the equations for calculating the maturity offset for boys and girls, respectively:

Boys

$$= -9.236$$

$$+ (0.0002708 \times (\text{leg length} \times \text{sitting height}))$$

$$- (0.001663 \times (\text{age} \times \text{leg length}))$$

$$+ (0.007216 \times (\text{age} \times \text{sitting height}))$$

$$+ (0.02292 \times (\text{mass} \div \text{height} \times 100))$$

Girls

$$= -9.376$$

$$+ (0.0001882 \times (\text{leg length} \times \text{sitting height}))$$

$$+ (0.0022 \times (\text{age} \times \text{leg length}))$$

$$+ (0.005841 \times (\text{age} \times \text{sitting height}))$$

$$- (0.002658 \times (\text{age} \times \text{weight}))$$

$$+ (0.07693 \times (\text{mass} \div \text{height}))$$

The standard errors associated with these equations for boys and girls, respectively, are 0.59 and 0.57 years. These figures translate to a standard error of about seven months, with a standard error providing a confidence interval of 68 percent. The standard error would need to be doubled in order to achieve a 95 percent confidence interval in the prediction.

Mirwald and colleagues (2002) suggested that the estimated maturity offset could be used to provide a maturational classification for use in research and in sporting contexts to match participants biologically rather than chronologically. Certainly, the method has been popular in pediatric research because it allows maturity to be calculated easily. When a youth fitness specialist does not feel confident about calculating the maturity offset, a quick web search will find an online calculator for this and other methods to estimate maturity. In addition, Moore and colleagues (2015) have recently presented simplified equations for predicting the maturity offset by using age and standing height:

$$\text{Boy's maturity offset} = -7.999994 + (0.0036124 \times \text{age} \times \text{height})$$

$$\text{Girl's maturity offset} = -7.709133 + (0.0042232 \times \text{age} \times \text{height})$$

For girls, an equation including height yielded the most accurate results (standard error = 0.53 yr). For boys, an equation using sitting height yielded the most accurate results, and where sitting height is not available a second equation using standing height demonstrated similar precision (standard error 0.51 versus 0.54 yr). Maturity offset provides an advantage over longitudinal monitoring insofar as it immediately identifies an individual as either pre-PHV (offset <0) or post-PHV (offset >0). A category of circa-PHV could also be introduced to denote an individual who is moving through the growth spurt; no established criteria exist for this category, but it is suggested that an adolescent who is within one year (before or after) PHV can be considered circa-PHV.

The limitations of maturity offset predictions include the level of error associated with these measurements and the sensitivity with which they can detect early- and late-maturing youth. Using skeletal age, Malina and colleagues (2012) classified 20 percent of a youth soccer population as late maturing and 29 percent as early maturing. However, when a maturity offset prediction was applied to the same population, only 2 percent were classified as late maturing and only 1 percent as early maturing (the remaining 97 percent were classified as average maturing). It has also been shown that predictions of age at PHV using both original (Mirwald et al., 2002) and modified equations

(Moore et al., 2015) are biased toward chronological age at the time of prediction in both boys and girls (Koziel & Malina, 2018; Malina & Koziel, 2014a, 2014b). This bias means that younger individuals are predicted to have an earlier age at PHV and older individuals to have an older age at PHV; moreover, the error increases with greater offsets.

Most recently, Fransen and colleagues (2018) extended the work of Mirwald and colleagues (2002) and proposed the maturity ratio as a new method for estimating somatic maturity. Fransen's group advocates using this new method as the standard practice for noninvasive maturity assessment in order to overcome some limitations of previous methods. Eminent statisticians, however, have criticized this new approach on the basis that it may be misleading or even fundamentally flawed, while also pointing out that the predictive equation could be simplified (Nevill & Burton, 2018).

Therefore, caution is called for when using anthropometric measures to estimate somatic maturity from methods that calculate a maturity offset. These equations may be most valid at the time around PHV, which may be a particularly useful period to identify. However, their validity becomes poorer in youth who are further away from PHV, and their ability to identify early- and late-maturing youth is questionable. Where possible, then, it is advisable to undertake some longitudinal monitoring of growth rates in order to provide a more comprehensive picture of somatic development.

One alternative assessment of somatic maturity focuses on percentage of predicted adult stature, which has been suggested to be reasonably well related to other direct measures of maturation, such as skeletal age (Bielicki et al., 1984). This method first predicts final adult stature, then expresses current stature as a percentage of adult stature. This approach can be used to compare the maturity status of youth who have the same chronological age. Specifically, those who have achieved a greater percentage of their adult stature are more mature than those who have achieved a lower percentage of their adult stature. For instance, consider two boys aged nine years old who are both 55 inches (140 cm) tall, a height that represents 75 percent of predicted adult stature for the first boy but 80 percent for the second. The second boy is more mature, because he is closer to his fully mature state, whereas the first boy has been predicted to achieve a greater adult stature (predicted adult height of 74 versus 69 in., or 187 versus 175 cm). In this way, the method can help differentiate between individuals who are tall due to advanced maturity and those who are tall due to genetic factors. The expected percentage of adult

TABLE 3.2 PERCENTAGE OF ADULT HEIGHT ATTAINED BY CHRONOLOGICAL AGE

Age (yr)	Boys (%)	Girls (%)
2	49	52
3	54	58
4	58	62
5	62	66
6	65	70
7	69	74
8	73	78
9	76	82
10	79	85
11	82	88
12	85	93
13	89	96
14	93	98
15	96	99
16	98	100
17	99	
18	100	

Data from CDC National Center for Health Statistics, Percentile Data Files with LMS Values (https://www.cdc.gov/growthcharts/percentile_data_files.htm).

height at different chronological ages is shown in table 3.2 based on population data from the Centers for Disease Control and Prevention.

DO YOU KNOW?

Attained percentage of predicted adult stature can be used as an indicator of maturity.

The data presented in table 3.2 are based on growth rates from the 50th percentile of the U.S. population, but the percentages are largely stable across all percentiles for all ages. Given that, on average, females reach their mature state two years before males do, their relative maturity at each chronological age is more advanced than that of males. This difference holds true even in early childhood, thus indicating that girls are biologically more mature than boys from a young age. Percentage of adult height has been used to categorize youth as early, average, or late maturing (Malina, Dompier, Powell, Barron, & Moore, 2007), though only limited data are available on which to base thresholds for making these classifications. Where sufficient data are available, these thresholds would be set by identifying youth who sit outside of plus or minus one standard deviation of the mean percentage of adult height for a given chronological age (Malina et al., 2005; Malina, Dompier, Powell, Barron, & Moore, 2007).

In a practice known as **bio-banding**, youth athletes are sometimes grouped on the basis of measures of size or maturity (rather than chronological age). For instance, percentage of adult height has been used to bio-band youth athletes into maturity groups for training and competition (Cumming et al., 2017). This technique may also be useful when comparing fitness scores between youth in cases where the youth fitness specialist would consider fitness for a given maturity status rather than for a given chronological age.

Various methods are available for predicting adult stature. Originally, predictions were based on measurement of skeletal age, but estimates based on somatic measures from an individual or parents have been shown to provide comparable reliability (Luo et al., 1998; Sherar et al., 2005). Adult height can be predicted from a growth chart, wherein a child's percentile for height is followed through to adult height; for example, a seven-year-old in the 75th percentile would be predicted to have an adult height that also falls in the 75th percentile. Cole and Wright (2011) provided such a chart and reported a standard error of prediction of 1.6 to 2 inches (4-5 cm), with improved accuracy outside of the pubertal years.

Adult height can also be estimated through the use of predictive equations. Given the genetic heritability of height, parental height is often used to predict the final adult height of offspring. Parental height can be measured directly or self-reported; in the latter case, youth fitness specialists should be aware of the tendency for parents to overestimate their height. To adjust for this overestimation, Epstein and colleagues (1995) provided the following corrective equations for self-reported height:

Man's adjusted height = 7.12 + (0.953 × reported height in cm)

Woman's adjust height = 5.88 + (0.955 × reported height in cm)

In another approach, Tanner and colleagues (1970) introduced the method of using midparental height to predict final adult height of children. This method is based on the genetic heritability of height and the observation of an average difference in height in the population of about 13 centimeters (5 in.) between men and women. Consequently, this approach calculates midparental height, then adds 6.5 centimeters for a boy and subtracts 6.5 centimeters for a girl:

Midparental height = (father's height + mother's height) ÷ 2

Boy's predicted adult height (cm) = midparental height + 6.5

Girl's predicted adult height (cm) = midparental height − 6.5

For example, if a father is 180 centimeters tall and a mother 160 centimeters tall, then the midparental height is 170 centimeters. In turn, a son would have a predicted adult height of 176.5 centimeters and a daughter a predicted adult height of 163.5 centimeters.

One criticism of this equation is that the predictive error is increased for a child if one or both parents are either very tall or very short, because the child is likely to regress toward the population mean. To help overcome this problem, other researchers developed additional methods and equations, such as those proposed by Luo and colleagues (1998):

Boy's predicted adult height (cm) = (0.78 × midparental height) + 45.99

Girl's predicted adult height (cm) = (0.75 × midparental height) + 37.85

Using the same example from before (father's height of 180 cm, mother's height of 160 cm), this method would predict a son to achieve an adult height of 178.6 centimeters and a daughter to achieve an adult height of 165.4 centimeters but with lower predictive error for children of parents who are either very tall or short. The standard error of estimation in this method is about 5 centimeters.

In both research and practice in youth sport, a popular method for estimating adult height (and current percentage of predicted adult height) has been the Khamis-Roche method (Khamis & Roche, 1994). Developed with reference to a sample of white American children, this method predicts adult height based on the child's age, height, and weight, as well as midparental height. Separate equations exist for each half-year increment in current chronological age from 4 to 17.5 years in both boys and girls. As with other methods, online calculators are widely available for predicting height using this method.

Maturity offset can also be used to predict adult stature in boys and girls aged 8 to 16 years. This method has been developed using the maturity offset prediction of Mirwald and colleagues (2002). It calculates the maturity offset, classifies the individual as early or average or late maturing, then adds a value for the estimated growth yet to come to the child's current stature. Sherar and colleagues (2005) describe the full method for this procedure and provide reference tables for predicting adult stature. This method is reported to have a standard error of about 3 centimeters, although, given the limitations of maturity offset (see earlier discussion), the error may be greater for early- and late-maturing youth.

Development of Physical Fitness

The growth curves presented earlier make it clear that growth and maturation follow a pattern of nonlinear development, wherein boys and girls experience a similar rate of development during childhood but boys then experience a more exaggerated increase in size during adolescence than girls do. This broad pattern of change can also be observed in the development of physical fitness. During childhood, boys and girls have similar physical abilities, which are underpinned by similar biological development. However, trends for boys to be more habitually active than girls in childhood (Griffiths et al., 2013) may promote greater physical fitness levels in boys and reflect the influence of environmental factors.

During infancy and early and mid-childhood, the central nervous system undergoes rapid growth and development. During this period, motor skills are quickly developed, as children learn to crawl, walk, balance, run, jump, climb, kick, catch, and throw; in addition, these skills are refined to perform more complex tasks. Having opportunities to practice and reinforce these skills with guidance and instruction from youth fitness specialists is important for children's motor skill development (Robinson et al., 2015; Society of Health and Physical Educators, 2014). In another indicator of the importance of this period, children's coordination patterns for locomotor skills are expected to develop fully by seven years of age (Whitall, 2003).

Unfortunately, evidence from both Australia (Hardy et al., 2010; Okely & Booth, 2004) and the United Kingdom (Stratton et al., 2009) suggests that children are not developing adequate mastery of fundamental movement skills. This finding raises concern because movement skills are associated with positive health development in youth (Lubans et al., 2010), whereas low proficiency in movement skills is associated with lower levels of physical activity in childhood (Fisher et al., 2005; Fransen et al., 2014; Lopes et al., 2011). Consequently, parents, school administrators, health care providers, and fitness professionals must provide opportunities for youth to be active and expose them to situations that promote skill development and enhance physical fitness.

DO YOU KNOW?

Children should develop their adult gait pattern by the age of seven years.

Rapid development and refinement of the central nervous system during childhood also enhance physical performance capabilities in tasks requiring strength, speed, power, endurance, or some combination of these factors; the rate of improvement slows in late childhood (Viru et al., 1999). With the onset of adolescence, sex differences in physical fitness become more apparent. In boys, adolescence is a period of rapid increases in stature, limb length, muscle mass, internal organ size (e.g., heart size), and blood volume—all of which positively influence physical fitness. Girls may experience similar positive adaptations during adolescence, but the changes are smaller and are accompanied by increasing fat stores.

Consequently, performance gains during adolescence are lower for females than for males, and females may find it more difficult to make gains in exercises in which body mass must be moved. For instance, both boys and girls demonstrate an increase in isometric strength during adolescence (Blimkie & Sale, 1998; Catley & Tomkinson, 2013), and peak rates of improvement are aligned with peak weight velocity in both groups (Blimkie & Sale, 1998). However, the peak rates are greater in boys (Blimkie & Sale, 1998); moreover, when body mass must be moved repeatedly during a push-up test, performance declines during the adolescent years for females but improves considerably for males (Catley & Tomkinson, 2013). Figure 3.8 shows that the rate of development of isometric strength in males and females is aligned with the timing of PHV and PWV.

Viru and colleagues (1999) performed an extensive review of developmental trends for improvements in strength, speed, power, and endurance throughout childhood and adolescence. Across a range of fitness components, they observed two clear phases that included periods of accelerated gains in physical fitness in both boys and girls. The first phase, termed the *preadolescent spurt*, occurred between the ages of 5 and 9 years, thus approximating mid-childhood, and was marked by improvements (attributed to rapid CNS development) in factors such as muscle recruitment and coordination. The second stage, or *adolescent spurt*, was aligned with maturation rather than chronological age. This pattern of change was recently confirmed for the development of speed in Japanese boys (Nagahara et al., 2018). The preadolescent spurt in sprint speed was observable from rapid gains in performance up

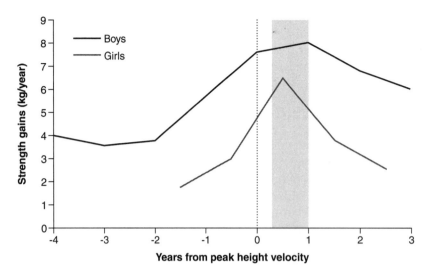

FIGURE 3.8 Rate of improvement in isometric strength in boys and girls around the time of peak height velocity (dotted line). The shaded area represents the approximate timing of peak weight velocity.

Adapted by permission from J.R. Blimkie and D.G. Sales, "Strength Development and Trainability During Childhood." In *Pediatric Anaerobic Performance*, edited by E. Van Praagh (Champaign, IL: Human Kinetics, 1998), 205.

until the age of 8.8 years, followed by a period with little further development until 12.1 years, and then a further rapid increase in speed that was likely attributable to an adolescent spurt (Japanese boys mature relatively early).

Although all fitness components are deemed to experience an adolescent spurt, the timing of this spurt varied slightly across components. Viru and colleagues (1999) reported that endurance experienced a spurt aligned with PHV, whereas the spurt for strength and power occurred slightly after PHV, which is most likely aligned to peak weight velocity. The adolescent spurt was attributed to the modulating effect of sex hormones on physical abilities.

Improvements in absolute fitness during development are largely influenced by changes related to growth and maturation, but they also require a child to be physically active. Without the stimulus of regular exercise, absolute gains in physical fitness may plateau or even decrease, particularly in girls, who experience increases in fat mass during adolescence. Fitness relative to size and body composition may remain fairly consistent throughout childhood and adolescence if growth-related changes can be appropriately accounted for. This process might include controlling for increases in body mass, lean mass, fat mass, height, limb length, and proportions. Expressing fitness relative to size may be useful when youth fitness specialists monitor fitness longitudinally, because it may help in partly distinguishing gains due to the effects of training over and above those experienced simply due to growth and maturation.

Controlling for body size may help to identify changes in fitness relative to size, but youth fitness specialists should be cognizant of appropriately controlling for changes in body size, proportions, and composition in order to make valid interpretations. For instance, although absolute aerobic power divided by body mass (mL · kg^{-1} · min^{-1}) is known to increase throughout childhood and adolescence, little change with age is found when aerobic power is scaled allometrically to account more appropriately for proportional changes in size (Armstrong & Welsman, 1994). Similarly, grip strength relative to body mass has been reported to increase in childhood and adolescence, with particularly large increases during adolescence for boys (Blimkie & Sale, 1998). However, when grip strength is normalized to forearm muscle volume, measured through resonance imaging, relative strength has been shown not to differ between children, adolescents, and adults (Tonson et al., 2008). Increases in sprint speed during adolescence can also be attributed partly to increased leg length (Meyers et al., 2017). Consequently, caution must be exercised when interpreting changes in fitness during childhood and adolescence; changes in fitness often result from increased size.

DO YOU KNOW?

Many gains in fitness during adolescence can be attributed primarily to increased size, particularly the addition of fat-free mass.

Once adolescence is reached, large performance gains are made, particularly in boys. However, physical education and youth sport are normally organized into chronological age groups, which presents a potential problem because biological age varies considerably across children of the same chronological age. It remains unclear whether being early- or late-maturing provides a performance advantage for females, and the answer is likely to depend on the demands of a particular sport. However, the more pronounced effect of adolescence on the physical fitness (e.g., speed, strength, power, endurance) of boys means that an early-maturing individual can enjoy a substantial physical advantage over average- or late-maturing peers of similar chronological age. Figure 3.9 shows the longitudinal development of muscular fitness in a group of Belgian boys tracked throughout their teenage years and then again at 30 years old. Longitudinal monitoring of stature was used to identify age at PHV and classify the boys into early-, average-, and late-maturing groups.

Peak height velocity typically occurs around 14 years of age in boys. At that age, as shown in figure 3.9, early-maturing boys are already well into their growth spurt and therefore hold a considerable advantage over the other groups in terms of muscular fitness (about 13% and 19% greater than average- and late-maturing boys, respectively). Early-maturing boys maintain a performance advantage in terms of strength and power throughout the teenage years, which means that they are more likely (and other groups less likely) to get selected for sport teams and

to enter sport development systems. However, when the groups are revisited at 30 years of age, not only have the early-maturing males lost their advantage but also the late-maturing individuals now demonstrate superior muscular fitness.

Reviewing data across a number of studies, Malina and colleagues (2004) reported similar results for boys across a range of fitness parameters, including grip, arm pull, vertical jump, shuttle run, maximal oxygen uptake, and plate tapping. That is, early-maturing boys consistently outperformed average- and late-maturing boys of the same chronological age. However, it is likely that if data had been collected into adulthood, then maturity-driven variability in physical performance around the teenage years would have disappeared later in life. In contrast, Malina and colleagues (2004) reported that girls of differing maturity status do not differ consistently across various measures of physical fitness. This finding likely derives from the fact that maturation aids performance in some aspects of physical fitness (e.g., absolute strength, power) but not others (e.g., movement of body weight).

Beunen and colleagues (1997) reported that vertical jump and other measures of physical fitness did not track well from the early and mid-teenage years to adulthood; rather, they showed generally weak to moderate correlations ($r \leq 0.52$). As a result, we cannot assume that a teenager with superior physical fitness will still display this characteristic as an adult. This finding may also explain the relative failure of many sporting systems to progress junior

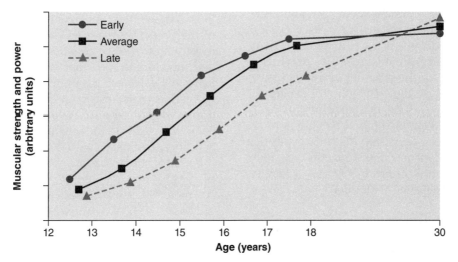

FIGURE 3.9 Average growth curves for physical fitness in a group of early-, average-, and late-maturing boys. Muscular strength and power are calculated from a composite score of strength (in the arm pull) and explosive power (in the vertical jump).

Adapted from Beunen, Ostyn, Simons, et al. (1997).

Teaching Tip

EARLY- VERSUS LATE-MATURING BOYS

At a given chronological age, early-maturing boys gain the clear advantages of increased body size and superior physical fitness as compared with their late-maturing peers. However, late-maturing boys eventually catch up, and when fully mature they can expect to have a level of physical fitness that is similar or even superior to that of their early-maturing peers. The effect of maturity on body size and physical fitness makes it difficult to predict adult fitness levels and sporting success based on performance during childhood and adolescence. Selecting early-maturing boys who are physically big, strong, and powerful may enable short-term success in age-specific competitions, but it is unlikely to create a system of long-term success. Instead, youth fitness specialists should focus on meeting long-term goals and working to ensure that all youth have the opportunity to flourish in sport.

competitors into the senior ranks; in other words, they bias selection of junior athletes toward those who are biologically advanced, but those individuals lose that advantage once their initially less mature peers reach adulthood.

Adolescent Awkwardness

One potential negative effect of the adolescent spurt on physical performance is the occurrence of **adolescent awkwardness**, which is defined as temporary disruption of motor control caused by rapid limb growth. This phenomenon can be observed in an adolescent who quickly grows tall and becomes clumsy while learning to coordinate the longer limbs. For instance, Philippaerts and colleagues (2006) observed a decline in the sprint speed of boys 12 months before PHV—a time when the limbs are likely to grow rapidly—and attributed the regression to adolescent awkwardness. Thankfully, the awkwardness should be temporary, and, with encouragement and instruction from a youth fitness specialist, adolescents can learn to coordinate their changing body dimensions. The prevalence of adolescent awkwardness is not known, but it is accepted that some portion of youth will experience some degree of disruption in sensorimotor mechanisms during adolescence (Quatman-Yates et al., 2012). It has also been suggested that this disruption may be more prevalent in females and may contribute to increased incidence of certain injuries in females around adolescence (Caine et al., 2014).

Relative Age Effect

When children are grouped into age categories, which are usually based on one-year intervals, one child may be meaningfully older than another in the same group. For instance, if the cut-off dates for an age-year group are January 1 and December 31, then group members can differ in age by almost a year. In this context, the term **relative age effect** (RAE) refers to a bias distribution of birth dates within an age-specific group of children (e.g., "under-11s"). The advantage of being born early (or sometimes late) in the season creates a situation where relatively older (or sometimes younger) individuals are overrepresented in a sport. RAE varies with sport, age group, level of performance, and sex; in addition, it is known to exist for boys across a range of sports, but the evidence is conflicting regarding its existence in girls (Stratton & Oliver, 2014).

Evidence of RAE has existed for a quarter of a century, and one of the earliest studies to report this phenomenon addressed its occurrence in youth ice hockey (Boucher & Mutimer, 1994). Despite awareness of RAE, no initiative has yet been able to overcome it. Indeed, it remains apparent in youth ice hockey (Sherar et al., 2007), and, as reported by Del Campo et al. (2010) and Deprez et al. (2013), more than 40 percent of youth soccer players were born in the first three months of the year and less than 14 percent in the last three months of the year. This pattern is attributed to the fact that those who are born earlier are likely to be more mature and therefore to have had more time to practice and learn skills. In fact, the point could be interpreted as indicating that those born earlier are likely to have a more advanced training age and higher technical competency due to the accumulation of more physical activity as compared with those born later in the year.

In another study, Romann and Cobley (2015) reported the existence of RAE in nearly 8,000 youth sprinters. Specifically, the researchers found that RAE increased with competitive level and that 45 percent of top athletes were born in the first quarter of the year. The authors also reported that RAE declined with advancing age. In particular, the effect of being born at the start or end of the season translated to a 10.1 percent difference in 60-meter sprint time in eight-year-olds but only 5.3 percent in 15-year-olds. The authors provided corrective equations based on sprint time and birth date to enable fairer comparison of performance across athletes born throughout the competitive season.

In boys, RAE is evident before puberty (Gil et al., 2014) but is still likely to reflect maturity to some degree given that biological age varies even in the prepubertal years. For girls, RAE is the subject of contrasting evidence, reflecting the smaller physical benefits that maturation brings to females as compared with males. In fact, for female figure skaters RAE is skewed to favor those born late in the year; specifically, 29 percent of singles skaters were born in the last three months of the year as compared with only 21 percent in the first three months (Baker et al., 2014). This differing profile may be attributed to the advantage conferred by maturing late and avoiding the added fat mass associated with adolescence. It has also been demonstrated that RAE exists in the general population, where those born early in the school year outperform those born later, both in physical fitness tests (Roberts et al., 2012) and in academic performance, though the advantage declines with advancing age (Navarro et al., 2015).

Summary

Considerable variation exists between individuals in levels of growth and in timing and tempo of maturation, and this variability exerts a profound effect on the development of physical fitness. Fitness levels diverge markedly between the sexes during adolescence, when males benefit from large increases in lean muscle mass while females develop increasing fat stores. Youth who mature early (particularly boys) see large increases in absolute fitness at a relatively younger chronological age than do their peers. However, any fitness advantage is only temporary, because average- and late-maturing individuals eventually catch up with their early-maturing counterparts. Thus youth fitness specialists should consider the maturity of children and adolescents and how it affects their physical fitness.

Biological age can be considered in terms of skeletal age, sexual age, and somatic age, which are interrelated but not the same. For instance, children may be considered sexually immature until the onset of puberty, but prepubescent children of the same chronological age can vary dramatically in skeletal age and maturity. Assessment of somatic age is the most accessible method for measuring maturity and is relatively easy because it requires little equipment or expertise. Somatic age can be measured through longitudinal monitoring of stature or estimated by means of a variety of methods. Although maturation is accompanied by changes in size, composition, and function that can profoundly affect physical performance, youth typically take part in sport and exercise through systems based on chronological-age groups. Therefore, we need to identify maturational status—as well as individuals who are early, average, or late maturing (e.g., based on somatic maturity)—in order to differentiate the physical abilities of youth of similar chronological age.

CHAPTER 4

Long-Term Athletic Development

CHAPTER OBJECTIVES

- Explain why early participation in physical activity is essential for long-term athletic development for all youth
- Understand why long-term athletic development programs should avoid early specialization and promote early diversification
- Critically analyze the benefits and limitations of existing talent and athletic development models for youth
- Understand why long-term athletic development programs should emphasize the development of muscular strength and motor skill competence early in life
- Explore the importance of adapting long-term athletic development programs for the developmental needs of children and adolescents

KEY TERMS

Introduction

The opening chapters of this book have examined fundamental principles of pediatric exercise science and discussed how growth and maturation can affect physical fitness. This chapter, in turn, demonstrates how youth fitness specialists can use these scientific principles to construct developmentally appropriate exercise strategies for the long-term athletic development of all youth. The chapter refers to a number of fitness components that youth fitness specialists should seek to develop in children and adolescents; however, specific training guidance for each of these components is examined later in the book.

Long-Term Athletic Development for All Youth

The notion of engaging children in exercise from an early age is not a novel concept. However, given ongoing developments in pediatric exercise science and continual advances in our understanding of **trainability**, youth fitness specialists should be able to adopt a contemporary and evidence-informed approach to exercise prescription. Unfortunately, despite increased interest in the trainability of youth, consensus has yet to emerge about the most appropriate training strategies for specific stages of development.

Enhancement of sporting talent is important and provides both athletes and coaches with a rich and rewarding experience. From the perspective of public health and fitness, however, we must ensure that development pathways are not reserved solely for the minority of young athletes but are structured, progressed, and integrated for youth of all ages and abilities. The prospect of working with elite athletes is alluring, but most youth either never succeed in reaching professional sport, or actually prefer to participate in noncompetitive sport or recreational physical activity, or simply lead a sedentary lifestyle. Therefore, long-term athletic development strategies should not be designed solely with the end goal of maximizing sporting potential in "talented athletes"; instead, they should provide all youth with the opportunity to develop requisite physical fitness qualities that enable a lifetime of engagement in sport and physical activity (Bergeron et al., 2015; Lloyd, Cronin, et al., 2016; Lloyd et al., 2015a).

DO YOU KNOW?

Depending on the sport, only 0.2 percent to 0.5 percent of high school athletes reach the professional level (Brenner & Council on Sports Medicine & Fitness, 2016).

Global statistics show that inactivity among children and adolescents has reached pandemic proportions (Barnes et al., 2013; Kalman et al., 2015); in addition, longitudinal data show that youth fitness levels have deteriorated over the past 20 to 30 years (Cohen et al., 2011; Moliner-Urdiales et al., 2010; Runhaar et al., 2010; Tomkinson, Leger, Olds, & Cazorla, 2003). Research also shows that pediatric injuries related to sport and physical activity continue to constitute a serious concern, especially among those who are ill prepared for the demands of physical activity (Bloemers et al., 2012; DiFiori et al., 2014). Consequently, greater efforts are needed from key stakeholders in order to maximize the many benefits of long-term approaches to athletic development in children and adolescents and to ensure that youth are suitably prepared for the demands of daily physical activity and sport.

Youth fitness specialists should adopt a well-rounded approach to the development of physical fitness in order to inspire youth to participate in a variety of physical activities from the earliest age possible. Doing so enables youth to develop positive health and fitness behaviors and reduce the injury risks associated with sport and physical activity (Lloyd et al., 2015a). The concept of a well-rounded approach to development is reflected in the term **holistic development**, which refers to a philosophy of simultaneously promoting physical, social, and psychological development in youth in order to inspire and motivate lifelong participation in physical activity.

The rationale for adopting a lifetime approach to athletic development is also grounded in the fact that children differ markedly in their physiology and psychosocial characteristics as compared with adults and that development occurs in a nonlinear manner. As is often stated, children are not miniature adults and therefore should not be prescribed adult-based training programs. Instead, youth fitness specialists should consider the biological processes that occur during the developmental years and how they can affect the growth, trainability, and recovery of youth. For example, children can resist fatigue more readily than adults during an acute bout of high-intensity exercise (Ratel, Duche, & Williams, 2006), but they require more time for rest and recuperation between demanding training sessions in order to minimize the accumulation of fatigue and allow normal growth processes to occur. Another complexity when training youth lies in the fact that the timing, tempo, and magnitude of maturation vary considerably among children and likely affect their physical fitness capacities and sensitivity to training-induced adaptations (Lloyd, Oliver, Faigenbaum, Myer, & De Ste Croix, 2014). Considering that young people also differ markedly from adults in psychological makeup and social behaviors, it is apparent that children and adolescents form a unique population with complex needs, interests, and abilities.

Another reason to implement a lifetime strategy for training youth is to ensure that short-term advances in fitness or performance (e.g., gains in muscular strength) are not pursued at the expense of **technical competence**. Rather, youth fitness specialists should use a long-term approach to physical development geared toward the evolution of a broad range of physical fitness qualities. This approach should be grounded in the development of a comprehensive repertoire of sound movement mechanics that can be performed repeatedly with control and in a range of environments. Concurrently, youth should be exposed to training methods that develop the relevant neuromuscular properties to facilitate movements that are strong, coordinated, and reproducible. Such an approach takes time, and the optimal strategy is to expose youth to a variety of physical activities early in childhood so they are prepared for more advanced training programs later in life. Youth fitness specialists should prescribe developmentally appropriate training regimens and coach and progress training in a child-friendly manner.

When Should Youth Begin to Exercise?

The physical activity guidelines presented in chapter 1 show that children should be encouraged to exercise from birth onward. However, due to previous misconceptions, conflicting assumptions persist about the age at which children should engage in formalized modes of training. Specifically, the appropriateness of resistance training (American, 1983) and prolonged aerobic exercise (Roberts, 2007) have previously been questioned due to fears about safety and damage to the immature skeleton. In addition, the suitability of high-intensity interval training has been debated due to a perceived lack of trainability in children before the onset of puberty (Katch, 1983). These myths have now been dispelled on the proviso that developmentally appropriate training programs are planned, delivered, assessed, and modified by a youth fitness specialist (Lloyd, Cronin, et al., 2016; Lloyd, Faigenbaum, et al., 2014; McNarry et al., 2014).

From a chronological perspective, no single age acts as a threshold at which children are deemed ready to begin formalized training. However, an international consensus statement on youth resistance training recently stipulated that children should be sufficiently mature to receive and comprehend instructions and should possess competent levels of balance and postural control before engaging in a training program (De Ste Croix, Priestley, Lloyd, & Oliver, 2014). To put it more simply, youth fitness specialists might assume that if children are old enough to play a sport (generally, age five or six years), then they are old enough to participate in some form of structured athletic development program.

The rationale for engaging youth in resistance training derives from physical activity guidelines stipulating that children should participate in weight-bearing exercise to improve bone health and muscle strength (World Health Organization, 2010). Resistance training should also be viewed as a lifelong component of an individual's physical activity profile; it should not be used merely as a short-term intervention within, say, an isolated block of a health-related exercise curriculum in school-based physical education. As compared with other activities, resistance training has high participation rates in adult populations, and it came in second only to cycling in a large-scale sport participation study from the United Kingdom (Stamatakis & Chaudhury, 2008; Thompson, 2016). As youth get older, they are more likely to gravitate away from free-play activities. Therefore, introducing children to resistance training at an early age would appear logical and beneficial in order to foster interest in this type of training as an ongoing lifestyle choice.

The need to engage youth in formalized preparatory conditioning is also supported by the increased and unpredictable loadings and stresses that youth are likely to experience during free play, recreational physical activity, and competitive sport as they get older. Such forces far exceed those that they will need to tolerate in a training environment that is developmentally appropriate, well controlled, and well supervised. In the case of youth who are sedentary, youth fitness specialists acknowledge the risk of "underuse" injury, as many inactive children simply do not possess the requisite motor skill competence or muscular strength to tolerate the rigors of competitive sport (Stovitz & Johnson, 2006). Therefore, from the perspective of long-term athletic development, youth should engage in developmentally appropriate training with technique-driven progression to foster competent and robust movement mechanics in a controlled environment *before* exposing these movements to more reactive and uncontrolled settings. Indeed, undertraining should be viewed in much the same way as overuse injury is viewed in elite sport—that is, as a "training load error" (Gabbett, 2016). Youth fitness specialists should consider this notion for long-term athletic development and should ensure that youth are exposed to appropriate training loads that can adequately prepare them for the demands of sport and exercise.

DO YOU KNOW?

Physical inactivity is a major risk factor for activity-related injuries in children.

Should Youth Sample or Specialize?

Sampling can be defined as an approach that encourages children to experience a number of different sports or activities with qualified instruction, or a number of different positions within a sport. Arguments in favor of sampling note that it does not restrict elite development in sports where peak performance is typically witnessed after maturation; it is associated with longer sporting careers and facilitates long-term participation in sport; it positively affects youth development; and deliberate play serves as a foundation for intrinsic motivation and provides a range of motor and cognitive experiences (Côté, Lidor, & Hackfort, 2009). In contrast, **early specialization** involves intensive year-round training in a single sport from a young age, which likely limits the child's exposure to a breadth of sporting activities (Brenner & Council on Sports Medicine & Fitness, 2016; DiFiori et al., 2014; LaPrade et al., 2016). Although researchers and youth fitness specialists have debated the advantages and disadvantages of both approaches for youth development, concerns are now growing about the inherent risks associated with early specialization (see figure 4.1) (LaPrade et al., 2016; Lloyd et al., 2015b; Myer et al., 2015).

Despite support for sampling, it is not uncommon for youth to specialize in a single sport from an early age (Brenner & Council on Sports Medicine & Fitness, 2016) where apparent benefits of early specialization are promoted. It is now acknowledged, however, that early specialization potentially increases injury rates, likelihood of burnout, and eventual disengagement from sport and physical activity (Capranica & Millard-Stafford, 2011; DiFiori et al., 2014; Feeley, Agel, & LaPrade, 2016). One particular concern focuses on the increasing incidence of overuse injuries related to participation in a single sport or a single position in a sport (DiFiori et al., 2014; LaPrade et al., 2016; Lloyd, Cronin, et al., 2016; Myer et al., 2015). Specialization subjects children to high volumes of repetitive training that promote the monotonous development of a narrow range of movement patterns and provides insufficient opportunities for rest, recovery, and adaptation. Such an approach to physical development can lead to repetitive submaximal loading of the musculoskeletal system, which may result in overuse injury (Brenner & Council on Sports Medicine & Fitness, 2016; DiFiori et al., 2014; Stein & Micheli, 2010). For example, research indicates that when a high volume of baseball pitching is completed in the absence of developmentally appropriate preparatory physical conditioning, the risk of overuse injury in the shoulder or elbow is likely to increase in young athletes (Fleisig et al., 2011; Iyer,

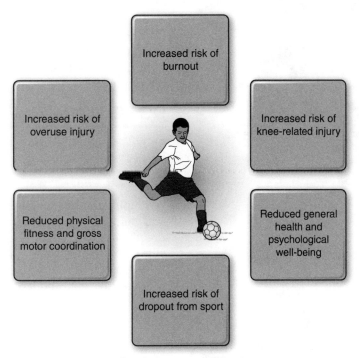

FIGURE 4.1 Potential negative consequences of early sport specialization.

Based on data from Jayanthi et al. (2011); Fleisig, Andrews, Cutter, et al. (2011); Barynina and Vaitsekhoskii (1992); Hall, Barber Foss, Hewett, and Myer (2015); Moesch, Elbe, Hauge, and Wikman (2011); Fransen, Pion, Vandendriessche, et al. (2012); Law et al. (2007); Gould et al. (1996); and Wall and Cote (2007).

Thapa, Khanna, & Chew, 2012; Olsen, Fleisig, Dun, Loftice, & Andrews, 2006).

Beyond the importance of sampling with qualified instruction to reduce the risks of overuse injury, sampling is also central to the development of athleticism. Fundamental movement skills and requisite levels of muscular strength serve as the building blocks for global, more complex movements at a later stage of development (Cattuzzo et al., 2016; Deli, Bakle, & Zachopoulou, 2006; Hulteen, Morgan, Barnett, Stodden, & Lubans, 2018; Lloyd, Cronin, et al., 2016). Therefore, for all children, possessing competence in a breadth of movement skills is more important than acquiring a depth of mastery in a very narrow range of skills.

For example, early-maturing children who are taller and stronger than peers may be encouraged to play the center position on a high school basketball team. However, even if they succeed, they risk developing only a finite number of movement competencies that are specific to that position if they engage only in sport-

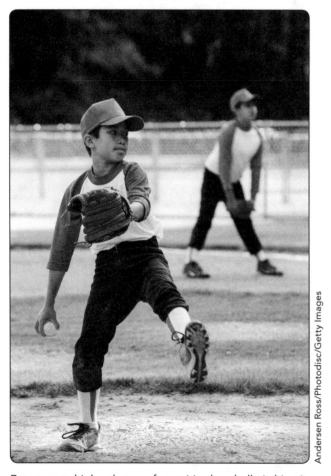

Exposure to high volumes of repetitive baseball pitching in the absence of rest, recovery, and preparatory conditioning can lead to overuse injury.

Andersen Ross/Photodisc/Getty Images

and position-specific practice sessions and competitive basketball matches from an early age. In addition, they will typically be at a heightened risk of developing muscular imbalances and asynchronous movement discrepancies, which, in the absence of targeted training programs to address neuromuscular deficiencies, will fail to prepare them for the demands of sport practice and competition. In such cases, though they may develop proficiency in basketball-specific skills, their athleticism and ability to use transferable motor skills in different positions, different sport environments, and different physical activities will likely be reduced, both on the playground and in sport settings.

We also find a need for sampling when we take a global health perspective on helping young people develop a broad range of movement skills in order to promote a satisfactory level of physical literacy. This notion is supported by research showing that children who possess, or perceive themselves as possessing, competent fundamental movement skills are more likely to engage in sport and physical activity, both throughout childhood (Fransen et al., 2014; Hardy, Reinten-Reynolds, Espinel, Zask, & Okely, 2012) and into adulthood (Lubans, Morgan, Cliff, Barnett, & Okely, 2010; Stodden, Langendorfer, & Roberton, 2009). In addition, motor skill competence has been shown to be inversely associated with overweight and obesity during childhood (D'Hondt et al., 2013; D'Hondt et al., 2014; Hardy et al., 2012; Lopes, Stodden, Bianchi, Maia, & Rodrigues, 2012). Moreover, motor skill competence appears to decline over time (D'Hondt et al., 2013; Robinson et al., 2015; Rodrigues, Stodden, & Lopes, 2016; Stodden, True, Langendorfer, & Gao, 2013), thus highlighting the critical importance of early engagement in appropriate training for long-term athletic development.

DO YOU KNOW?

Early specialization has been linked with increased injury risk and higher rates of dropping out of sport participation.

Empirical data have shown that specializing later and being exposed to lower volumes of deliberate practice early in life act as significant determinants of elite performance in adulthood (Moesch, Elbe, Hauge, & Wikman, 2011). Specifically, the authors collected retrospective data about the careers of a sample of 243 Danish athletes from sports measured in centimeters, grams, or seconds (e.g., track and field, weightlifting, swimming). The data showed that elite athletes (those who achieved a top-10 finish in a world championship or medaled at the European level) accumulated fewer hours of practice in their "main sport" during

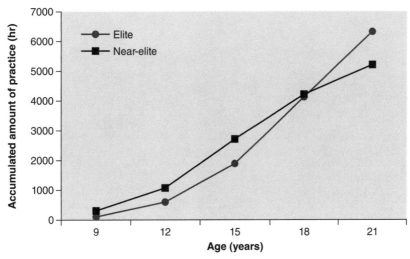

FIGURE 4.2 Comparison of accumulated hours of practice during childhood, adolescence, and early adulthood between elite and near-elite athletes.

Based on data from Moesch, Elbe, Hauge, and Wikman (2011).

childhood and adolescence than did near-elite athletes (see figure 4.2). In the study, age at the time of first competition was about 14.5 years for elite athletes and 12.4 years for non-elite athletes. Overall, the study indicates that athletes who accumulate more hours of specialized practice and focus on competitions at an earlier age may initially experience relative success yet be unable to maintain it as they grow older. The study also showed that elite athletes intensified their training toward the end of adolescence, which resulted in a higher accumulation of training hours around the time of early adulthood (Moesch et al., 2011).

Research also shows that greater sport diversification in early years and later specialization leads to improved physical fitness performance and superior gross motor coordination in 6- to 12-year-old boys (Fransen et al., 2012). In a sample of 735 boys, individuals were categorized as either single-sport or multisport participants. Across all three age groups (6-8, 8-10, and 10-12 years), boys involved in multiple sports spent more time on sport per week (on average, one or two additional hours). More specifically, the research reported two key findings for the 10- to 12-year-olds: Those who participated in more hours of sport per week performed better than those who participated only periodically, and those who specialized in a single sport performed significantly worse in terms of gross motor coordination and standing broad jump tests (see figure 4.3). Combined, these findings suggest that youth benefit from greater exposure to a variety of sport and physical activities (tempered with appropriate rest and preparatory conditioning) and that early specialization can lead to reduced physical performance and a blunting of motor coordination.

Teaching Tip

THINK LONG-TERM

Long-term athletic development models should be grounded in sampling during childhood. This approach develops physically literate individuals who possess a diverse range of movement skills that facilitate lifetime engagement in sport and physical activity. Too often, however, youth choose (or are encouraged by significant others) to focus solely on sport-specific skills from an early age, whether because of developmentally inappropriate programming or due to external factors, such as desire for team selection or the lure of a college scholarship or future professional contract. This approach can lead to intolerable workloads, increased risk of injury, overtraining, and potential burnout—and still it does not guarantee success. Consequently, the athletic development of youth must be viewed as a long-term process, and youth fitness specialists carry a responsibility to educate parents, coaches, and significant others about adopting an evidence-based approach to exercise programming that meets the needs of the individual child.

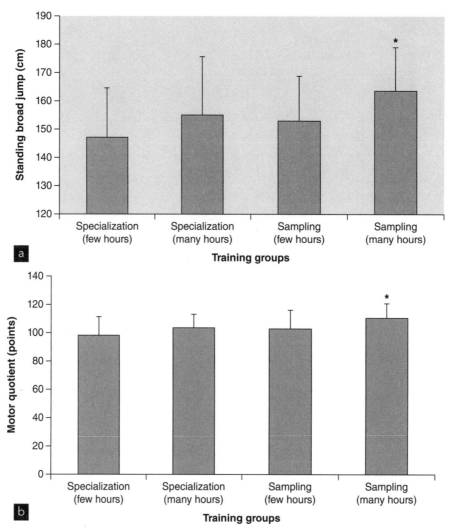

FIGURE 4.3 Performance in the standing broad jump (a) and motor skill quotient (b) for 10- to 12-year-old boys classified within either a specialization or a sampling cohort.

*Significant at $P < 0.05$

Data from Fransen, Pion, Vandendriessche, et al. (2012).

Aside from the potential benefits for physical performance, research has also shown that later specialization leads to reduced injury risk in adolescent females (Hall, Barber Foss, Hewett, & Myer, 2015). Hall and colleagues (2015) showed that in a sample of 546 female youth athletes (comprising middle and high school years), early specialization increased the relative risk of knee-related injury by a factor of 1.5. Diagnoses included patellar tendinopathy and Osgood-Schlatter disease, the latter of which showed a fourfold increase in relative risk in single-sport specialized athletes versus multiple-sport athletes. These data show that diversification appears to be beneficial not only for physical performance but also for reducing the relative risk of injury in youth. Consequently, it would seem prudent for any long-term athletic development model to accommodate a diversification approach that enables children to sample a range of activities and sports before specializing in a single sport or activity at a later stage of development.

Development Models: Talent Versus Athleticism

The need for a systematic and progressive approach to youth development has resulted in the creation of a number of **development models**. These models have been designed to provide theoretical frameworks that youth fitness specialists can either adopt or adapt to help structure the development pathways provided to children and adolescents in a given educational

Bringing Long-Term Athletic Development to the Forefront

Although previous literature has modeled the development of either talent (Bailey & Morley, 2006; Côté, Baker, & Abernethy, 2007; Gagné, 1993; Tinning, 1993) or athleticism (Balyi & Hamilton, 2004; Lloyd & Oliver, 2012), more recent publications have attempted to amalgamate existing knowledge into consensus statements (Bergeron et al., 2015) and position statements (Lloyd, Cronin, et al., 2016). In 2015, the International Olympic Committee (IOC) published a consensus statement on youth athletic development (Bergeron et al., 2015). Its mission was to critically evaluate relevant existing literature and provide an integrated and evidence-based approach to the development of youth athletes. The manuscript included a vast array of recommendations, covering issues related to coaching practice; conditioning, testing, and injury prevention; nutrition, hydration, and exertional heat illness; and sports medicine governance. Central to the consensus statement was the fact that practitioners and relevant governing bodies should acknowledge, embrace, and implement recommendations that align with key principles for growth and maturation, as well as pediatric exercise physiology, psychological and sociological influences, healthy lifestyle behaviors, and the safeguarding and well-being of youth.

Following the publication of the IOC statement, the National Strength and Conditioning Association published its inaugural position statement on long-term athletic development (Lloyd, Cronin, et al., 2016). This document was not compiled to serve as a set of specific training guidelines, or to provide a universal model for youth fitness specialists to simply copy and deliver verbatim. Rather, this landmark document focused on creating "10 pillars of successful long-term athletic development," which should be used by youth fitness specialists as a checklist to ensure that any development pathway facilitates a systematic approach to the long-term development of athleticism in youth of all ages, abilities, and aspirations (see figure 4.4).

FIGURE 4.4   THE NATIONAL STRENGTH AND CONDITIONING ASSOCIATION'S 10 PILLARS FOR SUCCESSFUL LONG-TERM ATHLETIC DEVELOPMENT

1. Long-term athletic development pathways should accommodate the highly individualized and nonlinear nature of the growth and development of youth.

2. Youth of all ages, abilities, and aspirations should engage in long-term athletic development programs that promote both physical fitness and psychosocial well-being.

3. All youth should be encouraged to enhance physical fitness from early childhood, with a primary focus on motor skill and muscular strength development.

4. Long-term athletic development pathways should encourage an early sampling approach for youth that promotes and enhances a broad range of motor skills.

5. Health and well-being of the child should always be the central tenet of long-term athletic development programs.

6. Youth should participate in physical conditioning that helps reduce the risk of injury to ensure their ongoing participation in long-term athletic development programs.

7. Long-term athletic development programs should provide all youth with a range of training modes to enhance both health- and skill-related components of fitness.

8. Practitioners should use relevant monitoring and assessment tools as part of a long-term physical development strategy.

9. Practitioners working with youth should systematically progress and individualize training programs for successful long-term athletic development.

10. Qualified professionals and sound pedagogical approaches are fundamental to the success of long-term athletic development programs.

Reprinted by permission from R.S. Lloyd, J.B. Cronin, A.D. Faigenbaum, et al., "National Strength and Conditioning Association Position Statement on Long-Term Athletic Development," *Journal of Strength and Conditioning Research* 30, no. 6 (2016): 1491-1509.

system or sport program. However, it is apparent that a number of these models relate to the development of "talented" athletes rather than being grounded in the process of developing physical fitness qualities in children of all ages and abilities.

Talent Development Models

Although talent development models typically do not promote exercise guidelines for long-term athletic development, they do provide some valuable insight into the learning and development processes for youth. Consequently, youth fitness specialists should be acquainted with their central philosophies in order to optimize a long-term and holistic approach to athletic development. The following discussion examines the most popular talent development models in the literature and highlights relevant information for youth fitness specialists to consider when designing long-term athletic development programs.

Pyramid Model of Sport Development

There are many versions of the model of sport development, which is a pyramidal approach to talent development (Tinning, 1993). Traditionally, it involves a broad introductory level designed to engage large numbers of participants in foundational activities. Going up the pyramid, participant numbers typically decrease as competition levels rise and performance standards improve (see figure 4.5). The model supposes that school-based physical education should serve as the vehicle for the introductory level of the pyramid and that the primary goal at this level should be to develop physical literacy. As children transition from the bottom of the pyramid toward the top (elite) sporting level, they are exposed to a more rigorous competitive schedule and greater focus on sport-spe-

cific training. Thus, although the model includes all youth at the initial stage, it fails to account for individual rates of development due to variations in growth and maturation. In another area of concern, data on the health and fitness of modern-day youth call into question whether existing school-based physical education structures develop physically literate children, especially during the elementary school years (Society of Health and Physical Educators, 2016).

Differentiated Model of Giftedness and Talent

The differentiated model of giftedness and talent, which originated in the educational sector, proposes that a child or adolescent needs to learn and practice skills methodically in order to translate an innate gift into a systematically developed talent (Gagné, 1993). The model implies that practice should increase in intensity over time and that children should be exposed to activities that promote development of intellectual, creative, socioaffective, and sensorimotor abilities in order to maximize talent (Gagné, 1993). Although the model provides no guidance in terms of physical fitness development, it does support the development of multiple abilities, which should be a central focus of any long-term athletic development pathway.

Model of Talent Development in Physical Education

Another structured pathway that was devised in the education domain is the model of talent development in physical education (Bailey, 2006). This model recognizes that talent is multifactorial and that attempts should be made to help young people develop psychomotor, interpersonal, intrapersonal, cognitive, and creative abilities. It features a focus on **deliberate practice**, which

---

Teaching Tip

TALENT IDENTIFICATION AND DEVELOPMENT

Talent identification is the process of identifying current participants who have the potential to excel in a given sport or activity. *Talent development*, on the other hand, involves providing the best learning environment and support systems to develop such talent (Vaeyens, Lenoir, Williams, & Philippaerts, 2008). Although many sporting structures incorporate talent identification programs into their development pathways, these systems encourage the early selection and deselection of children and adolescents, which typically leads to discrimination against later-maturing youth (see chapter 3). Therefore, youth fitness specialists should view the talent *development* philosophy as far more important and beneficial to youth. The International Olympic Committee supports this premise and views long-term athletic development as the process of developing healthy, capable, and resilient young athletes while also attaining widespread, inclusive, sustainable, and enjoyable participation and success for youth (Bergeron et al., 2015).

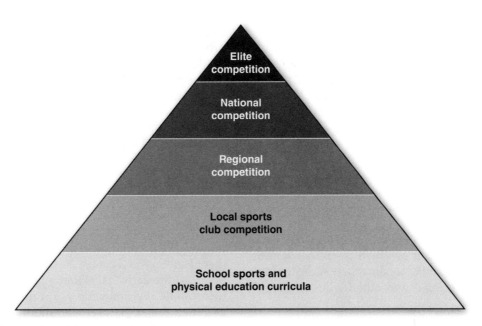

FIGURE 4.5 Pyramid model of sport development.

Reprinted by permission from UK Coaching (formerly Sports Coach UK). Reprinted from R.P. Bailey, D. Collins, D.P.A. Ford, et al., *Participant Development in Sport: An Academic Literature Review,* commissioned report for Sports Coach UK (Leeds: Sports Coach UK, 2010). Adapted from R. Tinning, D. Kirk, and J. Evans, *Learning to Teach Physical Education* (Sydney: Prentice-Hall, 1993).

is characterized by specific practice entailing both physical and cognitive contributions designed to improve performance and aid skill development (Ericsson, 2013). The model proposes that a child requires exposure to both general and specialized learning opportunities in order to develop talent(s); however, development should be pursued in a holistic manner to retain the child's interest and engagement with the chosen activity. Holistic development is an important concept for youth fitness specialists to consider when designing any long-term athletic development pathway, because physical fitness and skill acquisition should not be pursued at the expense of social and psychological well-being or sheer enjoyment of the exercise experience.

Developmental Model of Sport Participation

Perhaps the most prominent of the talent development models is the developmental model of sport participation (Côté et al., 2007), which distinguishes between three stages of development for youth. First, the model identifies the "sampling years" (6-12 years of age), during which youth are encouraged to experience a range of activities and sports and develop through exposure to **deliberate play**. Deliberate play differs from deliberate practice and reflects early exploratory activities that are intrinsically motivated and focused on maximizing enjoyment (Côté et al., 2007). It is an important construct for youth fitness specialists to consider, especially when developing physical devel-

opment programs for toddlers, young children, or inexperienced individuals who are new to the concept of athletic development.

Second, the model proposes the "specializing years" (13-15 years of age), during which the child begins to participate in a reduced number of sports and exhibits a more even ratio of deliberate play and deliberate practice. Finally, the model incorporates the "investment years" (16+ years), which are characterized by higher amounts of deliberate practice, less exposure to deliberate play, and, typically, investment in a single sport.

The notions of deliberate play and deliberate practice feature prominently in the talent development literature. But youth fitness specialists should also appreciate the value of **deliberate preparation**, which involves using developmentally appropriate training modalities to help prepare youth for the demands of both deliberate play and deliberate practice. Notwithstanding the potential value of deliberate play—which characterizes sporting activities that are unstructured, play-like, and enjoyable (Berry, Abernethy, & Cote, 2008)—there is a need for deliberate preparation characterized by qualified instruction and planned training in order to improve a youngster's motor skill competence and overall physical fitness. This approach also helps prevent an upsurge in neuromuscular deficits that can manifest during the growing years (Faigenbaum, Lloyd, MacDonald, & Myer, 2016).

Structured, organized training delivered by youth fitness specialists can be intrinsically motivating and stimulating, which encourages youth to engage in exercise and sport as an ongoing lifestyle choice (Holt, 2011). The primary aim of any exercise class or sport program should be to enhance participants' physical literacy by improving their ability to move with confidence and competence in a variety of physical activities and in multiple settings (Whitehead, 2001). The concept of physical literacy refers not only to the physical domain of performing a skill but also to the attitudes, motivations, and psychosocial skills needed for continued participation in exercise and sport (Edwards et al., 2018; Edwards, Bryant, Keegan, Morgan, & Jones, 2017).

Although talent models differ in terminology and design, they also exhibit common traits that youth fitness specialists should consider when designing and implementing long-term athletic development programs.

- Athletic development programs should foster positive learning processes and be driven by long-term holistic improvement rather than short-term gains in performance.

- Sampling and deliberate play, under the guise of developmentally appropriate instruction, provide the foundations for long-term athletic development and should be prioritized for young and inexperienced children.

- Youth should also be exposed to deliberate practice in order to provide sufficient opportunity for motor skill development.

- Deliberate preparation is a critical component of long-term athletic development intended to prepare youth for the rigors of sport and physical activity.

- Those responsible for designing and delivering athletic development programs for children and adolescents should be well versed in effective pedagogy and principles of pediatric exercise science.

Athletic Development Models

Whether the goal is to enhance sport performance or improve general health and well-being, the development of physical fitness in youth is a complex and dynamic process. Models designed to optimize talent and sporting success have been adopted by a number of sporting associations, national governing bodies, and educational sectors, but these models provide less focus on processes that foster the athletic development of youth. Consequently, youth athletic development focuses all too often on the outcome or product (i.e.,

indices of physical performance) rather than on the process (i.e., learning experience, technical competence).

Moreover, close inspection of the literature reveals that very few published athletic development models have successfully bridged the interaction between age, maturation, and training. The systems that appear most prominently in the literature are the long-term athlete development model (Balyi & Hamilton, 2004) and the youth physical development model (Lloyd & Oliver, 2012).

Long-Term Athlete Development Model

Although the concept of long-term athletic development is not novel (Bompa, 2000; Riordan, 1977), it was not until the early 2000s that attempts were made to incorporate the interaction of training with growth and maturation (Balyi & Hamilton, 2004). The model that first attempted to combine training prescription with the timing and tempo of maturation was the long-term athlete development (LTAD) model (Balyi & Hamilton, 2004). Using individual maturation rates (estimated from measures of peak height velocity and peak weight velocity), the model attempts to pair specific training-induced adaptations with the naturally occurring adaptive responses associated with growth and maturation. The model is viewed as an appealing concept and succeeded in advancing previous pediatric training practice, which was often based solely on chronological age. As often noted, the use of chronological age for training prescription is inherently flawed due to the potentially large variation in individual maturation status within a single age group (Lloyd, Oliver, et al., 2014).

The process of developing physical fitness in youth is made challenging by the unique demands surrounding the growth and maturation of anatomical, neurological, hormonal, and musculoskeletal systems in the developing child. Longitudinal data show that the natural development of physiological processes (e.g., height) and physical fitness measures (e.g., strength, power) follow a nonlinear pattern during childhood and adolescence. In this pattern, phases of little or no change are interspersed with periods of rapid development, often referred to as periods of **accelerated adaptation**. It is believed that during these accelerated periods, the neural, biological, and hormonal systems of youth are all sensitive to extraneous variables, such as nutritional intake, environmental factors, and physical training.

Previous developmental models have proposed that periods of accelerated adaptation should be viewed as specific "windows of opportunity" (Balyi & Hamilton, 2004), during which youth fitness specialists should provide a training stimulus matched to the adaptive processes resulting from growth and maturation. For example, the LTAD model proposes that suppleness should be targeted during early childhood, when the musculotendon properties of the child naturally facilitate a greater degree of stretching; similarly, it proposes that strength should be targeted after peak height velocity, when circulating hormonal concentrations enable increased gains in muscle strength and size (Balyi & Hamilton, 2004). Unfortunately, this theory and its associated time frames promote a narrow view of trainability in youth, thus leading youth fitness specialists to potentially veer away from a multifaceted approach to training prescription. Furthermore, the LTAD model states that failure to train the appropriate physical fitness component during a specific window of opportunity prevents the child or adolescent from reaching full athletic potential (Balyi & Hamilton, 2004). Ultimately, then, although the theory may seem appealing, there is a lack of longitudinal empirical evidence to support strict adoption of it in any long-term athletic development pathway (Ford et al., 2011).

Synergistic Adaptation

More recently, researchers have proposed a new training concept known as **synergistic adaptation** (Faigenbaum et al., 2016; Lloyd, Radnor, De Ste Croix, Cronin, & Oliver, 2016; Radnor, Lloyd, & Oliver, 2017). Like the windows theory, this approach posits a compatible relationship between specific adaptations to an imposed training demand and adaptations related to age and maturity (Lloyd, Radnor, et al., 2016). It does not, however, hold that youth are trainable only during specific periods. Rather, it adheres to the notion that while all fitness components are trainable irrespective of maturation, particular training stimuli may be preferable to complement particular adaptations occurring as a result of growth and maturation.

For example, research has shown that in a group of active school-age youth, boys who were pre– and post–peak height velocity were both able to make significant gains in jump and sprint performance following various forms of resistance training (plyometric training, traditional strength training, and a combination of the two) (Lloyd, Radnor, et al., 2016). However, boys who were pre–peak height velocity made the greatest gains from plyometric training, whereas boys who were post–peak height velocity appeared to benefit most from combined training. From the viewpoint of synergistic adaptation, plyometric training stimulates mainly neural adaptations, which mirror the nature of the naturally occurring adaptations prior to peak height velocity. In contrast, the combined training stimulus complements both the ongoing neural adaptations and the structural or architectural adaptations occurring after peak height velocity. Although the concept of synergistic adaptation is evolving, supporting evidence does exist in the literature related to developing both strength and power (Rumpf, Cronin, Pinder, Oliver, & Hughes, 2012) as well as speed (Behringer, Vom Heede, Matthews, & Mester, 2011; Chaouachi et al., 2014; Fathi et al., 2018; Meylan, Cronin, Oliver, Hopkins, & Contreras, 2014).

DO YOU KNOW?

Plyometric exercise appears to be an effective mode of training for children, especially during the initial stages of training.

Myth of the 10,000-Hour Rule

Another concern about previous developmental models focuses on the prominence given to the now-infamous 10,000-hour rule (Ford et al., 2011). This notion holds that an individual must acquire 10,000 hours of deliberate practice in order to attain mastery in a given sport or activity, which could also be viewed as dedicating specific practice to the same sport or activity for three hours per day for 10 years. This recommendation supposedly originated from the work of Ericsson and colleagues (Ericsson, Krampe, & Tesch-Römer, 1993), who examined the development of expert performance in elite musicians. However, Ericsson (2013) later suggested that their seminal work on expert

---

Teaching Tip

QUALITY NOT QUANTITY

Long-term athletic development should always emphasize the quality of practice rather than the quantity. Although repetition is necessary for development of motor skill, youth require training environments to be fun and interesting and to provide challenging learning experiences. Therefore, especially during childhood and early adolescence, youth fitness specialists should focus not on helping youth accumulate hours of sport-specific training but on providing exposure to a range of sports or activities as a composite measure of training workload.

performers had been misinterpreted and that they do not stringently subscribe to the 10,000-hour rule as first believed. Furthermore, some of their original data contradicted the rule (Ericsson, 2013). For example, some elite violinists had engaged in an average of only 5,000 hours of specific practice by the time they reached adulthood. Similarly, research by Moesch and colleagues (2011) showed that elite athletes accumulated only about 6,300 hours of deliberate practice by the time they reached adulthood.

Even on an intuitive level, it is simplistic to focus strictly on accumulating a set number of hours of practice in order to achieve expert performance. The development of any skill or innate ability is multifactorial and requires the intricate interaction of a number of constraints (Seifert, Button, & Davids, 2013). In addition, focusing only on accumulating an explicit volume of practice is likely to encourage youth to specialize early in a particular sport or activity, which may also encourage overtraining or lead to burnout in the quest to accumulate the 10,000 hours ahead of their peers. Instead, we should focus on providing children and adolescents with a breadth of experiences, including sampling different sports, activities, and training methods with guidance from qualified youth fitness specialists who understand the physical and psychosocial uniqueness of youth.

Youth Physical Development Model

Due to the lack of empirical evidence to support the LTAD model, researchers developed an alternative approach referred to as the youth physical development (YPD) model (Lloyd & Oliver, 2012) (see figure 4.6). This model was intended to provide a more realistic and evidence-based approach to long-term athletic development during childhood and adolescence. Its most novel aspect was the recognition that, in contradiction of the theory of windows of opportunity, all fitness components are trainable at all stages of development.

The YPD model underlines the importance of engaging youth in multifaceted training programs that incorporate a range of training methods to improve all physical attributes (e.g., speed, strength, power) irrespective of maturity stage. The model also provides a more comprehensive approach to developing physical fitness than did previous models, stipulating training rationales for agility, muscular power, and muscular hypertrophy—fitness components that had not previously received as much attention in the youth-based training literature.

In the YPD model, muscular strength and motor skill development are key priorities throughout both childhood and adolescence because they provide the foundations for other physical attributes (i.e., power, agility), enhance physical performance, and help reduce the risk of injury in sport and physical activity. Lloyd and Oliver (2012) suggested that other fitness components characterized by high neuromuscular demand (i.e., power, speed, agility) should also serve as training foci during childhood due to the neural plasticity associated with this stage of development. Providing that children remain within the development pathway, adolescence would then serve as an opportune time to use further neural gains in addition to structural and architectural adaptations to maximize physical development. For instance, during this stage of development, muscular hypertrophy was suggested as becoming a more important component of training programs to maximize muscle cross-sectional area and thus enhance force-producing capacities.

Mobility is defined as the integration of strength, power, and motor control to effectively move a joint or series of joints at the desired speed, in the proper sequence, at a specific time, and in a given direction for a particular movement (Sands & McNeal, 2013). Despite its importance for health and fitness, mobility is never viewed as a key training priority at any stage of development in the YPD model, but it is recognized as an underlying component of fitness that should always be addressed in any athletic development program.

The authors of the YPD model placed endurance and metabolic conditioning as a training priority for later in adolescence. This stance was rationalized on the grounds that youth are more likely to engage in endurance-related activities in physical education curriculums, whereas sport competitions and training sessions typically provide opportunities to develop sport-specific endurance. Consequently, it is suggested that if children are able to access developmentally appropriate training (e.g., small section of a physical education lesson, after-school fitness program, organized strength and conditioning sessions), they will benefit more from developing neuromuscular qualities (i.e., strength, speed, power, agility) than from having additional exposure to endurance-based training.

In summary, the YPD model was grounded in seven central postulates for the physical development of children and adolescents:

- *Trainability is possible for all.* All fitness components are trainable irrespective of stage of development; however, the mechanisms of adaptation could differ due to growth and maturation.

- *Start early.* Children should engage in physical activity and preparatory conditioning as soon as they are able to accept and follow instructions.

Youth physical development (YPD) model for males

Chronological age (years)	2	3	4	5	6	7	8	9	10	11	12	13	14	15	16	17	18	19	20	21+
Age periods	Early childhood			Middle childhood							Adolescence									Adulthood
Growth rate	Rapid growth ⟷ Steady growth ⟷ Adolescent spurt ⟷ Decline in growth rate																			
Maturational status	Years pre-PHV ⟵ PHV ⟶ Years post-PHV																			
Training adaption	Predominantly neural (age-related) ⟷ Combination of neural and hormonal (maturity-related)																			

Physical qualities:
- **FMS** / FMS / FMS / FMS
- SSS / SSS / **SSS** / **SSS**
- Mobility / **Mobility** / Mobility
- Agility / **Agility** / **Agility** / **Agility**
- Speed / **Speed** / **Speed** / **Speed**
- Power / **Power** / **Power** / **Power**
- **Strength** / **Strength** / **Strength** / **Strength**
- Hypertrophy / Hypertrophy / **Hypertrophy** / Hypertrophy
- Endurance and MC / Endurance and MC / Endurance and MC / Endurance and MC

Training structure	Unstructured	Low structure	Moderate structure	High structure	Very high structure

a

PHV-Peak height velocity   **FMS**-Fundamental movement skills   **SSS**-Sport-specific skills   **MC**-Metabolic conditioning

---

Youth physical development (YPD) model for females

Chronological age (years)	2	3	4	5	6	7	8	9	10	11	12	13	14	15	16	17	18	19	20	21+
Age periods	Early childhood			Middle childhood							Adolescence									Adulthood
Growth rate	Rapid growth ⟷ Steady growth ⟷ Adolescent spurt ⟷ Decline in growth rate																			
Maturational status	Years pre-PHV ⟵ PHV ⟶ Years post-PHV																			
Training adaption	Predominantly neural (age-related) ⟷ Combination of neural and hormonal (maturity-related)																			

Physical qualities:
- **FMS** / FMS / FMS / FMS
- SSS / SSS / **SSS** / **SSS**
- Mobility / **Mobility** / Mobility
- Agility / **Agility** / **Agility** / **Agility**
- Speed / **Speed** / **Speed** / **Speed**
- Power / **Power** / **Power** / **Power**
- **Strength** / **Strength** / **Strength** / **Strength**
- Hypertrophy / Hypertrophy / **Hypertrophy** / Hypertrophy
- Endurance and MC / Endurance and MC / Endurance and MC / Endurance and MC

Training structure	Unstructured	Low structure	Moderate structure	High structure	Very high structure

b

PHV-Peak height velocity   **FMS**-Fundamental movement skills   **SSS**-Sport-specific skills   **MC**-Metabolic conditioning

FIGURE 4.6   The youth physical development (YPD) model for (a) males and (b) females.

Reprinted by permission from R.S. Lloyd and J.L. Oliver, "The Youth Physical Development Model: A New Approach to Long-Term Athletic Development," *Strength and Conditioning Journal* 34, no. 3 (2012) 61-72.

- *Prioritize muscular strength and motor skill development.* All youth should be exposed to developmentally appropriate training that promotes development of muscular strength and motor skill competence.
- *Progress from fundamental to sport specific.* The emphasis of motor skill development should shift over time; fundamental movement skills should be prioritized during childhood, and greater focus should be given to sport-specific skills during adolescence.
- *Increase training structure over time.* Training programs should become more structured over time; however, experiential learning opportunities should be promoted wherever possible during early childhood.
- *Individualize training prescription.* Youth fitness specialists must modify training prescription to accommodate the specific needs of the individual, accounting primarily for technical competence but also for training age, biological maturation, and sex of the participant.
- *Youth fitness specialists are essential.* Those who design, deliver, and monitor long-term athletic development programs should be suitably qualified; specifically, they should possess relevant fitness qualifications, sound understanding of pediatric exercise science, and a strong pedagogical background.

Pulling It All Together: What, Why, and When to Train?

Having reviewed the talent and athletic development models, we can now consider how to collate this information in order to provide guidance for long-term athletic development. The following section discusses how training directives could be prescribed for an ideal case scenario, wherein a child enters a developmental program during early childhood and progresses along that pathway until the end of adolescence and the start of adulthood. We can also consider how to work outside of this idyllic model in a reality where adolescents routinely present with no training history and low levels of technical competence.

Childhood: Laying the Foundations

Due to the heightened neural plasticity associated with childhood, this stage of development should be viewed as an opportunity for youth fitness specialists to lay the foundations for long-term athletic develop-

ment. During the early phases of childhood (up to five years of age), children should engage in exercises and activities that develop fundamental motor skills and primal levels of athleticism (e.g., strength, power, balance, coordination) while simultaneously promoting cognitive development. For example, gymnastics and the martial arts provide excellent mediums through which to develop body-weight management, muscular strength, and coordination in a cognitively challenging environment.

The concept of training the developing brain (discussed in chapter 5) is intended to provide learning experiences that make use of the neuroplasticity and motor learning potential of youth (Myer et al., 2013). At this stage of development, youth fitness specialists typically need to help youth develop physical qualities and enhance movement competence within fun-based games or activities that kinesthetically challenge young children to manage body weight in space. For instance, exposing children to novel training challenges (e.g., obstacle courses) gives them opportunities to develop their movement capacities in fun and stimulating environments. Above all, young children should be exposed to a variety of training settings that

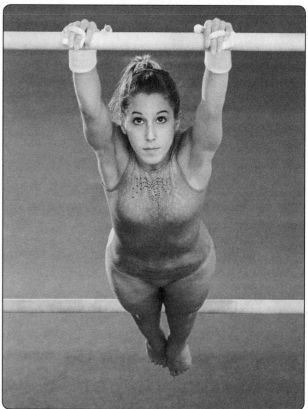

Gymnastics can serve as an excellent activity to develop coordination, motor skills, and basic levels of muscular strength.

facilitate experiential learning in a fun, challenging, and somewhat unstructured environment while promoting not only physical development but also key psychosocial benefits (e.g., social interaction).

Although performance outcomes do not form a key focus during early childhood, youth fitness specialists should view this stage of development as an opportunity to begin developing the young child's technical competence (i.e., movement performance quality) and **training age** (i.e., the number of years for which a child has participated in structured training). In particular, technical competence is the variable on which exercise prescription will largely be based for the remainder of a child's lifetime.

As a child transitions through childhood, the notion of sampling various sports and training modes should continue to be prioritized. Youth fitness specialists should retain a focus on training all components of fitness in an integrated manner, and training should begin to take on a more structured approach. Ideally, in the later years of childhood, children should be involved in a well-rounded and periodized exercise program to maximize their chances of developing the requisite levels of athleticism to facilitate lifetime participation in recreational physical activity or even future involvement in competitive or noncompetitive sport. From a psychosocial perspective, as youth enter adolescence, peer comparisons become more commonplace; consequently, among other parameters, youth fitness specialists should aim to prioritize each child's motivation, self-worth, and self-esteem and to encourage empowerment (Lloyd et al., 2015a).

DO YOU KNOW?

Training prescription and progression should be based on how technically proficient an individual is, not on how long someone has been involved in formalized training or sport.

Adolescence: Building on the Foundations

A child who has been involved in an appropriately structured and suitably coached long-term athletic development program from an early age should be physically literate by the end of childhood, especially toward the middle or later years of this developmental stage. Consequently, youth fitness specialists should view the ensuing stage, adolescence, as an opportunity to build on the foundations laid during childhood. Invariably, adolescence is a stage of development in which a number of youth who are engaged in competi-

tive sports will either begin to specialize in a particular sport or opt out of sport programs and transition to a pathway of recreational participation.

For youth who remain in sporting pathways, exercise prescription should be programmed with high relevance to their individual needs and the unique demands of the chosen sport. Irrespective of the sport in question, well-rounded physical training programs must be considered an essential component of the child's overall development program in order to enhance performance and minimize the risk of sport-related injury. Athletic development programs should not be viewed simply as optional additions to the program. Instead, structured training programs should include a variety of training modes designed to enhance multiple components of fitness throughout childhood and adolescence.

Similarly, youth who choose not to engage in competitive sport should still be encouraged to participate in well-rounded exercise programs. Moreover, such programs should enable them to develop, or at least maintain, the requisite levels of athleticism for participating in recreational sports and physical activity; help them accumulate the recommended amount of daily physical activity; and encourage them to engage in lifelong physical activity (Moesch et al., 2011). Whereas youth who are engaged in sport may receive psychosocial support from their coaches or other personnel in their associations or clubs, those who are not engaged in this manner should be encouraged by parents and youth fitness specialists to develop and maintain motivation for ongoing participation in daily physical activity.

Realities of Long-Term Athletic Development Models

Although the notion of development pathways appears to provide an attractive approach to long-term athletic development, youth fitness specialists should acknowledge and recognize the realities of working in accordance with such models. For example, children do not always engage in a highly organized, long-term program of training from a very young age. As a result, in many cases, youth fitness specialists train adolescents with very low training ages and low levels of technical competence. They may also be faced with groups of youth who have mixed abilities and are at various stages of maturation. Thus, it is imperative to view any developmental model as a flexible template that provides generic structure and guidance rather than a rigid, gold-standard blueprint that should be superimposed on everyone. Wherever possible, youth fitness specialists should be encouraged to design and (if appropriate) tailor generic guidelines to create specific, individualized strategies for the individuals with whom they work.

Figure 4.7 provides a basic decision-making framework for training prescription that could be used for a child or adolescent entering an athletic development program for the first time. The framework suggests that youth fitness specialists introduce the child to some form of physical activity or training to allow the child to sample a variety of related activities or training methods; assess the athlete's competence in the activity or training method; and modify program content based on the child's performance in the assessment. This simple approach can provide clarity and enable individual tailoring in youth-based training prescription.

The following scenarios have been designed to illustrate the realities and potential complexities of working with youth within the confines of long-term athletic development models. The scenarios highlight the need for youth fitness specialists to be flexible in approaching their work with children and adolescents.

Scenario 1: Mixed-Ability Group

The importance of flexibility is heightened when coaching youth who have different levels of technical competence, different stages of maturation, or both. Although many education systems and a number of sporting clubs and associations use chronological age to group youth into age-based teams or to identify talent, this approach

is inherently flawed due to the large individual differences present in biological maturation (Lloyd, Oliver, et al., 2014). Similarly, it is highly probable that a physical education class or sport team will be characterized by considerable variation in training history among those involved. As a result, youth fitness specialists need to differentiate accordingly.

For example, in a group of seventh-grade schoolchildren, some may have a training age of five years, be experienced in playing multiple sports, and possess a high level of technical competence in a range of exercise modalities (e.g., flexibility training, strength training, running mechanics). This profile contrasts sharply with that of individuals who have never experienced formalized training or played a single sport. In such an instance, the youth fitness specialist must realize that the children should not all be exposed to the same training program, that they will inevitably differ in their rates of progression in exercises or activities, and that they will need differentiated exercise prescriptions (e.g., exercise selections, volumes, intensities) if they are trained simultaneously in a large-group setting.

In a large-group training environment, the youth fitness specialist could design training programs that pursue common goals (e.g., developing speed and motor skill competence) but include different levels. For example, a bronze level could provide an introduction to the program, a silver level could offer intermediate programming, a gold level could incorporate more

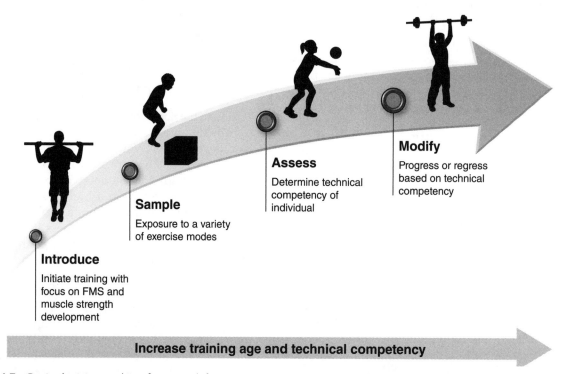

FIGURE 4.7   Basic decision-making framework for training prescription. FMS=fundamental movement skills.

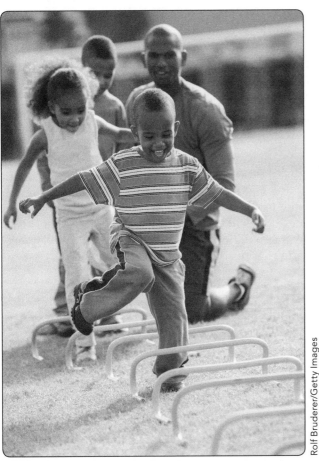

An obstacle course can provide a fun and engaging way for children to explore movement.

Rolf Bruderer/Getty Images

difficult programming, and a platinum level could offer the most advanced programming. This strategy would enable the youth fitness specialist to develop similar fitness qualities in all members of the group in a differentiated manner that is responsive to the ability levels of all involved. From a psychosocial perspective, children would be able to work with peers of similar ability, thus reducing the potentially negative consequences of peer comparison and maximizing enjoyment. In addition, by differentiating the program, the specialist would provide children with a motivational stimulus to reach the next level; for instance, upon becoming technically proficient at the silver level, a child could move to the gold level.

Scenario 2: Late Starter

Now consider an example in which an adolescent enters a developmental model having not been exposed to the early stages of training. As a result, the individual has missed out on critical opportunities to develop motor skill competence and associated neuro-

muscular qualities (i.e., strength, power, speed). In this situation, the individual should begin by mastering a range of fundamental motor skills and basic levels of muscular strength. Once that is achieved, the individual can engage in more advanced training techniques that may already be used by age-group peers who have accumulated a higher training age and can consistently demonstrate technical competence. In other words, individuals with this type of training history should not be accelerated through differentiated training programs without first demonstrating competence at more rudimentary levels.

Similarly, programming flexibility would be needed for an early-maturing 10-year-old girl who possesses outstanding levels of athleticism. She should not be restricted to introductory methods of training but instead should be allowed to progress to appropriate training strategies that are more advanced. As a caveat, youth fitness specialists should never increase training difficulty or progress an individual at the expense of technical competence. It is not uncommon for youth who have graduated to more advanced forms of training to need to revisit more fundamental levels of training in order to refine their technical competence.

Scenario 3: Late-Maturing Child

Flexibility would also be required in the case of a late-maturing child who does not show gains similar to those of earlier-maturing peers. For example, a 16-year-old basketball player who is late maturing may not demonstrate the same rate or magnitude of change in morphology and physical performance that is seen in the majority of teammates. As a late maturer, he has not yet experienced the rapid natural gains in muscle mass that result from the increase in hormonal concentrations associated with adolescence.

Given the demands of the sport, improving muscle mass might be identified as an important goal for the player. From an athletic development perspective, due to the lack of a muscle-building anabolic environment in the player's muscle cells, a youth fitness specialist would be well advised to prioritize strength- and power-based loading schemes instead of a hypertrophy-based prescription. The specialist should also work on relationship building and on reassuring the player that when the maturational process arrives, the training focus can transition toward hypertrophy in order to facilitate catching up with peers.

Summary

In order to maximize the number of youth who participate in sport (whether competitive or noncompetitive) and recreational physical activity, youth fitness specialists should adopt a long-term approach to athletic development. Due to the complexities of growth and maturation, as well as their potential interaction with training, long-term athletic development planning for youth requires a sound understanding of physical training and of the principles of pediatric exercise science. Youth fitness specialists should look to help youth develop physical fitness early in life within an integrated and holistic development program that accounts for individual differences and promotes development of a wide range of physical fitness qualities and movement skills.

All components of fitness are trainable in youth irrespective of the stage of maturation; therefore, training prescription should not be based on the notion of windows of opportunity. In order to make use of the heightened neural plasticity associated with childhood, and to foster healthy behaviors, it is critical to provide youth with opportunities for early engagement in physical activity that sets them up for effective long-term athletic development. In order to benefit physical performance, reduce injury risk, and promote general health and well-being, long-term athletic development pathways should avoid early specialization and encourage early sampling.

Because every individual is unique, it is imperative that youth fitness specialists design, teach, assess, and adapt long-term athletic development programs that fulfill the needs of individual participants. Any developmental model should focus not on short-term gains in performance but on long-term development and continued participation for all youth.

CHAPTER 5

Pedagogy for Youth Fitness Specialists

CHAPTER OBJECTIVES

- Discuss the theory and practice of teaching children and adolescents
- Understand the influence of cognitive age on engagement and participation
- Recognize instructional strategies that enhance the learning process
- Learn how to create a positive motivational climate
- Identify 12 fundamental principles of effective coaching

KEY TERMS

cognitive age (p. 87)

external focus (p. 90)

extrinsic motivation (p. 92)

internal focus (p. 89)

intrinsic motivation (p. 92)

modeling (p. 91)

pedagogy (p. 86)

physical literacy (p. 87)

scaffolding (p. 89)

Introduction

With guidance from youth fitness specialists who understand the importance of skillful teaching and active learning, children and adolescents can improve their physical fitness and enhance their athletic abilities while working toward a common goal in a supportive environment. Practitioners who model appropriate behaviors and develop a teaching philosophy that is consistent with the physical and psychosocial uniqueness of school-age youth are better prepared to design exercise programs and teach the technical aspects of complex exercises to the young people they hope to inspire. The most successful youth fitness specialists are effective teachers who understand the fundamental principles of pediatric exercise science and developmental physiology.

The term **pedagogy** refers to the theory and practice of education; literally, it means "to lead the child." Although the study and practice of effective pedagogy are often associated with academic subjects, sport and exercise pedagogy involves the educational aspects of teaching and coaching a diverse group of participants to move and learn with confidence and competence in a variety of settings and situations (Armour & Chambers, 2014). With the exception of physical education teachers, practitioners who work with youth in fitness centers and sport programs may not be educated in effective pedagogical strategies that specifically address the cognitive abilities and learning styles of all children and adolescents. Therefore, youth fitness specialists should gain practical experience in the field and work with seasoned professionals in order to genuinely appreciate the observable influence of effective pedagogy on the attitudes, behaviors, and actions of children and adolescents in exercise classes and sport programs. If youth participate in integrative training programs that are grounded in appropriate pedagogical strategies and effective group management skills, they will likely become independent learners who regularly engage in physical activity as an ongoing lifestyle choice.

DO YOU KNOW?

Young children of active parents are more likely to be active than are children of inactive parents.

Training the Developing Brain

Regular participation in well-designed exercise programs can enhance the health, fitness, and athletic performance of children and adolescents (Bond, Weston, Williams, & Barker, 2017; Faude et al., 2017;

Lloyd et al., 2014). However, youth fitness specialists need to be aware that training adaptations and adherence to an exercise class or sport program can both be influenced by the exercise instructions and feedback methods used. Therefore, when designing and implementing youth programs, we must consider the relationship between a participant's cognitive and physical development. As with classroom teaching of academic subjects, youth fitness specialists must use developmentally appropriate strategies that enhance learning, maximize engagement, and improve performance in the fitness center or sport venue. Enhanced physical education programs delivered by well-trained specialists have proven to be effective in schools (Faigenbaum et al., 2015; Mooses et al., 2017; Silva et al., 2018), and similar benefits can be expected in other settings, provided that instructional practices meet the needs of all participants.

DO YOU KNOW?

Adequate sleep keeps the mind alert, the body engaged, and the brain ready to learn.

Effective teaching strategies help youth acquire new skills and decision-making abilities, whereas ineffective teaching is unproductive and potentially injurious. When exercises or sport skills are learned and practiced incorrectly from the start, they become difficult to correct later in life. If you have ever taught an adult how to swing a golf club or perform a weightlifting movement, then you have witnessed support for the premise that the motor capabilities of youth are more pliable and therefore more responsive to skill-based training than those of older participants. Although adults certainly can learn complex sport skills and advanced exercises, brain development during the growing years likely corresponds to a period of time when the critical subsystems for skill development are most responsive to training (Myer et al., 2015; Thelen, 1995; Ungerleider, Doyon, & Karni, 2002).

Research on the plasticity of brain development during the early years of life suggests that the brain becomes less malleable and requires more effort to adapt with advancing age (Ismail, Fatemi, Johnston, 2017; Myer et al., 2015). As with learning how to play a musical instrument or speak a second language, an individual's potential for learning new physical skills and complex movements may be diminished once neural pathways have been established in the developing brain. As such, the timing of brain development and associated neuroplasticity are important considerations because an individual may find it more challenging to learn dynamic actions and master advanced sport skills if this opportunity is missed.

Youth fitness specialists can profoundly influence children's development, motivation, and lifelong well-being by increasing their exposure to various movement skills and behavioral strategies that support daily physical activity and enhance talent development (Chan, Lonsdale, & Fung, 2012; Collins, Macnamara, & McCarthy, 2016; McKenzie & Lounsbery, 2013). Interventions that include educational, curricular, and environmental components have been found to increase physical activity and provide youth with the knowledge and skills needed to maintain an active lifestyle (Institute of Medicine, 2013; United States Department of Health and Human Services, 2012). Within the school setting, we can increase physical fitness levels and improve brain health by providing youth with enhanced physical education curriculums and ongoing instruction that support the adoption and maintenance of physical activity throughout the day (ParticipACTION, 2018; United States Department of Health and Human Services, 2012). Collectively, these findings highlight the importance of social support and effective teaching strategies that are specifically designed to enhance participants' skills and their knowledge of how and why they should be active.

During the growing years, the brain reinforces neural pathways that get sufficiently used and prunes those that are underused (Johnson, Blum, & Giedd, 2009; Saxena & Caroni, 2007). Therefore, growth and maturation provide a unique opportunity to positively influence the structural development of the brain through developmentally appropriate exercise interventions; on the other hand, prolonged periods of inactivity and excessive sedentary behavior (e.g., screen time) may lead to changes in neural structure and function that may limit motor-skill development which underlie sustainable participation in exercise and sport activities (Gogtay et al., 2004; Myer et al., 2015; Zhou et al., 2011). Consequently, youth fitness programs that integrate multiple components of fitness and stimulate cognitive processes may provide a mechanism to develop, reinforce, and expand dynamic neural pathways that enhance motor skill development and increase physical activity early in life. Promising interventions for preschoolers (age 3-5 yr) include those that increase outdoor time, provide access to portable play equipment (e.g., balls, hoops, tricycles), and offer staff training in how to deliver structured physical activity sessions (De Bock, Genser, Raat, Fischer, & Renz-Polster, 2013; Pate et al., 2016; Robinson, Palmer, Webster, Logan, & Chinn, 2018).

DO YOU KNOW?

About half of the neurons in a child's brain do not survive to adulthood.

Although training experience should be considered, **cognitive age** can be equally important when designing youth fitness programs or teaching complex exercises. Cognitive age is a measure of one's ability to manage intellectual processes that require attention, alertness, memory, comprehension, application, judgment, and problem solving (Kushner et al., 2015; Myer et al., 2013). Youth think differently than adults do, and a participant's cognitive age can influence the safety and efficacy of a youth fitness program. Is a child willing and able to accept and follow safety rules in the fitness center? Does a teenager understand what it means to perform a triple extension, wherein the body explosively extends at the ankles, knees, and hips? A child must have the intellectual capacity to comprehend instructions and listen to constructive

Teaching Tip

CONTINUUM OF PHYSICAL LITERACY

The construct of *physical literacy* refers not only to physical competence but also to the motivation, confidence, knowledge, and understanding needed in order to value and take responsibility for engagement in physical activities throughout the life course (Whitehead, 2010). That is, as youth enhance their physical literacy, they become more able and willing to participate in a variety of physical activities in a range of situations and contexts. From this perspective, the journey of physical literacy can be viewed as occurring on a continuum, and it may be influenced either positively or negatively by life experiences and interactions with others (Faigenbaum & Rial Rebullido, 2018). Because youth can both progress and regress along the continuum, youth fitness specialists should inspire participants to use their minds as well as their bodies when teaching new games or progressing exercise programs. Again, physical literacy is not just a physical trait but also a behavior that needs to be developed, maintained, and embraced throughout the life course. Qualified instruction and education provided by youth fitness specialists can produce a physically literate individual who is prepared for a physically active lifestyle.

feedback about the performance of a skill or adherence to program guidelines. For example, the American Academy of Pediatrics states that children under the age of four years are not developmentally ready for structured swim lessons because they may lack the cognitive and physical readiness to comprehend swim instructions and perform relatively complex tasks safely and efficiently (Weiss & American Academy of Pediatrics Committee on Injury, Violence, and Poison Prevention, 2010).

Clearly, then, youth fitness specialists need to consider the cognitive age of each child in order to deliver information in a manner that enables real learning to occur. Table 5.1 presents selected milestones associated with certain periods of cognitive development (Centers for Disease Control and Prevention, n.d.; Hagan, Shaw, & Duncan, 2008; Wilks, Gerber, & Erdie-Lalena, 2010). Note that these age ranges are only guidelines along a continuum of cognitive development.

A child's ability to focus and follow directions influences the learning process and the ultimate success of a program. Consequently, youth fitness specialists need to match the physical and mental demands of an exercise session with the cognitive age of the participants. It is unrealistic, for example, to expect children to comprehend the complexities of periodization, but youth should understand safety rules and why they are being asked to perform a particular exercise or activity at a given stage of their training. Exercise classes that consider participants' training experience and cognitive age are more likely to produce desired changes in attention, attitude, and performance. When participants are given meaningful instruction and adequate time to practice and reinforce exercises and skills in a supportive environment, they learn to organize a connected network of physical, cognitive, sensory, and emotional subsystems that evolve throughout childhood and adolescence (Handford, Davids, Bennett, & Button, 1997; Myer et al., 2013; Thelen, 1995); see figure 5.1. Over time, learned skills become automatic as the movements become more accurate, efficient, and seemingly effortless even with less instructional feedback. True learning takes place when participants become aware of their own mistakes and are able to make proper corrections.

DO YOU KNOW?

A child's cognitive age is affected by both genetic and environmental factors.

Effective Pedagogy

The process of properly learning a new skill or exercise depends on regular practice and reinforcement of the desired movement pattern. With qualified instruction and guidance, the desired pattern becomes "hardwired" into participants' movement vocabulary. For example, when children learn how to perform a walking lunge while moving a medicine ball in various directions, they are challenged to maintain proper body control throughout the full range of motion. As they perform these movements correctly, they learn how to control their body through a constant interplay between imbalance and balance. Experiencing competence through good performance can enhance the learning process as participants find optimal solutions to unanticipated events (Chiviacowsky, Wulf, & Lewthwaite, 2012). Providing meaningful feedback during the initial stages of learning a new exercise can maximize the integration of physical and cognitive networks that support the development of efficient movement patterns, as well as continued participation in exercise and sport programs that are challenging, engaging, and rewarding.

TABLE 5.1   MILESTONES ASSOCIATED WITH COGNITIVE DEVELOPMENT IN CHILDREN AND ADOLESCENTS

Age (yr)	Milestones
5-6	Begin to reason and ask why; know left and right; categorize objects; sound out words, such as *jump*, *hop*, and *kick*; follow simple instructions.
7-8	Understand concept of space; accept more responsibility and follow instructions; take turns and play cooperatively.
9-10	Think more independently; exhibit improved decision-making and organizational skills; enjoy group activities; exhibit longer attention span.
11-12	Increase capacity for learning and abstract thinking; exhibit improved problem-solving abilities; show growing interest in community; enjoy displaying skills and talents.
13-17	Exhibit willingness to understand and consider other perspectives; demonstrate growing capacity for abstract reasoning; exhibit heightened self-consciousness.

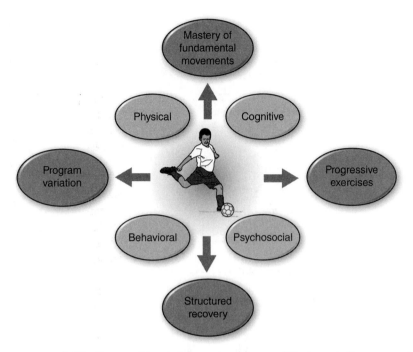

FIGURE 5.1   The cornerstone of effective teaching is instruction by a qualified youth fitness specialist who understands the influence of a participant's cognitive age and training age on physical literacy and performance.

Reproduced from *British Journal of Sports Medicine*, G.D. Myer, A.D. Faigenbaum, N.M. Edwards, et al., vol. 49, 1510-1516, 2015, with permission from BMJ Publishing Group Ltd.

Over time, similar or more advanced exercises and skills can be learned more efficiently with less instructional feedback because participants can build on pathways that exist from prior training. The instructional technique that connects past experiences to present actions is called **scaffolding**. As is done with physical scaffolding around a new building, youth fitness specialists can gradually remove instructional scaffolding when participants become aware of their own mistakes, self-correct training errors, and take increasing responsibility for their own learning. When an individual is learning a new exercise, the movements may initially appear constrained or feel awkward. As competence and confidence increase, each participant explores and discovers a new range of motion and a new level of neuromuscular control. During this phase of learning, the individual's ability to perform an exercise can be influenced both by visual and tactile feedback and by real-time feedback from youth fitness specialists who understand proper exercise technique and human kinetics.

Coaching Cues

As competence to perform an exercise or motor skill improves, a participant's attention begins to shift

---

Teaching Tip

APPROPRIATE TOUCH

Although the politics of touching youth participants during sport activities has affected the coaching experience, touch can still serve as a good teaching tool if used appropriately (Child Protection in Sport Unit, 2012; Heather, Garratt, & Taylor, 2013; Mesquita et al., 2015). For example, a gymnastics coach can physically support a child who is learning how to tumble properly, and a youth fitness specialist should spot the wrists of a young weightlifter who is unable to complete the last repetition of a dumbbell chest press. Physical contact in youth fitness and sport programs should always meet the needs of the child and should be used only to develop sport skills, treat an injury, prevent an injury, or meet the minimum requirements of the sport. Youth fitness specialists should receive guidance on appropriate touch for a range of sports and exercises and should use alternative pedagogical strategies when necessary.

TABLE 5.2   EXAMPLES OF VERBAL INSTRUCTIONS WITH AN INTERNAL FOCUS OR AN EXTERNAL FOCUS

Exercise	Instruction with internal focus	Instruction with external focus
Swimming	"Pull your hands back."	"Push water back."
Throwing	"Bend your wrist."	"Keep your eye on the target."
Vertical jump	"Jump as high as you can."	"Focus on reaching the rim."
Lunge	"Keep your front knee on top of your lead foot."	"Point your front knee toward a cone in front of you."
Sprint	"Extend your hips."	"Push the ground away."
Dumbbell curl	"Contract the biceps."	"Curl the weight."
Deadlift	"Don't round your back."	"Show me the logo on your shirt."

away from an **internal focus** (on the movement itself) and toward an **external focus** (on the outcome of the movement) (Benjaminse et al., 2015). Internal focus is invoked, for instance, by reminding a child to "keep your hips back" while learning how to perform the back squat, whereas external focus is invoked by asking the child to "imagine sitting in a chair." Although both types are meaningful, external focus in particular may enhance the learning process by helping the individual produce efficient movement patterns (Benjaminse et al., 2015; Kal, van der Kamp, & Houdijk, 2013; Wulf, Dufek, Lozano, & Pettigrew, 2010). If an individual focuses on a particular body movement during an exercise (i.e., asserts internal focus), then the movements may become less "automatic" (i.e., less efficient) as the person learns, for instance, to squat, jump, or sprint. Simple instructions work best, because complex directions can stifle motor learning and performance. Table 5.2 provides examples of verbal instructions with internal focus or with external focus.

When youth focus on an external object (e.g., a red line on a long-jump mat), they shift their attention away from their body, whereas internal instructions are directed toward their body (e.g., "jump as far as possible"). As a result, during the performance of the long-jump test, practitioners should mark every jump on the mat and encourage participants to jump farther

than the marked target. This type of feedback can improve skill performance and provide motivation that influences learning (Wulf, Shea, & Lewthwaite, 2010).

The learning process can be facilitated by both verbal and visual cues (Benjaminse et al., 2015; Valentini, 2004). Participants should observe a youth fitness specialist performing each exercise properly or watch a peer attempt a similar movement. Although watching a novice perform an exercise can highlight common errors and promote problem solving, watching an expert demonstrate an exercise correctly can enhance skill acquisition (Hodges & Franks, 2002; Laguna, 2008). Providing both visual cues and verbal instruction may offer the best approach for developing and retaining efficient movement patterns (Benjaminse et al., 2015; Janelle, Champenoy, Coombes, & Mousseau, 2003).

Listening and Learning

If participants do not listen to the instructor, they will not learn the desired exercise or game tactic. Consequently, participants need to pay attention and engage actively in the learning process. Certainly, there are times when youth fitness specialists need to provide direct instruction and guidance, but they should not overlook the importance of creating an environment

Teaching Tip

ACTIVE CUEING

Both visual demonstrations and verbal cueing can improve learning in the fitness center and in the sport venue. A visual demonstration can paint a picture of the proper movement pattern, and verbal cueing can guide the participant toward the desired outcome. As youth gain competence and confidence in their abilities to perform more complex exercises and skills, practitioners may be able to reduce instructional cueing as participants build on their experience and self-correct their movement errors. Youth fitness specialists should periodically refine visual demonstrations and verbal cueing to enhance the learning experience and, ultimately, the acquisition of desired movement patterns.

in which participants are engaged actively in learning (Fuller et al., 2015; Kibbe et al., 2011). Effective instructional strategies can increase activity time while still allowing needed opportunities to practice movement skills and learn complex exercises.

Most youth fitness specialists need to organize a group of participants in fitness classes or athletic programs. Although some may work one on one or in small groups, all practitioners who train youth in fitness centers or sport facilities need to be effective leaders who can help participants become aware of their weaknesses, mindful of their strengths, and engaged in the process of learning and discovery. The most effective youth fitness specialists are able to motivate youth in a manner that is consistent with the interests and abilities of each participant.

At the beginning of every lesson, participants need to understand what they will be doing and with whom. When youth fitness specialists clearly describe lesson objectives, equipment needs, and session format, participants know where the activity will take place, what they need in order to perform the activity, and when to start. It is also important to clearly define the boundaries in which the activity will take place and review safety guidelines. When working with a group of young children, it may be helpful to ask a child to demonstrate the desired actions. For example, after telling children to pick up two colored cones, ask one child to complete the task and move to the desired location. Another effective strategy involves **modeling** the desired behavior with visual cues so that participants can see what they should do, how they should do it, and where it should be done. Practitioners can also check for understanding by asking open-ended questions about the desired behavior to ensure that instructions have been heard and understood.

Mastery Motivational Climate

Youth fitness specialists should provide the required instruction for an activity or skill in a manner that

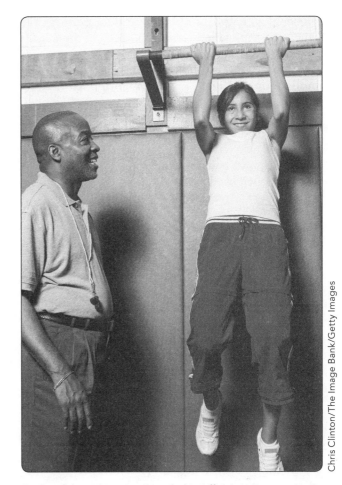

Chris Clinton/The Image Bank/Getty Images

Successful teaching is grounded in effective communication.

is positive, informative, and inspiring. Participants need to become partners in the learning process and feel good about what they are doing. They need to understand important concepts, learn new exercises, and practice sport skills with energy, interest, and enthusiasm in a mastery motivational climate (Ames, 1995; Haywood & Getchell, 2014; Parish & Treasure, 2003; Smith, Smoll, & Cumming, 2007). By focusing on

Teaching Tip

CHECK IN

In addition to using objective performance measures (e.g., heart rate, weight lifted), it can be helpful to ask youth how they feel before an exercise session begins. Subjective questions can provide useful information about health, motivation, training state, and personal issues. Moreover, asking youth to check in before an exercise session shows genuine interest in their well-being. In addition, by listening to individual feedback, youth fitness specialists can modify workouts to better develop physical qualities and enhance training outcomes. The long-term monitoring of stress and recovery may also help with early detection of excessive training, which is associated with decreased vigor, sore muscles, and performance decrements (Brink, Visscher, Coutts, & Lemmink, 2012; Saw, Main, & Gastin, 2016).

personal accomplishments rather than performance outcomes, less-skilled participants become more likely to work hard, show improvement, and stay engaged in the process of training and discovery. A mastery motivational climate provides an opportunity for youth to gain confidence and competence in their physical abilities as they learn new skills and experience success. Fostering a supportive environment in youth programs also reduces the likelihood of maladaptive responses and behaviors, including anxiety, stress, and burnout (Ommundsen, Roberts, Lemyre, & Miller, 2006; Roberts, Treasure, & Conroy, 2007).

The most successful youth fitness specialists find ways to create mastery motivational climates in which all participants—regardless of body size or physical ability—have an opportunity to participate in a variety of challenging activities, reflect on their performance, and develop confidence in their capacity to use learned skills. This approach to teaching and coaching can increase enjoyment, improve motor skills, and engage all participants in the learning process (Curran, Hill, Hall, & Jowett, 2015; Granero-Gallegos et al., 2017; Gutiérrez & Ruiz, 2009; Parish, Rudisill, & St Onge, 2007). Strategies for fostering a mastery motivational climate include teaching challenging skills, providing immediate feedback, rewarding effort, building confidence, and allowing participants to be part of the decision-making process (Collins et al., 2016; Epstein, 1989).

Creating a positive learning environment in which all participants can gain competence and confidence in their physical abilities is an important objective for youth fitness specialists. In this type of environment, participants are more likely to develop good sporting behavior, believe that success is related to effort, and generate high levels of **intrinsic motivation** because they are stimulated to participate and to improve their performance (Boixados, Cruz, Torregrosa, & Valiente, 2004; Treasure, 2001). Intrinsically motivating activities are characterized by challenge, curiosity, control, and creativity (National Association for Sport and Physical Education, 2011). In contrast, **extrinsic motivation** occurs when participants play a game or sport in order to win, say, an award or scholarship. Youth who are intrinsically motivated to participate accept responsibility for their own behavior and take a genuine interest in participating, learning, and improving.

There appears to be a motivational continuum for participation in sport (Vallerand & Losier, 1999), and excessive use of external rewards can weaken intrinsic motivation and lead to dependence on other factors to make participation habitual (Deci, Koestner, & Ryan, 1999; National Association for Sport and Physical Education, 2011). Although external rewards (e.g., certificates, trophies, praise from a parent or coach) can generate interest and serve as markers of achievement, the extent to which a child's participation is self-determined influences the child's quality of experience and interest in the activity. If a child gets an ice cream cone after every practice, or if a young athlete receives enthusiastic praise after every play (regardless of physical effort or skill proficiency), then the internal desire to participate with energy and enthusiasm begins to wane. Consequently, youth fitness specialists should create an environment in which external rewards are appreciated but internal rewards are prized. Fostering intrinsic motivation results in the best outcomes in children and adolescents who need to learn that effort and desire enhance performance (Jonsson, Berg, Larsson, Korp, & Lindgren, 2017; Karageorghis & Terry, 2011).

Instructional Strategies

Youth enjoy participating in challenging games and skill-building activities as they attempt to solve problems and overcome perceived barriers (Collins et al., 2016). When participants learn how to perform skills and exercises properly, they gain confidence in their physical abilities and are likely to take responsibility for

Teaching Tip

INSTANT ACTIVITY

Most youth come to exercise and sport programs ready to move (Graham, 2008). Therefore, instead of starting each session with a prolonged period of inactivity (which can be boring), we can use the first few minutes of an exercise class or sport practice to set the desired tone and tempo for the upcoming lesson. Instant activity can reduce discipline problems, encourage socialization, and reinforce desired movement patterns. Following dynamic warm-up activities, clearly and succinctly explain the purpose of the lesson; this explanation should stimulate interest in the class or practice session. Describe the exercises or activities that will be performed and outline a progression of tasks that should be accomplished in the session. In some cases, it may be appropriate to list the desired outcomes on a board or provide each participant with a card outlining the day's workout.

their actions. In turn, they are motivated to create new games, novel exercises, and original dance sequences.

At the same time, it can be challenging for youth fitness specialists to accomplish desired goals in a given period of time. For instance, it is unrealistic to expect a group of seven-year-olds to throw a ball with a mature pattern after one lesson or for adolescent athletes to master proper technique for a single-leg hop in 10 minutes. Even so, key components of these skills (i.e., learnable tasks) can be handled during each session as participants begin to learn how to move their body as a unit instead of as separate parts.

The following instructional strategies have proven to be effective when teaching exercise and sport to children and adolescents (Graham, Holt/Hale, & Parker, 2013; Martens, 2004).

Short and Simple

This guideline is commonly known as the KISS principle, for "keep it short and simple." If participants are given too much information, they simply won't remember everything. Therefore, youth fitness specialists should present one idea or concept at a time, so that participants can begin to perform the desired task correctly. Although a lesson may include information from previous sessions, the idea is to focus participants' attention on one skill or movement at a time and then progress based on observations and performance. For example, when instructing youth on proper technique for the squat jump, teach them to jump straight up while reaching as high overhead as possible. Encourage them to land softly on the same spot on the floor, while maintaining an upright posture. Finally, remind them to point their feet and knees forward and keep their arms to the outside of their legs. Presenting information in small, learnable nuggets throughout the lesson is far more effective than giving a 10-minute lecture on the biomechanics of the squat jump at the start of the practice session.

Show-and-Tell

Clear instructions supported by meaningful demonstrations form an effective instructional strategy. Although show-and-tell was originally designed to provide young children with a forum for speaking in class, it can also be used to demonstrate an exercise correctly while emphasizing a body part or muscle action that participants need to observe. This type of instruction is most effective for beginners, participants who are visual learners, and those who are not native speakers of the practitioner's language. To be most effective, stand in a location that all the participants can see, then demonstrate the entire exercise or skill so that participants can grasp the complete picture. Supplement demonstrations with a small number of verbal cues so that participants know exactly what to focus on as they watch the performance.

Spot Check

After explaining and demonstrating the exercise or skill, assess participants' comprehension of it to ensure that they are able to perform it correctly. Various techniques can be used, based on cognitive age, available time, and lesson content. Whatever option is chosen, a quick performance check can help determine what participants understand and what they can do; for example, ask them to demonstrate proper starting position for a push-up. When appropriate, check for understanding by asking relevant questions about the exercise or activity: Where should you place your hands on the barbell when performing the bench press? How should you move your arms when you jump? What are the safety rules in the fitness center? Such questions allow participants to explain in their own words what they know and why it matters.

Teaching Tip

TECHNOLOGY BYTES

Although technology is not essential for effective instruction, advances in electronic devices and associated software can help professionals teach exercises and sport skills. For instance, video analysis software (e.g., Coach's Eye, Ubersense, Dartfish) allows youth fitness specialists to record performance in the fitness center or sport facility and provide immediate feedback during practice or game situations. In particular, slow-motion playback and side-by-side comparisons may be valuable for teaching complex exercises or highlighting errors in sport skills that are performed at very high speeds. However, even if these programs enhance the learning experience for children and adolescents, they should not be viewed as substitutes for effective teaching by practitioners. We still need to develop the observational and auditory skills that are necessary to assess and monitor performance. Youth fitness specialists need to observe carefully and listen intently in order to identify subtle changes in performance, motivation, and behavior.

DO YOU KNOW?

Visual displays can promote retention of learning while providing a needed opportunity for children to understand what they should be learning.

Managing Behavior

Youth fitness specialists are commonly concerned about their ability to keep youth on task and engaged in the learning process. Unsurprisingly, the more

Keeping Your Practice Organized

The most effective youth fitness specialists organize practice sessions with clear objectives that are consistent with individual needs, abilities, and interests. Without a well-designed lesson plan, participants may be physically active yet still unengaged as learners. Although some practitioners do not start thinking about what they will do until practice begins, youth fitness specialists who are genuinely committed to learning and discovery devote considerable time to reviewing relevant material, talking with colleagues, and preparing

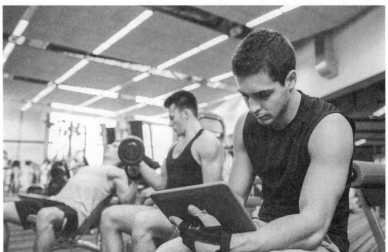

A workout log is a teaching tool that can help track progress and improve performance.

lessons that meet the needs and abilities of their participants. Such planning is particularly important due to the limited time available to most youth fitness specialists.

Given that most youth enjoy age-related games and sports, some practitioners may be tempted to avoid careful planning simply because participants prefer the sheer experience of moving. Unlike physical education teachers, most youth fitness specialists are not required to develop formal lesson plans, even though careful planning provides purpose and direction for both exercise programs and sport practices. However, notwithstanding the benefits of unstructured free play, structured exercise classes and sport practices both require thoughtful planning. Ideally, lesson plans outline both what participants should learn today and what they should be able to do when they leave the program (Graham, 2008). Although long-term (yearly) planning has traditionally been associated with sport development, a systematic approach to exercise training is important for all youth, regardless of athletic prowess (Haff, 2014; Lloyd et al., 2016).

Without a plan in place, youth fitness specialists may be inclined to view "activity time" as a marker of success, when in fact success should also be based on skill development, fitness achievement, and knowledge of behaviors that support a physically literate lifestyle. Moreover, practitioners who do not follow a predetermined lesson plan are more likely to spend time on less important topics and engage in unfocused discussions on irrelevant subjects that do not contribute to meeting desired objectives. Although all practitioners need to make adjustments when participants are struggling to learn a new skill or perform a complex exercise, it is also important to follow a plan in order to achieve desired outcomes. Planning provides an opportunity for youth fitness specialists to sensibly progress or modify exercises or activities based on each participant's attitude, affect, and skill level. For instance, providing each participant with a workout card and posting exercise guidelines in the activity space gives participants an idea of what they are learning and how they should follow the exercise program.

EXPECT THE UNEXPECTED

Youth fitness specialists should be prepared for unexpected events. Schedule changes, weather conditions, staffing issues, and variations in equipment availability can all exert an immediate effect on the safety and implementation of youth programs. For this reason, it is advisable to make a contingency plan laying out actions to be taken in order to ensure the safety of all participants while continuing the operations of the program. Contingency planning involves preparing for circumstances that might affect participant well-being or lesson design. For example, what steps should be taken if a child suffers an injury during an exercise class, or if the gymnasium is closed for a special event? Youth fitness specialists should identify major contingency events and be prepared with plans and strategies that serve the best interests of participants.

time children spend on task, the more time they spend actively involved in instructional activities with energy and interest. The most successful youth fitness specialists are able to keep the group alert and engaged by capturing their attention, maintaining it throughout the lesson, and refocusing it when it wanders off. Practitioners are more likely to keep all participants engaged in desired activities with energy and interest when they recognize that the learning process is a journey that takes time, patience, and a genuine understanding of developmentally appropriate pedagogical strategies. This is where the art of designing youth programs comes into play, because the physical demands of training must be balanced with appropriate strategies to effectively manage the attitudes and behaviors of all participants.

Even seasoned youth fitness specialists have to manage "off-task" behaviors, such as failing to follow instructions, seeking attention, interrupting, or just acting lazy. The reality is that most programs have a few participants who will disrupt class or training. In some cases, practitioners may need to review the lesson plan to see if off-task behavior is being invited by activities that are either too easy or too hard. If an exercise or game is too challenging for beginners, they will not have the skill level to succeed; conversely, simple exercises and activities are likely to bore trained youth. The key is to engage all participants with exercises, activities, and games that strike a balance between current skill level and challenge. However, even with well-designed classes and practice sessions, some youth may tend to engage repeatedly in off-task behavior due to personal issues. To help them become active participants, provide them with support and gentle encouragement (Graham, 2008).

There is no single strategy that will minimize off-task behavior in all youth. Therefore, youth fitness specialists need a variety of strategies that can be used in different situations. The most successful

practitioners proactively manage off-task behavior and seem to stop it before it gets out of control. These professionals become aware of such behavior as they teach and are able to minimize distractions while continuing to control the situation and keep participants focused on the task at hand. Effective management is not just about enforcing rules but also about liking participants and helping them understand what is expected of them in the program. Show genuine interest in participants, be fair, avoid unnecessary threats, and stay alert to what is happening in the exercise or activity area.

To help with managing or even preventing off-task behavior, the following paragraphs summarize a few proven strategies: back to the wall, proximity control, positive pinpointing, and active voice (Graham, 2008; Martens, 2004).

Back to the Wall

At any given time, youth fitness specialists should be able to see most if not all participants. If you stand with your back to the wall of the gymnasium or on the edge of the playing field, you will be able to see the participants and identify off-task behavior as soon as it begins. This awareness will likely prevent other participants from engaging in unwanted behavior. In contrast, if a practitioner stands in the middle of the gym or field, then only about half of the participants can be seen at once.

Proximity Control

While observing all participants, youth fitness specialists should move about the exercise area or playing field to enable proximity control. In this strategy, the practitioner simply walks in the direction of participants who are engaging in off-task behavior. By letting them know that their unwanted behavior has been noticed, the practitioner can prevent the situation from getting worse.

Positive Pinpointing

Though it is important to identify off-task behavior, youth fitness specialists should also recognize participants who consistently engage in positive behavior. Youth who model appropriate behavior and properly perform desired skills or exercises should be identified, or pinpointed, by the practitioner in front of other participants. To facilitate this strategy, it is useful to learn the names of all participants in the program.

Active Voice

Youth fitness specialists can use the tone, tempo, and magnitude of their words to send a message to participants. In some situations, silence may be appropriate to get the class's attention, but in other circumstances—for instance, if participants engage in risky or off-task behavior—then it may be best to deliver a forceful message. The style in which a message is delivered, along with the accompanying facial expressions and body language, influence how the message will be perceived by participants.

DO YOU KNOW?

The majority of communication is conveyed through nonverbal actions and expressions.

Direct Learning

The success of any youth fitness program depends on the leadership provided by the instructors, who should be knowledgeable about effective teaching and learning strategies. The exercise program will be less effective if too much emphasis is placed on exercise prescription and not enough on quality of instruction. The primary leaders in a youth program are the youth fitness specialists, and every decision they make can influence participants' training outcomes and psychosocial well-being (Oliver, Lloyd, & Meyers, 2011;

Weiss, 2011). Although program design and amount of instruction may differ between children and adolescents, all decisions should be made to enhance the learning process and help participants feel as though they are part of something special.

There are many models of effective teaching. One approach is the direct instruction model, which requires explanations, demonstrations, and practice sessions (Metzler, 2005) and is characterized by meaningful interactions between participants and qualified practitioners. More specifically, this model requires youth fitness professionals to explain procedures, demonstrate techniques, assess performance, correct mistakes, and provide individual and group feedback (see figure 5.2). The most successful youth fitness specialists assess performance and then progress or

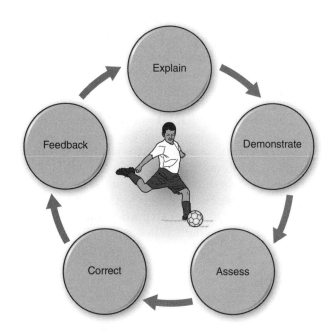

FIGURE 5.2   The direct instruction model is an engaging approach to teaching that requires meaningful interaction between instructor and participants.

Teaching Tip

STAY ON TASK

The most effective youth fitness specialists keep all participants on task and engaged in desired behaviors for the entire session. They capture the attention of all participants and use effective strategies to maintain interest and engagement. With a proactive strategy designed to keep participants on task, practitioners can increase the amount of time participants spend on physical activity and decrease the amount of time they spend on disruptive behavior. Practitioners should address participants by name, recognize good behavior, move around the exercise area, and allow children to serve as helpers. When practitioners partner with participants, they can establish a caring community in which all youth stay on task because they want to be part of a team.

regress each participant's program based on skill level, performance, behavior, and attitude.

Given the need to provide clear instructions, informative demonstrations, and direct feedback during every lesson, practitioners should know how to manage a group of participants, organize a lesson, and provide exemplary instruction (Tomporowski, McCullick, & Horvat, 2011). Practitioners must also attend to sex-related differences and the effect of instructor feedback on effort and performance. For example, in order to improve attitudes toward exercise in girls, youth fitness specialists should praise good effort, offer nonverbal support, and spend adequate time with the girls when providing feedback (Nicaise, Bois, Fairclough, Amorose, & Cogérino, 2007). Adults who do not have academic training and experience in youth fitness may be less able to create an instructional environment in which learning is engaging, enjoyable, and long-lasting for all participants. Practitioners can also enhance the learning experience, both for participants and for themselves, by engaging in ongoing assessment of and personal reflection about the planning and delivery of their programming.

Youth Coach's Dozen

Effective pedagogy lies at the heart of any successful youth program. Although knowledge of pediatric exercise science and developmental psychology remain necessary as prerequisites for effective teaching, youth fitness specialists ultimately need to design and implement instructional methods that enhance the process of learning and discovery. Research has enhanced our understanding of effective instructional practices in the classroom, but it is up to us to adapt these fundamental principles to the practice of pediatric exercise science. We can find a useful framework for discussing the characteristics of successful exercise and sport professionals in the 5 Cs perspective on positive youth development—namely, competence,

confidence, connection, character, and caring (Jones, Dunn, Holt, Sullivan, & Bloom, 2011; Lerner et al., 2005).

The coach's dozen is a list of 12 principles that youth fitness professionals should consider when teaching children and adolescents (Faigenbaum & Meadors, 2016). Some of these principles are well supported by research (Ames, 1995; Bulger, Mohr, & Walls, 2002; Schickedanz, Schickedanz, Forsyth, & Forsyth, 2000), whereas others are based on practical experience in working with school-age youth in schools, fitness centers, and sport programs. The list is not meant to be definitive or comprehensive; rather, it is a collection of principles to help youth fitness specialists promote learning through safe, effective, and enjoyable instructional methods.

1. Ensure a safe exercise environment.

The exercise area must be spacious, uncluttered, well ventilated, and well lit. Exercise equipment should be in good working order and appropriate for the smaller body size of children and adolescents; participants should not use broken or malfunctioning equipment. Loose equipment such as dumbbells, weight plates, and medicine balls should be stored in proper locations. Participants should dress appropriately for the session, and practitioners should periodically review safety rules.

2. Stay connected.

The success of any exercise class or sport program depends largely on the leadership provided by instructors and coaches, who should stay connected to the participants in the program. Take the time to learn every child's name, address individual concerns, and show genuine interest in every participant. A child who makes friends, plays fair, and feels connected to the instructor or coach cannot at the same time be a child who routinely disrupts the program or engages in negative behavior. Encourage participants to ask questions; never use sarcasm.

Teaching Tip

TEACHING BOYS AND GIRLS

Although both boys and girls can benefit from regular participation in well-designed fitness programs, their thoughts and feelings during exercise classes may differ. Therefore, teaching styles that enhance performance in boys may be suboptimal for girls, or vice versa. For some girls, the social and emotional aspects of training may be just as important as the physical skills (Barr-Anderson et al., 2008; Robbins, Wen & Ling, 2019). Accordingly, practitioners should realize that establishing trust with participants in a supportive environment can affect what they think and how they react. In addition, although coeducational exercise classes are beneficial, it may sometimes be appropriate to offer different classes for less-fit teenage boys and girls in order to reduce negative feelings and optimize adaptations.

Just like substitute teachers in the classroom, substitute coaches who do not form partnerships with participants will have a very difficult time teaching youth and inspiring them to achieve personal goals. The best approach is for professionals to develop a positive rapport with participants and show that they care.

3. Be enthusiastic.

Youth fitness specialists should be positive and passionate about exercise, fitness, and sport. If coaches are not enthusiastic about teaching, then children will not be enthusiastic about learning. Enthusiasm is contagious and contributes to a positive learning environment. In turn, a positive learning environment contributes to participants' success, which is a powerful motivator for engaging in the desired activities with energy and vigor. Inspiring practitioners generally possess content knowledge, instructional experience, and genuine interest in helping all participants perform to the best of their abilities.

4. Foster creativity.

Youth exercise programs should be both stimulating and engaging while providing an opportunity for participants to develop a positive sense of self. Creativity is associated with physical fitness in children (Latorre Román, Pinillos, Pantoja Vallejo, & Berrios Aguayo, 2017), and efforts to encourage creativity are needed in order to reclaim opportunities for children and adolescents to use their imagination, collaborate with peers, and release their creative energy. Sadly, creative thinking appears to be declining in children (Kim, 2011), which is all the more reason that participants should be given opportunities to create new games and exercises that are safe, stimulating, and fun. Notwithstanding the importance of education and instruction, the creation of new games and exercises contributes to a mastery-oriented climate in which participants control the type of task engagement and overcome self-determined challenges as they apply learned skills in novel situations. For example, participants might create a new exercise with medicine balls or modify a game of tag that requires speed and agility. This type of instruction can enhance the learning experience and promote physical engagement during exercise classes and sport programs.

5. Understand the process.

In addition to teaching participants about the quantitative aspects of the program (e.g., sets, repetitions, training intensity), youth fitness specialists should also engage participants in activities that are both physically and mentally challenging (Collins et al., 2016). That is to say, both the quantitative and the qualitative aspects of the movement experience should be considered when implementing and evaluating youth programs (Faigenbaum & Rial, 2018; Pesce, Faigenbaum, Goudas, & Tomporowski, 2018). Highly effective youth fitness specialists use instructional strategies that engage participants repeatedly throughout the practice session. When participants do something right, the practitioner should praise them; and if they do something wrong, the practitioner should help them understand that they are still liked as a person. The most important motives for youth are to demonstrate physical competence, gain social acceptance, and have fun.

6. Deliver clear instructions.

Successful youth fitness specialists are good listeners and exceptional communicators who understand individual needs and learning styles. In order to teach effectively, practitioners need to be concerned with how they deliver content to participants and how the participants react to that delivery. To help explain an exercise or game, a practitioner can use aids such as analogies, demonstrations, and coaching cues. The practitioner's tone, pronunciation, and choice of words can also influence participants' ability to understand lesson content. In some cases, it may be helpful to provide participants with an agenda for the activity period. Combining instructions with clear demonstrations and an organized lesson plan will likely yield the highest physical, cognitive, and affective benefits for participants (Tomporowski et al., 2011).

7. Diversify the portfolio.

The most stimulating youth programs encompass a variety of skills and activities that are developmentally appropriate, challenging, and fun. The outcome of a youth exercise program is determined by systematic and sensible progression of program variables over time, along with enthusiastic instruction. Most children find prolonged periods of monotonous aerobic exercise to be boring. Instead, youth should be exposed to an assortment of exercises and sport activities in a variety of settings with different people so that they can discover what they enjoy while maximizing their physical, psychological, and social development (Lloyd et al., 2014; Pesce et al., 2018).

8. Learn from mistakes.

Youth will inevitably make mistakes when they learn a new exercise or perform a complex skill.

Instead of being viewed in a negative light, mistakes should be recognized as valuable parts of the learning process that provide opportunities for participants to become aware of what they know and what they need to improve. When participants correct their own mistakes or offer constructive feedback to a peer, they become engaged learners who are able to think for themselves. Consequently, instead of merely recognizing the strongest participants, or those who perform a complex movement correctly, practitioners should also acknowledge participants who learn from their mistakes, ask for advice, and offer meaningful assistance to others. Collaborative learning provides an opportunity for youth fitness specialists and participants alike to share ideas, learn from each other, and work toward a common goal. This type of engagement can facilitate the acquisition of the necessary knowledge and skills to achieve long-term objectives.

9. Be patient.

Although it may be tempting to look for quick fixes and rapidly advance youth through exercise protocols, sustained participation in exercise and sport is built on a solid foundation of general preparation (Haff, 2014; Lloyd et al., 2016). Therefore, youth fitness specialists need to be patient in their practice so that participants have time to develop basic movement patterns before progressing to more complex skills and advanced training techniques. Practitioners should also recognize individual differences and realize that progression or regression should be based on skill proficiency, disposition, and understanding of training principles. Patience is needed in order to correct technical errors and develop physical skills that properly prepare youth for the enduring demands of exercise and sport. In contrast, an impatient approach to teaching and training increases the risk of injury and limits participants' long-term potential.

10. Maximize recovery.

Designing programs for youth of any age involves balancing the demands of training (required for adaptation) with the need for recovery (also required for adaptation) (Lloyd et al., 2016). Although any practitioner can make a child tired, successful youth fitness specialists understand and value the importance of developing high-quality movement patterns and enhancing the learning experience through less intense training sessions and appropriate recovery strategies. A training and recovery schedule that is well planned and well balanced improves participants' learning and the program's overall effectiveness. Practitioners need to attend to what is done between sessions as well as what is done during them. The importance of adequate recovery needs to be reinforced regularly because a "more is better" attitude is counterproductive. Related factors such as adequate hydration, proper nutrition, and sufficient sleep also promote well-being, which in turn enhances learning and on-task behavior during exercise sessions and sport practices (Oliver et al., 2011).

11. Think long-term.

Physical activity is a learned behavior; therefore, children and adolescents should be given ongoing opportunities to participate in exercise and sport programs. Without a long-term approach to physical development, boys and girls are less likely to reach their performance potential (Lloyd et al., 2016). Although some practitioners may want immediate results and quick-fix solutions to problems they encounter, a long-term approach is needed in order to optimize training adaptations and enhance the holistic development of all youth (Oliver et al., 2011). If the health-enhancing benefits of daily physical activity early in life are to be realized later in life, youth fitness specialists must know when to progress an activity and how to modify or even regress an exercise due to poor technique or inappropriate behavior. When practitioners help participants connect new information with what they already know, they encourage participants to think long-term about their education and training.

12. Enjoy the game.

The importance of having fun should not be underestimated when engaging youth in fitness, sport, and clinical exercise programs (Dishman et al., 2005; Visek et al., 2015; Watson, Baker, & Chadwick, 2016). When participants see others having fun and learning new skills, they are more likely to participate and become or remain engaged learners. Although encouragement and support from youth fitness specialists can influence exercise habits, the sheer enjoyment that a child experiences during an exercise session can facilitate sustainment of desired behaviors. In this vein, it is sometimes helpful for practitioners to remember what types of fitness activities they enjoyed as children. The most successful professionals maintain a balance between skill and challenge so that exercises and sport activities remain enjoyable. Participants who become proficient and perceive themselves as skilled are more likely to respond to effective teaching with a higher level of engagement and enjoyment.

DO YOU KNOW?

The best youth fitness specialists are often those who understand that each child is unique and learns in a distinctive way.

Summary

It is not enough merely to be a youth fitness specialist with exceptional motor skills, good intentions, and a desire to work with children and adolescents. To help youth become the best they can be, practitioners must also gain field experience, network with successful colleagues, and adapt training sessions to each individual's chronological age, developmental age, and training age. Effective teaching strategies help participants acquire new skills and physical abilities as they learn to organize physical, cognitive, sensory, and emotional subsystems and their movement patterns become more efficient. Without qualified instruction, youth are less likely to master desired movements and more likely to drop out. But with qualified instruction, they are more likely to engage in the learning process as they socialize with others, gain confidence in their abilities, and become skilled movers.

Effective pedagogy lays the foundation for long-term physical development. If participants are not actively engaged in the learning process, they will not learn the desired movement skills or exercises with energy and interest. The most successful youth fitness specialists are themselves lifelong learners who are willing to try new instructional methods and learn from others in the field. They explain procedures, demonstrate techniques, assess performance, correct mistakes, minimize off-task behaviors, and provide direct feedback during every class. Although research on coaching effectiveness continues to enhance our understanding of effective pedagogical practices, we must also prioritize interacting positively, communicating effectively, managing efficiently, and taking time to reflect on our own practice.

PART II

YOUTH FITNESS DEVELOPMENT

CHAPTER 6

Assessing
Youth Fitness

CHAPTER OBJECTIVES

- Discuss the potential advantages and disadvantages of assessing youth fitness
- Identify ways to make fitness assessment a positive and worthwhile experience for youth
- Evaluate the options for assessing movement skill competence
- Evaluate test batteries for assessing physical fitness
- Evaluate the options for assessing physical activity

KEY TERMS

construct validity (p. 109)

content validity (p. 109)

criterion validity (p. 109)

discriminative validity (p. 119)

ecological validity (p. 119)

ego orientation (p. 108)

goal orientation (p. 108)

health-related fitness (p. 104)

indirect calorimetry (p. 123)

peak oxygen uptake (p. 105)

physical fitness (p. 104)

reliability (p. 105)

skill-related fitness (p. 104)

task orientation (p. 108)

Introduction

Physical fitness, defined as a set of attributes that individuals either have or achieve, can be subdivided into two types: skill-related and health-related (Caspersen et al., 1985). **Skill-related fitness** is often associated with qualities of athleticism, such as speed, power, agility, coordination, and balance. **Health-related fitness**, as the name indicates, is associated with health, or health risk, and more specifically with qualities such as cardiorespiratory, muscular, and metabolic health (Institute of Medicine, 2012). As a result, skill-related and health-related fitness are often referred to as independent qualities, but they are not completely separate. For instance, cardiorespiratory fitness and muscular strength are each associated with both athleticism and health in youth. Practitioners can help youth develop skill- and health-related fitness by providing a varied exercise program—for instance combining elements of resistance training, vigorous exercise, dynamic stability, plyometric activities, agility exercises, and core exercises.

Fitness assessment of youth is not a new concept, and it is worth considering the history that has shaped current opinion and practice. Kraus and Hirschland (1954) first popularized the use of standardized, skill-related fitness test scores by providing markers of "minimal muscular fitness in children." The authors showed that only 9 percent of European children fell behind these standards, as compared with 58 percent of U.S. children. Shortly after that report was published, President Dwight D. Eisenhower established the President's Council on Youth Fitness, which required regular fitness testing of U.S. schoolchildren. Increasing the fitness of children was viewed as a key objective for ensuring the military preparedness of the young American population; in fact, President John F. Kennedy (1960) stated that lack of physical fitness was "a menace to security."

These events created an approach in which fitness testing was used to provide extrinsic motivation for children to become fit. For instance, the Presidential Youth Fitness Award honored those who scored at or above the 85th percentile on all of the tests, although very few youth met that standard (Pate et al., 2013). In addition, the focus on using normative comparisons for fitness test performance has been viewed as possibly contributing to negative characterizations of fitness testing in schools (Wiersma & Sherman, 2008), as well as creating demeaning and embarrassing experiences for many children (Rowland, 1995).

DO YOU KNOW?

The majority of U.S. states require schools to assess students' fitness levels (Society of Health and Physical Educators, 2016).

From the 1980s onward, opposition to performance-based testing of motor skills prompted a move toward assessment of health-related physical fitness (Pate et al., 2013). This effort shifted the emphasis from standardized testing of athletic attributes to assessing markers of fitness believed to be related to health. In the early 1980s in the United States, the Cooper Institute developed the FitnessGram battery and the notion of "healthy fitness zones" (Plowman et al., 2013). Simultaneously, other test batteries were developed around the world to measure common components of health-related fitness, and many of them included the same or similar tests (Safrit, 1990).

In the mid-1980s and early 1990s, the United States, Canada, Australia, and the United Kingdom all published large-scale national surveys of children's fitness, although they focused more on reporting physical activity than on fitness itself (Harris & Cale, 2006). The focus on physical activity and related behaviors derived from debate about which was more important—physical fitness or physical activity. Although that debate continues today, recent evidence has shown that both physical activity and physical fitness are independently associated with metabolic health in children (Ekelund et al., 2007; Gomes et al., 2016). It has also been suggested that being unfit confers greater health risks than does being fat in children and adolescents (Donaldson, 2010).

The evidence that physical activity and physical fitness both relate to childhood health has been used to argue for fitness assessment of children with the caveat that practitioners should not monitor fitness in isolation (Lloyd et al., 2010). Indeed, mounting evidence suggests that physical fitness, physical activity, fundamental motor skills, and knowledge are interrelated and that each element should be considered during any assessment (Lloyd et al., 2010). This understanding has led to the development of contemporary assessment tools that combine the measurement of interlinked variables associated with positive health and lifelong participation in physical activity.

Whereas fitness assessment focuses solely on physical qualities, physical literacy considers both physical competence and the motivation, confidence, and knowledge that are needed in order to take part in physical activity (Whitehead, 2016). To provide a more holistic approach, the Canadian Assessment of Physical Literacy (CAPL, 2017; Francis et al., 2016) assesses daily behavior, knowledge and understanding, motivation and confidence, and physical competence (see figure 6.1). Physical competence includes physical fitness and motor skill proficiency. Similarly, the recently developed Australian Physical Literacy Standard includes domains for the physical, psychological, social, and cognitive aspects, though

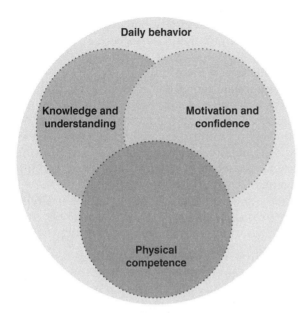

FIGURE 6.1   The four overlapping domains of assessment in the Canadian Assessment of Physical Literacy.

Reprinted by permission from C.E. Francis, P.E. Longmuir, C. Boyer, et al., "The Canadian Assessment of Physical Literacy: Development of a Model of Children's Capacity for a Healthy, Active Lifestyle Through a Delphi Process," *Journal of Physical Activity and Health* 13, no. 2 (2016): 214-222.

it currently uses quite subjective assessment criteria (Australian Sports Commission, 2018). These contemporary models recognize the need for youth fitness specialists to consider the multidimensional nature of fitness and its assessment in children and adolescents.

For any assessment to be worthwhile, the **reliability** and validity of its tests must be confirmed. Moreover, protocols that are routinely applied to adults cannot

be assumed to be appropriate for youth. Fortunately, contemporary research has established the reliability and validity of tests for movement competence and health-related fitness in children and adolescents (Castro-Piñero et al., 2010; Ortega et al., 2015; Ruiz et al., 2011; Williams et al., 2009). However, even when using appropriate assessment tools, considerable challenges remain in terms of creating a positive test environment that motivates children. In addition, meaningful interpretation of test scores can be problematic because relative age, growth, and maturation are all likely to influence performance throughout childhood and adolescence (see chapter 3). Thus, although fitness assessment may offer many benefits, youth fitness specialists must carefully consider what to assess, how to assess it, and how to use the information collected—all while ensuring that the entire process is a positive experience for each child.

To Test or Not to Test?

In schools around the world, there is little or no debate about the importance of assessing and evaluating in the cognitive domains (e.g., literacy, numeracy); however, assessment in physical education continues to be a contentious topic (Lloyd et al., 2010). It has been suggested that in order for physical literacy to achieve the same prominence as literacy and numeracy in the curriculum, it must be measured in order to improve standards (Lloyd & Tremblay, 2010). This viewpoint has been strongly opposed by others, who suggest that fitness assessment in children and adolescents will not improve health or lifelong engagement in physical activity (Cale et al., 2007; Naughton et al., 2006; Rowland, 1995). Although the debate has continued for many decades, it has done little to influence the

---

Teaching Tip

RELIABILITY AND VALIDITY OF FITNESS ASSESSMENT

Reliability refers to the consistency of a test. If a test is not reliable, then the practitioner cannot be confident that the results are accurate. Happily, many tests across many components of fitness have been shown to be reliable in children and adolescents. Validity, on the other hand, refers to the degree to which a test measures what it is supposed to measure. Thus, tests of health-related fitness should relate to underlying qualities of health, and field-based tests that estimate fitness qualities should be well related to robust criterion measures. For example, a direct measurement of **peak oxygen uptake** is considered a gold standard measure of cardiorespiratory fitness, but it requires access to laboratory equipment. Field-based tests, on the other hand, may be more accessible, and estimated cardiorespiratory fitness from a shuttle run test is well related to peak oxygen uptake; in turn, both of these measures have been shown to be associated with markers of cardiovascular health in youth (Castro-Piñero et al., 2010, Ruiz et al., 2016). To reiterate, in order for fitness assessment to be worthwhile, youth fitness specialists must select tests that are both reliable and valid for pediatric populations.

popularity of fitness testing in U.S. schools (Pate et al., 2013) or to change the global trend of increasing childhood and adolescent obesity (Ng et al., 2014).

Before using fitness assessment, youth fitness specialists must consider the purpose of assessment. Suggested reasons for assessing the fitness of children and adolescents include program and curriculum evaluation, motivation, identification of children in need of improvement, identification of individual fitness needs for exercise prescription and improvement, promotion of physical activity, goal setting, development of self-monitoring and self-testing skills, and cognitive and emotional learning (Harris & Cale, 2006). As this list makes clear, fitness assessment of youth is concerned not only with physical fitness outcomes but also with educational and psychosocial benefits.

DO YOU KNOW?

It can be useful to assess physical fitness, physical activity, and screen time—each of which is independently associated with level of health in children (Ekelund, Anderssen, et al., 2007; Ekelund, Brage, et al., 2006).

Consistent criticism has been directed at youth fitness testing for purportedly failing to achieve the stated purposes of assessment. In a seminal article, Rowland (1995) declared that if the (then) current understanding of the health–exercise link meant that exercise testing in schools was pointless, then the practice should be stopped. This position was based on the suggestion that the best preventive health strategy is not to increase cardiorespiratory fitness but to improve activity habits. However, the assumption that increased physical activity results in increased fitness has been called into question by suggestions that the relationship between these variables can be low in children (Harris & Cale, 2006). Indeed, the health outcome of fitness is influenced not only by physical activity but also by many other factors, such as oppor-

tunity for physical activity, heredity, maturation, age, nutrition, environment, socioeconomic status, and responsiveness to exercise and training (Presidential Youth Fitness Program, 2015).

Practitioners can influence certain modifiable factors in order to exert a positive influence on fitness in youth. These factors include increasing physical activity, providing more opportunity for physical activity, and improving nutrition. One way to evaluate the effectiveness of such efforts is to assess the fitness of youth.

In discussing the potential flaws of health-related fitness assessments for youth, Rowland (1995) identified four assumptions of field-based testing:

1. Physical fitness (e.g., strength, cardiorespiratory fitness) is linked to good health.
2. Markers of fitness can be reflected in field tests.
3. Performance on such tests can identify children who are at risk for poor health.
4. Deficient performance can be corrected by well-developed training programs.

Over the last quarter of a century, these assumptions have gained increasing credibility due to accumulation of supporting research. Regarding the first assumption, a body of evidence has been presented to demonstrate the association between physical fitness and health. Specifically, movement competence (Lubans et. al., 2010), strength (Lloyd et al., 2014), and cardiorespiratory fitness (Boreham & Riddoch, 2001; Ortega et al., 2008) in children and adolescents have all been associated with improved markers of health. Research has also shown a relationship between fitness test performance and neurocognitive performance in children (Hillman, Catelli, et al., 2005; Hillman, Pontifex, et al., 2014). Regarding the second assumption, it is only recently that researchers have systematically examined the validity of field-based measures of health and fitness in youth populations. Castro-Piñero and

Teaching Tip

ADULT VERSUS CHILD FITNESS ASSESSMENT

Silverman and colleagues (2008) point out that adults are free to choose whether or not they want their fitness assessed and that those who opt for fitness testing already have an attitude that supports engagement in physical activity. In contrast, in the context of physical education, youth do not have a choice about whether to participate in fitness assessment; to the contrary, they are required to do so within the remit of the educational curriculum. In addition, whereas adults are often assessed individually or in small groups and can stop the assessment at any time, children are normally assessed in large groups and may perceive that they are required to complete all tests. These conditions may create an assessment environment that is demotivating and counterproductive for some youth.

colleagues (2010) reviewed the criterion-related validity of field tests in youth and concluded that strong evidence supports the validity of various tests—the 20-meter shuttle run; tests for handgrip strength; and measures of BMI, waist circumference, and skinfold thickness—as indicators of an individual's level of health-related fitness.

It is more difficult to evaluate the third assumption—that is, the ability to identify children at risk from poor fitness—and this is where most of the contention persists. In particular, it is difficult to identify evidence-based criterion scores demonstrating that a given threshold is associated with health risk. In this vein, the manual for the popular FitnessGram test battery states that identifying criterion scores for health-related fitness is a "combination of art and science" (Morrow et al., 2013, pp.4-3), thus implying that precise thresholds are not known.

Nonetheless, in a recent systematic review, Ruiz and colleagues (2016) stated that cutoffs for peak oxygen uptake of 35 mL · kg^{-1} · min^{-1} for girls and 42 mL · kg^{-1} · min^{-1} for boys are associated with cardiovascular disease. Based on these cutoffs, nearly all 9-year-olds are considered to be healthy, but the proportion classified as healthy declines by 3 percent to 8 percent per year in boys and by 7 percent to 10 percent per year in girls; as a result, as little as half of the population would be considered healthy by age 17 (Tomkinson, Carver, et al., 2017; Tomkinson, Lang, et al., 2016). It is debatable whether this drop-off can be fully attributed to reduced fitness and health; for one thing, it is due at least in part to the fact that peak oxygen consumption is expressed as a ratio scale relative to body mass. This scaling method reduces the scores of larger (and therefore older) individuals relative to the scores of smaller (and therefore younger) individuals, and the effect is exaggerated where body composition changes to include a greater proportion of fat with maturation,

as it does in girls (Armstrong & Welsman, 2000). Consequently, although practitioners can view a low test result for cardiorespiratory fitness as a red flag, they should exercise caution in using current cutoff values.

The fourth and final assumption identified by Rowland (1995) is that deficient fitness performance can be corrected through training interventions. On this point, accumulated evidence now demonstrates that children do improve their fitness with training (see chapters 2 and 7 through 11). More specifically, cardiorespiratory fitness, strength, and body composition have all been established as valid markers of health-related fitness (Castro-Piñero et al., 2010), and systematic reviews have found each of these components to be responsive to training in youth (Armstrong & Baker, 2011; Atlantis et al., 2006; Baquet et al., 2003; Behringer et al., 2010, Lesinki et al., 2016).

For fitness assessment results to be valid, each child must be motivated to provide best effort on a given test. However, large-scale fitness testing can reinforce the belief that physical activity is competitive, which can be unpleasant for some youth participants (Naughton et al., 2006). This effect can be detrimental to children and their future level of physical activity (Silverman et al., 2008); it may even create a dislike for physical activity (Pate et al., 2013). This scenario may demotivate the very youth who most need encouragement to engage in physical activity (Rowland, 1995), such as those who are currently involved in little or no physical activity, who have poor fitness, or who are overweight. Dislike of fitness assessment can also lead to deliberately unmotivated responses in children (Naughton et al., 2006), which makes it difficult to interpret test scores. Despite concerns about the potential for negative experiences and negative consequences as a result of youth fitness assessment, many believe that if assessment is effectively delivered by qualified professionals, it can be engaging, motivating, and empowering for

Teaching Tip

USING FITNESS TEST SCORES TO MOTIVATE YOUTH

Using fitness test scores to provide a grade or to make comparisons with standardized norms (e.g., of a state, region, or country) should be avoided because it can be a demotivating experience. Although some children thrive on the belief that fitness assessment is a competition, many others find such an approach unpleasant. Therefore results should be kept private to each child rather than openly posted for comparison between individuals. In addition, although achieving high fitness scores should be praised, the major focus should be on empowering youth to understand and take responsibility for monitoring their fitness over time. Youth fitness specialists play an important role in this process by facilitating physical activity opportunities that allow all youth to experience and observe improvements in fitness scores over time. This feeling of individual success should increase perceived physical competence and help youth remain engaged in physical activity (Silverman et al., 2008).

all youth, irrespective of fitness levels or tendency to exercise regularly (Silverman et al., 2008; Society of Health and Physical Educators, 2010; Wiersma & Sherman, 2008).

Motivation and maturation both exert substantial influence on fitness test performance. In the worst-case scenario, fitness testing does nothing more than distinguish mature and motivated individuals from immature and unmotivated ones (Armstrong, 1995). Although maturation can be accounted for when interpreting test scores, practitioners must ensure that all participants are equally motivated to give a full effort during each fitness test; they should also consider each individual's **goal orientation**—that is, what motivates the individual (Wiersma & Sherman, 2008). Youth with a **task orientation** are motivated by personal improvement and task mastery, whereas those with an **ego orientation** are motivated by social comparisons with others (Lochbaum et al., 2017). Some evidence also suggests that one's predisposition toward either task or ego orientation in youth sport remains unchanged throughout childhood and adolescence (Lochbaum et al., 2017). Youth who are ego oriented may be naturally motivated to perform well in fitness testing and may enjoy comparing their results with percentile ranks and standardized scores; the same approach, however, may be demotivating for those individuals who are task oriented, especially for youth with low skill or low fitness (Silverman et al., 2008).

Providing a test environment that is task oriented and allows participants to recognize personal improvements over time will increase their sense of competence and encourage them to continue engaging in physical activity. Competence motivation can be reinforced through positive external feedback—that is, feedback provided by others, such as teachers, coaches, and peers. Perceived competence can be reinforced even more powerfully if we help children give themselves internal feedback by self-assessing their abilities, but this process can be difficult for younger children and requires refinement with maturity (Oliver et al., 2014; Wiersma & Sherman, 2008). Reinforcing a task mastery climate in physical activity is associated with positive outcomes, such as increased enjoyment and belief that effort leads to success (Oliver et al., 2014). Therefore, youth fitness specialists should provide positive instructions and developmentally appropriate assessment feedback focused on process goals and individual development to promote task orientation.

DO YOU KNOW?

Lack of knowledge about fitness assessment has been shown to influence youth motivation and performance during testing (Silverman et al., 2008).

In summary, youth fitness assessment has the potential to be a positive experience, provide useful information, and encourage lifelong participation in physical activity and sport. Figure 6.2 provides recommendations for practitioners to consider when implementing fitness assessment in order to make it a worthwhile process for all involved.

FIGURE 6.2   RECOMMENDATIONS FOR EFFECTIVE IMPLEMENTATION OF YOUTH FITNESS ASSESSMENT

1. Fitness assessment should promote learning and positive attitudes about being active.
2. Establish a positive and motivating measurement environment for students.
3. Where possible, administer testing in small groups (e.g., use stations); certainly avoid formats that might embarrass some individuals.
4. Promoting task mastery and competence should allow all participants to be motivated and challenged.
5. Provide ongoing measurement to allow monitoring of personal fitness and progress toward activity goals.
6. Keep results and feedback confidential to each individual; do *not* make results public.
7. Assessment should focus not on comparison with others but on personal improvement over time.
8. Use of criterion-referenced standards is associated with health and should be achievable for the vast majority.
9. "Very low fit" youngsters should be provided with sensitive remedial support and encouragement.

Adapted from Cale and Harris [2005] and the Society of Health and Physical Educators—Shape America [2010]. *Appropriate uses of fitness measurement position statement*

What and When to Assess?

Practitioners must decide thoughtfully which components of fitness to assess, how to assess them, and at what age to begin doing so. Myriad fitness tests and test batteries are available for youth fitness, and choosing what is most appropriate can be a difficult task. On the other hand, it should be easy to appreciate that fitness is influenced by a number of factors; indeed, movement skills, physical fitness, and physical activity knowledge and behavior all relate to one another and are worthy of assessment (Lloyd et al., 2010). As for when to initiate fitness assessment, there is no golden rule, and the appropriate age depends on the nature of the test. In younger children, there may be a need to assess fitness in order to identify poor movement competence, low fitness, or high body fat and thus allow for early intervention.

DO YOU KNOW?

A health-related fitness battery has been developed for use in three- to five-year-olds (Ortega et al., 2015).

Assessing Motor and Movement Skills

As discussed in earlier chapters, the development of motor and movement skills mirrors the rapid development of the central nervous system from birth through childhood. During this period, individuals are expected to master fundamental movement skills associated with locomotion, stabilization, and manipulation. Establishing proficient movement skills is associated with increased levels of physical activity and health in youth (Lubans et al., 2010), whereas a lack of motor skills can lead to a "proficiency barrier" that restricts one's ability to engage in physical activities requiring the use of more complex skills (Seefeldt, 1980). Given the importance and early development of motor skills, practitioners should prioritize the assessment of movement competencies, particularly in young children.

Ideally, the assessment of movement competence should address not only the product (test outcome) but also the process of movement. For instance, the primary objective is not to assess how fast a child can run or how far a child can throw; rather, it is to determine how the child coordinates body segments to produce a movement. A number of protocols exist for directly measuring motor skill competence in children. In a review of four established tests of motor development, Wiart and Darrah (2001) identified potential issues relating to reliability and validity of the Bruininks-Oseretsky Test of Motor Proficiency, the Movement Assessment Battery for Children, and the Peabody Developmental Motor Scales while noting some evidence of validity for the Test of Gross Motor Development (TGMD). The TGMD has since been updated in a second edition (TGMD-2; Ulrich, 2000) and more recently a third edition (TGMD-3; Ulrich et al., 2019).

The TGMD is designed to assess gross motor function in children of ages 3 to 10 years; specifically, the test administrator rates the quality of movement across a number of motor tasks. The TGMD-2 manual touts the protocol as having good **content validity, construct validity**, and **criterion validity**, as well as good reliability, as evidenced by consistency of scores over repeated measures ($r > 0.85$) and excellent interrater agreement ($r = 0.98$) (Ulrich, 2000). Published research supports acceptable interrater reliability and validity for the TGMD-2 (Barnett et al., 2014; Farrokhi et al., 2014) and the TGMD-3 (Ulrich et al., 2019); the TGMD-2 has also been shown to detect longitudinal changes in motor skill competence of five-year-old children following various physical education curriculums (Lemos et al., 2012).

The TGMD-2 assesses six locomotor skills and six object control skills. Participants are scored on a number of performance criteria relating to how each skill is executed. Each participant performs two trials of each skill, scoring one point for each criterion passed and zero for each criterion failed on each attempt. Scores can then be summed to give a total score for each skill, a score for each subset of skills (locomotor or object control), and an overall score. The components (number of criteria) assessed for locomotor skills include sprinting (4), galloping (4), hopping (5), a leap (3), a horizontal jump (4), and lateral sliding (4). Components for object control include striking a stationary ball (5), stationary one-handed dribble (4), two-handed catch (3), kicking a stationary ball (4), an overhand throw (4), and an underhand throw (4). As an example, during sprinting, criteria relate to arm position and movement, observation of an airborne period, foot placement when landing, and support leg position. Full details on the TGMD-2 criteria and scoring are widely available elsewhere. Administering the test takes about 20 minutes per child and requires a space of 60 by 30 feet (18 by 9 m) with a wall. Each task should be explained and demonstrated, and each participant should complete at least one practice attempt before performance is rated.

The total score for both locomotion and object control can be compared with normative data, such as average scores across a range of ages, as shown in table 6.1 (the scores are representative of children on the 50th percentile). Comparing a child's score with the data presented in table 6.1 will give an indication of whether the child's locomotor and object control skills are at the expected level for chronological age. For instance, a six-year-old girl who scores 21 for object control could be considered to be behind the expected rate of motor skill development, because her score is at the level of an average four-year-old. Ulrich (2000) also provides TGDM-2 scores across a range of percentiles and a standardized total score adjusted for age and performance. However, a more informative use of the assessment results is to consider performance in each individual skill, refer to this information when planning future exercise programming, and monitor the progress of motor skill development over time.

A screen similar to the TGMD was developed by the New South Wales (NSW) Department of Education and Training (2000) for its Get Skilled: Get Active campaign. In this assessment, children complete a number of movements (e.g., run, leap, gallop, kick), for each of which five or six criteria are assessed. This approach is distinguished by the fact that the movement skills differ with advancing age to reflect changes in the physical education curriculum; as a result, the curriculum determines progression rather than individual mastery, which perhaps is not an ideal scenario given the individual nature of motor learning trajectories. In

this screen, children are considered to have mastered a movement if all criteria are passed or to have nearly mastered it if all but one criteria are passed (Okely & Booth, 2004). An adapted version of the NSW screen has also been used in research with schoolchildren in the United Kingdom (Foweather, 2010; Stratton et al., 2009).

Given the greater detail in the TGMD-2's scoring system when compared to other movement screens, the body of evidence supporting its reliability and validity, and the availability of resources to support practitioners who use it, the TGMD-2 is recommended as a suitable assessment tool for youth fitness specialists. The TGMD-2 test manual is available through the website of the Centers for Disease Control and Prevention. The TGMD-3, which provides a slightly altered selection of skills and performance criteria, was released only recently; therefore, more research is needed to confirm its usefulness.

Detailed assessment of movement competence can be time-consuming. Alternative approaches require children to complete an obstacle course involving a variety of skills. Time to complete the obstacle course has been used as an indirect measure of movement skill based on the assumption that individuals with greater movement competence can complete the course more quickly. In one example, Zuvela and colleagues (2011)

TABLE 6.1 AVERAGE SCORES* ON THE TGDM-2

Age (yr)	Locomotor (male and female)	Object control (female)	Object control (male)
3.0	19	15	19
3.5	22	18	20
4.0	25	21	23
4.5	29	24	27
5.0	32	26	30
5.5	35	28	33
6.0	38	30	36
6.5	40	31	39
7.0	41	34	41
7.5	41	37	42
8.0	43	39	43
8.5	43	39	43
9.0	44	41	44
9.5	44	41	44
10.0	44	42	44

*Based on the 50th percentile in data collected from n = 1208 American children; both locomotor and object control have a maximum total score of 48.

Data from Ulrich (2000).

developed FMS-POLYGON, a fundamental movement skills test in which participants bounce a volleyball against a wall six times, run 15 meters while clearing three hurdles, place two medicine balls on a platform, and then sprint 20 meters. The test was shown to have good levels of reliability and validity, and a strong relationship was found between the Polygon test and the criterion measure of the TGDM-2. This type of approach may be useful when a practitioner must assess a large group of children with limited time and resources.

The Canadian Agility and Movement Skill Assessment (CAMSA) is part of the Canadian Assessment of Physical Literacy (CAPL) test battery. CAMSA requires children to perform two- and one-footed jumps, lateral sliding, catching, throwing, hopping, and kicking. Instructions and the layout of the test are provided in the CAPL manual for test administration (CAPL, 2017). Performance is scored with equal weighting of time to complete and use of correct movement pattern during each exercise. Children are awarded 14 points for completing the test in less than 14 seconds, 13 points for completing it in 14 to 14.9 seconds, and so on (the number of points awarded decreases by 1 for each additional second used). Children are then awarded up to 14 points for 14 different skills that are assessed on a pass/fail basis during the circuit.

The test has been shown to be a valid component of physical literacy in 8- to 12-year-old children (Longmuir et al., 2015), but debate continues about the appropriateness of the scoring system (Francis et al., 2016), in which movement proficiency is estimated partly from a performance outcome. Longmuir and colleagues (2015) reported that the time to complete the obstacle course was highly reliable (ICC = 0.99), although performance improved significantly from trial 1 to trial 2. The Longmuir results also showed that ratings of skill execution were less reliable within (ICC = 0.52) and between (ICC = 0.69) raters when compared with performance times. Collectively, these findings suggest the need to fully familiarize children with an obstacle course before testing in order to remove any learning effects; they also suggest that performance times are likely to be more reliable than ratings of skill execution during such tests.

Assessing movement competence may also be important for youth who are involved in sport. To this end, the fundamental movement screen developed by Cook and colleagues (2006) has been shown to relate to physical performance of young soccer players (Lloyd et al., 2014). Similarly, youth rugby players with low physical competence have been reported to have lower speed, power, and endurance than their more physically competent counterparts (Parsonage et al., 2014).

It has also been shown that movement competence is generally low in Australian rules football and soccer players in talent development programs (Woods, et al., 2016), which suggests that we should not assume that talented athletes are necessarily "good movers." This finding may result from specialization, in which youth athletes spend most of their time developing a narrow range of movement skills.

Lubans and colleagues (2014) developed the Resistance Training Skills Battery for adolescents, a screen that assesses resistance training skill competence during a squat, push-up, lunge, suspended row, overhead press, and front support with chest touches. The format and scoring system are similar to those of the TGMD in that participants are given two trials and a pass/fail mark for a number of criteria for each exercise. Each participant completes four repetitions of each movement and is scored on the best repetition during each trial. The totals can be summed to provide an overall total for the screen, which is referred to as the resistance training skills quotient (Lubans et al., 2014). The screen has been reported to have good levels of reliability and validity (Lubans et al., 2014; Barnett et al., 2015) and may provide a useful tool for determining whether youth possess the technical competence to engage in resistance training. A link to a score sheet for administering the resistance skills training battery was provided in the original study describing the screen (Lubans et al., 2014). Recently, the Athlete Introductory Movement Screen (AIMS) adapted the Resistance Training Skills Battery for use in emerging junior athletes, removing the suspend row and overhead press but slightly extending the scoring range for the four remaining movements (Rogers et al., 2019). Initial research on the AIMS has reported acceptable levels of intra and interrater reliability (Rogers et al., 2019).

Assessing Health-Related Fitness

Health-related fitness assessment assumes that some measures of physical fitness reflect underlying health qualities. Although this concept has been debated over the years, systematic examination of an accumulation of evidence has provided support for an association between physical fitness and health in youth (Ortega et al., 2008). As shown in figure 6.3, health-related fitness has traditionally been viewed as consisting of five components (Caspersen et al., 1985; Society of Health and Physical Educators, 2010).

A number of assessment batteries have been developed to measure the components of health-related fitness, and many of them include the same or similar tests (Safrit, 1990). Table 6.2 provides an overview of prominent health-related fitness testing batteries

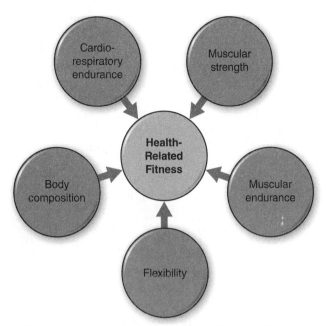

FIGURE 6.3 Components traditionally considered to comprise health-related fitness.

from around the world, as well as the tests included in those batteries for assessing various components of fitness. As the table shows, practitioners can choose from a large collection of existing batteries or from different tests for any given component of fitness. When choosing the most appropriate tests to use, youth fitness specialists should consider whether a given test is reliable, whether the test is a valid indicator of health, whether a field-based test gives a valid representation of criterion measures (e.g., laboratory test), whether the test is practical to administer in a given situation, what supporting resources are available, and whether the data gathered can be interpreted and used meaningfully.

Table 6.2 provides an indication of the lack of consensus regarding which components of health-related fitness should be assessed and with what protocols. Cardiorespiratory fitness is most commonly measured by means of a progressive 20-meter shuttle run or the progressive aerobic cardiovascular endurance run (PACER), which is also normally completed over 20 meters but can be completed over a 15-meters course with younger children or when necessary due to space restrictions. A progressive test may be considered preferable to a timed distance run because youth may not have the capacity to adequately pace themselves in the latter option (Castro-Piñero et al., 2010). Pacing in a progressive test is controlled by audible beeps, and young children can be assisted if an administrator runs with them during the test and instructs: "Run with me—don't run faster!" (Ortega et al., 2015). Progressive tests also allow the least fit children to withdraw first;

as a result, they do not have to exercise for a long time and do not experience the embarrassment of finishing far behind their peers as they might during a timed run over a given distance.

Muscular strength is most commonly measured using a handgrip test, in which a nondigital dynamometer may be needed in order to allow detection of low strength measures in young children (Ortega et al., 2015). Grip span should be adjusted to the size of the child's hand according to the following equations, where x (in cm) is the maximal width between the thumb and the small finger with the hand spread out:

Children, Aged 6 to 12

Female grip span = 0.3x − 0.52

Male grip span = (x ÷ 4) + 0.44

Adolescents, Aged 13 to 18

Female grip span = (x ÷ 4) + 1.1

Male grip span = (x ÷ 7.2) + 3.1

From España-Romero, Artero, Santaliestra-Pasias, et al. (2008).

Measurement of handgrip strength is a readily accessible method; requires minimal equipment that is relatively inexpensive; and provides an easy, low-skill test for children and adolescents to complete. Alternatives are available but are not included in popular test batteries. Similar to handgrip strength, an isometric mid-thigh pull or isometric squat can provide a low-skill, static measurement of strength. These options offer the advantage of measuring the strength of a large muscle mass working around multiple joints, and they are likely to be more ecologically valid because they assess the musculature that is most often used during exercise (e.g., running, jumping, hopping). Peak force in an isometric mid-thigh pull test has been shown to have good levels of reliability in 15-year-old boys (Secomb et al., 2015) and in both prepubertal and postpubertal girls (Moeskops et al., 2018). Figure 6.4 shows front and side views of a child performing an isometric mid-thigh pull. The participant stands with the feet hip-width apart, the adjustable bar positioned at mid-thigh level, the torso upright, the spine in a neutral position, and the knees and hips slightly flexed. Where possible, it is advisable to use lifting straps to help the child grasp the bar in order to ensure that grip strength does not become the limiting factor of performance (Moeskops et al., 2018).

As indicated in table 6.2, there is no single field-based measure of strength endurance used consistently across assessment batteries, which may reflect the difficulty and usefulness of measuring this component of fitness. The influence of fatigue on the ability to maintain correct technical form makes it problematic

TABLE 6.2 PROMINENT ASSESSMENT BATTERIES FOR HEALTH-RELATED FITNESS IN YOUTH

Assessment battery		FitnessGram	Canadian Assessment of Physical Literacy health-related fitness test	Assessing Levels of Physical Activity health-related fitness test battery	PREschool FITness testing battery	EuroFIT	YMCA Youth Fitness Test	Health-Related Fitness Test	New Zealand Fitness Test	Australian Fitness Education Award
		USA	CAN	EU	EU	EU	USA	USA	NZ	AUS
Age range (yr)		5-17	8-12	6-18	3-5	6-18	6-17	5-18	6-12	9-19
Cardiorespiratory fitness	20 m shuttle run/PACER	×	×	×	×	×				×
	1 mi (1.6 km) run/walk	×					×	×		
	Cooper test							×	×	
	9 min run							×	×	×
	Handgrip strength		×	×	×	×				
	Trunk lift					×				
Strength	Bent-arm hang	×				×				
	Pull-up	×								
Strength endurance	Modified pull-up	×					×			
	Push-up	×								
	Sit-up					×		×		
	Curl-up	×					×		×	×
	Prone plank		×							
	Basketball throw									×
	Medicine ball throw								×	
Explosive strength (power)	Sand ball throw								×	
	Shot put								×	
	Standing long jump			×	×	×			×	
	Sit-and-reach		×			×	×	×	×	×
	Back-saver sit-and-reach	×								×
Flexibility	Shoulder stretch	×								
	Height and weight	×	×	×		×	×	×	×	
	BMI	×	×	×						×
Body composition	Skinfold thickness	×		×		×	×	×	×	
	Waist circumference		×	×						
	10 × 5 m shuttle run					×				
	4 × 10 m shuttle run			×	×					
Motor skill	Plate tapping					×				
	Flamingo/single-leg balance	×			×					

Data from Castro-Piñero et al. (2010).

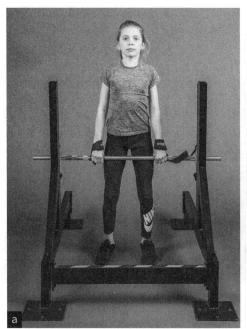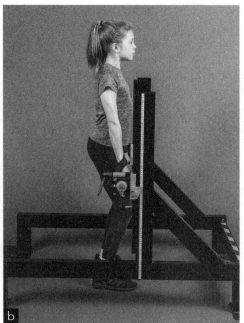

FIGURE 6.4 Isometric mid-thigh pull.

to use tests of the maximal number of repetitions (e.g., push-ups in 30 seconds). In addition, the results of muscle endurance tests, in which body mass must be held or repeatedly moved, have been viewed as being determined primarily by body fat and body weight rather than by fitness; as a result, it has been suggested that exercises such as the bent-arm hang, push-up, and pull-up are not valid measures of muscle endurance in youth (Castro-Piñero et al., 2010; Woods et al., 1992). Alternatively, a prone plank hold can be achieved by nearly all children and has been shown to be both reliable and valid (Boyer et al., 2013); therefore, as a simple, low-skill exercise, it may provide a suitable method for testing muscle endurance.

Flexibility is most commonly measured using a sit-and-reach test; however, youth fitness specialists should be aware of the influence of growth and maturation on test performance. Sit-and-reach performance

can be affected by growth spurts independent of any "real" change in flexibility, as performance decreases with a growth spurt in the legs and improves with a growth spurt in the trunk due to the influence of these spurts on reach distance (Malina et al., 2004).

Body composition is most commonly assessed using height and weight, which allows the calculation of body mass index; some batteries also include waist circumference. These are simple and accessible measures, although youth fitness specialists should be mindful of following established techniques to ensure that results are accurate. The use of skinfold measurements is also a popular method for estimating body fat in children and adolescents. However, this technique should be undertaken only by practitioners with the necessary skill and experience and should follow established procedures set out by the International Society for the Advancement of Kinanthropometry. Although it can

Teaching Tip

USING ONE-REPETITION-MAXIMUM (1RM) TESTS OF STRENGTH

Many myths and controversies have existed in regard to strength and resistance training in children and adolescents, and they are dispelled in chapter 9. Strength training is not only safe and beneficial for youth but also can be used to test strength by means of a one-repetition maximum effort with a resistance machine or free weights. Healthy children can safely perform a 1RM test if they are properly supervised, possess the necessary skill to perform the movement, are able to follow instructions, and, most important, are supervised by an appropriately qualified and experienced youth fitness specialist (Faigenbaum et al., 2003; Lloyd et al., 2014).

seem relatively easy to take a skinfold measurement, it is in fact quite difficult to obtain accurate results, and the stakes are significant. Incorrectly reporting that a child is excessively fat, or has gained a large amount of fat, based on erroneous skinfold measures could carry serious negative implications.

Table 6.2 also shows two other components of fitness that are included in some test batteries but traditionally have not been considered to be health-related fitness measures: explosive strength and motor skill. Explosive strength, most commonly measured by means of a standing long jump, has been shown to be associated with cardiovascular diseases in children and adolescents (Ortega, et al., 2008). Motor skill tests may be more closely associated with movement competence or skill-related fitness, depending on the design of the individual test, but there is some suggestion that such tests are also directly relevant to bone health (Ruiz et al., 2011).

The majority of tests identified in table 6.2 may be considered reliable provided that test procedures are accurately followed and participants are adequately familiarized with each protocol. However, an important consideration remains: whether all components of health-related fitness are valid markers of health. Ortega and colleagues (2008) reviewed existing evidence and concluded that physical fitness was a powerful marker of health in childhood and adolescence. According to the authors, the evidence demonstrated that cardiorespiratory fitness was associated with fatness, cardiovascular disease, and mental health,

whereas muscular fitness was associated with cardiovascular disease and skeletal health. Castro-Piñero and colleagues (2010) provided the first systematic review of the criterion-related validity of field-based tests for health-related fitness in youth. Their study showed the validity of cardiorespiratory fitness, muscular strength, and body composition measurements in the field but found only limited evidence to support the assessment of muscular endurance and flexibility. The same group of researchers also found some limited evidence that assessment of motor skills by means of a speed and agility test may provide an important marker of bone health (Ortega et al., 2008, 2015; Ruiz et al., 2011).

Collectively, this research was used in developing the Assessing Levels of Physical Activity and Fitness (ALPHA-FIT) test battery for children and adolescents aged 6 to 18 years. Figure 6.5 shows the fitness components along the top row and their respective tests underneath. Components and tests shown in boxes with a solid outline are included in the high-priority version of the battery, whereas those in open boxes are included only in the extended version. Shaded boxes indicate tests supported by strong evidence of criterion-related validity, and lightly shaded boxes indicate tests for which evidence is limited. A later extension of the ALPHA-FIT came in the form of the Preschool Fitness testing battery (PRE-FIT) for three- to five-year-olds (Ortega et al., 2015).

Table 6.3 summarizes the advantages and disadvantages of four popular test batteries for health-related fitness: FitnessGram, the Canadian Assessment of

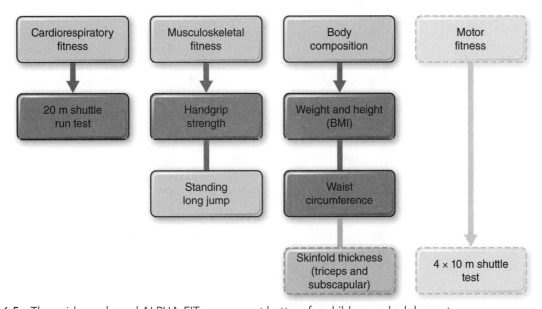

FIGURE 6.5   The evidence-based ALPHA-FIT assessment battery for children and adolescents.
Adapted from ALPHA Consortium, *The ALPHA Health-Related Fitness Test Battery for Children and Adolescents* (2009), accessed May 6, 2019, http://www.ugr.es/~cts262/ES/documents/ALPHA-FitnessTestManualforChildren-Adolescents.pdf, by permission of Manuel J. Castillo Garzón.

TABLE 6.3   ADVANTAGES AND DISADVANTAGES OF FOUR POPULAR TEST BATTERIES FOR HEALTH-RELATED FITNESS

	Advantages	Disadvantages
FitnessGram	• Lots of supporting resources are available. • Is reported to be reliable and valid (Plowman & Meredith, 2013). • Requires minimal equipment. • Should allow large groups of children to be assessed. • Fitness standards are provided for children aged 5-17 years. • Provides standards for healthy fitness zones. • Assessment of physical activity can be included.	• Does not include measures of strength or power. • Includes only limited tests of movement skill. • Strength endurance tests may not be valid. • Healthy fitness zones are based on a combination of "art and science" (Morrow et al., 2013). • Scoring considers only a single snapshot in time, not individual progress.
Canadian Assessment of Physical Literacy	• Lots of supporting resources are available. • Is reported to be reliable and valid (Larouche et al., 2014; Longmuir et al., 2015). • Requires minimal equipment. • Should allow large groups of children to be assessed. • Provides standards for beginning, progressing, achieving, and excelling. • Complete assessment includes a circuit to assess fundamental movement skills and assessment of physical activity.	• Does not include a measure of power. • Flexibility test may not be valid. • Fitness standards are provided only for children aged 8-12 years. • Lacks evidence to support fitness standards. • Scoring considers only a single snapshot in time, not individual progress.
ALPHA-FIT for children and adolescents	• Supporting resources are available. • Is reported to be reliable and valid (Castro-Piñero et al., 2010; España-Romero et al., 2010; Ruiz et al., 2011). • Requires minimal equipment. • Should allow large groups of children to be assessed. • Provides standards for very low, low, average, high, and very high fitness. • An adapted version (PRE-FIT) exists for preschool-age children. • Assessment of physical activity can also be included.	• Does not include measures of strength endurance, balance, or flexibility. • Includes only limited tests of movement skill. • Fitness standards are provided only for children aged 13-17 years. • Fitness standards are based on a relatively small sample of Spanish children. • Scoring considers only a single snapshot in time, not individual progress.
EUROFIT	• Supporting resources are available. • Most of the tests are reliable in children (Fjortoft, 2000) and adolescents (Mac Donncha et al., 1999). • Includes tests for most aspects of health- and skill-related fitness. • Requires minimal equipment. • Should allow large groups of children to be assessed. • Normative data are available from a large sample (Tomkinson et al., 2017).	• Does not include tests of movement skill. • Does not include a measurement of physical activity. • Some tests may not be reliable. • Some tests may lack validity. • No standards are provided for health-related fitness. • Scoring considers only a single snapshot in time, not individual progress.

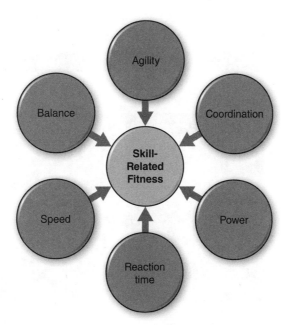

FIGURE 6.6 Components traditionally considered to comprise skill-related fitness.

Physical Literacy (CAPL), ALPHA-FIT, and EUROFIT. These batteries share the advantage of being supported by resources to help demonstrate the reliability and validity of their test measures, to help with test administration, and to help with interpretation and feedback. However, each battery also has disadvantages, such as the absence of some important measures of fitness and a focus on interpreting fitness through a single snapshot in time rather than considering individual development. Therefore, although practitioners may choose to use one of these batteries, they should be aware of the limitations and consider the possible need to incorporate additional tests (e.g., movement screening, strength testing).

Assessing Skill-Related Fitness

Skill-related fitness has been defined as including the components of physical fitness that relate to enhanced performance of sport and motor skills (Corbin et al., 2000). As shown in figure 6.6, skill-related fitness has traditionally been considered to consist of six components (Caspersen et al., 1985).

The definition of skill-related fitness is somewhat misleading, in that most or all components of health-related fitness would also positively influence athletic abilities. For instance, greater endurance capacity and increased strength would likely enhance motor skill and sport performance. Similarly, the skill-related components of speed, agility, and power have been suggested as markers of health-related fitness (Ortega et al., 2008; Ruiz et al., 2011). In addi-

tion, agility, balance, and coordination are included as components of skill-related fitness but would also be considered in assessing motor skill competence, which in turn is associated with health outcomes in children and adolescents (Lubans, et al., 2010). The overlapping nature of heath- and skill-related fitness means that these constructs may be better considered together and alongside movement competence to provide an overview of athleticism. Table 6.4 provides a composite youth physical fitness test battery that incorporates components of both health- and skill-related fitness.

The assessments for cardiorespiratory fitness, muscle strength, muscle endurance, body composition, flexibility, agility, power, and balance are all included in prominent health-related fitness assessment batteries (refer back to table 6.2 on page 113), and these qualities also contribute to athletic ability. The prone plank is included to assess muscular endurance because it has been shown to be a valid and reliable test with children (Boyer et al., 2013). The back-saver sit-and-reach is included as a measure of flexibility because it has been shown to be a valid measure of hip and lower-back flexibility in adolescents (Chillón et al., 2010). Given the potential for measurement error, skinfold measurements were not included as a measure of body composition; however, they could be included if the administrator is well practiced in this technique. A 30-meter sprint is included as a measure of linear speed and would allow for measures of both acceleration (10 m) and speed (30 m). A sprint test is easy to administer, can be performed with minimal

TABLE 6.4 SUGGESTED YOUTH PHYSICAL FITNESS ASSESSMENT BATTERY TO MEASURE HEALTH- AND SKILL-RELATED FITNESS

Component	Test
Cardiorespiratory fitness	20 m shuttle run test (PACER)
Muscle strength	Handgrip (a) OR Isometric mid-thigh pull (b and c)
Muscle endurance	Prone plank hold
Body composition	BMI and waist circumference
Flexibility	Back-saver sit-and-reach
Agility	4 × 10 m shuttle sprint
Speed	30 m sprint

Component	Test
Power	Standing broad jump
Balance	Single-leg balance

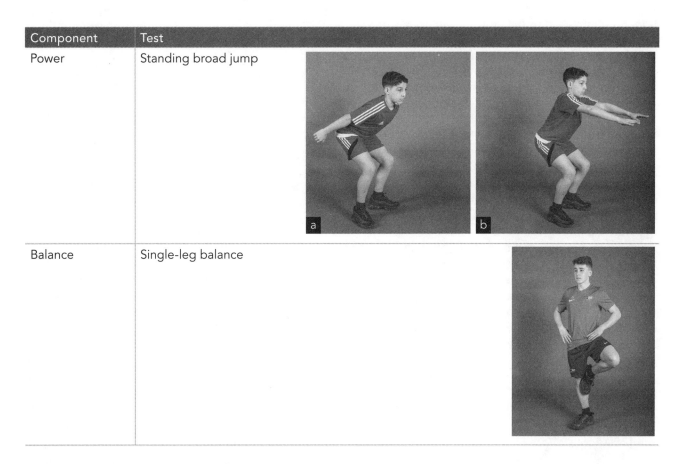

equipment indoors or outdoors, and, like jumping, is both a natural activity for youth and typical of many athletic activities (Tomkinson & Olds, 2008).

Although a generic assessment battery can be used to provide an indication of health-related fitness and athleticism, sport-specific assessments may be required for the development of youth who are involved in sport. Although the assessment batteries should be specific to the demands of the sport, the process of selecting appropriate tests follows established principles; any test must be reliable and valid. When working with young athletes, the choice of tests also depends on the resources and expertise available. The test battery presented in table 6.4 is suitable for testing the general population; it can be implemented with large groups using relatively little equipment, and measurement and interpretation of results are simple. Practitioners who work with youth athletes may have the opportunity to undertake more detailed tests. For example, strength and jump tests performed on force plates can provide in-depth information about ability to produce and direct force and power; skinfolds collected by experienced kinanthropometrists can provide greater insight into body composition; and custom-made agility tests can be used to assess change-of-direction speed in movements replicating the demands of a given sport. This in-depth assessment can help practitioners develop more specific and individualized training programs for their athletes.

When choosing appropriate fitness tests for a given sport, two key considerations are **ecological validity** and **discriminative validity**. Ecological validity requires the demands of a test to reflect the demands of the sport, whereas discriminative validity requires that a test distinguish between more and less successful athletes. In soccer players, for instance, cardiorespiratory fitness is often measured using a yo-yo intermittent-recovery test. This is a progressive test similar to a PACER but including a brief rest period after each shuttle, which is thought to more closely reflect the demands of intermittent team sports. The yo-yo test has been found reliable and shown to correlate significantly with the distances typically covered in match play in elite youth soccer (Castagna et al., 2010), and test performance has been shown to discriminate between elite and non-elite youth soccer players (Deprez et al., 2014). Therefore, a yo-yo test may be considered as providing a valid measurement of cardiorespiratory fitness in youth soccer players.

Practitioners must be able to interpret fitness test

performance and provide participants with meaningful feedback. To help with interpretation, an abundance of data and resources are available. As shown in table 6.3, FitnessGram, CAPL, and ALPHA-FIT all provide performance standards to classify youth into fitness categories, although the age ranges differ. In addition, normative data on EUROFIT has been provided by Tomkinson and colleagues (2017) from more than two million tests, thus establishing percentile norms based on sex and age. Reference data on health-related fitness tests are also available for Australian children (Catley & Tomkinson, 2013) and for U.S. children of mixed ethnicity (Laurson et al., 2016). The thresholds or percentiles provided by established health-related fitness batteries can be used to provide a traffic light approach. That is, scores indicative of poor fitness and health act as a red light and require immediate action; scores approaching an undesirable level act as a yellow light and need careful monitoring and potential intervention; and scores indicative of good health act as a green light.

All health-related fitness standards and percentiles are subject to the limitation that they rely on age-based bandings, an approach that ignores the profound influence of growth and maturity on physical fitness. Therefore, rather than simply relying on comparison with age-related norms at one snapshot in time, practitioners are encouraged to consider how the fitness of each child progresses over time. Talent identification initiatives and sport systems often fall into the trap of taking a short-term view and selecting youth athletes into or out of a system based on a single snapshot that is compared with data for youth of similar chronological age. Figure 6.7 shows the fitness performance of a youth athlete. The scores have been converted into a standardized format to allow comparisons with a population (e.g., teammates) and to show results that would otherwise be expressed in different units, such as kilograms, seconds, or centimeters. Standardized Z scores are reported, wherein an individual's results are expressed relative to the overall performance of a group using the following equation:

(Individual performance − mean group performance) ÷ group standard deviation

A score of zero would reflect an individual whose score is exactly the same as the group mean, whereas a score of plus (or minus) two lies at the very upper (or lower) end of the population. In figure 6.7, the black line shows the traditional approach, in which a young athlete's performance is compared with those

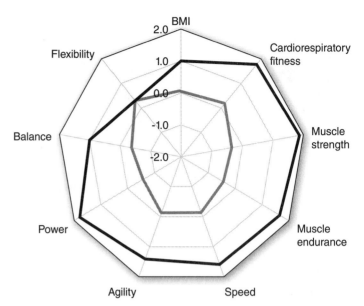

FIGURE 6.7   Radar plot showing fitness test performance of an individual child relative to peers. The black line represents the traditional approach of comparing an individual with age-group peers (e.g., an under-12 team). The gray line represents fitness of the individual relative to peers of similar maturity status (e.g., 92%-95% of predicted adult height). Fitness is reported in terms of standardized Z scores, where zero indicates a score that is the same as the group average.

of other athletes of the same age. In that approach, the participant scores very positively on most components of fitness; is considerably stronger, faster, and fitter than age-group peers; and is more likely to be selected into a sport. The gray line in the figure shows fitness performance for the same individual with results standardized to a group of youth athletes of similar maturity—the process referred to as bio-banding (Cumming et al., 2017). Now, all test scores move inward, suggesting that the individual is largely an average performer when compared with others of similar maturity (e.g., those at 92%-95% of predicted adult height). Thus the individual outperforms age-matched peers due to being biologically advanced, but that advantage is lost when the individual is considered relative to others of similar maturity. In this way, the comparison in figure 6.7 illustrates the shortcomings of considering fitness solely in relation to age group and highlights the need to consider maturity as well (for information on measuring maturity, see chapter 3).

Rather than considering fitness from a single snapshot in time, a more informative approach focuses on personal improvement over time. This approach helps promote engagement in physical activity and facilitates a task mastery climate. Fitness assessment should be used to guide exercise prescription, and physical activity opportunities must be provided so that fitness can develop over time. Figure 6.8 shows an example of change in a child's fitness between two assessment

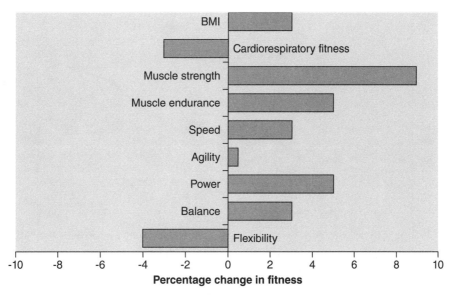

FIGURE 6.8 Change in fitness performance of a child between two test occasions.

points. The change has been standardized to the percentage change in performance, which is a simple and intuitive variable that children, parents, educators, and coaches can understand; it also allows for direct comparison of test results measured in different units. The approach can be used over a short time frame (e.g., two or three months) if the goal is to evaluate the success of a specific intervention. However, to promote a sense of perceived competence, it is advisable to make comparisons over a longer term (at least three months) to allow individuals the opportunity to improve fitness between test occasions.

Change in performance should still be considered in the context of growth and maturation. For example, in figure 6.8, BMI may have increased due to growth-related gains in muscle mass, which may have facilitated improvements in strength and power; at the same time, the increased mass may have exerted a small negative effect on cardiorespiratory fitness.

The overall goal is to use fitness assessment to promote long-term development of both athleticism and health. The most powerful approach for practitioners is to consider the fitness progression of a child over a number of years. To that end, figure 6.9 provides a sample plot of the development of cardiorespiratory fitness in an individual between the ages of 10 and 15 years. Absolute fitness, measured as number of laps completed, improves over time, which would be expected due to the interaction of growth, maturation, and an active lifestyle. In contrast, fitness relative to body mass—expressed as estimated peak oxygen uptake calculated from age, body mass, and speed at the end of a 20-meter shuttle run test (Leger et al., 1988)—shows a more undulating response with an overall slight improvement. Converting scores to a measure relative to body size can help account for some of the changes in performance that occur as a result of maturity; in figure 6.9, absolute fitness is increasing, driven largely by positive changes in size (results relative to body size show a more blunted response).

Figure 6.9 also shows that individual development is rarely a smooth, continual process; instead, it is marked by peaks and troughs. These natural developmental variations will be missed if a practitioner considers only one snapshot in time, or even two consecutive test occasions. A period of little change may be preceded by a period of rapid change, or vice versa, and these sequences may relate to periods of rapid growth and maturation.

Youth fitness specialists should not view large improvement over the short term as the ultimate goal; nor should a short-term decrease or plateau in performance be viewed as a dire outcome. Instead, practitioners should consider whether youth are making consistent, long-term gains in fitness that are at or above the level expected with an active lifestyle and growth and maturation. Intervention is most needed when an individual falls below a healthy level of fitness or when fitness consistently declines over multiple test sessions. Figure 6.9 shows a healthy cutoff threshold for peak oxygen uptake, although, as discussed earlier, such thresholds should be used with caution. The child moved downward toward this threshold at age 10.5 years but then exhibited improved fitness, which suggests that the child remained healthy. Thus, relative fitness tended to move up and down, but over the long-term we see a slight upward trend.

It is difficult to understand how much value has been

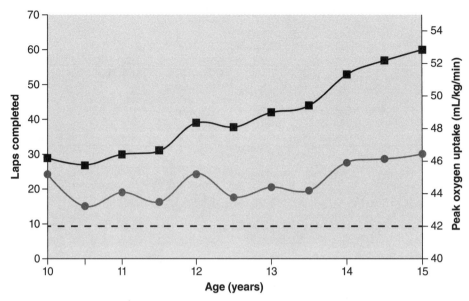

FIGURE 6.9   Change in the cardiorespiratory fitness of a boy tracked over a number of years. The black line represents total laps completed on a 20-meter shuttle run test. The grey line represents predicted peak oxygen uptake scores. The dashed line represents a suggested minimum healthy threshold for cardiorespiratory fitness.

added by a youth fitness specialist because it is hard to distinguish training gains from those that occur naturally as a result of growth and maturation. In research, changes in performance with training would be compared with data from a control group, but this approach is not practical for youth fitness specialists. Instead, practitioners can consider an individual's long-term development against expected trends in the general population. For instance, based on the data in figure 6.9 and normative data provided by Ruiz et al. (2016), the child moves from a score around the 40th percentile for cardiorespiratory fitness at age 10 to the 60th percentile at age 15, although this change may derive partly from the timing of growth and maturation. It has also been shown that sprint speed and jump height improve at annual rates of just below 3 percent and 7 percent,

respectively, in 11- and 16-year-old boys (Williams et al., 2011). Programs that demonstrate consistent long-term gains above these levels may be considered to be promoting development over and above that which is expected through growth and maturity alone.

Assessing Physical Activity

Some debate has existed about whether it is more worthwhile to assess physical fitness or physical activity in children (e.g., Rowland, 1995). It has also been suggested that physical fitness and physical activity are partly related and should both be considered as part of any assessment—a philosophy shared by the Canadian Assessment of Physical Literacy (Lloyd et al., 2010) and the scientific advisory board of FitnessGram (Welk et al., 2013). Physical fitness is influ-

Teaching Tip

THREE KEY QUESTIONS WHEN INTERPRETING FITNESS SCORES

Youth fitness specialists can consider a number of key questions when interpreting a child's results: Does this represent a healthy fitness score? Is fitness developing as it should be? Are there any confounding factors that help explain the results? The primary goals for youth fitness specialists should be to enable youth to obtain a healthy level of fitness, improve their athleticism, and experience improvements in fitness over time. Where these goals are not achieved, practitioners should consider possible confounding factors, such as degree of maturation, level of physical activity, and lifestyle behaviors. For example, a girl who is going through puberty and naturally gaining fat mass may struggle to make gains in some measures of fitness, particularly where body mass has to be moved.

enced by a number of factors that lie beyond a child's control. Incorporating physical activity assessment allows children to learn that they have some control over their physical activity behavior and that their choices can influence their health (Welk, 2008). Youth who are physically active and demonstrate positive behaviors and awareness of the health benefits may be considered to be physically educated. Those who are inactive, have limited motivation to exercise, and possess only poor knowledge of the benefits of exercise can be identified as having exercise deficit disorder (Faigenbaum & Myer, 2012).

DO YOU KNOW?

Youth fitness specialists should be able to directly promote and influence physical activity behavior, which is more amenable to change than is fitness itself (Welk et al., 2013).

Assessing physical activity can be challenging given that youth are often involved in varied, spontaneous, and intermittent activity throughout the day. Sirad and Pate (2001) classified physical activity measurement into three categories:

1. Primary measures, including **indirect calorimetry** and direct observation
2. Secondary measures, such as heart rate and the use of accelerometers and pedometers
3. Subjective measures, such as self-reporting and interviews

Primary measures may be the most valid measures of physical activity; however, the money, resources, and expertise needed to use these techniques are prohibitive for most people, and their application may therefore be limited to research. Secondary measures are more accessible, but issues can arise with their sensitivity and ability to detect various types and intensities of physical activity. Self-report measures may be limited by perception bias, but subjectivity could also provide the advantage of enabling insight into individual responses to physical activity (Welk et al., 2013).

Table 6.5 presents advantages and disadvantages of the most prominent techniques for monitoring physical activity. One consideration involves the information to be captured. Youth fitness specialists should choose different tools for assessing different outcomes, such as whether a child is meeting physical activity guidelines or how well youth are maintaining a training regime. Understanding the strengths and limitations of various measures will help practitioners decide which tools are most useful in which conditions.

During direct observation, an observer codes the type and intensity of activity performed and captures information about behavior and environmental factors; this information is often processed with the assistance of software (McKenzie, 2002). Direct observation has been shown to have a stronger association with body fatness in children as compared with the indirect methods of heart rate monitoring and self-reporting (Rowlands et al., 2000). However, cost and time requirements make this type of assessment practical only for research (Welk et al., 2013). A simplified method for assessing levels of physical activity in a group or class setting is the System for Observing Play and Leisure Activities in Youth, or SOPLAY (McKenzie et al., 2006). With this system, the observer scans from left to right once per minute and records the number of children who are sedentary, walking, or very active. This approach allows the practitioner to gauge activity levels during, say, a group training session or physical education class.

Heart rate monitors, accelerometers, and pedometers can all be used to provide an assessment of physical activity. Each may also offer educational benefits, such as demonstrating the link between exercise and cardiovascular health (heart rate monitor) and showing how activity can be accumulated over a day or an even longer duration (accelerometer and pedometer). However, these methods also have their limitations, which are identified in table 6.5. A GPS device can also be used to provide a measure of physical activity, although this approach shares some of the disadvantages of using a heart rate monitor or accelerometer. In research where GPS has been used to assess children's physical activity, the measurements have been coupled with either heart rate (Duncan et al., 2009) or use of an accelerometer (Cooper et al., 2010).

A self-report is subjective and requires that the user be able to recall information and complete a report. Despite these limitations, the self-report is the most commonly used method for collecting information about physical activity. Its low cost, ease of use, and educational potential make this method well suited for use with large groups of children, providing that they possess the cognitive ability to complete the report accurately (Welk et al., 2013). A self-report may require a child to recall physical activity over a set period (e.g., a week), complete detailed activity logs over one or more days, or answer general questions about typical exercise behavior. Children generally find it easier to recall activity from a previous day rather than over a longer period of time.

Many questionnaires exist to allow youth to self-report their understanding of, and involvement in, physical activity. In a systematic review, Chinapaw and colleagues (2010) identified 61 versions of self-report questionnaires used to assess the physical activity of

TABLE 6.5   COMPARISON OF THE MOST COMMON METHODS FOR ASSESSING PHYSICAL ACTIVITY

Type of measure	Data collection	Outcomes captured	Other considerations
Direct observation	• Trained observers needed • Can only observe a few participants at a time • Time-consuming	• Can document both quantitative and qualitative results	
Heart rate monitor	• Time-consuming • Response lags behind movement • Influenced by age, maturation, and environmental factors	• Reliably measures physical activity • More applicable to aerobic activity	• Good educational opportunity • High cost
Accelerometer	• Time-consuming • Challenging to assess large numbers of participants	• Reliably measures physical activity • Cannot capture certain movements well (e.g., walking uphill, bicycling)	• Good educational opportunity • High cost
Pedometer	• Easy to use	• Only records quantity (volume) of movement • May not detect some movements • May detect some "false" movements	• Low cost
Self-report	Easy to administer to large groups Requires ability to objectively self-report	Can assess frequency, intensity, time, and type Potential reliability and validity issues	Good educational opportunity Low cost

Adapted from Welk and Wood (2000) and Welk, Mahar, and Morrow (2013).

children and adolescents. This range highlights the absence of an established gold standard questionnaire and the difficulty involved in comparing findings across studies. One example is FitnessGram, which provides the option for participants to complete the ActivityGram, in which physical activity from the previous day is recalled in 30-minute blocks. Specifically, activity is recorded for the whole day (from 7 a.m. to 11 p.m.), and the child indicates the predominant type of activity during each 30-minute block, as well as the intensity of the activity and whether it was done all, most, or some of the time during that block. Welk and colleagues (2004) previously showed ActivityGram to be a valid measure of physical activity in children. It has been suggested that ActivityGram can be used from age 9 upward but with improved accuracy for age 11 and above (Welk et al., 2013).

In another example, the ALPHA project supports the use of the Physical Activity Questionnaires for children and adolescents (PAQ-C and PAQ-A, respectively), which are nine- or eight-item questionnaires that ask individuals to rate how active they have been over the past seven days. The PAQ-C and PAQ-A were devel-

oped and validated in the late 1990s (Crocker et al., 1997; Kowalski, Crocker, & Faulkner, 1997; Kowalski, Crocker, & Kowalski, 1997) in studies suggesting that they had acceptable levels of reliability and moderate levels of validity. However, a similar questionnaire has recently been reported to be poorly related to direct measures of physical activity (Hagströmer et al., 2008). Even so, the use of the PAQ-C and PAQ-A has received support from experts in the field (Biddle et al., 2011).

In the CAPL, physical activity is measured by a combination of pedometer use and self-reporting. Participants complete a physical activity questionnaire, which includes 21 questions examining the amount of time spent being physically active versus being sedentary. The battery also assesses knowledge and understanding of physical activity, as well as motivation and confidence to engage in physical activity. Such questioning can provide the youth fitness specialist with useful information for understanding physical activity behaviors, but time restrictions may mean having to prioritize decisions about which questions to ask (and, similarly, which aspects of fitness to assess).

The general FitnessGram fitness test battery

includes three questions about physical activity behavior (Meridith & Welk, 2013):

1. *Aerobic activity.* On how many days in the past week have you participated in physical activity for a total of 30 to 60 minutes over the course of the day? This includes moderate activities (e.g., walking, slow bicycling, outdoor play) as well as vigorous activities (e.g., jogging; active games; and sports such as basketball, tennis, and soccer).

2. *Muscle strength and endurance.* On how many of the past seven days did you do exercises to strengthen or tone your muscles? This includes exercises such as push-ups, sit-ups, and weight-lifting.

3. *Flexibility.* On how many of the past seven days did you do stretching exercises to loosen or relax your muscles? This includes exercises such as toe touches, knee bending, and leg stretching.

Unfortunately, the test manuals (Meridith & Welk, 2013; Plowman & Merideth, 2013) do not provide detail about how answers to these questions are used to determine whether or not a child is sufficiently active; rather, this feedback is automatically generated by a software algorithm. However, answers to questions 1 and 2 could be compared with guidelines to determine whether a child is sufficiently active. It is suggested that children and young people aged 5 to 18 years should engage in moderate- to vigorous-intensity physical activity for at least 60 minutes every day and incorporate vigorous weight-bearing activities to strengthen muscle and bone on at least three days per week (World Health Organization, 2011).

The CAPL consists of four component parts designed to assess physical literacy (see figure 6.1 on page 105), and assessing each of these components requires considerable time. As shown in figure 6.10, a quick initial screening procedure has been developed by CAPL (2015) to identify children who may be struggling to develop physical literacy.

If a child indicates a score of 5 or more on the physical activity question, then further testing is probably not required. Those who score less than 5 move on to step 2 to be rated for movement competence. A child who achieves a rating of 3 or 4 probably does not require more in-depth assessment. A child who achieves a score of 1 or 2 would need more detailed assessment, which would include completing the entire CAPL screen of motor skills, physical fitness, physical activity behavior, and knowledge and understanding. Based on this approach, it is claimed that 90 percent of children who pass the test and 80 percent of children who do not pass the test will have been screened correctly (CAPL, 2015). This process demonstrates that youth fitness specialists may be able to use quick initial screening procedures to identify children who are most in need of additional support, which may be particularly useful in a large-group setting. There is some risk, however, of not correctly identifying all children who should be classified as having suboptimal physical literacy.

Summary

Assessment can provide youth fitness specialists with useful information for understanding how a child's fitness is developing. Careful consideration must be given to how assessment is undertaken and how results are used in order to make the process positive and worthwhile for youth. Practitioners should educate children about the benefits of assessment and ensure that assessment is delivered in a positive environment that motivates all children to perform well. Fitness assessment should be used to promote task mastery, and practitioners should provide appropriate physical activity opportunities to allow children to experience improvement in fitness over time.

Movement skills are fundamental to developing the ability to engage in physical activity. Therefore, it is recommended that youth fitness specialists assess movement skills in order to understand whether a child has the competence to be active. Various methods are available for screening movement competence, and practitioners should choose the method that is most appropriate for their situation in terms of available time and resources and the needs of the child. Existing batteries for monitoring health-related fitness include ALPHA-FIT, EUROFIT, FitnessGram, and the Canadian Assessment of Physical Literacy. Evidence of test reliability and validity has been provided, and supporting material is available to help with test administration and data interpretation.

Although health- and skill-related fitness are often considered independently, many components overlap, and a single battery has been presented that would allow simultaneous measurement of both health- and skill-related fitness (see table 6.4). Rather than considering fitness test scores only at a single moment in time or in reference to standards, practitioners should take a long-term view and use assessment to understand how fitness is developing over time. Measurement of physical activity behavior can also provide both the practitioner and the child with an appreciation of how lifestyle, growth, and development influence movement competence and physical fitness, and vice versa.

FIGURE 6.10   CANADIAN ASSESSMENT OF PHYSICAL LITERACY INITIAL SCREENING TEST

Step 1: Physical Activity Question

Compared with other kids your age, how active are you?

A lot less active   Same   A lot more active

| 1 | 2 | 3 | 4 | 5 | 6 | 7 | 8 | 9 | 10 |

Step 2: Movement Competence Test

Run forward seven meters and then backward seven meters between two cones.

Rating 1

- Stumbles, trips, or slips.
- Transitions are not smooth.
- Movement is disjointed.
- Steps over the line at the cone.
- Runs slowly.

Rating 2

- Arms and legs are not always in sync.
- Stops by sliding or shuffling.
- Makes a long stop at the cone.

Rating 3

- Runs in a straight line.
- Maintains good speed (jog or run).
- Running backward is not as good as running forward.
- Uses mature running form.

Rating 4

- Sprints to cone
- Accelerates rapidly
- Decelerates at cone
- Runs backward efficiently, turns head to face direction of movement
- Arms and legs are used purposely

Adapted from CAPL (2013).

CHAPTER 7

Dynamic Warm-Up and Flexibility

CHAPTER OBJECTIVES

- Differentiate between dynamic warm-up procedures and preevent static stretching
- Explain the physiological and psychological benefits of warming up
- Discuss the effects of different types of flexibility training on fitness performance
- Provide an overview of dynamic warm-up procedures for children and adolescents
- Design a dynamic warm-up for children and adolescents

KEY TERMS

active warm-up (p. 129)

autogenic inhibition (p. 145)

ballistic stretching (p. 131)

dynamic stretching (p. 131)

dynamic warm-up (p. 128)

flexibility training (p. 128)

general warm-up (p. 129)

mobility (p. 128)

passive warm-up (p. 129)

postactivation potentiation (p. 130)

proprioceptive neuromuscular facilitation (p. 141)

reciprocal inhibition (p. 145)

specific warm-up (p. 129)

static stretching (p. 128)

Introduction

A dynamic warm-up can prepare children and adolescents both physically and mentally for the demands of exercise and sport. In addition to elevating oxygen uptake kinetics, increasing muscle temperature, and improving joint range of motion, a dynamic warm-up can boost fitness performance and reduce injury risk by enhancing motor unit excitability, improving kinesthetic awareness, and maximizing strength and power (Behm, Blazevich, Kay, & McHugh, 2016; Emery, Roy, Whittaker, Nettel-Aguirre, & van Mechelen, 2015; McGowan, Pyne, Thompson, & Rattray, 2015). A **dynamic warm-up** involves a series of preparatory activities and whole-body movements that are purposely designed to prepare the body for exercise and sport (Faigenbaum, 2012; Jeffreys, 2007). Instead of focusing on individual muscles, a dynamic warm-up consists of low-, moderate-, and higher-intensity exercises that emphasize specific movement patterns. Moreover, a well-designed dynamic warm-up can set the desired tone for upcoming activities and establish an upbeat tempo for practice and games. Youth fitness specialists should consider a dynamic warm-up to be an integral part of every exercise class or sport event.

It is important to distinguish a dynamic warm-up from **static stretching** activities. Static stretching is a type of **flexibility training** that is used to increase joint range of motion by slowly lengthening a muscle to an elongated position and then holding this position for a predetermined period of time (e.g., 10 to 30 sec) (Apostolopoulos, Metsios, Flouris, Koutedakis, & Wyon, 2015; Sands & McNeal, 2014). Although preevent static stretching is a common practice in some sport programs (Popp et al., 2017; Slauterbeck et al., 2017), the potential benefits of this type of warm-up for fitness performance, injury risk reduction, and muscle soreness have been questioned (Behm et al., 2016; Hammami, Zois, Slimani, Russel, & Bouhlel, 2018; Laursen, Bertelsen, & Andersen, 2014; Simic, Sarabon, & Markovic, 2013). At present, there is little scientific evidence that a bout of preevent static stretching enhances anaerobic performance in school-age youth or prevents sport-related injuries in young athletes (Emery et al., 2015; Laursen et al., 2014; Sugimoto, Myer, Barber Foss, & Hewett, 2015). Thus the distinctions between dynamic warm-up protocols and preevent static stretching are important due to their apparently different effects on fitness performance and injury risk reduction.

DO YOU KNOW?

The most flexible child is not always the most athletic.

Notwithstanding the desired effects of flexibility training on joint range of motion, it is advantageous to perform dynamic activities rather than static stretching alone immediately before exercise and sport (Behm et al., 2016; McCrary, Ackermann, & Halaki, 2015; McGowan et al., 2015). Although a few minutes of low-intensity aerobic exercise can increase heart rate, blood flow, and body temperature (as evidenced by the onset of sweating), a well-designed series of dynamic warm-up exercises can also "turn on" the neuromuscular system and maximize active ranges of motion. That is to say, dynamic movements such as lunge patterns, squatting, and twisting focus on activating and mobilizing key muscle groups and joint structures. The concept of **mobility** refers to moving freely and effectively through an uninhibited range of motion with adequate flexibility, stability, and motor control (Jeffreys, 2007; Sands & McNeal, 2014). Although mobility is influenced by flexibility, these concepts are not synonymous, because the fluidity of movement patterns is also influenced by other factors, including strength, balance, and coordination.

Youth fitness specialists should understand the acute and chronic effects of different warm-up procedures on performance. They should also be knowledgeable of program design considerations for developing warm-up protocols that enhance the physical and psychological preparedness of youth for exercise and sport. Since age- and sex-associated changes in

Teaching Tip

TIME MANAGEMENT

Although most warm-ups last only 10 or 15 minutes, the cumulative effects of dynamic warm-up protocols can result in positive changes in performance. If children perform a dynamic warm-up on four or five days per week, before every exercise session or sport practice, they can accumulate an additional hour or so of weekly training that is designed to target neuromuscular deficits and reinforce desirable movement patterns. Thus a dynamic warm-up can be a time-efficient method for enhancing fitness performance and reducing sport-related injuries in youth.

flexibility are observable during the growing years (Malina, Bouchard, & Bar-Or, 2004), it is important to appreciate the unique benefits of different warm-up procedures and stretching techniques for children and adolescents. In addition, practitioners should not overlook the long-term benefits of well-designed warm-ups for injury risk, motor skill development, and fitness performance (Richmond, Kang, Doyle-Baker, Nettel-Aguirre, & Emery, 2016; Rössler, Donath, Bizzini, & Faude, 2016; Zarei et al., 2018).

Types of Warm-Ups

Warm-ups can be broadly categorized as either active or passive. An **active warm-up** involves exercises and movement patterns that increase body temperature, blood flow, heart rate, and respiration rate. The two types of active warm-ups are general and specific. A **general warm-up** involves several minutes of low-intensity aerobic exercise, such as slow jogging, whereas a **specific warm-up** consists of movement patterns that are similar to the upcoming sport or activity (Ratamess, 2012). In contrast, **passive warm-up** techniques (e.g., hot shower, sauna, or heat application) may increase body temperature without increasing metabolic demands, but this type of warm-up by itself may not be practical or optimal for activating the neuromuscular system, developing fundamental movement skills, or enhancing physical fitness in youth (Brunner-Ziegler, Strasser, & Haber, 2011; McGowan et al., 2015). Using passive techniques such as heated garments during the transition phase between the completion of the warm-up and the start of a sporting event may attenuate the decline in body temperature (Russell et al., 2015; Silva et al., 2018). Notably, postwarm-up performance in children and adolescents who are not involved in competitive sport may also be influenced by the design, progression, and intensity of the warm-up protocol.

Broadly speaking, active warm-ups that include general and specific exercises may last 10 to 15 minutes, but the specific exercises and movement patterns may vary considerably depending on participants' needs, goals, and physical abilities. Therefore, youth fitness specialists need to carefully consider the design and structure of active warm-up protocols in order to optimize both short-term and long-term training outcomes. A dynamic warm-up is a type of active warm-up that consists of specific exercises chosen to prepare participants for the demands of the upcoming activities. The physiological and psychological responses to a dynamic warm-up are shown in figure 7.1 (McGowan et al., 2015; Ratamess, 2012). A well-designed dynamic warm-up can improve performance and enhance psychological readiness to perform—if it allows participants to begin the subsequent task in an "activated" but relatively unfatigued state (Behm & Chaouachi, 2011; Faigenbaum et al., 2010; Faigenbaum, McFarland, et al., 2006).

One way to develop effective dynamic warm-up activities is to use a novel conception referred to as the RAMP approach (Jeffreys, 2007). As reflected in the acronymic name, the key elements of a RAMP protocol are to raise body temperature, activate the neuromuscular system, mobilize joints, and potentiate the neuromuscular system (Jeffreys, 2007; Jeffreys, 2019). Practitioners should extend the acronym to RAMPED by focusing also on engaging all participants and developing movement skills. Because adherence to any intervention will influence training outcomes, practitioners need to deliver technique-driven progression and enthusiastic instruction in order to keep the warm-up challenging and the young participants engaged as they gain competence and confidence in their physical abilities. Thus, a RAMPED approach to warming up reinforces important elements of youth fitness programming, which include having fun with friends and learning something new (see figure 7.2).

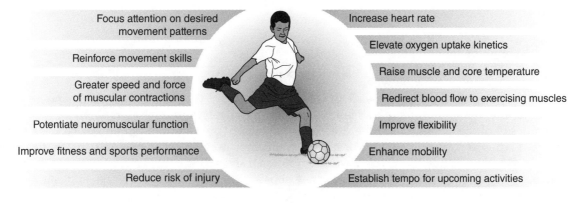

FIGURE 7.1   Potential benefits of warming up for children and adolescents.

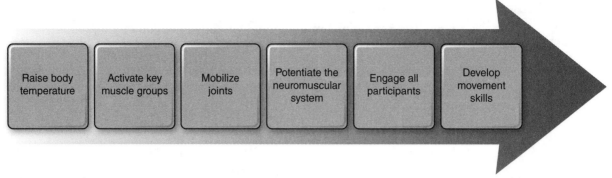

FIGURE 7.2   The RAMPED warm-up continuum.
Adapted from Jeffreys (2007).

A warm-up can be viewed as a continuum that begins with lower-intensity exercises to raise body temperature and progresses to higher-intensity dynamic movements designed to potentiate the body by increasing the strength of nerve impulses and optimizing force and power production (Jeffreys, 2007). The concept of potentiation refers to an enhanced state of muscle functioning that occurs shortly after a well-designed dynamic warm-up (Ratamess, 2012). Hence, the term **postactivation potentiation** is often used to describe the acute enhancement of muscle function as a direct result of its contractile history (i.e., previous contractions) (Robbins, 2006; Seitz & Haff, 2016; Wilson et al., 2013). This approach to designing warm-up protocols can enhance performance in children and adolescents provided that the cumulative effects of fatigue are minimized (Allen, Hannon, Burns, & Williams, 2014; Ayala et al., 2016; Faigenbaum, Bellucci, Bernieri, Bakker, & Hoorens, 2005; Faigenbaum et al., 2010; Faigenbaum, McFarland, et al., 2006; Needham, Morse, & Degens, 2009). As a result, critical factors in the design of dynamic warm-up protocols include the intensity and duration of the warm-up exercises, as well as the length of the recovery interval between the warm-up and the start of the training session or sport competition.

Dynamic Warm-Up and Performance

Dynamic warm-up protocols that include movement patterns typical of sport and daily life are becoming more popular in youth fitness and athletic development programs. Research in the fields of exercise science and sports medicine continue to highlight the potential benefits of well-designed dynamic warm-up protocols for fitness performance and sport-injury reduction (Behm et al., 2016; Emery et al., 2015; Silva, Neiva, Marques, Izquierdo, & Marinho, 2018; Rössler, et al., 2018; Zarei et al., 2018). High adherence to warm-up protocols that include dynamic movements has been found to enhance functional performance, decrease the risk of sport-related injury, and reduce health-care costs in young athletes (LaBella et al., 2011; Rössler, et al., 2019; Steffen et al., 2013; Sugimoto et al., 2015; Waldén, Atroshi, Magnusson, Wagner, & Hägglund, 2012; Zebis et al., 2016). These findings highlight the importance of introducing school-age youth to dynamic warm-up protocols early in life so that they can develop favorable movement patterns and learn to appreciate the importance of a proper warm-up before bad habits develop and become more difficult to address later in life.

Teaching Tip

JUMP START

A dynamic warm-up satisfies the need for youth to be active at the start of the session and helps to focus their attention on listening, learning, and receiving task-relevant coaching cues. By manipulating the intensity of the activities and the duration of the warm-up period, practitioners can use many different types of dynamic warm-up protocols to enhance performance while keeping participants active and engaged. The design of a warm-up protocol should be influenced by the training experience of the participants and the nature of the subsequent activity (e.g., physical education class, sport competition).

Elements of a Dynamic Warm-Up

A dynamic warm-up typically includes a series of movements at low, moderate, and high intensity that are designed to increase core temperature, enhance motor unit excitability, develop kinesthetic awareness, and maximize active ranges of motion. Instead of slowly stretching individual muscles or muscle groups, a dynamic warm-up emphasizes various movement patterns and muscle actions. As a result, it is often referred to as **dynamic stretching**. This type of movement preparation involves actively moving through a full range of motion without relaxation or holding of body positions (Behm et al., 2016; Ratamess, 2012). Although static stretching and proprioceptive neuromuscular facilitation stretching (discussed later in this chapter) provide a stimulus to chronically increase range of motion (ROM) around a joint or series of joints, youth fitness specialists often incorporate dynamic stretching into well-designed warm-ups in order to acutely increase ROM. Dynamic stretches can be performed either while standing in place (e.g., forward and backward arm circles) or in a series covering a specific distance (e.g., walking lunges). Table 7.1 outlines several static and dynamic stretches for the upper body, trunk, and lower body.

Dynamic stretching does not involve the rapid or bouncing movements that are characteristic of **ballistic stretching**; instead, it uses controlled elongations of selected muscle groups. A traditional concern associated with ballistic stretching is that it could invoke the myotatic stretch reflex and consequent muscle contraction (Sands & McNeal, 2014). Although preevent ballistic stretching has been found to improve jumping and sprinting performance in adults (Maloney, Turner, & Fletcher, 2014), only limited data are available regarding the effects of ballistic stretching on youth. The results from one study found that a preevent warm-up that included ballistic stretching was not optimal for enhancing dart-throwing accuracy in school-age boys (Frikha et al., 2016).

During a dynamic stretch, the muscles are actively stretched to a new range of motion as the desired action is performed in a controlled and purposeful manner. For example, during a walking lunge the muscles are actively engaged as the participant lengthens each stride and maintains proper body control throughout the exercise. Although different dynamic stretches and movement patterns can be incorporated into a dynamic warm-up, it is best practice to progress from dynamic movements that are less intense to more intense activities or small-sided games that resemble upcoming fitness exercises and sport activities. Throughout the warm-up period, youth fitness specialists should emphasize proper technique in order to reinforce appropriate movement patterns and optimize skill development.

DO YOU KNOW?

Dynamic stretching offers the time-saving advantage of warming up several muscle groups simultaneously.

The choice of warm-up exercises and movement patterns should be consistent with participants' needs and abilities because preevent protocols that are too challenging or fatiguing will result in suboptimal performance. Although higher-intensity movements are needed in order to "turn on" the neuromuscular system and optimize performance (Rassier & MacIntosh, 2000; Tillin & Bishop, 2009), practitioners must also attend to the recovery interval between the end of the dynamic warm-up and the start of the exercise or sport session (Abade et al., 2017; Faigenbaum et al., 2010). If the recovery interval is too short, the lingering effects of fatigue will adversely affect subsequent performance; if, on the other hand, the recovery interval is too long, the potentiating effects of the dynamic warm-up will begin to disappear. In addition, youth fitness specialists may need to modify warm-up procedures when children and adolescents exercise in hot and humid conditions in order to avoid thermal intolerance and adverse consequences (Bergeron et al., 2015). In this case, the warm-up not only provides an opportunity to monitor performance and assess skill technique but also time to look for signs or symptoms of exertional heat illness, which may include weakness, dizziness, and decreased muscle coordination (American College of Sports Medicine, 2018).

Different types of dynamic warm-ups can be used to create an optimal environment for exercise and sport. As noted earlier, a well-designed dynamic warm-up can result in a phenomenon called postactivation potentiation (PAP), which can enhance subsequent muscle performance (Robbins, 2006; Seitz & Haff, 2016; Wilson et al., 2013). Although additional research is needed to determine the precise mechanisms of PAP in youth, this potentiation phase of the warm-up is grounded in the fact that the response of skeletal muscle to the demands placed on it is influenced by its contractile history (Robbins, 2006). Proposed neuromuscular mechanisms of PAP include enhanced central output to motor neurons, increased synaptic excitation within the spinal cord, and increased phosphorylation of myosin regulatory light chains within the muscle, all of which can increase muscle force and rate of force development in the involved muscle groups (Lorenz, 2011; McGowan et al., 2015).

TABLE 7.1   EXAMPLES OF STATIC AND DYNAMIC STRETCHES

Target zone	Static		Dynamic	
Upper body	Standing chest stretch		Arm circle	
	Shoulder stretch		Shoulder circle	
	Triceps stretch		Arm swing	
	Kneeling forearm stretch		Wrist circle	

Target zone	Static		Dynamic	
Trunk	Side bend		Medicine ball rotation	
	Standing rotation		Medicine ball diagonal chop	
	Knee to chest		Sitting T-spine rotation	
	Figure-four stretch		Walking lunge with rotation	

(continued)

TABLE 7.1 (CONTINUED)

Target zone	Static		Dynamic	
Lower body	Quadriceps stretch		Standing lunge	
	Hamstring stretch		Inchworm	
	Butterfly stretch		Forward crawl	
	Wall calf stretch		Bunny hop	

DO YOU KNOW?

The potentiating effects of dynamic exercises, such as squat jumps and plyometric push-ups, may persist for several minutes if the movements are performed explosively.

A series of progressive dynamic warm-up exercises (e.g., moderate- and high-intensity jumping, throwing, squatting, and sprinting) can enhance the overall effectiveness of the warm-up, whereas continued stimulation without adequate recovery can impair performance. Because potentiation and fatigue can coexist in skeletal muscle during the warm-up period and for some time afterward, there seems to be an optimal time when the body has recovered from the PAP stimulus but is still potentiated (Bazett-Jones, Winchester, & McBride, 2005; Faigenbaum et al., 2010; Kilduff et al., 2007). Youth fitness specialists must be aware of the interaction between PAP and fatigue when designing and implementing dynamic warm-up protocols, because the net difference between these two phenomena will influence the outcome of the preevent protocol (Wilson et al., 2013).

Although it is important to carefully consider the choice of warm-up activities and the recovery interval, youth fitness specialists should also consider the training experience of the participants. Data gathered on adults suggest that stronger individuals tend to perform better after shorter rest intervals, whereas weaker participants may need longer rest intervals (Seitz & Haff, 2016). These findings suggest that the level of potentiation may depend on the intensity and design of the preevent stimulus, the length of the transition period, and the training experience of the participants. Thus practitioners need to consider many factors when designing dynamic warm-up protocols for youth with different needs, goals, and abilities.

Designing a Dynamic Warm-Up

A dynamic warm-up typically takes less than 15 minutes and should include a variety of exercises for strength, power, speed, and balance that are sensibly progressive over time. Not only does this approach make efficient use of time, but it can also enhance compliance and promote the development of proper technique, because exercises are performed in a less-fatigued state. As noted earlier, an effective dynamic warm-up can be developed using the RAMPED framework. This approach includes three key phases of an effective warm-up—(1) raise, (2) activate and mobilize, and (3) potentiate (Jeffreys, 2007; Jeffreys, 2019)—and subsequent performance and adherence can be further enhanced by also engaging all participants and developing movement skills as part of the process.

If a warm-up is slow and monotonous, then the performance that follows may fall short of what is desired. But if youth fitness specialists develop time-efficient warm-ups that are dynamic, diverse, and engaging, then performance during the exercise class or sport practice is likely to meet or exceed expectations. For instance, a dynamic warm-up of body-weight calisthenics, medicine ball exercises, mini-band routines, footwork patterns, and sprint drills can set the pace for the upcoming activities and make a valuable contribution to the overall conditioning process. In addition, most youth enjoy dynamic warm-ups because task-oriented movement skills require participants to think about what they are doing and how they are moving.

One fundamental principle of dynamic warm-ups involves a focus on performing large-muscle-group activities. Participants can perform different movements in place for a certain number of repetitions (e.g., 8 to 12 repetitions of a body-weight squat) or cover a predetermined distance (e.g., walking knee grabs for 10-20 m). Although six to eight patterns may be

Teaching Tip

HALFTIME STRATEGIES

Most team sports use a halftime break of 10 to 20 minutes. During this period, young athletes typically rehydrate, address injury concerns, and receive feedback from coaches about game tactics and strategies. Yet the passive nature of halftime breaks has been found to adversely affect performance in elite adult athletes (Edholm, Krustrup, & Randers, 2014; Silva et al., 2018), and similar effects have been observed in younger athletes (Abade et al., 2017). Therefore, strategies are needed to maintain body temperature and "prime" the neuromuscular system for the second half. To this end, and notwithstanding the importance of player–coach interactions during the halftime break, a dynamic re-warm-up lasting about 5 minutes should be a routine part of halftime procedures.

appropriate for beginners, more advanced participants may benefit from additional exercises progressing from relatively simple movements to more complex exercises relevant to the movement patterns that will be performed during training or competition.

In addition to calisthenics and body-weight movements, a warm-up protocol for children and adolescents can incorporate exercises that use elastic bands, medicine balls, and weighted vests (Faigenbaum & McFarland, 2007; Faigenbaum, McFarland, et al., 2006; Mediate & Faigenbaum, 2007). These exercise modalities not only add variety to the preevent stimulus but also can be used to activate, mobilize, and potentiate key body zones. Medicine balls are available in a variety of sizes, and exercises that use them can be performed in various movement patterns to address specific body zones. For example, warm-up exercises such as the medicine ball diagonal chop can be used to activate the upper body, torso, and lower body (see figure 7.3). Participants can start with a 1-kilogram (2.2 lb) medicine ball over the right shoulder, lower the body into the squat position as the ball is pulled toward the left ankle, and then stand back up while pulling the ball back over the right shoulder. The movements should be performed forcefully but with control for the desired number of repetitions on each side.

Medicine balls provide a unique type of unguided resistance that can be used for any number of beginner and advanced warm-up exercises performed at differ-ent movement speeds (Mediate & Faigenbaum, 2007). For example, youth can perform a series of movements with a medicine ball that involve pressing, twisting, rolling, catching, squatting, and lunging. When participants are able to perform body-weight movements properly, practitioners can ensure progressive overload by sensibly incorporating exercises with light external loads into the routine. For instance, performing a walking lunge while moving a medicine ball in different rotational and diagonal movement patterns can be a challenging activity that requires participants to control their center of gravity. Likewise, a medicine ball squat toss can be used to turn on the neuromuscular system and engage more advanced participants as they interact with each other (see figure 7.4). In fact, medicine balls are so versatile that they can be used to replicate an unlimited number of movement patterns and sport actions.

If a dynamic warm-up is consistent with the skill level and fitness background of the participants, then this type of preevent stimulus can contribute to motor skill development and general conditioning in a time-efficient manner (Richmond et al., 2016; Rössler et al., 2016; Steffen et al., 2013; Zebis et al., 2016). During the performance of dynamic movements, the muscles not only lengthen but also contract and move through a new range of motion. This type of movement-based training can provide an opportunity for participants to develop kinesthetic awareness, maximize active

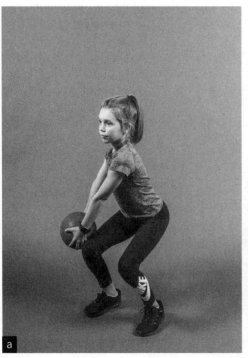
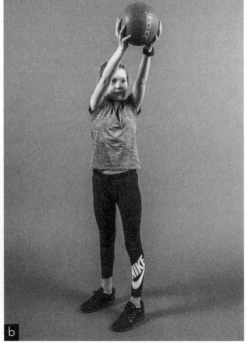

FIGURE 7.3   Medicine ball diagonal chop.

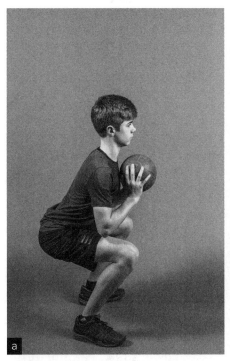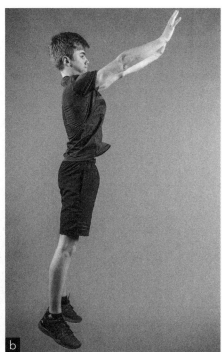

FIGURE 7.4   Medicine ball squat toss.

ranges of motion, and gain competence and confidence in their ability to perform a variety of movement skills.

Due to the established efficacy of injury prevention strategies in youth sport, researchers and practitioners have purposely designed structured warm-up programs to reduce sport-related injuries and enhance performance in young athletes (Foss, Thomas, Khoury, Myer, & Hewett, 2018; Olsen, Myklebust, & Engebretsen, 2005; Owoeye, Akinbo, Tella, & Olawale, 2014; Rössler et al., 2016; Rössler et al., 2018; Sakata et al., 2018; Waldén et al., 2012). The incidence of injury in youth sport can be reduced by targeting neuromuscular deficits with well-designed interventions. In one study that included nearly 1,900 females athletes (13 to 17 years of age), researchers reported that the risk of injury could be reduced by about one-third and severe injuries by one-half through regular participation in dynamic warm-ups that included running, strength, balance, and jumping exercises (Soligard et al., 2008). Others found that neuromuscular training prevented injury in school-age basketball and volleyball players and that the greater protective effect related to knee injuries in the younger athletes (Foss et al., 2018). The FIFA 11+ kids program has been found to enhance physical performance in youth (Rössler et al., 2016; Zarei et al., 2018), and these improvements may also contribute to a reduction in injury risk if the program is implemented correctly (Silvers-Granelli, Bizzini, Arundale, Mandelbaum, & Snyder-Mackler, 2017; Rössler

et al., 2018). Collectively, these observations highlight the importance of incorporating dynamic warm-ups into youth programs and designing integrative and progressive protocols that target neuromuscular deficiencies.

Youth fitness specialists may need to modify established dynamic warm-up protocols to add variety, generate progression, and address the individual needs of participants (O'Brien, Young, & Finch, 2016). High interest and adherence to dynamic warm-up protocols are needed in order to enhance performance and reduce injury risk (Hägglund, Atroshi, Wagner, & Waldén, 2013; Steffen et al., 2013). Therefore, concerted efforts are needed to develop child-friendly versions of adult warm-up strategies in ways that are fun, engaging, and challenging while also consistent with the ever-changing needs, abilities, and interests of youth (Keats, Emery, & Finch, 2012; Kilding, Tunstall, & Kuzmic, 2008; Rössler et al., 2016). Long-term adherence may be enhanced by varying warm-up activities, sensibly progressing exercises, and incorporating games and activities into the routine. For example, young children may enjoy a dynamic warm-up full of animal games and activities that include bunny hops, crab walks, and bear crawls (Faigenbaum & Bruno, 2017).

Continuing education during academic courses and coaching workshops may help youth fitness specialists improve delivery, enhance adherence, and ensure that evidence-based injury prevention guidelines are followed (Steffen et al., 2013). Although further study is warranted, youth fitness programs that are delivered early in life (e.g., during primary school) may be the ideal time to optimize reduction of injury risk while reinforcing the importance of warming up by integrating developmentally appropriate activities (Myer, Sugimoto, Thomas, & Hewett, 2013). Regardless of age or athletic ability, however, practitioners need to provide feedback about proper exercise technique so that participants can learn and practice the appropriate movement patterns while gaining competence and confidence in their physical abilities.

DO YOU KNOW?

A well-designed dynamic warm-up is a time-efficient strategy for enhancing performance and reducing injury-related health care costs in children and adolescents.

Whereas youth in a fitness class may perform a series of dynamic exercises for the upper body, lower body, and trunk, young athletes could progress from lunges to power skips and sprint drills in order to be better prepared to perform at maximal levels during sport practice and competition. For example, incorporating plyometric jumps and power exercises with medicine balls during the latter part of the warm-up could ensure that youth are physically and mentally prepared for an upcoming training session. With this possibility in mind, the sample dynamic warm-up protocols outlined in tables 7.2 and 7.3, respectively, should be viewed as general guides to help youth fitness spe-

cialists design warm-up protocols for beginners and participants with higher levels of training. Progression should be based first on technical skill competence, then on the intensity of the subsequent exercise or sport session. Thus, regardless of chronological age or maturity status, inactive children or adolescents should start with the beginner program.

Flexibility and Performance

Flexibility refers to the range of motion about a joint or series of joints and is recognized as a health-related fitness component in youth exercise programs (National Association for Sport and Physical Education, 2011). Although optimal levels of flexibility allow the body to move freely and are important for sports and activities such as dance, gymnastics, and the martial arts, adequate levels of strength and motor control are also needed in order to efficiently move a joint or series of joints at a desired speed and in a given direction for a particular movement. Thus extreme levels of flexibility without sufficient strength and mobility are unnecessary and potentially harmful. Furthermore, evidence is limited for a direct association between flexibility and sport performance outcomes in young athletes (Geladas, Nassis, & Pavlicevic, 2005; Stodden, Fleisig, McLean, Lyman, & Andrews, 2001).

Flexibility during childhood and adolescence is determined by a number of factors, including age (flexibility tends to decrease during the growing years), sex (girls tend to be more flexible than boys), genetics, joint structure, muscular imbalances, and activity level

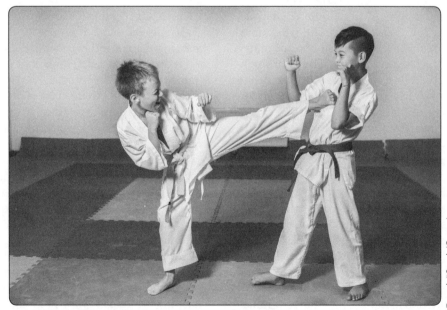

Adequate levels of strength, motor control, and flexibility are needed in order to perform complex movements efficiently.

7stock/iStock/Getty Images

TABLE 7.2   SAMPLE 15-MINUTE RAMP WARM-UP FOR BEGINNERS

Phase	Exercise	Volume (sets × time/distance/reps)	Intensity	Time	Total phase time
Raise	Stuck in the mud	3 × 30 sec	Body weight	120 sec	4 min
	Bear crawl tag	3 × 20 sec	Body weight	120 sec	
Activate and mobilize	Single-leg T-balance	2 × 10 reps (5 each leg)	Body weight	60 sec	9 min
	Squat with arms overhead	2 × 10 reps	Body weight	60 sec	

(continued)

TABLE 7.2   (CONTINUED)

Phase	Exercise		Volume (sets × time/ distance/reps)	Intensity	Time	Total phase time
Activate and mobilize (continued)	Walking lunge		2 × 10 m	Body weight	90 sec	
	Inchworm		2 × 10 m	Body weight	60 sec	
	Glute bridge		2 × 10 reps	Body weight	90 sec	
	Medicine ball rotation		2 × 10 reps (5 each side)	1-2 kg (2.2-4.4 lb)	90 sec	

Phase	Exercise	Volume (sets × time/ distance/reps)	Intensity	Time	Total phase time
Activate and mobilize (continued)	Medicine ball diagonal chop	2 × 10 reps (5 each direction)	1-2 kg (2.2-4.4 lb)	90 sec	
Potentiate	Squat jump	2 × 5 reps	Body weight	2 min	2 min

(Malina et al., 2004; Sands & McNeal, 2014). Youth fitness specialists should consider these factors when designing youth exercise programs. Children tend to enjoy stretching exercises because improvements in flexibility occur rapidly, but the reduction of flexibility due to structural changes with increasing age (and growth) can increase stiffness (Sands & McNeal, 2014). Therefore, childhood may be an opportune time to enhance flexibility, whereas adolescence may be a time to focus on maintaining it.

Various stretching methods can be used to modify musculoskeletal stiffness and improve the ability to move through a range of motion. Static stretching is characterized by slow and controlled stretching of target muscle groups (American College of Sports Medicine, 2018; Medeiros, Cini, Sbruzzi, & Lima, 2016). Youth should stretch until mild tension is felt in the target area; stretching to the point of pain means that the movement has gone too far. Static stretching is most effective when muscle temperature is increased through general warm-up activities such as slow jogging (Garber et al., 2011). Static stretching should be performed at least twice per week, although more frequent training sessions with additional stretching exercises may be more effective for children and adolescents (Kamandulis, Emeljanovas, & Skurvydas, 2013; Santonja Medina, Sainz De Baranda Andújar,

Rodríguez García, López Miñarro, & Canteras Jordana, 2007). In some cases, daily stretching may be needed in order to maintain training-induced improvements in flexibility. General guidelines for static stretching are outlined in figure 7.5 on page 144.

DO YOU KNOW?

Children can enhance flexibility faster than adolescents and adults.

Another stretching technique to enhance range of motion is **proprioceptive neuromuscular facilitation** (PNF). Although PNF stretching was first used as a therapeutic aid to treat neuromuscular dysfunction, it is now used by athletes to enhance functional ROM (Akbulut & Agopyan, 2015; Dallas et al., 2014). A variety of PNF protocols exist, and one common approach is the contract–relax (or active assisted) method (Hindle, Whitcomb, Briggs, & Hong, 2012). This technique involves placing a muscle in a static stretched position, then, after about 10 seconds, contracting the target muscle isometrically for about 6 seconds against a fixed object. Following a short recovery of 1 or 2 seconds, another passive stretch is performed, potentially at an increased range of motion.

TABLE 7.3   SAMPLE 15-MINUTE RAMP WARM-UP FOR MORE ADVANCED YOUTH

Phase	Exercise	Volume (sets × time/ distance/reps)	Intensity	Time	Total phase time
Raise	Jump-rope skipping	2 × 30 sec	Body weight	90 sec	4 min
	Pogo hop	3 × 10 m	Body weight	90 sec	
Activate and mobilize	Four-point grid hop and stick	4 × 2 circuits (2 each leg)	Body weight	60 sec	4 min
	Walking lunge to knee lift	2 × 10 m	Body weight	60 sec	

Phase	Exercise			Volume (sets × time/ distance/reps)	Intensity	Time	Total phase time
Activate and mobilize (continued)	Reverse lunge			2 × 10 m	Body weight	90 sec	
	Overhead dowel squat			2 × 10 reps	Body weight	60 sec	
	Single-leg glute bridge			2 × 10 (5 each leg)	Body weight	90 sec	
	Medicine ball squat toss			2 × 5 reps	2-10 kg (4.4-22 lb)	90 sec	

(continued)

TABLE 7.3   (CONTINUED)

Phase	Exercise	Volume (sets × time/ distance/reps)	Intensity	Time	Total phase time
Activate and mobilize (continued)	T-spine windmill 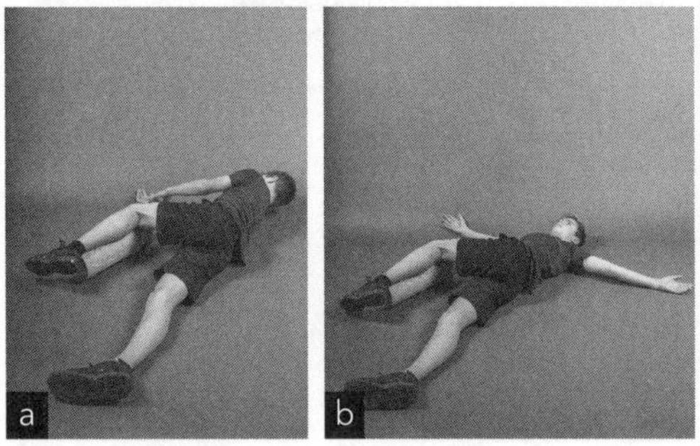 	2 × 10 reps (each side)	Body weight	90 sec	
Potentiate	Countermovement jump to box 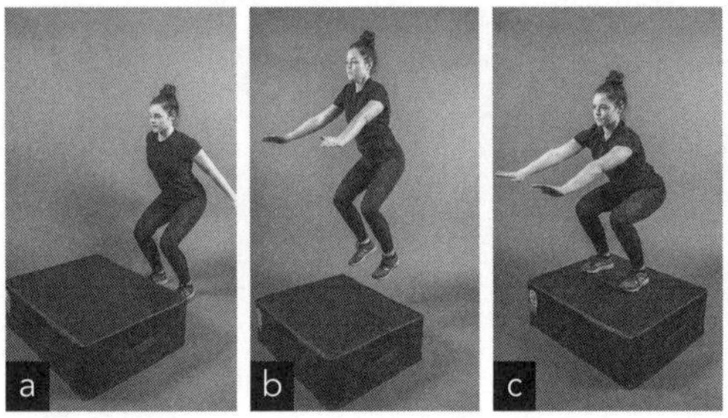 	3 × 3 reps	Body weight	3 min	3 min

---

FIGURE 7.5   YOUTH STATIC STRETCHING GUIDELINES

1. Static stretching should be preceded by at least 5 minutes of general aerobic activity.
2. Perform each stretch in a slow and controlled manner and avoid bouncing or jerking.
3. Stretch to the point of mild muscle tightness, then back off slightly. Breathe normally.
4. Hold each stretch for 10 to 30 seconds, relax briefly, and then repeat 2 to 4 times.
5. Stretch all major muscle groups.
6. Stretch at least twice per week, preferably on most days of the week.
7. It may be ideal to perform static stretches during the cool-down period.

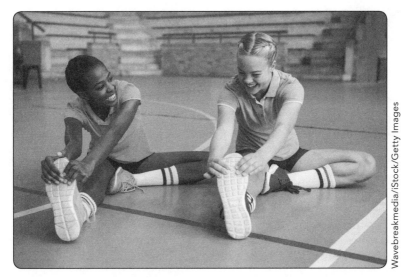

Static stretching should be preceded by at least 5 minutes of general aerobic activity.

Although PNF stretching may enhance a participant's stretch tolerance, any increase in ROM following PNF results largely from neuromuscular mechanisms, including **autogenic inhibition** and **reciprocal inhibition** (Hindle et al., 2012; Ratamess, 2012). Autogenic inhibition involves reflex relaxation in an agonist muscle group following a muscle contraction, whereas reciprocal inhibition involves relaxation in an antagonist muscle group from contracting the agonist muscle group. For example, autogenic inhibition can occur during a PNF hamstring stretch when the target muscle exerts a maximal isometric contraction. This type of muscle action stimulates the Golgi tendon organ (GTO), which subsequently protects the hamstrings by causing the muscle to relax. The GTO is a sensory organ in the muscle that prevents overactivity of nerve fibers innervating the target muscle. During a PNF hamstring stretch, reciprocal inhibition can occur during active flexion of the hip because contraction of the quadriceps causes a reflex relaxation of the hamstrings, which allows for a greater ROM. These two neuromuscular mechanisms can act synergistically during PNF stretching techniques to allow a target muscle to move through a greater ROM.

PNF stretching can be performed with a partner in a fitness class or alone with straps (Akbulut, 2015; Maddigan, 2012). Either way, participants must be instructed on appropriate procedures for safely performing PNF stretches. Improper PNF techniques can overstretch a muscle and be injurious. For this reason, youth fitness specialists should have experience implementing PNF stretching methods and should take the time to ensure that participants understand the instructions for each exercise. When training with a partner, youth need to listen carefully to the partner throughout the performance of every PNF movement. Unless there are specific reasons to perform PNF stretching as part of rehabilitation or sport training, it may be more appropriate for children and adolescents to perform dynamic warm-up activities or static stretching until more research becomes available on PNF stretching in youth.

Notwithstanding the chronic benefits of flexibility training, most exercise scientists and fitness practitioners propose that stretch-and-hold techniques should either be excluded from the general warm-up, performed within a warm-up that includes additional post-stretching dynamic activities, or performed during the cool-down period or as part of a separate exercise session (Maddigan, 2012; Peck, 2014; Behm, 2016; Opplert & Babault, 2018). A growing body of evidence indicates that warm-up static stretching of the prime movers may negatively affect force production, power production, and sprint speed in youth (Faigenbaum et al., 2005; Faigenbaum, Kang, & McFarland, 2006; Faigenbaum, McFarland, et al., 2006; McNeal & Sands, 2003; Paradisis et al., 2014; Siatras, Papadopoulos, Mameletzi, Gerodimos, & Kellis, 2003). In addition, preevent static stretching may not offer a protective effect against sport-related injuries in young athletes (Lauersen et al., 2014; Zakaria, Kiningham, & Sen, 2015).

In one investigation that examined the acute effects of static stretching on fitness performance, researchers reported a significant decrease in jump height and sprint speed in children (Faigenbaum et al., 2005).

Teaching Tip

STRETCHING EDUCATION

Because misperceptions persist, youth fitness specialists should consider prior beliefs and perceptions about the purported benefits of preevent static stretching (McKay, Steffen, Romiti, Finch, & Emery, 2014; Slauterbeck et al., 2017). In some cases, participants, parents, and coaches may need to be educated about current research and the desirable effects of preevent dynamic warm-ups on athletic performance and injury risk. Practitioners should sensibly introduce dynamic activities into the warm-up routine of young athletes who have strong beliefs about the value of preevent static stretching.

Other researchers reported that preevent static stretching negatively affected balance, agility, explosive force, and speed development in youth (Chatzopoulos, Galazoulas, Patikas, & Kotzamanidis, 2014; McNeal & Sands, 2003; Siatras et al., 2003). In support of these observations, an acute bout of static stretching enhanced sit-and-reach flexibility performance in boys and girls but hindered 20-meter sprint time and countermovement jump height by 2.5 percent and 6.3 percent, respectively (Paradisis et al., 2014). These small but significant decrements in performance following preevent static stretching can make a noticeable difference in the outcome of a fitness test or athletic event. The adverse effects of preevent static stretching on performance may relate to a decrease in neural activation, reduced musculoskeletal stiffness, or a combination of neural and muscular factors (Behm et al., 2016; Kallerud & Gleeson, 2013; Kay & Blazevich, 2012). Therefore, youth fitness specialists should consider both the immediate and the long-term effect of warm-up procedures on fitness performance, whether in the training center or the sport facility.

This is not to say that PNF or static stretching should be eliminated from a fitness class or sport practice. Rather, stretch-and-hold techniques should be sensibly incorporated into the exercise session because chronic stretching can benefit range of motion (Behm & Chaouachi, 2011; Kokkonen, Nelson, Eldredge, & Winchester, 2007). The American College of Sports Medicine (2018) now recommends that individuals perform static stretching exercises following cardiorespiratory or resistance training or as a separate program. It may be worthwhile for children and adolescents to perform flexibility exercises as part of cool-down activities at the end of an exercise class or sport practice to improve or in some cases maintain their flexibility. Even young athletes who compete in sports that require a high degree of flexibility should consider both the immediate effects of static stretching on strength and power performance and the potential benefits associated with dynamic warm-up procedures (Chaouachi et al., 2010; Taylor, Sheppard, Lee, & Plummer, 2009). For example, it may be desirable for young gymnasts and martial artists to perform preevent static stretching after a general warm-up, provided that they perform a series of dynamic activities and sport-specific movements prior to training or competition.

Summary

A well-designed dynamic warm-up can prepare children and adolescents physically and mentally for the demands of the upcoming exercise class or sport competition. Various types of flexibility training, including static and PNF stretching, can be used to increase joint ROM, but the purported benefits of preevent static stretching have been questioned. In contrast, active warm-ups that include dynamic stretching have been found to raise body temperature, activate key muscle groups, mobilize joints, potentiate the neuromuscular system, and develop desired movement skills. Furthermore, engaging youth in fitness programs that begin with a progressive series of dynamic movements favorably influences long-term development of athleticism. Youth fitness specialists should plan warm-up activities with the same energy and interest they invest in planning the main exercise or sport session.

CHAPTER 8

Motor Skill Training

CHAPTER OBJECTIVES

- Define and understand the classifications of motor skills
- Critically analyze the determinants of motor skill performance
- Examine how motor skill performance develops naturally as a result of growth and maturation
- Critically analyze the trainability of motor skills in children and adolescents
- Discuss relevant training strategies for motor skill development, as well as the process of manipulating training variables for long-term adaptation

KEY TERMS

Introduction

Running, crawling, skipping, jumping, and catching are often viewed as natural movements that children should be able to perform innately as they grow up. More generally, the acquisition of motor skills is viewed as a key developmental milestone for youth, because these skills enable children to experience their environmental surroundings and interact with others. However, competence in these skills is often substandard in modern-day youth due to habitual levels of physical inactivity (Hardy, Reinten-Reynolds, Espinel, Zask, & Okely, 2012; Lopes, Stodden, Bianchi, Maia, & Rodrigues, 2012); in fact, only about 50 percent of children can demonstrate competence in basic motor skills (Bryant, Duncan, & Birch, 2014; Hardy, Barnett, Espinel, & Okely, 2013). Moreover, because motor skill competence has been associated with long-term engagement in physical activity (de Souza et al., 2014; Fransen et al., 2014; Lopes, Rodrigues, Maia, & Malina, 2011; Loprinzi, Davis, & Fu, 2015), failure to appropriately develop motor skill proficiency early in life may lead to reduced levels of physical activity during adulthood. To address this problem, youth fitness specialists must do the following: (1) recognize the importance of motor skill competence; (2) understand the key determinants of motor skill performance; (3) appreciate how motor skill performance can be affected by growth, maturation, and training; and (4) be able to design, implement, and modify appropriate training programs for long-term motor skill development.

The association between motor skill competence and physical activity levels in youth hinges in part on **perceived competence** (Robinson, 2011b). Children with high motor skill proficiency typically perceive themselves as being "good movers" and are more likely to engage in higher levels of physical activity. In contrast, children with low levels of motor skill competence are likely to perceive themselves as being "poor movers" and are less likely to participate in physical activity. This effect may be relatively mild during early and middle childhood, but as children approach early adolescence, their tendency for peer comparison increases and they become far more critical of their own capabilities.

At this point, children may go in one of two directions, which lead to vastly different outcomes: (1) a **positive spiral of engagement**, wherein "good movers" are more likely to engage in physical activity and thus have greater opportunities for further motor skill development; or (2) a **negative spiral of disengagement**, wherein "poor movers" are less likely to participate in physical activity and thus are

not exposed to opportunities to improve their motor skills (Crane, Naylor, Cook, & Temple, 2015; Faigenbaum & Myer, 2012; Gallahue, Ozmun, & Goodway, 2012; Malina, Cumming, & Coelho, 2016; Robinson et al., 2015; Stodden, Gao, Goodway, & Langendorfer, 2014; Stodden, Langendorfer, & Roberton, 2009). These divergent scenarios highlight the critical importance of early investment in motor skill development during childhood to foster positive physical activity behaviors. These scenarios also underscore the critical role of youth fitness specialists. Aside from technical knowledge, practitioners need effective pedagogical skills in order to maintain the interest and enthusiasm of youth who are in a positive spiral of engagement and to inspire inactive youth to reverse the negative spiral by engaging in physical activity.

DO YOU KNOW?

Children with low levels of motor skill competence are less active than children with high proficiency, and in the absence of targeted interventions this trend continues into adolescence and adulthood.

Motor Skills and the Process of Learning

In broad terms, motor skills develop from complex interactions between the nervous and muscular systems to produce skilled and coordinated movement. They are typically subdivided into two distinct categories: **gross motor skills** and **fine motor skills**. Gross motor skills involve whole-body movements or movements of large body parts, as in locomotive tasks. Fine motor skills, on the other hand, typically involve movements that require accuracy and dexterity—for example, manipulative tasks. Although certain tasks may require the independent use of gross or fine motor skills (e.g., gross motor in sprinting, fine motor in gripping a tennis racket), many tasks require a combination of the two (e.g., running toward and then catching a batted baseball). Consequently, youth fitness specialists should appreciate that the goal of motor skill development is to develop a broad range of skills that can be adapted and used in a variety of environments. For example, though it is necessary for a child to learn to jump and land correctly, it is also important for the child, with sufficient practice and by using a variety of training environments, to be able to jump and land on different surfaces, in response to different stimuli, and in reactive and unanticipated game situations—all with appropriate technique and neuromuscular control.

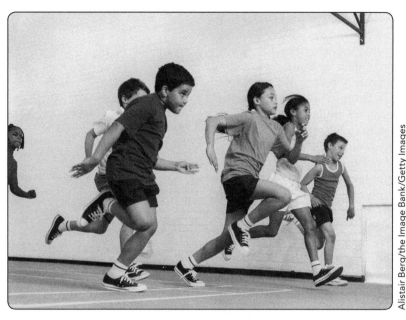

Alistair Berg/the Image Bank/Getty Images

Sprinting is an example of a gross motor skill.

As a result, youth fitness specialists should focus not only on the **product of motor skill performance** (e.g., how far a child can jump) but also on the **process of motor skill performance** (e.g., whether the child can demonstrate technical proficiency when jumping). This dual approach requires patience because children develop motor skills in a nonlinear fashion and are likely to experience both progression and regression as they learn to move competently. Thus, while it may be rewarding to see children jump farther or squat with heavier weights than in previous sessions, practitioners should never seek these improvements at the expense of technical competence. The process of teaching correct movements, giving children time to practice these movements, reflecting on performance, and then progressing or regressing exercises as appropriate takes time and requires a sound understanding of child pedagogy.

The manner in which children learn and adapt their motor skill strategies is influenced by the interaction of various constraints, which are often categorized as either individual, environmental, or task constraints (Gallahue et al., 2012).

• **Individual constraints** can be either *structural* (e.g., height, weight) or *functional* (e.g., motivation, fear). Structural constraints take a longer time to evolve, whereas functional constraints can fluctuate more rapidly. For example, though it takes many years for a child to reach adult height, the child's motivation and confidence may change following the outcome of a single event. This consideration emphasizes the need for youth fitness specialists to design, deliver, and refine programs on an individualized basis. For instance, regular monitoring of somatic measures can help explain how structural constraints affect disruptions of motor control in a child experiencing the growth spurt. Similarly, the ability to communicate effectively with children can help alleviate the potential negative effect of shorter-term functional constraints. Verbal reassurance, for example, if delivered by a practitioner in a softly spoken and empathetic manner at eye level, may be just what is needed to help a child who experiences a short-term loss in confidence after a poor performance in a motor skill challenge or competitive match.

• **Environmental constraints** exist outside of the body and can be easily manipulated to make a motor skill task more challenging. For example, if a child is performing a horizontal jumping and landing task in a school gymnasium, then introducing a more compliant surface (e.g., pliable gymnastics matting) will make the task more demanding.

• **Task constraints** allow practitioners to modify motor skill demands by manipulating the rules, degree of challenge, or type of equipment involved in a given movement or activity. For example, asking a child to kick a ball for distance versus kicking to a specific target will influence the selected movement pattern, whereas changing the size of the ball involved in a combined running and catching task will likely affect the child's ability to catch and grasp.

The interaction of various constraints is what ultimately leads to within- and between-individual variation in motor skill performance, as well as differences in rates and magnitude of development. Acquisition of **motor skill competence** is a crucial process for physical development in youth. Thus it is imperative that youth fitness specialists understand the interactive nature of a constraints-led approach to motor skill development when designing and implementing training programs for youth (see figure 8.1). Practitioners who try to manipulate too many constraints at once may risk overcomplicating a particular exercise or simply making the task too difficult, which could demotivate a young child. However, ongoing progression and variation in motor skill tasks constitute an important programming variable in order to progressively overload a young child and elicit ongoing physical adaptation.

The Language of Movement

Although children require opportunities for experiential learning and exposure to free play in order to refine motor skill patterns, it is often mistakenly thought that children will innately develop motor skill proficiency simply as a result of growth and development. In reality, existing data show that many children are not competent in a range of motor skills (Bryant et al., 2014; Hardy et al., 2013), which increases their likelihood of living in a sedentary manner. Thus it is clear that motor skills need to be taught, and teaching effectively means using appropriate pedagogy (Logan, Robinson, Wilson, & Lucas, 2012; Palmer, Chinn, & Robinson, 2017). Although multiple factors play a role in the process of learning new skills, we should not underestimate the importance of providing developmentally appropriate instruction during childhood (Foulkes et al., 2015; Lubans, Morgan, Cliff, Barnett, & Okely, 2010). Much in the same way that children require support

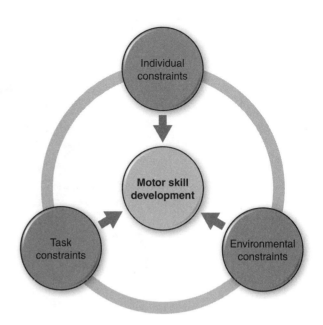

FIGURE 8.1   Newell's constraints model.

Adapted from Newell (1986).

and guidance from teachers in order to learn to read or play a musical instrument, they also need youth fitness specialists to teach them to move correctly. Indeed, developing a vocabulary of rudimentary and fundamental motor skills early in life should be viewed as the foundation for more specialized motor skills at a later stage of development. Pedagogically, the crucial skill of the youth fitness specialist is to say the right thing to the right individual at the right time in order to foster a positive learning environment for the child, which helps guide the child toward competence in a range of motor skills.

Achievement goal theory describes the goals and attributions that individuals embrace in the learning

Teaching Tip

MUSCULAR STRENGTH AND MOTOR SKILL COMPETENCE

The ability to perform motor skills requires effective use of the neuromuscular system. In order to carry out different forms of locomotion, stabilize the body in space, or manipulate objects, sufficient force must be produced to overcome the inertia of the body or object. Accordingly, research has shown that muscular strength is a determinant of motor skill performance (Comfort, Stewart, Bloom, & Clarkson, 2014; Lloyd, Oliver, Radnor, Rhodes, & Faigenbaum, 2015; Tveter & Holm, 2010), and the ability to produce force should be viewed as a critical component of motor skill competence. Indeed, coordination and muscular strength should be viewed not as separate entities but as synergistic components of motor skill performance (Cattuzzo et al., 2016). In combination, coordination and muscular strength should enable a child to perform a range of motor skills with energy, vigor, and proficiency and thereby facilitate engagement in physical activity as a lifetime choice.

process and that ultimately influence the way in which they approach and engage with their learning environment (Palmer et al., 2017). The literature indicates that learners typically assume either a **mastery orientation** or a **performance orientation** in regard to the process of learning (Ames, 1992; Palmer et al., 2017; Robinson, 2011a). Fostering a mastery-oriented climate to learning encourages youth to engage in learning for intrinsic value and to judge improvement against self-referenced standards (e.g., how much better is one's motor skill performance now than it was in the previous session). In contrast, a task-oriented climate leads the child to try to prove competence, avoid failure, and judge successful learning against norm-referenced standards (e.g., how much better is a child's motor skill performance than that of others in the group).

Within the education literature, research shows that adopting a mastery-oriented learning climate leads to greater intrinsic interest and more time spent on task (Butler, 1987; Meece, Blumenfeld, & Hoyle, 1988), belief in the notion that effort leads to success (Ames, 1992; Nicholls, Patashnick, & Nolen, 1985), positive attitudes toward learning (Ames, 1992), and greater resilience in the face of challenges (Elliott & Dweck, 1988). In addition, recent systematic review data have shown that adopting a mastery-oriented climate leads to improved motor skill competence in young children (Palmer et al., 2017); more specifically, studies have shown enhanced competence in object control (Robinson,

2011a; Robinson, Palmer, & Bub, 2016; L.E. Robinson, Veldman, Palmer, & Okely, 2017) and locomotive skills (L.E. Robinson et al., 2016; Robinson, Webster, Logan, Lucas, & Barber, 2012). From a holistic perspective, practitioners should promote intrinsic motivation in youth in order to encourage children and adolescents to participate, improve, and develop skills while also reducing the risk of being driven solely by external rewards such as trophies.

Natural Development of Motor Skills

A talented 17-year-old performing a complex sport skill might seem to exhibit fluent and natural movement, but youth fitness specialists must remain aware that successful performance of such skills involves an evolutionary process. It takes many years for youth to develop their capacity to perform complicated movements, and this process should include the initial development of a broad range of **fundamental motor skills** before focusing on more **specialized motor skills** at a later stage of development (Lloyd & Oliver, 2012). Practitioners must also remember that the process of acquiring motor skill competence begins at birth (Malina, 2004) and follows a developmental continuum of stages (see figure 8.2). Stage 1 is characterized by the spontaneous, **reflexive movements** seen in young babies, which develop into rudimentary motor skills during stage 2. In the presence of

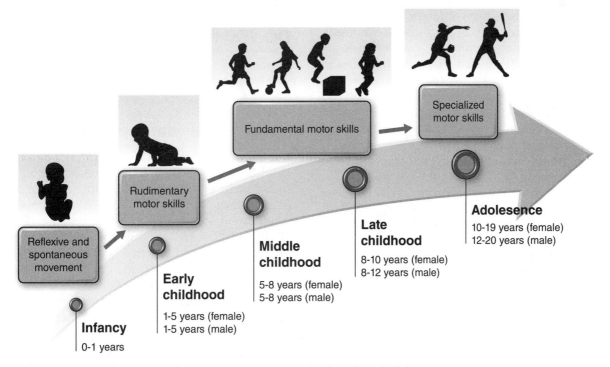

FIGURE 8.2 Stages of motor development across infancy, childhood, and adolescence.

appropriate instruction, guidance, and encouragement, these **rudimentary motor skills** transition in stage 3 into fundamental motor skills, which can then be developed into more specialized motor skills during the fourth and final stage of development. Thus, the first three stages serve as building blocks on which more sophisticated motor skills can be built.

Stage 1: Reflexive and Spontaneous Movements

Although youth fitness specialists are unlikely to work with infants, they need to appreciate that the early movement experiences occurring during this stage are vital for the subsequent development of rudimentary motor skills. During infancy (the first year of life), a typically developing child demonstrates a number of innate reflexes and spontaneous movements. These actions are involuntary and are controlled subcortically. At first, reflexive movements appear random and sporadic; collectively, however, they are instinctively linked to survival, help provide young children with information about the environment and their own body, and provide a foundation for motor skill execution at a later stage of development.

For instance, young babies display primitive reflexes such as sucking and rooting as survival mechanisms for feeding, and their postural reflexes appear to mirror more complex, voluntary motor skills that develop later in life. The stepping reflex closely resembles the walking gait pattern, and the palmar grasp reflex mirrors the voluntary grasping and releasing action seen in later stages of development. By either observation or stimulus, these reflexes are tested in newborns by pediatricians and other health care providers. For example, the Moro reflex test, which assesses a newborn's response to a sudden and brief loss of head support, should result in the child abducting and then quickly adducting and flexing the upper extremities (Zafeiriou, 2004).

Even though babies spend a large proportion of time sleeping, parents should not undervalue the importance of physical activity in the first few months of life. For example, infants who present with developmental delays are more likely to spend time in a supine position, spend insufficient time in the "prone play position," and exhibit lower activity levels (Hutchison, Stewart, & Mitchell, 2009). It has been suggested that when these factors are combined they may lead to inadequate neck strength and upper-body coordination, which can increase the risk of positional head deformation (Hutchison, Stewart, & Mitchell, 2011; Hutchison, Thompson, & Mitchell, 2003). Thus, developmentally appropriate physical activity for

motor skill development should begin at birth and become a habitual part of everyday life.

Stage 2: Rudimentary Motor Skills

As an infant develops and approaches the second year of life, primitive and postural reflexes become inhibited, but with practice and exposure to varied stimuli the infant begins to gain more voluntary control over movement. This increased control enables more coordinated and concerted neuromuscular function, which naturally leads to increased force output and heightened motor skill competence. During this stage of development, children cultivate a range of rudimentary motor skills, which can be assigned to three broad categories: **manipulation**, **stabilization**, and **locomotion**. As an example, table 8.1 presents an outline of the process of rudimentary motor skill development leading to proficiency in independent walking.

Crawling, rolling, sitting, standing with correct posture, and walking on all fours—these actions may appear to be elementary movements that all youth should be able to perform, but a number of contemporary youth struggle to demonstrate competence in such basic motor skills (Bryant et al., 2014; Hardy et al., 2013). Moreover, these rudimentary motor skills lay the foundation for more advanced skills developed later in childhood. Consequently, youth fitness specialists should routinely revisit rudimentary motor skills during childhood and adolescence as part of a training program, especially for adolescents who have not previously engaged in developmentally appropriate training.

DO YOU KNOW?

Most children should be able to demonstrate proficient walking gait by the age of 16 months.

Stage 3: Fundamental Motor Skills

During early childhood (1-5 yr), typically developing children build on their foundation of rudimentary motor skills and begin to develop a broader range of fundamental motor skills in the three domains of stabilization, locomotion, and manipulation (Lubans et al., 2010). Table 8.2 on page 154 presents examples of locomotive, manipulative, and stabilizing skills. In most instances, this stage of motor skill development is also the time when children start engaging in some form of formalized physical activity, most likely through a basic physical education curriculum in a primary school, sport club, or after-school physical activity program. Consequently, this stage is likely to provide the earliest opportunity for a youth fitness

TABLE 8.1   CHRONOLOGICAL AGE (MONTHS) AT WHICH HEALTHY, FULL-TERM INFANTS ATTAIN DEVELOPMENTAL MILESTONES LEADING TO INDEPENDENT WALKING

DEVELOPMENTAL MILESTONE	BOYS PERCENTILES			GIRLS PERCENTILES		
	10	50	90	10	50	90
Roll to supine	3.7	5.0	6.2	3.8	5.2	6.7
Roll to prone	4.8	6.0	8.8	4.6	6.0	8.7
Pivot	5.0	6.4	8.6	4.7	6.8	8.8
Crawl on stomach	6.1	7.0	8.7	5.8	6.9	8.9
Creep on hands and knees	6.8	8.3	10.4	6.5	8.8	11.8
Creep on hands and feet	8.1	9.0	11.8	7.7	9.6	11.9
Sit up	7.3	9.1	11.8	6.8	8.9	11.5
Stand at rail	7.4	8.4	9.8	7.1	8.7	10.5
Pull to stand	7.5	8.5	11.3	7.3	8.9	11.5
Cruise at rail	8.0	9.5	11.7	8.0	9.8	11.8
Stand momentarily	9.9	12.4	15.6	9.8	12.5	14.9
Walk with one hand held	9.2	11.5	13.0	9.5	11.8	13.5
Walk alone	10.8	13.0	15.9	11.0	13.1	15.7
Walk up and down stairs	16.2	18.9	23.7	16.0	19.7	23.8

Reprinted by permission from M. Malina, C. Bouchard, and O. Bar-Or, *Growth, Maturation, and Physical Activity*, 2nd ed. (Champaign, IL: Human Kinetics, 2004), 200. Data from R.H. Largo, L. Molinari, M. Weber, et al., "Early Development of Locomotion: Significance of Prematurity, Cerebral Palsy and Sex," *Developmental Medicine and Child Neurology* 27 (1985): 183-191.

specialist to introduce a child to developmentally appropriate training within the broad construct of a long-term athletic development pathway.

Fundamental motor skills, which are more complex forms of rudimentary motor skills, are developed as children explore their environment and use, refine, and manipulate their motor control strategies. Acquiring proficiency in fundamental motor skills during this stage of growth and development is often viewed as one of the more important developmental milestones during childhood (Cools, Martelaer, Samaey, & Andries, 2009; Iivonen et al., 2013; Malina, Bouchard, & Bar-Or, 2004). Children may well develop a rudimentary level of fundamental motor skill competence as a result of natural development; however, this level of skill will not automatically lead to mastery of movement. Research findings suggest that although a large proportion of youth attain the recommended levels of daily physical activity, the type and quality of physical activity is potentially insufficient to promote highly competent levels of fundamental motor skill (Foulkes et al., 2015). Therefore, in order to reach higher levels of competence, children must be given opportunities to practice motor skills in positive learning environments and must receive encouragement, constructive feedback, and developmentally appropriate instruction (Lubans et al., 2010).

Fundamental motor skills serve as the building blocks for future skill development and ensure that youth can move safely and efficiently (Logan, Ross, Chee, Stodden, & Robinson, 2017). Despite the acknowledgment that proficiency in fundamental motor skills is an important feature of childhood development, a number of modern-day youth fail to demonstrate competence across a range of fundamental motor skill tests (Booth et al., 1999; Hardy et al., 2012; Okely & Booth, 2004). Fundamental motor skill competence has also been associated with higher levels of engagement in sport and physical activity throughout childhood (Fransen et al., 2014; Laukkanen, Pesola, Havu, Saakslahti, & Finni, 2014; Wrotniak, Epstein, Dorn, Jones, & Kondilis, 2006), adolescence (Barnett, Van Beurden, Morgan, Brooks, & Beard, 2008), and adulthood (Lloyd, Saunders, Bremer, & Tremblay, 2014; Stodden, Gao, et al., 2014; Stodden, Langendorfer, & Robertson, 2009). Although epidemiological data provide useful information related to the quantity of time that youth spend in low-, moderate-, and vigorous-intensity physical activity, we must also attend to the quality of the movement experience in order to adequately prepare youth for ongoing participation in a variety of physical activities and sports.

Classic literature in the field shows that most children should be able to show proficient movement in a

TABLE 8.2   EXAMPLES OF FUNDAMENTAL MOTOR SKILLS

Locomotion	Manipulation	Stabilization*
Walking	Catching	Turning
Running	Pushing	Twisting
Bounding	Pulling	Bending
Hopping	Dribbling	Landing
Leaping	Carrying	Stretching
Jumping	Bouncing	Extending
Rolling	Trapping	Flexing
Galloping	Throwing	Hanging
Climbing	Kicking	Bracing
Sliding	Striking	Rotating
Skipping	Collecting	Hanging

*These movements are performed both dynamically and statically in place.

number of key fundamental motor skills by the age of 8 to 10 years (Malina et al., 2004). For example, mature kicking technique should be present by 7 or 8 years of age in boys and girls, respectively, and skipping technique should be competent by about 6 years of age in both sexes. However, in order to acquire competence in fundamental motor skills, children invariably progress along a common continuum of staged development, albeit at different rates. Similarly, rates of progression can also vary in the attainment of competence in different motor skills by a single individual.

Stage 4: Specialized Motor Skills

Once youth have gained competence and confidence in their ability to perform a broad range of fundamental motor skills, they are positioned to use these refined movement patterns in a variety of contexts (e.g., competitive sport, recreational physical activity, physical education class, free play). In order to execute highly coordinated specialized movements, children require a combination of fundamental motor skills. For example, a jump shot in basketball requires the following:

- *Manipulative skills:* catching, holding, and shooting the ball
- *Locomotive skills:* running around the court; jumping to take a shot
- *Stabilizing skills:* using postural stability for bending and stretching when jumping; using dynamic stability upon landing

Breaking down a motor skill to this basic level shows how important it is for youth fitness specialists to help children become proficient in a wide range of such skills. In the case of the jump shot, a child who cannot catch the ball competently is unlikely to ever be in a position to shoot, whereas failure to demonstrate dynamic stability upon landing increases the risk of

landing with a potentially injurious movement pattern. When a child is unable to make a successful transition to the final stage of motor skill development (i.e., to specialized motor skills), this failure may be explained in part by the **proficiency barrier** hypothesis (Seefeldt, 1980). This hypothesis posits that early deficiency in fundamental motor skill competence likely impedes progression to the learning of more complex movement patterns later in life (Hulteen, Morgan, Barnett, Stodden, & Lubans, 2018; Robinson et al., 2015; Stodden et al., 2014).

The development of specialized motor skills (e.g., double somersault diving technique, volleyball spike technique) is highly variable among individuals due to the interaction of individual, task, and environmental constraints. There are no definitive ages at which specialized motor skills are deemed mature, and a number of individuals have demonstrated competence in highly complex skills from an early age. For example, at age 15, three-time Olympic gold medalist Naim Suleymanoglu set his first weightlifitng world record; at age 14, Nadia Comaneci became the first Olympian to be awarded a perfect score of 10; and while still in childhood, now-four-time major winner Rory McIlroy was famed for his early mastery of the golf swing. Irrespective of these extraordinary cases, youth fitness specialists should look to provide all children and adolescents with the opportunity to practice and reinforce fundamental motor skill competence before seeking mastery of more advanced skills.

Trainability of Motor Skills in Youth

Research has shown that children and adolescents can make improvements in locomotive skills (e.g., running, jumping, hopping), stabilizing skills (e.g.,

Teaching Tip

GOOD ATHLETES ARE NOT ALWAYS GOOD MOVERS

As discussed in chapter 4, specializing in a single sport from an early age will likely limit a child's development of multiple motor skill abilities. For example, though a highly skilled tennis player can toss and strike a ball competently, the same player may be unable to demonstrate competence in a wide range of locomotive tasks (e.g., running, skipping) or stabilizing tasks (e.g., bracing, dynamic stability). In such an instance, the youth fitness specialist may need to address these motor skill limitations by revisiting the fundamental level of skill development as part of a long-term athletic development program. At first, this process may seem overly basic; however, correcting weaknesses and imbalances in fundamental motor skills will pay dividends for long-term development and engagement in the chosen sport.

balance, core stability), and manipulative skills (e.g., throwing, catching) when exposed to developmentally appropriate training programs (Christou et al., 2006; Ericsson & Karlsson, 2014; Faigenbaum et al., 2011; Faigenbaum et al., 2007; Granacher, Muehlbauer, Doerflinger, Strohmeier, & Gollhofer, 2011; Logan et al., 2012; Robinson et al., 2016). Such programs typically do not focus solely on practicing motor skills per se; rather, they tend to align with the concept of **integrative neuromuscular training**, which incorporates a variety of motor skill exercises, resistance training, coordination training, and exercises geared toward developing speed and agility (Myer et al., 2011).

A meta-analysis of 11 studies showed that motor skill interventions are effective in improving fundamental motor skills in children; specifically, locomotive and manipulative skills both showed improvement from pre- to post-intervention (Logan et al., 2012). These findings were corroborated by a more recent meta-analysis of 22 studies, which concluded that despite a relatively high risk of bias in the studies analyzed, motor skill interventions significantly improved fundamental motor skill proficiency in youth (Morgan et al., 2013). This review highlighted the fact that quality of instruction and time spent in practice are critical factors in the success of any motor skill training intervention.

Due to the heightened **neural plasticity** associated with childhood (Casey, Giedd, & Thomas, 2000; Casey, Tottenham, Liston, & Durston, 2005; Myer et al., 2015; Piek, Hands, & Licari, 2012), it is accepted that the earlier children engage in skill-building athletic development programs, the more likely they are to develop motor skill proficiency and enhance overall physical fitness (Faigenbaum, Lloyd, MacDonald, & Myer, 2016; Lloyd & Oliver, 2012). Encouraging evidence indicates that motor skill development programs can be successfully integrated into the curriculum with preschool children (aged 3-5 yr). One study reports

significant improvements in leaping ability following a 6-month training intervention that took place five days per week for 30 minutes per day (Alhassan et al., 2012). This study also showed that children who engaged in the training program significantly reduced their time spent in sedentary activity. In addition, a one-year intervention has shown that children of about five years of age made greater improvements in motor skill competence when they followed a structured physical education curriculum delivered by a qualified physical education teacher than when they received recreational physical education delivered by a classroom teacher (Lemos, Avigo, & Barela, 2012). These findings underline the critical role that qualified instruction plays in motor skill development.

DO YOU KNOW?

Current research shows that children as young as two years of age demonstrate substandard levels of motor skill competence; therefore, early intervention is critical.

Research has also examined the effectiveness of an integrative neuromuscular training intervention on measures of physical performance and motor skill function in seven-year-old children (Faigenbaum et al., 2011). The study showed that children made significant gains in curl-up and push-up performance (increased muscular strength and endurance) and in long jump and single-leg hop performance (motor skill) following an eight-week training program that took place twice weekly in 15-minute sessions (Faigenbaum et al., 2011). During this study, all of the children used a durable punch balloon as a form of resistance when performing various exercises. Although the study measured the product of motor skill performance rather than the process, it highlighted the benefits of including motor skill training as a component of an integrative training program. It also demonstrated the benefits that young

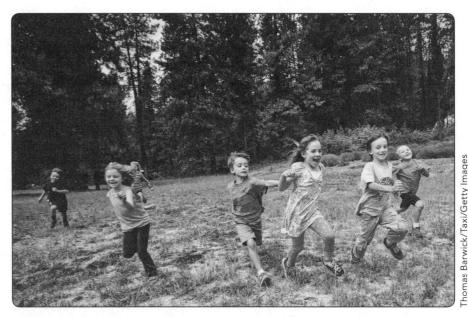

Thomas Barwick/Taxi/Getty Images

Motor skills can be developed following exposure to appropriate training interventions, which should help children move more competently during free-play activities, such as a game of "tag."

children can gain from just 15 minutes of training twice weekly and the fact that an effective youth-based training program can be implemented with minimal equipment. A follow-up study showed that after an eight-week detraining period, the training-induced gains were maintained in curl-up and single-leg hop performance (i.e., muscular strength and endurance) but significantly decreased in the long jump (i.e., motor skill) (Faigenbaum, Farrell, et al., 2013). Thus it was suggested that in order for youth to maintain training-induced adaptations in motor skill function, they require continual participation in developmentally appropriate training.

The importance of qualified supervision was highlighted by findings from a SCORES (Supporting Children's Outcomes using Rewards, Exercise, and Skills) trial that was randomized and controlled (Cohen, Morgan, Plotnikoff, Callister, & Lubans, 2015). The trial used a 12-month, multicomponent exercise intervention intended to enhance fundamental movement skill competence in some 200 primary school children aged eight to nine years. Results showed that children who were involved in the targeted intervention made significantly greater improvements in fundamental movement skill competence than did children in the control group, who simply followed their usual physical education curriculum.

Research has also examined the effects of a year-long, after-school training intervention for fundamental motor skills (known as the A-Class Project) on the technical performance of a range of locomotive skills (vertical jump, leap) and manipulative skills (kick,

throw, catch) in eight- to nine-year-old children (Stratton et al., 2009). The authors reported that children who were exposed to the intervention increased locomotive and manipulative skill competence by more than 15 percent and 30 percent, respectively, and that these improvements were significantly greater than those in the control group. Therefore, the study showed that both locomotive and manipulative skills were very responsive to appropriately designed training interventions delivered in both boys and girls. At the same time, however, girls showed reductions in their perceived competence throughout the intervention, possibly due to the typical social dynamics at this stage of development, which involve a greater degree of peer comparison with respect to body attractiveness and physical competence. Combined, the study findings support the benefits of well-designed integrative training on motor skill competence, but youth fitness specialists are encouraged to be thoughtful about timing, tempo, and magnitudes of individual progress wherever possible.

Research (Ericsson & Karlsson, 2014) tracked motor skill competence in youth from 7 to 9 years of age until 16 years of age. The study showed that those who received daily exposure to physical education (5 × 45 min per week) in addition to supplementary motor skill training (1 × 60 min per week) achieved significantly greater levels of motor skill competence than did the members of a control group, who received only the standard physical education provision of two 45-minute classes per week. It remains unclear whether the improved adaptation resulted directly from the targeted motor skill training or simply reflected the increased exposure to physical education. This is one of the few studies to examine the long-term effect of a motor skill training intervention.

DO YOU KNOW?

All youth can improve motor skill competence following training, but it is naive to think that children innately learn how to kick, catch, and throw proficiently without suitable guidance and instruction.

Although these studies have shown positive outcomes for motor skill training interventions, youth fitness specialists are particularly interested in the trainability of motor skills during the stages of childhood and adolescence. In this vein, a meta-analysis of 19 school- and community-based interventions for fundamental movement skills revealed large effect sizes for overall gross motor skill proficiency and locomotive skill competence, as well as a medium effect size for object control skill proficiency (Morgan et al., 2013). The A-Class project report mentioned earlier stated that the compliant aspect of children's health was their motor skill competence, which was reflected by the fact that children in the intervention group demonstrated large changes in manipulative and locomotive skills (Stratton et al., 2009). In addition, a review of 34 studies, which each included some form of resistance training, found that children achieved training-induced gains in motor skills that were about 50 percent greater than those achieved by adolescents (Behringer, Vom Heede, Matthews, & Mester, 2011). Collectively, these data suggest that there likely exists an optimal period before adolescence in which specific motor skills are more trainable in response to appropriate exercise interventions, including resistance training.

Altogether, the motor skill training literature suggests that early engagement in developmentally appropriate exercise, including resistance training, will enhance motor skill competence and increase levels of habitual physical activity among youth. Children as young as three years of age have been shown to make training-induced gains in motor skill competence in response to skill training effectively integrated within curriculum time or in after-school settings by qualified personnel. In order to maintain training-induced gains in motor skill competence, youth need to engage routinely in developmentally appropriate programs. Therefore, long-term motor skill function may be aided by exposure to physical education and motor skill training throughout the childhood years.

DO YOU KNOW?

As with learning music and language, it is easier to learn new fundamental motor skills in childhood than later in life.

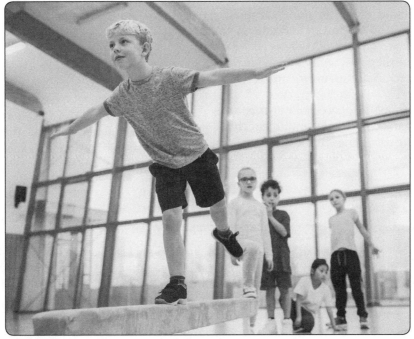

Westend61/Getty Images

Being able to maintain balance is recognized as an important skill for children to display competence in for overall motor skill development.

Training Prescription for Motor Skill Development

It is widely acknowledged that an integrative approach to training provides an optimal stimulus for motor skill development. Therefore, practitioners should aim to incorporate a variety of training modes, including resistance training, plyometrics, speed and agility training, and coordination and balance exercises. When focusing specifically on fundamental motor skill training, youth fitness specialists should try to plan and manipulate relevant training prescription variables in order to maximize the chances of continual adaptation.

Exercise Selection

When selecting appropriate exercises, youth fitness specialists should first consider the experience and technical competence of the child. Children with little or no training history and poor motor skill competence should focus on developing correct movement skills and improving basic levels of muscular strength. Over time, the level of exercise complexity can be increased in accordance with the individual's increased training experience and motor skill ability. Pedagogically, the challenge for practitioners when working with young children is to design training sessions that are engaging, fun, and interactive yet also contain key exercises that improve overall motor skill competence. For example, obstacle courses can be used both to challenge children's motor abilities (e.g., running, rolling, hopping, jumping) and to add a fun and engaging element to training. Even during this type of activity, practitioners still have the opportunity to provide relevant feedback and technical cues in order to develop technical competence.

Training sessions should also incorporate a mixture of simple exercises that provide opportunities for children to enhance their confidence in their movement abilities and complex movements that provide greater physical challenge. When working with large groups of children, practitioners should also be able to regress or progress exercises in order to differentiate between children with different levels of motor skill ability or to make a particular task easier or more difficult for a child. This approach helps cultivate a mastery-oriented environment for motor skill development, which encourages intrinsic motivation and a sense of learning based on personal achievement rather than peer comparison (Palmer et al., 2017).

DO YOU KNOW?

Fun depends on a balance between skill and challenge, and youth fitness specialists need to strike that balance in order to maximize motor skill development.

When planning a motor skill training session, it is beneficial to use a range of games and exercises that will target and subsequently develop a number of key movement patterns. This is especially true when working with very young and inexperienced children, for whom monotonous repetition and loading schemes that target a small range of specific movement patterns will typically be ineffective and demotivating. Although both the academic and the coaching literature often discuss fundamental motor skills in the context of generic gross or fine movements, some literature has identified a more sophisticated level of movement proficiency analysis termed **athletic motor skill competencies** (Moody, Naclerio, Green, & Lloyd, 2013). Figure 8.3 presents an overview of the athletic motor skill competencies, which reflect targeted movements that act as component parts of more specialized motor skills and serve as the foundations for advanced training methods at a later stage of development.

To maximize performance and minimize injury risk, it is recommended that athletic motor skill competence should be integrated into any youth-based

---

Teaching Tip

DON'T FORGET THE CONCRETE

When working with children or adolescents, youth fitness specialists should try to develop both the process and the product of motor skill function. Conceptually, this approach can be viewed much like the process of building a house. Although it is important to dig the foundations in a linear fashion so that the house is built accurately, it will not withstand the load of the house unless concrete is first poured in. In terms of motor skill development, practitioners must remember that although it is important for a child to move correctly (i.e., to lay the foundation), the child also requires sufficient levels of muscular strength (i.e., concrete) in order to safely produce and attenuate forces.

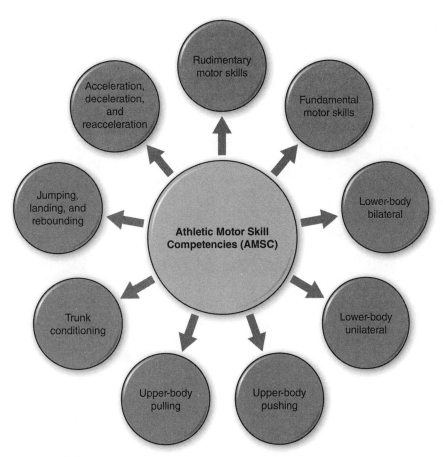

FIGURE 8.3   Athletic motor skill competencies.

Adapted by permission from J.A. Moody, F. Naclerio, P. Green, and R.S. Lloyd, "Motor Skill Development in Youths," in *Strength and Conditioning for Young Athletes: Science and Application*, edited by R.S. Lloyd and J.L. Oliver (Oxon, UK: Routledge), 49-65.

training program at some level (Myer, Lloyd, Brent, & Faigenbaum, 2013), whether in a 15-minute warm-up or a full 60-minute training session. Although children entering an athletic development program for the first time may be exposed to a wider variety of athletic motor skill competencies, their training will likely need to become more targeted as they become more proficient in order to address specific individual weaknesses. The ultimate goal for youth fitness specialists is to ensure that all youth are able to show proficiency across the full spectrum of athletic motor skill competencies.

DO YOU KNOW?

The most successful training programs place a high priority on developing youth who are competent in a large range of athletic motor skill competencies.

Volume and Intensity

For young children embarking on an integrative motor skill training program, the volume and variety of exercises is typically higher than is prescribed for older and more experienced youth. This difference derives primarily from the need to introduce children to a broad range of tasks and skills in order to maintain their enthusiasm and engagement. In addition, the greater volume of exercises reflects the relatively lower impact forces and joint loadings experienced during basic locomotive exercises, manipulative skills, and stabilization tasks. The numbers of recommended sets and repetitions are dictated largely by the nature of the selected exercises. For example, a group warm-up for young children might involve a series of fun animal-shape games that indirectly challenge multiple motor skills and encourage exploratory movement (e.g., crab walks, as shown in figure 8.4). Such a sequence might require children to work for a specific period of time (e.g., one set of five 10- to 20-second repetitions). However, if prescribing a more advanced exercise, such as a box jump (figure 8.5), then the target training volume may be in line with more recognized prescription guidelines (e.g., two to four sets of four to six repetitions).

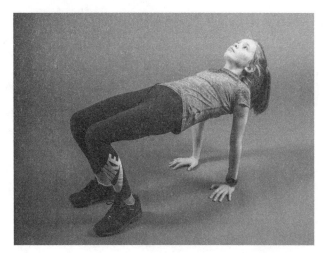

FIGURE 8.4   Crab walk as part of an animal-shape warm-up activity.

Practitioners will need to be flexible in their approach to prescription, especially when working with young children of varying abilities. Specifically, the requirement for children to explore movements and develop motor skill strategies needs to be balanced with the need for developmentally appropriate feedback in order to improve technique. In order to strike this balance, training prescription may need to vary, either within a session or between sessions. For example, a practitioner might provide minimal feedback during the fun-oriented animal-shapes warm-up but then provide relevant cueing on every repetition for the box jump exercise. This flexible approach to planning and delivery of training sessions reflects the need to blend the art of coaching with the science of training prescription.

Traditionally, resistance training prescription often bases intensity either on a percentage of one-repetition maximum (Fry, 2004) or on movement velocity (Gonzalez-Badillo & Sanchez-Medina, 2010), whereas endurance training prescription for adults commonly uses percentage of maximum heart rate or maximal oxygen consumption (ACSM, 2014; Seiler & Kjerland, 2006). Motor skill training intensity is more challenging to govern, because children will typically be working only against gravitational forces in addition to their own body weight when performing tasks that vary in nature (i.e., tasks that use a combination of locomotive, stabilizing, and manipulative skills). One option is to base training intensity on the complexity or intensity of the exercise or game. In this vein, the theory of **degrees of freedom** reflects the number of independent elements or components of a given task—in particular, any directions in which independent movement can occur (Gallahue et al., 2012). This theory supposes that an increase in task complexity (degrees of freedom) also brings an increase in the number of potential motor control strategies that can be employed by the participant's central nervous system.

Figure 8.6 shows how a unilateral lower-limb exercise can be progressed by gradually increasing the associated degrees of freedom. First, a child can perform a static split-squat exercise (figure 8.6*a*), which can then be advanced by instructing the child to perform a number of walking lunges (figure 8.6*b*), followed by walking lunges with a twist (figure 8.6*c*), and finally walking lunges while receiving a tennis ball to catch (figure 8.6*d*). The progressive intensity of this sequence begins by initially stressing only

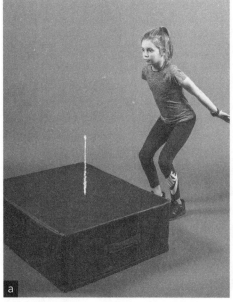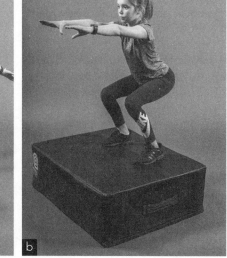

FIGURE 8.5   Box jump exercise.

locomotive coordination, then gradually introduces dynamic stabilization requirements, and finally adds a manipulative skill demand. This approach to exercise prescription enables youth fitness specialists to progress or regress training for each individual, as well as differentiate the technical competence levels of all youth in the program. As with other training modalities, in the event that a child is unable to maintain technical competence during a more advanced progression of a particular exercise, the practitioner should offer corrective feedback and, if necessary, provide an alternative exercise that reinforces the desired movement patterns.

DO YOU KNOW?

Youth fitness specialists should not increase the complexity of exercises at the expense of technical competence.

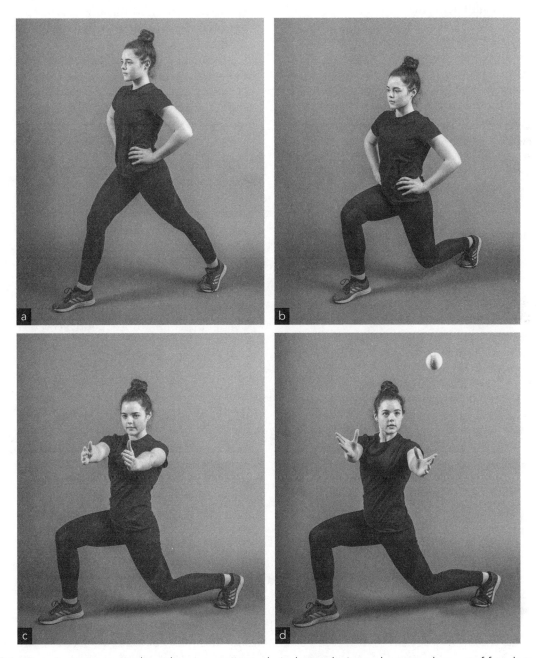

FIGURE 8.6 Exercise progression based on increasing technical complexity and greater degrees of freedom as a child moves from (a) an initial split-squat exercise to (b) walking lunges, (c) walking lunges with a twist, and finally (d) walking lunges with a tennis ball catch.

Repetition Velocity

The speed at which motor skill exercises should be performed depends on a number of factors, including the complexity of the exercise, the technical ability of the child, and the phase and goal of the training session. When working with novice individuals of limited technical competence, the exercises will likely need to be performed slowly and with control in order to learn correct movement patterns (Lloyd, Oliver, Meyers, Moody, & Stone, 2012). Similarly, when revisiting motor skill performance with more experienced youth, slower movement speeds might be used to reemphasize key technical points and highlight relevant coaching cues. However, irrespective of the capabilities of the child, practitioners also need to program exercises that teach the child to move explosively. Both of these outcomes will likely be enhanced by the neural plasticity associated with this stage of development (Myer et al., 2015).

DO YOU KNOW?

A mixed-methods approach to prescribing repetition velocities should ensure that a child develops the ability to move correctly and with high rates of force development.

In-Session Recovery

Children naturally engage in brief and intermittent recreational play activities (Bailey et al., 1995), and they are able to recover more quickly than adults from high-intensity exercise (Ratel, Williams, Oliver, & Armstrong, 2006). They are also less likely to suffer muscle damage following bouts of exercise, due to their increased muscle and tendon pliability (Eston, Byrne, & Twist, 2003). Cumulatively, these data suggest that youth fitness specialists should predominantly prescribe shorter training sessions (e.g., less than 45

minutes), inclusive of intermittent bouts of high-intensity exercise, interspersed with rest periods of about 1 minute. This approach has proven effective in pediatric settings, where training interventions of just 20 minutes per session, integrated at the start of physical education classes, have produced significant gains in both skill- and health-related components of fitness (Faigenbaum, Bush, et al., 2015; Faigenbaum, Farrell, et al., 2011, 2013). As children become more proficient and their exercises become more complex and more difficult, practitioners may need to use longer recovery periods, both to allow for sufficient rest and to provide opportunities for constructive feedback. Furthermore, though it is known that children and adolescents recover quickly from high-intensity exercise, technical competence should always be monitored during a training session in order to avoid deterioration of technique due to accumulated fatigue, reduced attention, or boredom.

Training Frequency

The optimal training frequency (i.e., number of training sessions per week) for motor skill development remains unclear. However, leading guidelines suggest that youth should participate in at least 60 minutes of moderate to vigorous physical activity per day (World Health Organization, 2010) and that this activity should encompass elements of skill development and muscle strengthening (Faigenbaum, Lloyd, & Myer, 2013; Lloyd et al., 2016; Lloyd, Faigenbaum, et al., 2014; Myer et al., 2015). Consequently, youth could engage in some form of daily motor skill training delivered by a youth fitness specialist through a physical education curriculum, organized sport participation, or recreational physical activity.

Training Program Duration

Although existing meta-analyses show that improvements in fundamental motor skill performance fol-

---

Teaching Tip

DAILY MOTOR SKILL TRAINING FOR YOUTH

In spite of the substandard levels of current health and fitness in modern-day youth, there remains a lack of robust governmental strategies for targeted, integrative physical activity in the educational sector (Weiler, Allardyce, Whyte, & Stamatakis, 2014). Furthermore, many U.S. states allow schools to use waivers, exemptions, and substitutions for physical education (Society of Health and Physical Educators, 2016). Therefore, whenever a youth fitness specialist has training time with children or adolescents, high priority should be placed on enhancing motor skill competence and requisite levels of muscle strength by means of creative programming that is safe, fun, and effective (Lloyd, Oliver, Faigenbaum, et al., 2015b).

lowing training interventions are not significantly associated with training program duration (Behringer et al., 2011; Logan et al., 2012; Morgan et al., 2013), this finding likely results from the fact that a number of studies fail to report training program length and dosage. Irrespective of the lack of association between training program duration and improvements in motor skill function, it is recognized that children should engage in developmentally appropriate training programs as part of a lifetime strategy for general health and well-being (Bergeron et al., 2015; Lloyd et al., 2016; Lloyd, Oliver, Faigenbaum, et al., 2015a). Although the amount of time devoted specifically to improving motor skills will likely decrease as children become older and more skilled, some amount of time should always be devoted to maintaining motor skill competence in an integrated training program.

Sample Training Programs

When programming motor skill training sessions for children or adolescents, practitioners should base training prescription primarily on the technical competence of the individual or group of individuals. Other factors to consider include age, stage of maturation, sex, and phase of the training program. Tables 8.3 and 8.4 provide sample training sessions with developmentally appropriate motor skill exercises for two children of differing technical ability. In either case, the opening section of the training session involves animal-shape warm-up activities designed to expose the child to key athletic motor skill competencies in the form of fun-based games. Next, **body management** training is designed to enhance the child's ability to orient and manage body weight, including a key focus on developing whole-body range of motion, stability, and basic strength. The final phases of the sessions involve exercises that target specific athletic motor skill competencies and introduce more recognizable resistance training exercises.

As the technical competence of the participant improves, the youth fitness specialist should introduce sensible progressions in motor skill training sessions to offer continual challenge and maintain enthusiasm. An example of this strategy is reflected in tables 8.3 and 8.4, wherein the beginner is prescribed simple variations of each exercise (e.g., alligator crawl, front-support "gorilla slap," and push-up) and the more experienced youth is provided with more challenging versions of each exercise (e.g., alligator crawl with roll, front-support step-up, and resistance band press). Depending on the quality of motor skill performance observed, the practitioner should be prepared to progress or regress exercises in a fluid and responsive manner, either within or between sessions. In addition, the naming of exercises and the nature of cueing should be developmentally appropriate wherever possible. The sessions presented in tables 8.3 and 8.4 are merely examples, and practitioners should design and deliver sessions that are relevant to the unique characteristics of the youth with whom they work and in accordance with their own unique situational environment (e.g., in terms of space, equipment, and available time).

Summary

Although childhood is the opportune time to develop rudimentary and fundamental motor skills, evidence shows that many children and adolescents worldwide are lacking in motor skill proficiency. Due to the heightened neural plasticity associated with childhood, it is a crucial time in which to develop motor skill proficiency through the use of integrative training methods. Although fundamental motor skills are traditionally characterized by locomotive, stabilizing, and manipulative tasks, all youth should seek to develop a broad range of athletic motor skill competencies in order to enable more advanced training at later stages of development.

Research shows that motor skills can be enhanced throughout childhood and adolescence; however, children may be more receptive than adolescents to training-induced adaptations due to their heightened neural plasticity. In any motor skill training program, exercises should be prescribed and instructed by a youth fitness specialist who is cognizant of the physical and psychosocial uniqueness of youth. Programs should progress from basic to complex by gradually increasing in degrees of freedom in order to continually challenge children with the demands of the movements. Over time, practitioners should routinely manipulate key training variables such as exercise selection, volume, and intensity as part of an integrative, long-term training program that is engaging, progressive, and enjoyable for all participants.

TABLE 8.3   SAMPLE BEGINNER TRAINING SESSION FOR MOTOR SKILL DEVELOPMENT

Phase	Exercise		Volume (sets × reps)	Intensity	Interset rest (sec)
Warm-up	Crab walk		2 × 15 seconds	Body weight	30
	Bear crawl		2 × 15 seconds	Body weight	30
	Bunny hop		2 × 15 seconds	Body weight	30
	Alligator crawl		2 × 15 seconds	Body weight	30
	Small-group crab-walk ball toss		2 × 30 seconds	Body weight	30
	Team obstacle course challenge		3 × 3	Body weight	30

Phase	Exercise	Volume (sets × reps)	Intensity	Interset rest (sec)
Body management	Dish-to-arch roll	2 × 10 m	Body weight	30
	Tuck roll to stand	2 × 5	Body weight	30
	Straddle teddy-bear roll	2 × 6 (3 each side)	Body weight	30
	Front-support "gorilla slap"	2 × 10 (5 each side)	Body weight	30
Athletic motor skill competencies	Body-weight "prisoner" squat	2 × 10	Body weight	30-45

(continued)

TABLE 8.3 *(CONTINUED)*

Phase	Exercise	Volume (sets × reps)	Intensity	Interset rest (sec)
Athletic motor skill competencies *(continued)*	Walking lunge	2 × 10 (5 each leg)	Body weight	30-45
	Glute bridge	2 × 10	Body weight	30-45
	Push-up	2 × 10	Body weight	30-45
	Supine row	2 × 10	Body weight	30-45

Phase	Exercise	Volume (sets × reps)	Intensity	Interset rest (sec)
Athletic motor skill competencies *(continued)*	Jump-to-box	2 × 5	Body weight	30-45
	Dead bug	2 × 5	Body weight	30-45

TABLE 8.4   SAMPLE ADVANCED TRAINING SESSION FOR MOTOR SKILL DEVELOPMENT

Phase	Exercise	Volume (sets × reps)	Intensity	Interset rest (sec)
Warm-up	Crab walk with pincer reach	2 × 15 seconds	Body weight	30
	Bear crawl with squat-to-roar	2 × 15 seconds	Body weight	30
	Bunny hop with fence jump	2 × 15 seconds	Body weight	30
	Alligator crawl with roll	2 × 15 seconds	Body weight	30
	Small-group crab-walk soccer	2 × 30 seconds	Body weight	30
	Team obstacle course challenge	3 × 5 circuits	Body weight	30

Phase	Exercise	Volume (sets × reps)	Intensity	Interset rest (sec)
Body management	Front-side-back support sequence 	2 × 4 (2 each way)	Body weight	30
	Back-to-back squat 	2 × 8	Body weight	30
	Partner box 	4 × 10 seconds	Body weight	30
	Front-support step-up 	2 × 8 (4 each arm)	Body weight	30

(continued)

TABLE 8.4 *(CONTINUED)*

Phase	Exercise	Volume (sets × reps)	Intensity	Interset rest (sec)
Athletic motor skill competencies	Overhead squat	3 × 8	Olympic barbell	30
	Walking lunge with ball catch	3 × 8 (4 each leg)	Body weight	30
	Band-resisted hip thrust	3 × 8	Band resistance	30
	Resistance band press	3 × 8	Band resistance	30

Phase	Exercise	Volume (sets × reps)	Intensity	Interset rest (sec)
Athletic motor skill competencies (continued)	Resistance band pull-down	3 × 8	Band resistance	30
	Jump with band perturbation	2 × 6	Band resistance	30
	Jackknife	2 × 8	Body weight	30

CHAPTER 9

Strength and Power Training

CHAPTER OBJECTIVES

- Identify misconceptions associated with strength and power training in youth
- Examine the physiological mechanisms for training-induced gains in strength and power during childhood and adolescence
- Review the health-, fitness-, and performance-related benefits of youth strength and power training
- Discuss training strategies used to enhance strength and power in youth
- Design strength and power training programs for children and adolescents

KEY TERMS

Introduction

Observing children and adolescents on a playground or sport field supports the premise that muscular strength and power are prerequisites for ongoing participation in physical activities that are developmentally appropriate and enjoyable. If youth are unable to push, pull, lift, and jump, it is unlikely that they will be able and willing to participate in play, games, and sport activities with energy and vigor. There is strong evidence and acceptance that regular participation in structured exercise programs designed to enhance muscular strength and power offer observable health and fitness benefits for children and adolescents (Behm et al., 2017; Faigenbaum, Lloyd, MacDonald, & Myer, 2016; Garcia-Hermoso, Ramirez-Campillo, & Izquierdo, 2019; Lloyd et al., 2014; Smith et al., 2014). As mentioned in chapter 4, enhancing muscular strength and power early in life should be viewed as a cornerstone of lifetime health and wellness.

Years ago, some observers were concerned that "lifting weights" would be harmful to the developing skeleton of young lifters, or that this type of exercise would be ineffective without adequate levels of circulating testosterone. Although these misconceptions swayed some observers from encouraging youth to participate in this type of training, a number of coaches, clinicians, and pediatric researchers continued to explore the safety and efficacy of youth resistance training (Micheli, 1988; National Strength and Conditioning Association, 1985; Rians et al., 1987; Westcott, 1979). Over the past two decades, the emergence of evidence-based guidelines from international organizations has influenced the acceptance of supervised resistance training for children and adolescents (American College of Sports Medicine, 2018; Australian Strength and Conditioning Association, 2007; Behm, Faigenbaum, Falk, & Klentrou, 2008; Bergeron et al., 2015; Faigenbaum, Kraemer, et al., 2009; Lloyd et al., 2014). Collectively, these guidelines highlight the need to increase opportunities for children and adolescents to engage in supervised training programs that enhance muscular strength and power as part of a long-term approach to physical development, health enhancement, and fitness improvement.

Nowadays, a growing number of schools and fitness centers offer exercise programs that target strength deficits, and public health objectives now aim to increase participation in activities that enhance both cardiorespiratory and muscular fitness (American Council on Exercise, IHRSA, & Club Intel, 2015; Bangsbo et al., 2016; Society of Health and Physical Educators, 2014; World Health Organization, 2010). In addition, the practice of developing muscular strength and power early in life to enhance athleticism, improve performance, and reduce the risk of sport-related injury is now considered foundational for long-term athletic development (Behm et al., 2017; Bergeron et al., 2015; Granacher et al., 2016; Lloyd, Cronin, et al., 2016). Youth fitness specialists need to be aware of resistance training guidelines for youth with various needs, goals, and abilities, as well as the potential benefits and risks associated with this type of exercise.

Concerns and Misconceptions About Youth Resistance Training

Although a compelling body of research indicates that supervised resistance exercise can be a safe and effective method of training for children and adolescents (Behringer, Vom Heede, Matthews, & Mester, 2011; Behringer, Vom Heede, Yue, & Mester, 2010; Faigenbaum & Myer, 2010b; Granacher et al., 2016; Lloyd et al., 2014), traditional concerns and misconceptions persist (Fröberg, Alricsson, & Ahnesjö, 2014; McGladrey, Hannon, Faigenbaum, Shultz, & Shaw, 2014; ten Hoor et al., 2015). One of the most common concerns associated with youth resistance training relates to the potential for injury to the **physis** or growth plate located near the ends of long bones (see figure 2.5 in chapter 2). The physis is an area of cartilage located between the **metaphysis** (widened part of the bone shaft) and the **epiphysis** (end of long bone). Unlike adult bone, the physis in youth has not yet ossified (hardened) and is susceptible to injury. Although a small number of fractures to the physis were reported in young weightlifters in the 1970s and 1980s (Gumbs, Segal, Halligan, & Lower, 1982; Jenkins & Mintowt-Czyz, 1986; Rowe, 1979; Ryan & Salciccioli, 1976), these reports were case studies and involved improper lifting techniques or the performance of heavy lifts in unsupervised settings.

In contrast, growth plate fractures have not been reported in any prospective youth resistance training study that was well designed and supervised by qualified professionals (Faigenbaum & Myer, 2010b; Lloyd et al., 2014; Malina, 2006). If participants are taught how to properly perform resistance training, and if progression is based on technical competence rather than amount of weight lifted, then the risk of injury to the growth plate is minimal. Moreover, the sport-specific forces placed on the developing skeleton of young athletes who participate in sports such as gymnastics and rugby are likely to be greater both in magnitude and duration than those resulting from resistance training (Malina, Baxter-Jones, et al., 2013; McNitt-Gray, Hester, Mathiyakom, & Munkasy, 2001). Even the weight-bearing jumping and hopping commonly seen on school playgrounds can place

Defining Terminology

By definition, **muscular strength** is the maximal amount of force that can be generated at a specified velocity, whereas **muscular power** refers to the rate of performing work (Fleck & Kraemer, 2014). Since power is the product of force and velocity, muscular strength is an integral component of power development (Suchomel, Nimphius, & Stone, 2016). **Local muscular endurance** refers to the ability of specific muscle groups to sustain repeated actions for a given time period. The broader term **muscular fitness** incorporates the domains of muscular strength, muscular power, and local muscular endurance.

Resistance training is a collective term that refers to methods of conditioning that involve the progressive use of a wide range of resistive loads, different movement velocities, and a variety of training modalities. Methods of resistance training include the use of body weight, free weights (barbells and dumbbells), weight machines, elastic bands, medicine balls, and manual resistance. The term *resistance training* should be distinguished from the sport of **weightlifting**, which involves performing the snatch and clean-and-jerk lifts in competition. The term **weight training** refers to a variety of multijoint movements, including modifications of weightlifting exercises.

Plyometric training is a specialized type of resistance training that consists of quick, powerful actions that involve muscle lengthening immediately followed by rapid shortening of the same muscle. Examples include explosive jumps, hops, and throws that use the stretch-shortening cycle.

---

demands on the musculoskeletal system that exceed the physical stress caused by resistance training (McKay et al., 2005). Thus the belief that participation in a well-designed resistance training program will harm the growing skeleton is inconsistent with the needs of modern-day youth and the documented benefits associated with weight-bearing physical activities (Behringer, Gruetzner, McCourt, & Mester, 2014; Gómez-Bruton, Matute-Llorente, González-Agüero, Casajús, & Vicente-Rodríguez, 2017; Larsen et al., 2018; Specker, Thiex, & Sudhagoni, 2015).

DO YOU KNOW?

Childhood is the opportune time to build bone mass and enhance bone structure by participating regularly in weight-bearing physical activity.

Another traditional misconception holds that gains cannot be induced by resistance training during childhood because children have insufficient levels of circulating androgens. Although this contention was supported by results from several early studies (Docherty, Wenger, & Collis, 1987; Vrijens, 1978), the data interpretation may have been influenced by methodological limitations including short study duration, low training volume, and lack of adequate control for growth and learning. In addition, follow-up investigations—which used higher training intensities and volumes—continue to provide strong evidence that training-induced gains are indeed possible throughout childhood and adolescence (Alves, Marta, Neiva, Izquierdo, & Marques, 2016; Chaouachi, Hammami, et al.,

2014; Faigenbaum, Zaichkowsky, Westcott, Micheli, & Fehlandt, 1993; Faigenbaum, Loud, O'Connell, Glover, & Westcott, 2001; Larsen et al., 2018; Lloyd, Radnor, De Ste Croix, Cronin, & Oliver, 2015; Pfeiffer & Francis, 1986; Ramsay et al., 1990). Although training outcomes are influenced by internal factors, such as individual genetics and personal motivation, untrained youth who participate in well-designed programs can generally be expected to experience gains in muscular strength of about 30 percent to 40 percent following the first two or three months of resistance training (Faigenbaum, Kraemer, et al., 2009; Lloyd et al., 2014).

If provided with ongoing instruction and technique-driven progression, youth who engage in resistance training are more likely to exhibit better muscular strength and power performance at any age than their age-matched peers who do not participate in this type of training (Behringer et al., 2011; Behringer et al., 2010; Lloyd et al., 2014). In addition, these training-induced adaptations will likely set the stage for even greater gains in strength and power later in life (Behm et al., 2017; Faigenbaum, Lloyd, & Myer, 2013; Lloyd, Cronin, et al., 2016). Furthermore, early exposure to strength-building exercises and positive learning experiences may lead to regular participation in resistance training activities as an ongoing lifestyle choice.

Trainability of Strength and Power

Training-induced gains in strength and power during childhood appear to derive primarily not from hypertrophic factors but from neuromuscular mechanisms.

Teaching Tip

WINDOW OF ADAPTATION

At the beginning of a resistance training program, the window of adaptation (i.e., opportunity for change) is relatively large, and participants are likely to experience impressive gains in any performance variable. During this time, youth fitness specialists need to provide all participants with an opportunity to develop good training habits through basic education about weightroom behavior, proper use of equipment, and sensible starting weights. It is prudent for beginners to learn correct exercise and practice proper training before developing bad habits that are difficult to correct later in life.

Because children lack adequate levels of circulating androgens to stimulate increases in muscle size, they appear to experience more difficulty than older populations in increasing their muscle mass following resistance training (Granacher et al., 2011; Ozmun, Mikesky, & Surburg, 1994; Ramsay et al., 1990). In order to fully distinguish the effects of resistance training on muscle mass from expected gains due to growth and maturation, we may need to design more advanced training protocols, observe longer training periods, and develop more sensitive measuring techniques that are ethically appropriate for youth. As of now, however, it appears that children's potential for strength and power gains induced by resistance training depend primarily on neuromuscular factors rather than hypertrophic factors.

Specifically, without corresponding increases in muscle mass, the available data indicate that gains induced in children by resistance training relate primarily to increases in motor unit activation and changes in motor unit coordination, recruitment, and firing frequency (Granacher et al., 2011; Ozmun et al., 1994; Ramsay et al., 1990). Other neuromuscular influences that may contribute to observed gains in strength and power in youth include a decrease in electromechanical delay (i.e., time between onset of muscle activity and production of force) and improvements in stiffness properties defined as the ratio between peak forces and deformation of the material (i.e., leg, joint, or tendon stiffness) (Lazaridis et al., 2013; Lloyd, Oliver, Hughes, & Williams, 2012; Waugh, Korff, Fath, & Blazevich, 2014). In addition, given that measured improvements in muscle strength following resistance training are typically greater than the changes observed in neuromuscular activation patterns, training-induced adaptions may also be influenced by improvements in motor skill performance and the coordination of involved muscle groups (Ozmun et al., 1994; Ramsay et al., 1990). Collectively, these findings are supported by research indicating significant improvements in muscular strength and power during childhood without corresponding gains in gross limb morphology as compared with age-matched controls (Faigenbaum et al., 1993; Granacher et al., 2011; Lillegard, Brown, Wilson, Henderson, & Lewis, 1997; Ramsay et al., 1990).

During and after puberty, testosterone secretion in males is associated with observable gains in fat-free mass and linear growth (Malina, Bouchard, & Bar-Or, 2004). During this developmental period, resistance training-induced gains in muscular strength and power may be associated with changes in hypertrophic factors due to testosterone and other hormonal influences (Kraemer, Fry, Frykman, Conroy, & Hoffman, 1989; Malina et al., 2004). However, the internal hormonal milieu can differ greatly between adolescents of the same chronological age; therefore, youth fitness specialists should expect interindividual differences in muscle size before and after resistance training in young lifters. In females, the smaller amount of testosterone limits the magnitude of gains in muscle mass following resistance training, and other growth factors and hormones such as estradiol may be at least partly responsible for resistance training-induced adaptations in adolescent females (Malina et al., 2004). If practitioners understand the mechanisms and endocrine profiles responsible for gains induced by resistance training during childhood and adolescence, then they will be better positioned to establish realistic goals for males and females.

Detraining and the Persistence of Strength and Power Gains

At some point, children and adolescents are likely to undergo periods of reduced training or inactivity due to program design factors, sport schedules, travel plans, academic calendars, decreased motivation, or injury. Therefore, it is important to evaluate and monitor temporary or permanent reduction of the training stimulus, or **detraining** (Faigenbaum et al., 1996). The concept of detraining in youth is relatively complex

Teaching Tip

GIRL POWER

During childhood, training-induced gains in muscle strength and power result primarily from neuromuscular adaptations and skill development. During adolescence, however, males may develop larger muscles due to the robust effects of anabolic hormones, whereas females can make remarkable improvements without corresponding gains in muscle size. Because some females may be dissuaded from resistance training for fear that they will develop "bulky muscles," youth fitness specialists should reassure them that they can achieve significant benefits from resistance training without observable changes in muscle mass. Educating youth and their parents about resistance training can help practitioners dispel myths and boost participation in this type of exercise, which offers distinct health and fitness benefits for female youth (Moran et al., 2018; Sommi, Gill, Trojan, & Mulcahey, 2018).

because any loss of muscular strength or power due to a reduction in training may be masked by concomitant growth-related gains in muscle performance (Faigenbaum, Farrell, et al., 2013; Faigenbaum et al., 1996; Meylan, Cronin, Oliver, Hopkins, & Contreras, 2014). Available research indicates that training-induced gains in muscular strength and power during childhood and adolescence are impermanent and that individuals tend to regress toward untrained control-group values during a detraining period (Faigenbaum, Farrell, et al., 2013; Faigenbaum et al., 1996; Ingle, Sleap, & Tolfrey, 2006; Meylan et al., 2014; Tsolakis, Vagenas, & Dessypris, 2004). In one report, the effects of an eight-week resistance training program followed by a detraining period of equal duration were evaluated in children aged 7 to 12 years (Faigenbaum et al., 1996). Following the training period, significant gains in upper- and lower-body strength were reported, but the gains regressed toward untrained control-group values during the detraining period at a rate of 3 percent per week. Observed differences in the magnitude of strength regressions in the upper body (−19 percent) and lower body (−28 percent) highlight the complexity of the detraining response, which may relate to the developing musculature of the upper and lower body in youth (Faigenbaum et al., 1996).

The precise physiological mechanisms responsible for the loss of muscular strength and power during detraining in childhood and adolescence remain uncertain, but possibilities include changes in neuromuscular functioning and loss of motor coordination. Detraining regressions may also be influenced by maturity status and the design of the training program (Faigenbaum, Farrell, et al., 2013; Meylan et al., 2014). Although further study is warranted, some of the neuromuscular adaptive mechanisms that underpin changes in performance during detraining may vary depending on the type of exercise (e.g., strength or power), the complexity of the motor skill

(e.g., single-leg or double-leg hop), and the musculature involved in the movement (e.g., upper body or lower body) (Chaouachi et al., 2018; Faigenbaum, Farrell, et al., 2013). These observations suggest that the phenomenon of detraining during childhood and adolescence is characterized by different regressions in strength and power performance that seem to be influenced by the design of the training program. Figure 9.1 illustrates the complexity of the detraining response in youth following different resistance training programs.

Youth fitness specialists should recognize the necessity of regular training throughout childhood and adolescence. Discontinuing structured resistance training reduces the likelihood that desired adaptations in fitness measures will continue to be observed. Notably, a once weekly maintenance training program was found to be just as effective as a twice-per-week program in retaining strength gains after 12 weeks of preseason resistance training in young athletes (DeRenne, Hetzler, Buxton, & Ho, 1996). Other researchers have reported that young athletes were able to maintain training-induced gains in muscular fitness following several weeks of reduced training that included sport practice (Diallo, Dore, Duche, & Van Praagh, 2001; Santos & Janeira, 2009). Therefore, in order to develop, maintain, and enhance muscular strength and power, young athletes should participate in some type of ongoing resistance training in addition to their sports practice.

Potential Benefits of Youth Resistance Training

Certain levels of force production and force attenuation are prerequisites for sustainable and enjoyable participation in playground games and competitive sports. Toward this end, youth can obtain benefits for both fitness and health through regular participation

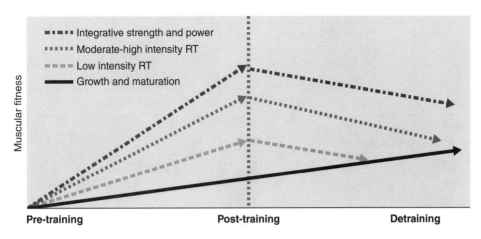

FIGURE 9.1 Theoretical model of the effects of training and detraining on muscular fitness in youth. RT=resistance training.

Teaching Tip

USE IT OR LOSE IT

Regardless of age, maturity status, and program design, resistance training-induced adaptations tend to regress toward untrained values during a detraining period. Therefore, an ongoing commitment to resistance training is needed in order to maintain or improve strength and power performance. Incorporating resistance exercises into fitness workouts and sport practice may maintain training-induced adaptations, but youth also need regular participation in year-round resistance training with systematic variation in training load and volume in order to optimize adaptations and long-term performance.

---

in exercise programs that include strength and power exercises, provided that the program is carefully prescribed, gradually progressed, and consistent with each participant's needs, goals, and abilities (Faigenbaum & Myer, 2010a; Garcia-Hermoso, Ramirez-Campillo, & Izquierdo, 2019; Granacher et al., 2016; Smith et al., 2014). More specifically, new insights into the design of resistance training programs for youth continue to highlight the unique benefits of resistance training early in life for improving physical activity trajectories and enhancing long-term health and well-being (Behm et al., 2017; Faigenbaum, Lloyd, et al., 2013; Lloyd, Cronin, et al., 2016; Smith et al., 2019). In addition to enhancing muscular fitness and reducing the risk of sport-related injuries, regular resistance training can increase bone mineral density, reduce cardiovascular risk factors, fuel metabolic health, facilitate weight control, enhance psychosocial well-being, and support ongoing participation in moderate and vigorous intensity physical activities including sport (Faigenbaum et al., 2016; Garcia-Hermoso, Ramirez-Campillo, & Izquierdo, 2019; Laursen, Bertelsen, & Andersen, 2014; Lloyd et al., 2014; Schranz, Tomkinson, Parletta, Petkov, & Olds, 2014; Smith et al., 2019).

Potential benefits of resistance training in youth are also described in figure 9.2.

Children and adolescents with inadequate levels of muscular strength and motor skill may be less able and less willing to engage in exercise and sport activities with energy and vigor (Cattuzzo et al., 2016; Fransen et al., 2014; Robinson et al., 2015). Moreover, youth with low levels of habitual physical activity and weak muscle strength appear to have the highest risk of injury during physical education, leisure activities, and sports (Augustsson & Ageberg, 2017; Bloemers et al., 2012; Laursen et al., 2014). When youth do not have regular opportunities to engage in planned exercise programs targeting the development of muscular strength and power, they may be more likely to experience negative health outcomes and less likely to optimize their long-term physical development (Faigenbaum, Lloyd, et al., 2013; Lloyd, Cronin, et al., 2016; Smith et al., 2019).

The term **dynapenia** (*dyna* for "power" and *penia* for "deficiency") was originally proposed to highlight the observable effect of muscle weakness and dysfunction on functional disability and mortality in older adults (Clark & Manini, 2008). However, the

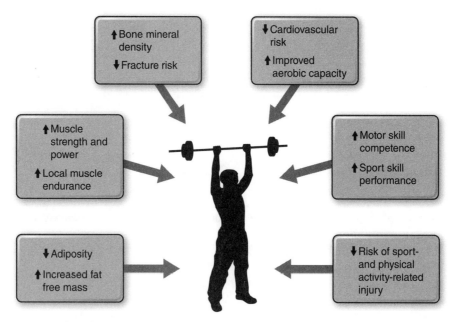

FIGURE 9.2   Potential benefits of resistance training in youth.

Adapted by permission from A.D. Faigenbaum and R.S. Lloyd, "Resistance Training," in *Oxford Textbook of Children's Sport and Exercise Medicine*, 3rd ed., edited by N. Armstrong and W. van Mechelen (Oxford: Oxford University Press, 2017), 493-506. Reproduced with permission of the Licensor through PLSclear.

life-changing consequences of low muscle strength are not limited to older populations. In a prospective study of more than a million male adolescents who were followed over a period of 24 years, low muscle strength was identified as an emerging risk factor for major causes of death, including cardiovascular disease (Ortega, Silventoinen, Tynelius, & Rasmussen, 2012). Others have reported that muscular weakness in adolescence is associated with disability 30 years later (Henriksson, Henriksson, Tynelius, & Ortega, 2018). Thus the construct of dynapenia should be expanded to include youth (Faigenbaum & Bruno, 2017), and the term *pediatric dynapenia* highlights an identifiable and treatable condition characterized by low levels of muscle strength and power and consequent functional limitations not caused by neurologic or muscular disease (Faigenbaum & MacDonald, 2017). These findings emphasize the importance of identifying inactive youth early in life and incorporating resistance exercise into school- and community-based fitness programs for youth.

Bone Health

Traditional fears that resistance training would be harmful to the developing skeleton have been replaced by reports indicating that childhood may be the opportune time for the bone remodeling process to respond to the tensile and compressive forces associated with weight-bearing exercise (as discussed in chapter 2) (Behringer et al., 2014; Ishikawa, Kim, Kang,

& Morgan, 2013). In all likelihood, regular participation in a variety of weight-bearing activities, including resistance training, can maximize bone mineral density during the growing years if the training program is well designed and participants follow nutrition recommendations (e.g., adequate intake of calcium and vitamin D). Moreover, no evidence indicates that participation in resistance training during childhood and adolescence will have a detrimental effect on linear growth (Falk & Eliakim, 2003; Malina, 2006; Malina, Baxter-Jones, et al., 2013).

The compressive and tensile muscle forces that act on bone to perform desired movements can provide a potent stimulus for osteogenesis, or new bone formation (Fritz, Rosengren, Dencker, Karlsson, & Karlsson, 2016; Kindler, Lewis, & Hamrick, 2015; Larsen et al., 2018). With developing muscular capacities, it is possible to augment the osteogenic response to resistance training by placing even greater demands on skeletal structures with heavier loads. Indeed, the bone mineral density of Junior Olympics weightlifters who train and compete with relatively heavy loads has been shown to surpass reference norms (Conroy et al., 1993; Virvidakis, Georgiu, Korkotsidis, Ntalles, & Proukakis, 1990). In addition, adolescent combat sport athletes (Nasri et al., 2013) and gymnasts as young as six years old have been found to have greater bone mass, size, and strength than age-matched controls (Burt, Ducher, Naughton, Courteix, & Greene, 2013).

Childhood represents an opportune time for the processes of bone modeling and remodeling to respond to the mechanical loading of weight-bearing physical activities (Francis, Morrissey, Letuchy, Levy, & Janz, 2013; Janz et al., 2014; Weaver et al., 2016). For instance, although training-induced responses to resistance training vary among individuals, it appears that if training is characterized by periodic bouts of high-impact loading, then skeletal adaptations early in life may exert a positive influence on bone health later in life, (Ferry, Lespessailles, Rochcongar, Duclos, & Courteix, 2013; Klentrou, 2016; Zouch, Vico, Frere, Tabka, & Alexandre, 2014). Therefore, youth fitness specialists incorporate different types of weight-bearing activities, including resistance training, into their fitness programs. Failure to maximize the development of bone mass and improve skeletal health early in life may predispose individuals to poor bone health and fractures later in life (Gunter, Almstedt, & Janz, 2012; Tveit, Rosengren, Nilsson, & Karlsson, 2015; Weaver et al., 2016).

DO YOU KNOW?

Swimming is a beneficial and enjoyable activity for boys and girls, but weight-bearing sports and activities such as gymnastics, soccer, and weightlifting are more likely to increase bone strength and bone size in youth.

Cardiovascular and Metabolic Health

As physical inactivity and obesity become more prevalent among children and adolescents worldwide, cardiovascular and metabolic ailments are appearing at an increasing rate (Bass & Eneli, 2015; Lobstein et al., 2015; Mayer-Davis et al., 2017). Notwithstanding the observable value of aerobic games and activities, a growing body of research supports the utility of resistance exercise for enhancing cardiovascular and metabolic health in youth (Bea, Blew, Howe, Hetherington-Rauth, & Going, 2017; Gomes, Dos Santos, Katzmarzyk, & Maia, 2017; Gordon, Dolinsky, Mughal, Gordon, & McGavock, 2015; Tarp et al., 2019). Resistance training has proven to be an effective nonpharmacological intervention for children and adolescents who have abnormal amounts of lipids in the blood (Fripp & Hodgson, 1987; Sung et al., 2002; Weltman, Janney, Rians, Strand, & Katch, 1987) and research findings suggest that muscular fitness also seems to play a protective role against the risk of elevated blood pressure (Cohen, López-Jaramillo, Fernández-Santos, Castro-Piñero, & Sandercock, 2017; Hagberg et al., 1984). In addition, in overweight and obese youth, resistance training seems to be associated with favor-

able changes in body composition, insulin sensitivity, and endothelial dysfunction (Dias et al., 2015; Sigal et al., 2014; Van der Heijden et al., 2010); for more on this topic, see chapter 14.

Along with traditional risk factors for disease, low levels of muscular strength early in life have been identified as an emerging risk factor for cardiometabolic disease (Cohen et al., 2014; Fraser et al., 2016; Gomes et al., 2017; Grøntved et al., 2015; Peterson, Zhang, Saltarelli, Visich, & Gordon, 2016). Based on a sample of 378 children aged 9 to 11 years, the "active and strong" group had the best metabolic risk profile, whereas the insufficiently active and low-strength group had the worst (Gomes et al., 2017). Other research found that low levels of muscular fitness during childhood and adolescence were independently associated with cardiometabolic risk, even after adjusting for cardiorespiratory fitness (Fraser et al., 2016; Peterson et al., 2016). These findings highlight the importance of identifying and treating low levels of muscular fitness early in life (i.e., pediatric dynapenia) in order to protect against cardiometabolic disease later in life.

Research has shown that regular participation in youth fitness programs designed to enhance muscular fitness may improve the metabolic efficiency of muscle (i.e., lipid oxidation, glucose transport capacity) and increase physical activity (Dias et al., 2015; Garcia-Hermoso, Ramirez-Campillo, & Izquierdo, 2019; Meinhardt, Witassek, Petrò, Fritz, & Eiholzer, 2013; Racil et al., 2016; Smith et al., 2019). Following 19 weeks of structured resistance training, spontaneous physical activity (measured by accelerometry) increased by 10 percent from baseline in boys, and the least active participants made the greatest gains (Meinhardt et al., 2013). Thus, the first step toward enhancing cardiovascular and metabolic health in inactive youth may be to increase their competence and confidence in performing a variety of resistance exercises; this foundation, in turn, may lead to improvements in daily participation in moderate to vigorous physical activity and associated cardiometabolic benefits.

The American College of Sports Medicine suggests that in the early stages of an exercise program, muscle-strengthening exercises may need to precede aerobic training in frail seniors (American College of Sports Medicine, 2018). In the same vein, resistance training may be needed in order to "activate" inactive youth. Although no single program offers proven efficacy to optimize cardiometabolic health in all youth, the effects of resistance training, either alone or in combination with other types of training, provide a worthwhile alternative to focusing only on continuous aerobic exercise of moderate intensity.

Teaching Tip

PUMP IT UP

Although traditional aerobic exercises such as running and cycling are recognized as moderate to vigorous physical activities, resistance training can also offer cardiometabolic benefits. For example, exercising with medicine balls and battling ropes has been found to provide a moderate to vigorous cardiometabolic stimulus in children (Faigenbaum, Kang, Ratamess, Farrell, Ellis, et al., 2018; Faigenbaum, Kang, Ratamess, Farrell, Golda, et al., 2018). Thus, while bearing in mind that responses to any type of training can be influenced by complexity, intensity, cadence, and rest intervals, practitioners should recognize the potent cardiometabolic responses to different types of resistance exercise.

Motor Skill and Sports Performance

Researchers and practitioners are increasingly interested in the potential effects of structured resistance training on motor skill and sport performance in children and adolescents. Youth who exhibit muscle weakness and low levels of motor skill performance participate less in sport and are often unable to perform desired movement patterns, demonstrate proper technique, or maintain adequate physical fitness (De Meester et al., 2018; Fransen et al., 2014; Ruas, Punt, Pinto, & Oliveira, 2014). Without early interventions to address strength deficits, neuromuscular limitations become ingrained as suboptimal motor control patterns are reinforced over time. Moreover, new insights into the design of long-term physical development plans continue to highlight the importance of improving muscular strength and motor skill performance early in life in order to give children the best possible chance of participating persistently and successfully in exercise and sport activities (Behm et al., 2017; Faigenbaum et al., 2016; Lesinski, Prieske, & Granacher, 2016; Lloyd, Cronin, et al., 2016). Indeed, developing skills that build a strong movement foundation have been found to be positively associated with multiple aspects of physical health and psychological well-being that strengthen with increasing age (Babic et al., 2014; Cattuzzo et al., 2016; Robinson et al., 2015; Utesch, Bardid, Büsch, & Strauss, 2019).

The literature has examined the influence of muscular strength on various specific factors associated with athletic performance (Faigenbaum et al., 2016; Granacher et al., 2016; Suchomel et al., 2016). Meta-analytical findings indicate that resistance training is an effective tool for enhancing general sport skills (e.g., jumping, running, throwing) during childhood and adolescence (Behringer et al., 2011; Harries, Lubans, & Callister, 2012). Due to the neuromuscular plasticity associated with the growing years, there appears to be a unique opportunity to enhance muscular fitness early in life and thereby set the stage for even greater gains in motor skill and sport performance later on (Faigenbaum et al., 2016; Myer, Faigenbaum, et al., 2015).

For example, regular participation in a two-year periodized program of resistance training improved sprint speed by up to 6 percent in elite youth soccer players as compared with a group of age-matched players who participated only in soccer training (Sander, Keiner, Wirth, & Schmidtbleicher, 2013). Others reported favorable adaptations induced by resistance training in age-group swimmers (Blanksby & Gregor, 1981), rhythmic gymnasts (Piazza et al., 2014), and adolescent distance runners (Blagrove et al., 2018), as well as young athletes who play badminton (Ozmen & Aydogmus, 2016), basketball (Santos & Janeira, 2008), handball (Ignjatovic, Markovic, & Radovanovic, 2012; Mascarin et al., 2016), and tennis (Behringer, Neuerburg, Matthews, & Mester, 2013; Fernandez-Fernandez, de Villarreal, Sanz-Rivas, & Moya, 2016).

Because sport participation alone does not ensure that young athletes will attain sufficient physical fitness to optimize athletic performance and reduce injury risk (Guagliano, Rosenkranz, & Kolt, 2013; Leek et al., 2010; Ridley, Zabeen, & Lunnay, 2018), structured resistance training is needed in order to optimize gains in muscular strength and power in young athletes. In fact, available data underline a potential synergistic adaptation wherein the stimulus of resistance training complements naturally occurring adaptations throughout the growing years (Faigenbaum et al., 2016). Resistance training has proven to be an effective strategy for enhancing motor skill performance in youth (Behringer et al., 2011), and these training-induced gains may support the acquisition of more complex sport tactics as one's competence and confidence to perform resistance exercise develops over time. Specifically, dose–response relationships for key training parameters indicate that the most effective approach for improving physical performance measures in young athletes is to perform dynamic muscle actions with free weights, multiple sets, and a training intensity of 80 percent to 89 percent of 1RM (Lesinski et al., 2016). However, progression toward targeted resistance training loads should always be technique-driven and consistent with each participant's abilities.

Injury Reduction in Youth

In addition to eliciting gains in muscular fitness, regular participation in a youth resistance training program has been found to enhance movement mechanics and improve functional abilities (Behm et al., 2017; Richmond, Kang, Doyle-Baker, Nettel-Aguirre, & Emery, 2016; Sugimoto et al., 2016). These training outcomes reduce the incidence of sport-related injuries in young athletes (Campbell et al., 2014; Emery, Roy, Whittaker, Nettel-Aguirre, & van Mechelen, 2015; Laursen et al., 2014; Owoeye, Palacios-Derflingher, & Emery, 2018; Sugimoto, Myer, Barber Foss, & Hewett, 2015). Youth who do not address neuromuscular deficits or enhance their muscular strength may be more likely to suffer a sport-related injury because both force production and force attenuation are required in order to perform all athletic movements. The importance of implementing injury prevention interventions with at-risk individuals is highlighted by the increasing incidence of anterior cruciate ligament (ACL) tears in school-age youth over the past 20 years (Beck, Lawrence, Nordin, DeFor, & Tompkins, 2017).

DO YOU KNOW?

Resistance training is a critical component of injury prevention for young athletes.

Athletes of any age who build and maintain their **strength reserve** (i.e., enhance their ability to produce force) are better prepared for the physical demands of sport training and competition (Faigenbaum, MacDonald, & Haff, 2019). A strength reserve refers to a special type of resource that can be used (or not) to overcome physical challenges. From this perspective, the lack of a strength reserve can be considered a vulnerability that may impede a child's ability to perform physical activities or overcome adverse events. Regular exposure to preparatory conditioning that builds a strength reserve has been found to significantly reduce both acute and overuse sport-related injuries (Laursen et al., 2014). This type of training may be particularly beneficial for young athletes who specialize in a single sport at an early age at the expense of enhancing muscular fitness (Myer, Jayanthi, et al., 2015). Research indicates that injury risk in adolescent athletes is reduced by training interventions that include progressive strengthening exercises, proprioceptive training, and instruction on proper landing and cutting techniques (Emery et al., 2015; Sugimoto, Myer, Foss, & Hewett, 2015; Webster & Hewitt, 2018). Although additional research is needed on age-related injury prevention, it is possible that similar effects would be observed in younger athletes provided that the training program is developmentally appropriate, supervised by qualified professionals, and driven by technical competence (Foss, Thomas, Khoury, Myer, & Hewett, 2018; Richmond et al., 2016; Thompson-Kolesar et al., 2018). The International Olympic Committee recommends that injury prevention programs start at the age of 6 to 10 years in some sports (Renstrom et al., 2016).

Without regular participation in recreational activities and planned exercise programs that enhance

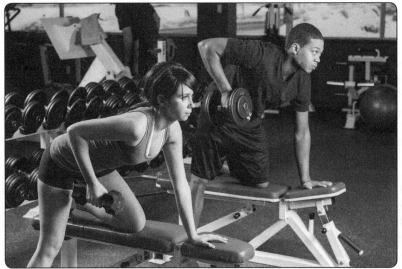

Resistance training helps teenagers improve fitness performance and maintain a healthy body composition.

FatCamera/E+/Getty Images

muscular strength and power, the divergence in performance between stronger and weaker youth may persist into adulthood and those with lower levels of muscular fitness may not catch up with their peers. Although practitioners should consider intrinsic risk factors such as growth, maturation, body composition, and previous injury, they should also recognize the importance of targeting neuromuscular deficits early in life as a cost-effective method to enhance performance and reduce injury rates (Marshall, Lopatina, Lacny, & Emery, 2016; Renstrom et al., 2016). As discussed in chapter 7, time-efficient injury prevention strategies can be incorporated into warm-up routines in physical education classes and sport practices.

DO YOU KNOW?

Injury prevention programs in youth sport can reduce the burden of injury and significantly reduce health care costs as compared with standard practice.

Youth Resistance Training Guidelines

Children and adolescents can make significant gains in muscular strength and power above and beyond growth and maturation by participating regularly in a well-designed resistance training program (Behringer et al., 2010; Faigenbaum & Myer, 2010b; Lloyd et al., 2014). Ongoing research indicates that a wide variety of training modalities and various combinations of sets and repetitions can provide adequate stimulus for enhancing muscular strength and power in youth, provided that the program is consistent with the needs and abilities of the participants (Granacher et al., 2016; Lesinski et al., 2016; Lloyd et al., 2014). Although there is no evidence-based minimum age for participation in a youth resistance training program, most seven- and eight-year-old boys and girls are ready to accept and follow instructions and participate in some type of structured resistance training as part of fitness classes or sport training (Faigenbaum, Kraemer, et al., 2009; Lloyd et al., 2014). Younger children may benefit from strength- and skill-building games and activities that are developmentally appropriate and enjoyable (Annesi, Westcott, Faigenbaum, & Unruh, 2005; Duncan, Eyre, & Oxford, 2017; Faigenbaum & Bruno, 2017; Robinson, Veldman, Palmer, & Okely, 2017).

Training outcomes can be influenced by various factors, such as heredity, nutrition, and sleep. However, the fundamental elements that determine the safety, effectiveness, and sustainability of youth resistance training programs are the interrelated principles of progression, regularity, overload, creativity, enjoy-

ment, socialization, and supervision (Faigenbaum & McFarland, 2016). These principles can be remembered acronymically as the PROCESS of youth resistance training (see figure 9.3). Although the time-honored tenets of progression, regularity, and overload affect the rate and magnitude of training-induced adaptions, youth fitness specialists should not overlook the importance of making friends, having fun, being creative, and teaching children something new.

In order to succeed, a training program needs to be built on a strategy of systematic and deliberate training characterized by qualified instruction in a socially supportive environment. Such a program can enhance participants' skill development, prevent the accrual of neuromuscular deficiencies, create a positive motivational environment, and help maintain adherence. Table 9.1 lists modifiable risk factors associated with youth resistance training that can be reduced (or eliminated) with qualified supervision and instruction (Faigenbaum, Myer, Naclerio, & Casas, 2011). Remember that youth with preexisting medical conditions (e.g., cancer, cardiomyopathy, seizure disorder) should receive medical clearance before participating in a resistance training program (American Academy of Pediatrics, 2008).

In order to engage in formalized training, youth should understand safety rules, be willing and able to follow exercise instructions, and be able to choose to participate in such training. Children in primary school have safely participated in supervised exercise interventions that included resistance training, and significant gains in performance measures have

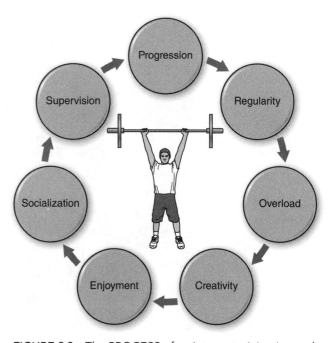

FIGURE 9.3   The PROCESS of resistance training in youth.

TABLE 9.1   MODIFIABLE RISK FACTORS ASSOCIATED WITH YOUTH RESISTANCE TRAINING

Risk factor	Modification by qualified professional
Unsupervised training area	Supervision by youth fitness specialist
Unsafe exercise environment	Adequate training space and proper equipment layout
Improper equipment storage	Proper and secure storage of exercise equipment
Unsafe use of equipment	Instruction on safety rules in the exercise area
Excessive load or volume	Gradual progression of the exercise program
Poor exercise technique	Clear instruction and feedback regarding exercise movements
Poor trunk control	Targeted core training
Previous injury	Communication with treating clinician; program modification
Growth process	Modification of training to address specific needs and abilities
Inadequate recuperation	Inclusion of less intense training sessions
Chronic fatigue	Consideration of lifestyle factors (e.g., nutrition, sleep)

Adapted by permission from A.D. Faigenbaum, G.D. Myer, F. Naclerio, and A.A. Casas, "Injury Trends and Prevention in Youth Resistance Training," *Strength and Conditioning Journal* 33, no. 3 (2011): 36-41.

been reported (Duncan et al., 2017; Faigenbaum et al., 2015; Faigenbaum et al., 2011; Löfgren, Daly, Nilsson, Dencker, & Karlsson, 2013). Youth fitness specialists should recognize children's ability to adapt to resistance training; understand the individual responses to different forms of exercise; and realize that no single combination of exercises, sets, and repetitions is optimal for all participants.

In addition to traditional strength-building exercises (e.g., squat, bench press), plyometric exercises and weightlifting have been found to enhance strength and power in youth (Channell & Barfield, 2008; Chaouachi, Hammami, et al., 2014; Faigenbaum, McFarland, Keiper, et al., 2007; Lloyd, Radnor, et al., 2015; Rumpf, Cronin, Pinder, Oliver, & Hughes, 2012; Thomas, French, & Hayes, 2009). With ongoing instruction and informed practice sessions focused on exercise technique, participants can begin to master the performance of multijoint exercises and complex movement patterns before neuromuscular deficiencies emerge. These observations underscore synergistic adaptations wherein training-induced gains in measures of muscular strength and power complement naturally occurring improvements in general physical abilities (Faigenbaum et al., 2016; Peitz, Behringer, & Granacher, 2018).

Although it is advantageous to integrate strength and power exercises into well-designed exercise programs, the most important considerations are technique-driven progression of program variables and close monitoring of skill development. As discussed in chapter 6, the concept of **resistance training skill competence** (RTSC) refers to the process of developing and assessing movement patterns that are essential to mastery of a specific exercise (Barnett et al., 2015;

Lubans, Smith, Harries, Barnett, & Faigenbaum, 2014). Notwithstanding the importance of providing constructive feedback and improving exercise technique, the construct of RTSC also relates to a participant's ability to focus, follow instructions, and cooperate with others. Consequently, RTSC relates to one's exercise performance, general demeanor, and willingness to learn.

If youth fitness professionals assess movement mechanics and provide meaningful feedback during training sessions, then participants have an opportunity to learn task-related activities and enhance their RTSC. Focusing on RTSC, rather than on the amount of weight lifted, helps reinforce the importance of proper exercise technique and highlights the significance of movement skill proficiency as the criterion measure.

To enhance the learning experience, youth fitness professionals should provide meaningful feedback about the quality of exercise performance as well as the participant's ability to focus, follow instructions, and accept constructive feedback. In addition to assessing exercise technique by means of accepted commonalities of resistance exercise performance, youth should earn the right to progress by demonstrating a positive demeanor characterized by responsibility, resourcefulness, and respect. This type of instruction can lay the foundation for enduring participation in resistance training by maximizing skill competence, reducing the risk of training-related injury, and optimizing exercise adherence. Although beginners may perform a range of basic exercises (e.g., squatting, pushing or pulling movements), youth with high RTSC will need a more advanced program to optimize adaptations. A strategy for enhancing RTSC is outlined in figure 9.4.

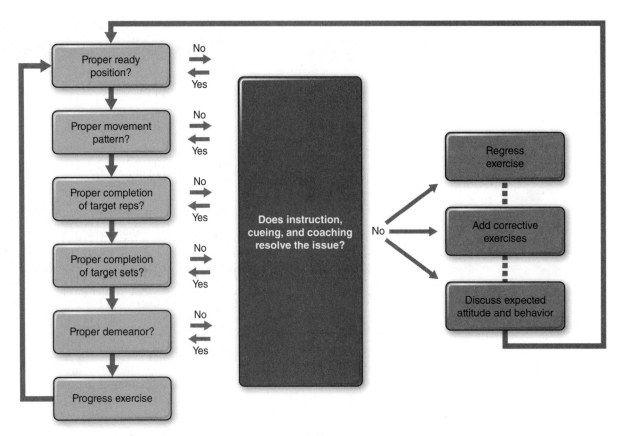

FIGURE 9.4   Strategies to develop resistance training skill competence.

Resistance Training Program Variables

Resistance training program variables need to be properly prescribed and carefully manipulated over time in order to optimize adaptations, interest, and adherence. Youth fitness specialists need to determine individual goals and establish realistic performance standards that are developmentally appropriate and meaningful. An "overdose" of resistance training at any stage of development increases the likelihood of injury, illness, or burnout (Difiori et al., 2014; Matos, Winsley, & Williams, 2011). Proper prescription is particularly important for untrained youth, who may overestimate their physical abilities and may be unaware of the inherent risks associated with resistance exercise. Consequently, in order to maximize adherence and long-term adaptations, practitioners should progress program variables in a stepwise fashion and monitor each participant's exercise technique and stress tolerance. They should assess performance, provide real-time feedback, and, when appropriate, make necessary modifications in the program.

Participants should receive basic education about safety concerns, including sensible starting weights,

appropriate spotting procedures, and proper maintenance and storage of equipment. Youth should be encouraged to embrace self-improvement, feel good about their performances, learn from their mistakes, and gain understanding of the benefits of resistance exercise. This is where the art of youth resistance training comes into play, because the physical demands of training need to be balanced with effective instructional strategies that provide an opportunity for all participants to have fun, make friends, and learn something new. The best approach to teaching maximizes enjoyment, fosters socialization, stimulates creativity, and sparks an ongoing interest in resistance training.

As shown in table 9.2, the program variables that should be considered when designing resistance training programs include choice and order of exercises, training intensity and volume load, rest intervals between sets and exercises, repetition velocity, and training frequency (Fleck & Kraemer, 2014; Ratamess, 2012).

Choice and Order of Exercises

Youth fitness specialists should select exercises that are consistent with each participant's body size, fitness level, and resistance training experience. Youth pro-

TABLE 9.2   RESISTANCE TRAINING PROGRAM VARIABLES

Variable	Specifics
Choice of exercises	Body weight or external load; single or multijoint exercise
Order of exercises	Large muscle group followed by smaller muscle group; complex exercise followed by simpler exercise
Number of sets	Single or multiple sets; number of sets per exercise and per muscle group
Training intensity (resistance)	Percentage of 1RM (RM target zone); repetition range
Rest intervals	Short or long rest interval (between sets, between exercises)
Repetition velocity	Moderate or high velocity; rate of force development
Training frequency	Training days per week; training sessions per exercise

grams have successfully used body-weight exercises, weight machines, free weights, elastic bands, medicine balls, and manual resistance (Dorgo et al., 2009; Faigenbaum et al., 2015; Faigenbaum, McFarland, Johnson, et al., 2007; Faigenbaum & Mediate, 2006; Faigenbaum et al., 1993; Lloyd, Radnor, et al., 2015; Meylan et al., 2014; Rivière, Louit, Strokosch, & Seitz, 2016). Although each training method has advantages and disadvantages, it is reasonable to start with basic movement patterns (e.g., jumping), unloaded exercises (e.g., squatting), or assisted exercises with light loads (e.g., elastic band press), then progress gradually as competence and confidence improve. Long-term athletic development models tend to employ systematic progression of exercise variables that emphasize specific outcomes along the developmental journey from foundational to high performance (Granacher et al., 2016; Hulteen, Morgan, Barnett, Stodden, & Lubans, 2018; Lloyd, Oliver, et al., 2015).

Youth with low levels of muscle strength and skill competence may need to begin resistance training with elastic bands, medicine balls, or weight-machine exercises that allow the use of relatively low resistance. In addition, at the start of a resistance training program, some participants may need assistance and cueing to ensure proper exercise technique. Body-weight exercises performed in a controlled and coordinated fashion can help youth build muscular fitness and develop requisite levels of balance and stability for meeting the demands of external loading as the program progresses. That said, multijoint exercises with free weights (e.g., squats) and dynamic whole-body movements (e.g., plyometrics) are particularly beneficial for enhancing motor skill performance and muscle power in youth (Channell & Barfield, 2008; Chaouachi, Hammami, et al., 2014; Faigenbaum, McFarland, Keiper, et al., 2007; Ramírez-Campillo et al., 2014). They should, of course, be targeted to each participant's competence and confidence to perform resistance exercises at any given time.

Exercises that improve strength of the core musculature (i.e., pelvis, abdominals, hips, trunk) may enhance performance while preparing youth for the high forces generated during recreational and sport activities (Allen, Hannon, Burns, & Williams, 2014; Contreras et al., 2017; Granacher et al., 2014; Prieske et al., 2016). During the period of peak height velocity, rapid growth of the tibia and femur initiate stature increases that concurrently increase the height of the center of mass, thus making muscular control of the trunk more challenging (Hewett, Myer, & Ford, 2004; Myer, Chu, Brent, & Hewett, 2008). Consequently, the potential benefits of integrating core exercises into youth fitness and sport programs are likely synergistic with other types of training and may help to prepare youth for the high forces generated distally during athletic movements (Chaouachi, Othman, Hammami, Drinkwater, & Behm, 2014; Prieske et al., 2016; Sugimoto, Myer, Barber Foss, et al., 2015). For example, the ABC push-up is designed to improve core strength and stability (see figure 9.5). To perform the exercise, maintain a push-up position with the body in a straight line, touch your chest with your right hand and say A, return the right hand to the starting position, and then repeat the movement with your left hand and say B. Try to complete the alphabet (or your first and last name).

There are many ways to order exercises in a resistance training program, and session design should be dictated by training goals. Since most youth will perform total-body workouts several times per week as part of a fitness class or sports training program, a variety of exercises that include whole-body movements should be performed in each session. In most cases, it is desirable to perform multijoint exercises early in the workout, when the neuromuscular system is less fatigued (Balsamo et al., 2013). Thus, if a child is learning how to perform the back squat, it should be performed at the start of the workout so that the child can practice the desired movement pattern without

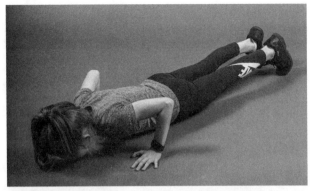

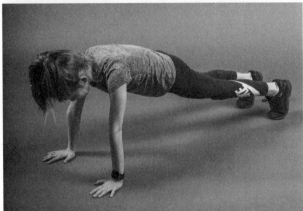

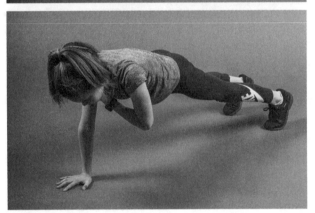

FIGURE 9.5   ABC push-up.

undue fatigue. In addition, if the goal of the session is to enhance muscular power, it is beneficial to perform plyometrics and weight training at the beginning of the session in order to reinforce proper training techniques and optimize training adaptations.

Training Intensity and Volume Load

Resistance training-induced adaptations are influenced heavily by the training intensity and volume load. Intensity is determined by the amount of weight lifted for a specific exercise and is typically expressed as a percentage of either the one-repetition maximum (1RM; e.g., 60 percent of 1RM) or the repetition range (e.g., 8RM-10 RM). Volume load, on the other hand, is a measure of the total workload and can be calculated by multiplying the load lifted by the total number of sets and repetitions performed during a workout. For example, if a child performs 2 sets of 10 repetitions with 30 kilograms in the squat exercise, then the volume load is 600 kilograms (2 sets × 10 repetitions × 30 kg). Both training intensity and volume load significantly influence the outcome of resistance training programs in youth (Lesinski et al., 2016; Lloyd et al., 2014).

Higher training intensities and volume loads are associated with greater gains in muscular strength and motor skill performance in youth (Behringer et al., 2011; Behringer et al., 2010; Lesinski et al., 2016). However, loads that require higher levels of neuromuscular activation and force expression also require higher levels of resistance training skill competence. Therefore, to optimize performance gains and reduce the risk of unexpected events, all participants must first learn how to perform each exercise correctly with a light load and then gradually progress the training intensity, volume load, or both, depending on needs, goals, and abilities. This deliberate approach is particularly important when youth are learning how to perform multijoint exercises and during periods of rapid

Teaching Tip

SAFETY FIRST

The injury risk associated with supervised resistance training is not greater than that of other sport or recreational activities in which children and adolescents regularly participate. Nonetheless, youth fitness specialists need to ensure that the training environment is safe and that participants follow established guidelines. Accidental injuries have been reported in relation to dropping weights on toes and pinching fingers (Myer, Quatman, Khoury, Wall, & Hewett, 2009). Common risk factors include inadequate supervision and aggressive progression of training loads. Without guidance from qualified practitioners, youth are more likely to suffer injury as a result of unsafe behavior or improper exercise technique.

growth, which naturally require youth to relearn skills due to the awkwardness associated with growing. Two ways to help youth develop correct movement skill patterns are to limit the number of repetitions and to provide real-time feedback after each repetition. Once youth can properly perform an exercise with light and moderate loads, the training program can be sensibly progressed over the next few weeks and months, so long as the participant maintains technical competence when heavier loads are introduced. This type of technique-based progression gives youth an opportunity to reinforce proper motor patterns while reducing injury risk and optimizing training outcomes.

Youth should begin resistance training with one or two sets of light intensity (<60 percent 1RM) on 6 to 10 exercises. Although 1RM testing has proven to be safe and reliable for youth (Faigenbaum et al., 2012; Faigenbaum, Milliken, & Westcott, 2003), it is labor-intensive and time-consuming when properly administered (see chapter 6). In addition, less-skilled participants will need to be familiarized with the testing procedures. Therefore, youth fitness specialists should prescribe basic exercises and light training loads for beginners, then adjust the load as necessary depending on their resistance training skill competence. Although the repetition range may vary, it is reasonable for beginners to perform 6 to 12 repetitions per set. When youth are initially learning a multijoint exercise (e.g., squat), the number of repetitions should be limited (to six or fewer) in order to safely develop and reinforce proper movement patterns.

Exercise choices and training loads can be progressed over time as youth gain competence and confidence in their physical abilities and exhibit desired behaviors in the fitness center. Research findings indicate that in order to optimize strength gains, youth resistance training programs should progress to two to three sets of 8 to 15 repetitions with loads up to 80 percent of 1RM (Behringer et al., 2010). If, on the other hand, the goal is to improve athletic performance, then dose–response relationships for resistance training parameters indicate that five sets of 6 to 8 repetitions at a training intensity of 80 percent to 89 percent of 1RM may be most effective (Lesinski et al., 2016). Exercises need not all be performed for the same number of sets

and repetitions in a given session. General recommendations for youth resistance training programs are outlined in table 9.3.

Plyometric training should not be viewed as a stand-alone entity but rather as a meaningful component of youth programs that link strength with speed and power (Chu & Myer, 2013; Peitz, Behringer, & Granacher, 2018). As discussed in chapter 11 plyometric exercises are characterized by a muscle pattern known as the **stretch–shortening cycle**, which involves a specific sequence of eccentric, isometric, and concentric muscle actions that enhance concentric force output (Komi, 2003). Due to the large neuromuscular demands of plyometric training and naturally occurring adaptations throughout childhood and adolescence, potential synergistic adaptations have proven to be beneficial for youth (Assunção et al., 2018; Faigenbaum, Farrell, et al., 2009; Lloyd et al., 2012; Lloyd, Radnor, De Ste Croix, Cronin, & Oliver, 2016; Rumpf et al., 2012).

The intensity of plyometric training is controlled not by amount of weight lifted but by type of exercise performed (Chu & Myer, 2013; Lloyd, Meyers, & Oliver, 2011). The continuum of plyometric exercises progresses from low intensity (e.g., squat jumps) to moderate intensity (e.g., box jumps) to high intensity (e.g., drop jumps). Youth fitness professionals should consider the eccentric load of each plyometric exercise and sensibly progress from minimal eccentric loading to higher eccentric loading. Moreover, the logical progression of plyometric training should be technique driven, and participants should be able to repeatedly demonstrate proper form on lower-intensity exercises before progressing to higher-intensity plyometrics. Successful performance of a plyometric exercise requires high movement velocity and proper body control on all repetitions in a set. Due to the neuromuscular demands inherent in plyometric training, practitioners should provide clear instructions and adequate recovery time between sets and between exercises in order to optimize adaptations. Child-friendly cues such as "land light as a feather" can support proper landing mechanics, which include triple flexion at the ankle, knee, and hip.

Although the volume of plyometric training has been discussed in relation to the total number of foot

TABLE 9.3   GENERAL RESISTANCE TRAINING GUIDELINES FOR PRIMARY EXERCISES

Training status	Sets	Repetitions	Load
Beginner	1 or 2	Varied	<60% 1RM
Basic	1 or 2	8-12	60%-70% 1RM
Intermediate	2 or 3	4-8	70%-80% 1RM
Athlete	3-5	2-8	80%-95% 1RM

Teaching Tip

WEIGHTLIFTING KID-STYLE

Weight training includes exercises such as modified cleans, pulls, and presses that involve explosive but highly controlled movements that require a high degree of technical skill. With qualified instruction on proper lifting technique and safety procedures (e.g., how to correctly miss a lift), youth can learn how to perform these lifts effectively by using a wooden dowel or light barbell. Youth fitness specialists should be aware of the time required to teach these lifts and should be knowledgeable of the progression from basic exercises (e.g., front squat) to skill-transfer exercises (e.g., overhead squat) and finally to competitive lifts (e.g., snatch). Since the performance of explosive movements can be influenced by fatigue, it is important to focus on movement speed and efficiency and allow for adequate recovery between sets. Providing real-time feedback after each repetition can help participants develop proper movement patterns.

contacts during a single session (Bedoya, Miltenberger, & Lopez, 2015), it is more important to consider the quality of the movement pattern. Youth with low plyometric skill competence should begin with basic exercises, such as standing jumps. After they learn how to perform an exercise correctly at a controlled movement speed, youth fitness specialists should provide clear instructions for increasing repetition velocity. Regardless of the exercise, the emphasis of plyometric training should be placed on proper body control followed by short ground contact time and use of the stretch reflex. That is, youth should first learn how to perform an exercise correctly, then try to maximize repetition velocity without compromising technique. It is reasonable to begin with a single set of 6 to 10 repetitions of low-intensity exercises and then progress to multiple sets of 6 to 10 repetitions of higher-intensity plyometrics. As with any type of resistance exercise, practitioners should progress plyometrics at a deliberate pace in order to minimize injury risk and maximize performance potential.

DO YOU KNOW?

Integrative training programs that include plyometric and resistance exercises may result in the greatest gains in muscular power performance in youth.

When designing plyometric training programs, practitioners should balance the neuromuscular demands of each exercise with the need to maintain proper technique and speed of movement. In some circumstances, beginners may need to focus on enhancing strength competencies before performing plyometric exercises. Participants who are unable to perform a plyometric exercise correctly (e.g., due to poor landing mechanics) should regress to a less intense exercise in order to enhance movement mechanics. In contrast, participants who are able to

demonstrate proper plyometric exercise technique should advance to more intense exercises. Since the performance of any plyometric exercise is negatively affected by fatigue, all participants should be afforded adequate recovery time between sets and between exercises (Faigenbaum, McFarland, Keiper, et al., 2007; Lloyd et al., 2012). Guidelines for youth plyometric training are outlined in table 9.4.

Regardless of participants' fitness goals and level of resistance training experience, youth fitness specialists should closely monitor exercise technique and perceived exercise exertion in order to ensure that the prescribed training intensity and volume load are consistent with each participant's stress tolerance. In addition, practitioners should remember that different combinations of exercises, sets, and repetitions have proven to be effective in youth resistance training program (Faigenbaum et al., 2016; Lloyd et al., 2014). If a training program is varied to include periods of light, moderate, and higher-intensity training, then long-term performance gains will be optimized and the risk of overtraining will be reduced (Haff, 2014; Moraes, Fleck, Ricardo Dias, & Simão, 2013). With a systematic prescription of program variables, the resistance training stimulus will remain effective and the effort-to-benefit ratio will be maximized.

Rest Interval Between Sets and Exercises

The length of the rest interval between sets and between exercises is an important variable that can influence acute force output, power production, and cardiometabolic demand. Whereas adults require rest intervals of three to five minutes in order to recover from heavy resistance training (de Salles et al., 2009), maturational differences mean that youth require less time (Falk & Dotan, 2006). Youth can resist neuromuscular fatigue

TABLE 9.4   YOUTH PLYOMETRIC TRAINING GUIDELINES

TRAINING VARIABLE	PLYOMETRIC TRAINING EXPERIENCE		
	Low	Moderate	High
Exercises per session	2-4	4-6	6-8
Repetitions per exercise	8-10	4-8	4-6
Sets	1 or 2	2 or 3	2-4
Exercise intensity	Low	Moderate	High
Sample exercises	Squat jump, medicine ball chest pass, low box jump	Forward jump, medicine ball push-up, box jump	Lateral cone jumps, plyo push-up, drop jump

to a greater extent than adults during several repeated bouts of resistance exercise, and the ability to recover quickly seems to be most pronounced in children (Bottaro et al., 2011; Faigenbaum et al., 2008; Murphy, Button, Chaouachi, & Behm, 2014; Tibana et al., 2012).

More specifically, a recovery interval of about one minute may be adequate for youth when performing a moderate-intensity resistance training program. As the intensity of the training program increases, longer rest intervals (2-3 min) may be needed, especially if the program involves multijoint exercises that require a high degree of technical skill (e.g., weight training). Nevertheless, within-session resistance training performance should be monitored by youth fitness specialists who provide real-time feedback to ensure that proper exercise technique is maintained throughout the performance of every set. Extreme cardiometabolic resistance training protocols with very short rest intervals have been found to adversely affect exercise technique in adults (Hooper et al., 2014), and it is unlikely that this type of programming would optimize resistance training skill competence and exercise adherence in youth.

Repetition Velocity

Adaptations to a training program can also be affected by the repetition velocity or cadence at which a resistance exercise is performed (Lloyd, Radnor, et al., 2016; Loturco et al., 2015; Rivière et al., 2016). A moderate training velocity may be recommended for untrained youth who are learning novel exercise techniques in order to ensure correct posture and limb alignment; however, participants also need to improve their ability to move quickly and efficiently in order to develop motor unit recruitment patterns and firing frequencies in the neuromuscular system (Lloyd et al., 2014). Enhancing the ability to perform controlled movements at a high velocity may be especially beneficial during childhood, when neural plasticity

and motor coordination are most sensitive to change (Casey, Tottenham, Liston, & Durston, 2005; Myer, Faigenbaum, et al., 2015).

As part of an integrative training program, resistance exercises performed at different movement velocities may provide an effective training stimulus (Cormie, McGuigan, & Newton, 2011; Haff & Nimphius, 2012). For example, the jump squat is a low force–high velocity exercise, whereas the back squat is a high force–low velocity exercise. For traditional resistance exercises that involve squatting, pressing, and pulling, the velocity at which the movement is performed is determined by the mass of the load. Still, some weightlifting movements, such as the power clean, should be performed as fast as possible with proper technique in order to promote neuromuscular adaptations while maximizing the transfer of the training effect to sport performance. Although practitioners should consider each participant's resistance training experience and strength level, they must also remember that optimizing performance requires integrating different repetition velocities into a training cycle (Haff & Nimphius, 2012).

Training Frequency

Training frequency is measured in terms of the number of training sessions per week. Most children and adolescents benefit from engaging in resistance training two or three times per week on nonconsecutive days (Behringer et al., 2010). Although training frequency is significantly correlated with resistance training adaptations in youth (Behringer et al., 2010), the prescribed training frequency must provide adequate time for rest and recovery. Young athletes who play on several sport teams and those who participate in resistance training programs with a higher training frequency (e.g., split-routine training) should be monitored closely for early signs of stress intolerance, including sore muscles and decreased motivation.

Periodization of Resistance Training for Youth

Youth fitness specialists need to periodically manipulate and progress training programs over time in order to optimize gains in muscular fitness, maintain exercise adherence, avert boredom, and reduce the risk of **overtraining**. The concept of systematically changing the training stimulus over time is known as **periodization**. This concept has been part of adult training programs for many years (Bompa & Haff, 2009), and the importance of dividing training programs into smaller segments is supported by research evidence and observations from practitioners (Haff, 2014; Moraes et al., 2013). Youth fitness specialists need to manage the overall workload placed on youth because prolonged periods of excessive physical exertion with inadequate levels of rest and recovery can result in undesirable consequences, including overtraining, injury, and illness (Difiori et al., 2014). To reduce the risk of such events and to make training more effective, resistance training should be sensibly integrated into a weekly exercise plan along with adequate time for rest and recovery. The demands of resistance training need to be balanced with efforts to develop other facets of physical fitness, including balance, speed, agility, and endurance.

Periodization is relevant not just for young athletes but also for all youth participating in a resistance training program. Without properly changing training variables, it is impossible to make continual gains in strength and power over long-term training. Once the body adapts to a resistance training stimulus, no further improvements in performance will be realized unless the training program is altered. By periodically varying program variables such as exercise selection, order of exercises, number of sets, training loads, or any combination of thereof, practitioners can optimize long-term gains in strength and power (Haff, 2014; Harries et al., 2012).

For example, at the beginning of a training program, the youth fitness specialist needs to focus on resistance training skill competence and general demeanor. The volume and intensity of training should be relatively low because participants need to develop proper movement patterns, enhance muscular fitness, and improve tissue tolerance. During this introductory phase, the importance of maintaining proper exercise technique may be reinforced less by the amount of weight lifted and more by the perception of resistance training skill competence. Participants should be given specific feedback related to their technical performance and their readiness to learn during every training session. This type of assessment can provide a unique opportunity for all participants to become aware of their mistakes and monitor their own progress as they work toward clearly defined goals. Participants with low RTSC may need two to three months of regular training in order to develop proper movement patterns in a variety of exercises and thereby gain confidence in their physical abilities.

When participants enhance their resistance training skill competence and begin to build a strong foundation, the volume and intensity of training can be gradually increased as participants adapt to the training stimulus and enter the next phase of

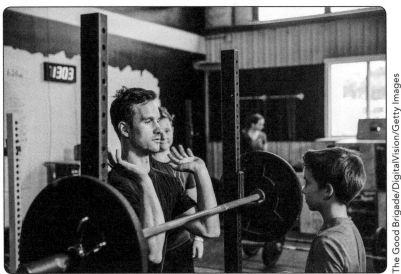

The Good Brigade/DigitalVision/Getty Images

Qualified supervision and instruction are foundational to youth resistance training programs.

training, which focuses on general strength. In the strength phase, structural multijoint exercises can be performed for multiple sets at moderate intensity. This phase may last one to three months, depending on participants' needs, goals, and abilities. The next phase is designed to optimize gains in muscular strength and power through higher-intensity training, fewer repetitions per set, and additional power exercises. A requisite level of RTSC and muscular strength should be attained before beginning the strength-and-power phase of training. This phase is important because it enables young athletes to translate training-induced gains in muscular strength into high power development (Haff, 2014).

Although the strength phase and the strength-and-power phase optimize performance gains, less-intense sessions of resistance training should still be incorporated into the long-term plan in order to reinforce proper technique and minimize the risk of overtraining. In other words, not every training session during a strength phase or a strength-and-power phase needs to involve moderate or high intensity. In addition, to allow for physical and psychological recovery from resistance training, the program should include periodic stints of active rest (about two weeks) throughout the school year (e.g., between sport seasons). During these times, young athletes should be encouraged to participate in recreational activities but should avoid structured training. Although additional research is needed on the efficacy of different types of periodized resistance training in children and adolescents, youth fitness specialists should appreciate the importance of systematically varying the resistance training program in order to keep the stimulus safe, effective, and fun.

Sample Training Programs

Since no single combination of acute program variables will optimize training adaptations in all participants, practitioners must assess each individual's health history, fitness level, and resistance training experience. This section of the chapter outlines resistance training programs that are designed for healthy youth without significant medical conditions. The beginner program includes body-weight exercises that use medicine balls and elastic bands. As participants improve their resistance training skill competence, they can use more complex exercises and higher training intensities to increase the neuromuscular demands of the training program. Recall that resistance training should be preceded by a dynamic warm-up (see chapter 7).

Beginner Program

Body-weight exercises can be used to stress the major muscle groups while using an individual's body mass as the source of resistance. The use of lightweight (1-2 kg) medicine balls and elastic bands provides a type of unguided resistance that can be used for different movement speeds and an unlimited number of dynamic movements (e.g., pulling, pushing, throwing, catching, rotating). This type of whole-body training should be performed two or three times per week on nonconsecutive days. In general, at least two or three months of basic training may be needed in order to enable youth to develop physical and technical abilities.

At the start of the program, participants can perform one or two sets of 8 to 12 repetitions for each exercise. As participants enhance their skill competence, the intensity of program can be controlled by either progressing the exercises or increasing the weight of the ball or the type of elastic band used. In order to maintain proper exercise technique when exercise intensity is progressed, the number of repetitions can be reduced. Table 9.5 outlines a sample resistance training session based on exercises using body weight, medicine balls, and elastic bands.

Advanced Program

As participants build a strong foundation and enhance their resistance training skill competence, the design of the resistance training program can be advanced to create a more challenging and more effective training strategy. Although advanced training is typically prescribed for young athletes, children or adolescents with a high level of RTSC and a growing interest in resistance training can certainly participate in this type of conditioning with a youth fitness specialist. The training session presented in table 9.6 starting on page 194 includes multijoint free-weight exercises, although body-weight exercises (with or without medicine balls or elastic bands) can certainly be part of a more advanced resistance training program. Participants should be able to perform the minimal number of repetitions for the desired number of sets with proper technique before progressing to heavier loads or more advanced exercises. A repetition range of 6 to 10 is typical, although a lower number of repetitions is appropriate for weightlifting movements.

Depending on program design, more advanced training can be performed two or three times per week; resistance training sessions should be separated by at least one day of active rest. Although the training and

TABLE 9.5 SAMPLE BEGINNER SESSION FOR RESISTANCE TRAINING IN YOUTH

Exercise	Volume	Intensity	Rest (min)
Goblet squat	2 × 8	Body weight, kettlebell, or medicine ball	1
Overhead squat	2 × 8	Dowel or junior barbell	1
Step-up	2 × 6 (each leg)	Body weight, dowel, or junior barbell	1
Monster band push press	2 × 8	Light band	1

Exercise	Volume	Intensity	Rest (min)
Monster band pull-down	2 × 8	Light band	1
Elevated push-up	2 × 8	Body weight	1
Suspended supine pull-up	2 × 8	Body weight	1
Plank variation (prone or side)	2 × 30 sec	Body weight	1

TABLE 9.6 — SAMPLE ADVANCED SESSION FOR RESISTANCE TRAINING IN YOUTH

Exercise	Volume	Intensity (body weight or % 1RM)	Rest (min)
Power clean	3 × 3	85%	2
Front squat	3 × 5	85%	2
Barbell step-up	3 × 5 (each leg)	85%	2
Pull-up	3 × 6	Body weight	2

Exercise	Volume	Intensity (body weight or % 1RM)	Rest (min)
Behind-the-neck press	3 × 6	85%	2
Elevated push-up	2 × 8	Body weight	2
Barbell roll-out	2 × 8	Body weight	1

recovery days can be structured in various formats, youth fitness specialists need to monitor participants' ability to tolerate the volume, intensity, and frequency of training used during this phase.

Summary

Regular participation in youth resistance training programs can offer observable benefits to children and adolescents in terms of health, fitness, and performance. Youth fitness specialists should dispel the misconceptions associated with resistance exercise and provide reassurance that regular participation in a supervised and well-designed resistance training program can be a safe, effective, and enjoyable method of conditioning for children and adolescents. With qualified instruction from youth fitness specialists, youth can gain competence and confidence in their ability to perform a variety of resistance exercises using different types of equipment. The foundational development of muscular fitness and movement skill can set the stage for ongoing participation in exercise and sport activities as a lifestyle choice. With systematic integration of technique-driven progression and effective pedagogical practices, participants can build a strong foundation for ongoing participation in exercise and sport activities.

CHAPTER 10

Speed and Agility Training

CHAPTER OBJECTIVES

- Define classifications of speed and agility
- Analyze key determinants of speed and agility performance
- Examine how growth and maturation influence the natural development of speed and agility
- Analyze the trainability of speed and agility in children and adolescents
- Discuss training strategies for speed and agility development and the process of manipulating training variables for long-term adaptation

KEY TERMS

acceleration (p. 197)

agility (p. 208)

change-of-direction speed (p. 208)

change-of-direction speed training (p. 212)

deceleration (p. 197)

first-step quickness (p. 197)

fundamental motor skill training (p. 212)

maximal velocity (p. 197)

perceptual and decision-making processes (p. 208)

reactive agility training (p. 212)

spring-mass model (p. 199)

sprint performance (p. 197)

stride frequency (p. 197)

stride length (p. 197)

Introduction

Observations of free-play activities typically show that children naturally engage in exercise with intermittent bouts of high-intensity jumping, running, and throwing (Cooper, 1995). Playground games often require participants to rapidly accelerate, decelerate, and change direction, all of which are normally performed when responding to an external stimulus (i.e., opponent or object). The most common forms of locomotion, namely sprinting and running, are commonly viewed as key fundamental motor skills that serve as building blocks for more complex movement skills at later stages of development. Similarly, research has shown that running, sprinting, and agility are key physical attributes of sporting success and are often included in testing batteries used to identify potentially talented athletes or to assess the fitness of youth (Reilly, Williams, Nevill, & Franks, 2000). Irrespective of whether a child participates in competitive sport or engages in recreational physical activity, competence in sprinting and agility-based movements is essential for all youth and should be developed within a multifaceted training program.

Speed

In its simplest form, running speed can be defined as the product of **stride length** and **stride frequency** (Hunter, Marshall, & McNair, 2004). Within that broad definition, **first-step quickness** can be viewed as the time required to cover the first five meters of a sprint (Cronin & Hansen, 2005). Thus it is considered to be part of **acceleration**—the phase of running that ends when the individual reaches maximum velocity, which in youth typically occurs after 15 to 30 meters (Meyers, Oliver, Hughes, Cronin, & Lloyd, 2015). Acceleration is governed by the individual's ability to apply high amounts of ground reaction forces relative to body weight in the horizontal direction (Buchheit et al., 2014; Morin et al., 2012). **Maximal velocity** occurs at the point where external forces are no longer changing velocity, which means that the individual is no longer accelerating. In the scientific literature, acceleration and maximal velocity are often addressed together in the term **sprint performance**, which replaces references to the independent phases of sprinting. Depending on the nature of the sprint, **deceleration** follows either the acceleration phase or the maximal velocity phase and is characterized by a percentage decrease in velocity until the conclusion of the sprint (Rumpf, Cronin, Oliver, & Hughes, 2011). Due to the lack of research regarding deceleration, it is considered within the confines of agility in this chapter.

Natural Development of Maximal Speed in Youth

Despite the fact that sprinting is viewed as a critical component of a child's fundamental movement skill portfolio (Lubans, Morgan, Cliff, Barnett, & Okely, 2010), there is a surprising lack of research studies directly examining the natural development of sprint performance in children and adolescents. The resulting lack of understanding is even more surprising in light of the fact that research has identified sprinting as both an important determinant of performance in youth sport (Mendez-Villanueva et al., 2011; Reilly et al., 2000) and a commonly used tool in talent identification systems (Reilly et al., 2000).

Available evidence suggests that sprint performance develops similarly in boys and girls during childhood, wherein both sexes experience noticeable spurts in performance improvement between the ages of 5 and 9 years—a trend referred to as the *preadolescent spurt* (Viru et al., 1999). This rapid improvement in sprint performance likely results from the rapid neural development that occurs during childhood (Gogtay et al., 2004; Malina, 2004). Peak brain maturation rates are experienced at 7.5 years of age in girls and at 10 years of age in boys (Lenroot & Giedd, 2006), and mature running gait cycles are established between 7 and 14 years of age in boys and girls (Hausdorff, Zemany, Peng, & Goldberger, 1999). As children transition into adolescence, noticeable improvements in sprint performance occur due to the *adolescent spurt*, during which males typically make greater gains than females; in addition, progression rates slow markedly in females starting at age 12 (Whitall, 2003).

Large-scale data on more than 85,000 children aged 9 to 17 years have shown that boys are faster than girls for any given percentile (Catley & Tomkinson, 2013). The same data also show that girls exhibit accelerated gains in sprint performance before 12 years of age, whereas boys demonstrate more rapid development after age 12. The sex-related differences that appear during adolescence derive largely from the fact that females experience increases in fat mass but do not experience the same degree of neuromuscular spurt that males experience, all of which leads to a reduction in the relative force production required for maximal speed performance. However, practitioners can attempt to induce a neuromuscular spurt in girls by prescribing appropriate exercise (Myer, Ford, Brent, & Hewett, 2007).

Acceleration Versus Maximal Velocity: Spot the Difference

Youth fitness specialists should be aware of, and be able to coach, technical characteristics of both the acceleration phase and the maximal velocity phase of sprinting. As depicted in figure 10.1, acceleration includes the following elements:

- Forward lean
- Long, high arm swings
- Positive shin angles at contact
- Powerful triple extension at the ankle, knee, and hip through the stance leg
- Powerful "piston-like" drive down and back by the leg in flight
- Foot of the leg in flight travels below the line of the knee of the stance leg

In contrast, the maximal velocity phase includes the following elements:

- Upright running position
- Smaller, more relaxed arm swing
- Neutral shin angles at contact
- "Stiff" stance leg to minimize collapse of the center of mass
- Leg in flight tucked underneath hips and minimal thigh swing behind torso
- Foot of the leg in flight travels above the line of the knee of the stance leg

Although it can be challenging to develop these techniques in youth, practitioners can optimize the process by prescribing appropriate exercises and using developmentally appropriate cues.

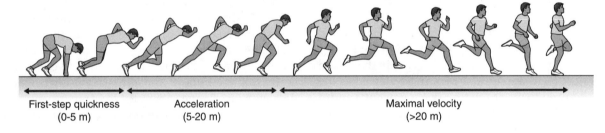

First-step quickness (0-5 m)   Acceleration (5-20 m)   Maximal velocity (>20 m)

FIGURE 10.1 Technical differences between acceleration and maximal velocity sprinting. Note the greater forward lean during acceleration as compared with the more upright alignment during maximal velocity sprinting.

DO YOU KNOW?

Differences between males and females in the timing of rapid-development periods for sprint performance highlight a maturational effect on speed development.

Longitudinal research that examined the development of maximal running velocity in a small sample of boys suggested that peak gains in speed occurred during the early phase of the growth spurt (Yague & De La Fuente, 1998). In contrast, research that examined physical performance in male youth soccer players showed that peak gains in sprint performance coincided with peak height velocity (PHV; Philippaerts et al., 2006). In that study, however, boys became slower in the 18 months preceding peak height velocity, and the "spurt" in speed may have simply reflected a natural long-term correction. These findings were corroborated in a large-scale, cross-sectional study of school-age boys, which showed that maximal running velocity remained relatively stable leading up to peak height velocity but increased markedly from the peak onward (Meyers, Oliver, Hughes, Cronin, et al., 2015). Overall, although current literature implies that a maturational influence exists on the development of maximal running velocity, the time at which youth experience peak gains remains unclear.

As mentioned earlier, running speed is a product of stride frequency and stride length (Hunter et al., 2004).

Stride frequency is a function of ground contact time and flight time, whereas stride length is a function of the distance covered during ground contact and when in flight. Given the dynamic nature of growth during childhood and adolescence, practitioners who want to optimize the training response need to understand how stride frequency and stride length change in response to natural development (Meyers, Oliver, Hughes, Lloyd, & Cronin, 2017). Cross-sectional data from 336 school-age boys showed that stride frequency decreased while stride length significantly increased from pre– to post–peak height velocity, resulting in increased maximal speed (Meyers, Oliver, Hughes, Cronin, et al., 2015). The data also showed that flight times remained consistent irrespective of maturation stage. Thus, during adolescence, boys appear to increase ground contact time, thereby reducing stride frequency, but compensate for this change by means of relatively larger increases in stride length. Further research has emphasized the influence of maturity on maximal speed in boys by showing that stride frequency accounted for 58 percent of speed variability in pre-PHV boys and that stride length explained 54 percent of maximal speed variability in boys who were circa- or post-PHV (Meyers, Oliver, Hughes, Lloyd, & Cronin, 2015).

The ability to express high amounts of relative force in a short time is desirable for sprint performance (Weyand, Sternlight, Bellizzi, & Wright, 2000). Previous research on adults has shown that athletes with less strength typically rely on stride frequency, whereas those with more strength rely more on stride length (Salo, Bezodis, Batterham, & Kerwin, 2011). Intuitively, this notion can be applied to the development of maximal running velocity in youth. Specifically, children with a well-developed central nervous system but smaller muscle mass and lower relative strength appear to rely more on stride frequency, thus requiring a faster gait turnover in order to generate speed. In contrast, adolescents appear to rely more on stride length thanks to their increased ability to produce larger relative forces, which derives from maturity-associated developments in strength and power (Forbes et al., 2009).

Relative force production has been shown to increase in accordance with stride length and maximal speed when comparing boys from pre-, circa-, and post-PHV maturity cohorts (Rumpf, Cronin, Oliver, & Hughes, 2015); comparable data for girls, however, remain scarce. The force-producing capacities that develop as a result of growth and maturation can likely be augmented by developmentally appropriate training interventions that include strength and power training (Meyers et al., 2017; Vanttinen, Blomqvist, Nyman, & Hakkinen, 2011; Wrigley, Drust, Stratton, Atkinson, & Gregson, 2014). Notwithstanding the importance of relative force production, research has shown that indices of strength and power can explain the majority of maturity-related improvements in 20-meter sprint times before peak height velocity but can explain only some improvements after peak height velocity (Meylan, Cronin, Oliver, Hopkins, & Pinder, 2014). These findings suggest that additional contributing factors should be identified and tracked for long-term development of sprinting in youth.

The importance of relative strength and power for sprint performance in youth is also emphasized when considering how the neuromuscular and skeletal systems are required to resist gravitational forces acting on the body during ground contact. In this vein, vertical and leg stiffness measures are often calculated in terms of the **spring-mass model** (Farley & Gonzalez, 1996), in which the spring is the lower limb and the mass is the center of mass (see figure 10.2). High amounts of stiffness are required in order to absorb ground reaction forces and to store and reuse elastic energy (Kuitunen, Avela, Kyrolainen, Nicol, & Komi, 2002) and have been associated with faster running speeds (Bret, Rahmani, Dufour, Messonnier, & Lacour, 2002; Chelly & Denis, 2001; Meyers et al., in press; Stefanyshyn & Nigg, 1998).

Conceptually, if mass is increased, as happens naturally through growth and maturation, then the force available to counteract the mass (and gravitational pull) must also increase; otherwise, the individual's ability to react explosively with the ground will be hampered. In fact, research shows that increasing body mass with advancing maturation is associated with prolonged ground contact times and reduction in stride frequency (Meyers, Oliver, Hughes, Cronin, et al., 2015). However, increased relative strength, stature, and leg length could all combine to compensate for the negative effects of body mass. Specifically, increased relative strength would help the individual reduce the yielding of the leg spring on ground contact (Meyers et al., in press), whereas increased leg length would allow the individual to cover more distance while in contact with the ground, as has been suggested in adult populations (Weyand, Sandell, Prime, & Bundle, 2010).

Trainability of Speed in Youth

Evidence suggests that both children and adolescents can make training-induced gains in sprint performance, although the mechanisms that drive such adaptations are likely to differ according to the stage of maturation (Lloyd & Oliver, 2012; Rumpf, Cronin, Pinder, Oliver, & Hughes, 2012). When seeking to develop sprint performance in youth, practitioners can choose from numerous training modes, including free

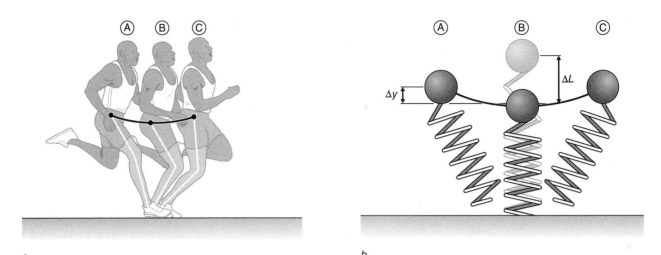

FIGURE 10.2   The use of leg stiffness at the (A) start, (B) middle, and (C) end of ground contact during the running cycle, represented by *(a)* a free body diagram and *(b)* the spring-mass model. In the figure, ΔL represents the peak displacement of the leg spring and Δy represents the vertical displacement of the center of mass.

sprinting and technical running drills, resisted and assisted sprinting, and complementary forms of training (e.g., for strength, power, and mobility). According to research on adults, the most effective training modes for speed development are free, resisted, and assisted sprinting, which offer greater performance improvements than do strength and power training in isolation (Rumpf, Lockie, Cronin, & Jalilvand, 2016). However, despite the simplicity of free, assisted, and resisted sprinting—as well as their high degree of training specificity—their efficacy in youth has been addressed by a surprisingly small amount of empirical research.

Although a small number of interventions to improve speed have incorporated sprint training as part of the training program (Marques, 2013; Kotzamanidis, 2005), most research has relied on strength training, power training, or a combination of both, which have often led to positive results. For example, a six-week program that combined sprint and jump training was found to improve 30-meter sprint performance in a cohort of 13-year-old soccer players (Marques, 2013). Similarly, a 12-week intervention that combined strength and power training significantly improved 10-meter and 30-meter sprint times in a group of under-14 soccer players (Wong, Chamari, & Wisloff, 2010). The advantages offered by a combined training approach are also evident in other studies. For example, research on a group of 17-year-old boys showed that a 13-week intervention combining resistance and sprint training achieved significantly greater improvements in 30-meter sprint performance than did resistance training only (Kotzamanidis, 2005). Also, combined plyometric and balance training has been found superior to a plyometrics-only intervention in improving 10-meter sprint performance in 13-year-old boys (Chaouachi, Hammami, et al., 2014).

Practitioners must attend to the interaction between training, growth, and maturation. A systematic review examined the effectiveness of different training methods for developing sprint performance in male youth (Rumpf et al., 2012). Analysis of the resulting data revealed that plyometric training exerted a large effect on boys who were pre-PHV and circa-PHV, whereas combined strength and plyometric training exerted a large effect on boys who were post-PHV. Moreover, despite design limitations in several reports (e.g., including measures of both acceleration and maximal running velocity, failing to directly measure maturation), findings from Rumpf and colleagues (2012) suggest that youth of different maturity stages may benefit from slightly different training stimuli, thus highlighting the complex interaction between training, growth, and maturation. Meta-analytical data have shown that sprint training (whether performed in isolation or in combination with resistance exercise) is more effective for developing sprinting velocity in male youth who are post- or circa-PHV than in boys who are pre-PHV (Moran, Sandercock, Rumpf, & Parry, 2016). However, the meta-analysis itself was subject to some limitations. Specifically, the categories used to account for biological maturity were based on chronological age, the final analysis included only 14 studies, a large degree of sample heterogeneity characterized the studies, and longitudinal studies were distinctly absent. Thus it remains unclear how growth, maturation, and training interact to influence overall trainability.

The interactions between age, maturation, and training have been examined directly in research (Lloyd, Radnor, De Ste Croix, Cronin, & Oliver, 2016; Meylan, Cronin, Oliver, Hopkins, & Contreras, 2014; Radnor et al., 2017; Rumpf, Cronin, Mohamad, et al., 2015). For

COMBINED TRAINING FOR SPEED DEVELOPMENT: MORE BANG FOR YOUR BUCK

Research has examined individual responsiveness to various forms of resistance training in a sample of 80 school-age boys (Radnor, Lloyd, & Oliver, 2017). The six-week study showed that combined strength training and plyometric training was more effective in eliciting improvements in sprint performance than either training mode in isolation. Specifically, the study reported that combined training led to worthwhile improvements in acceleration and maximal velocity for 90 percent of boys who were pre–peak height velocity. Similar improvements were seen in boys who were post–peak height velocity for acceleration (100% of the group) and maximal velocity (80% of the group). Although multiple training modes are available to youth fitness specialists who seek to enhance sprint performance, available research points to combined training as a highly potent stimulus in youth.

example, Meylan and colleagues (2014) reported that gains in sprint speed in response to an eight-week strength training program were smaller in pre-PHV boys (2.1%) than in boys who were either circa-PHV (3.6%) or post-PHV (3.1%). Rumpf and colleagues (2014) demonstrated that younger boys (about 10 years old) did not make significant improvements in sprint speed during a six-week sled-towing intervention; however, older boys (about 15 years of age) showed significant improvements in sprint speed and associated sprint characteristics (e.g., stride frequency, stride length, power production). Practitioners should consider, however, that pre-PHV youth are slowed to a greater extent than those who are post-PHV when pulling equal loads relative to body mass (Rumpf et al., 2014). Therefore, the results of Rumpf and colleagues (2014) may reflect a biologically immature state and consequently lower strength levels in the less mature subjects.

The transfer of training effect was highlighted in the study by Lloyd and colleagues (2016), who showed that both pre- and post-PHV boys made significant gains in flying 20-meter sprint performance with a six-week intervention of either plyometric training or combined strength and plyometric training. However, no gains in sprint performance were reported for either maturity group in the strength training or control group following the intervention period. Cumulatively, these data suggest that although improvements in sprint speed can be achieved by both children and adolescents, maturity status will likely influence the magnitude of improvement and to some extent determine the most efficacious training mode for developing sprint performance.

DO YOU KNOW?

Youth should work on acceleration and maximal running velocity at regular intervals in their training program in order to develop or retain technical competence and to condition their bodies for maximal effort sprinting.

Training Prescription for Speed Development

Youth fitness specialists need to consider a range of prescription variables when designing and implementing speed training programs for children and adolescents. Those variables include exercise selection, volume and intensity, recovery, and frequency.

Exercise Selection

Exercise selection for speed training can be categorized into three general groups: speed work and technical drills; resisted and assisted sprint drills; and strength, power, and mobility training. The apportioning of training time to exercises from each of these categories depends on the needs, goals, and aspirations of the individual. The youth fitness specialist should understand the specifics of each category in order to optimize the training response for each individual.

Speed Work and Technical Drills   The primary training method for speed development involves executing sound running technique. Developmental literature suggests that as a consequence of natural development, mature running gait will be evident from about seven years of age (Hausdorff et al., 1999); therefore, instead of teaching novel techniques, youth fitness specialists should typically focus on fine-tuning existing movement patterns and correcting technical faults (e.g., rotating arm swing around the longitudinal axis). Technical drills (e.g., A-skips, B-skips, high-knee cross-overs) can be integrated into the warm-up and performed linearly at a submaximal intensity requiring the athlete to focus on coordination and correct technique (e.g., short ground contact times, postural alignment).

Although technical drills hold anecdotal value for skill development, such benefits remain unproven through empirical research, especially in youth populations. In addition, careful, linear technical work can become repetitive and seem mundane to young children, which can lead to a lack of focus when performing the drills. To counter this risk, youth fitness specialists can integrate technical drills into challenging, gamelike activities or use criterion-based assessments that reward technical quality (Faigenbaum & McFarland, 2014) rather than a certain outcome (e.g., how quickly a drill is completed). In addition, practitioners can use novel cues and introduce a constraints-led approach to develop and reinforce good technique during more focused speed work, which involves maximal effort-sprints over a set distance (e.g., 30 m) and requires the participant to coordinate running gait near or at full speed. Distances can be set to develop different classifications of sprinting (e.g., 0-5 m for first-step quickness, 0-20 m for acceleration, or longer for development of maximal running velocity).

DO YOU KNOW?

Practitioners should not assume that youth know how to sprint properly; instead, they should provide opportunities to practice the skill of sprinting.

Resisted and Assisted Sprint Training Resisted sprint training uses an external source of resistance to increase the vertical and horizontal forces that the participant must overcome. Perhaps the most common method of resisted sprinting is sled towing (see figure 10.3); however, sled pushing, sprinting with a parachute, and uphill running are also options for the youth fitness specialist. The available literature shows that resisted sprint training can improve acceleration and maximal speed, albeit in adult populations (Rumpf et al., 2016). Earlier research indicated the use of an external load of about 13 percent of body mass or a decrement in running velocity of less than 10 percent (Alcaraz, Palao, & Elvira, 2009; Harrison & Bourke, 2009; Lockie, Murphy, & Spinks, 2003) in order to minimize interference with running technique. However, if resisted sprinting is viewed as a physical stimulus to promote horizontal force production, then heavier external loads may elicit greater adaptations. This notion has been supported by more recent evidence suggesting that external loads of 20 percent to 30 percent of body mass are superior to lighter loads for increasing acceleration and horizontal force orientation (Bachero-Mena & Gonzalez-Badillo, 2014; Kawamori, Newton, & Nosaka, 2014). In addition, a recent systematic review showed that sprints with very heavy external resistance (>30% of body mass) were most effective in eliciting adaptations in acceleration, albeit in experienced adult populations (Petrakos, Morin,

& Egan, 2016). It remains unclear whether the same trend exists in pediatric populations, and youth fitness specialists should consider the fact that a spectrum of light to heavy loads will likely promote desirable adaptations in sprint performance in untrained youth.

Assisted sprint training most often uses external assistance (e.g., stretch harnesses), high-speed treadmills, or downhill sprinting to elicit an "overspeed" effect. Assisted sprinting focuses primarily on increasing stride frequency and encouraging rapid horizontal force application. Youth fitness specialists should apply the external assistance with caution due to the risk of promoting a rearward torso lean, which can cause increased breaking forces to be applied during sprinting.

Strength, Power, and Mobility Training Both vertical and horizontal force production are required in order to sprint effectively (Morin et al., 2012; Morin, Edouard, & Samozino, 2011; Weyand et al., 2010; Weyand et al., 2000). The ability to exert force against resistance quickly (i.e., to apply power) is governed by maximal strength (Cormie, McGuigan, & Newton, 2011b) and effective functioning of the stretch–shortening cycle (Cormie, McGuigan, & Newton, 2011a), both

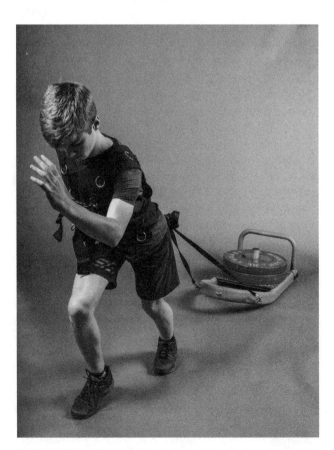

FIGURE 10.3   Resisted sprinting using sled towing.

of which are enhanced through strength and power training. Although free, resisted, and assisted sprinting are the most specific training modalities for speed development, youth fitness specialists should also view strength and power training as a means for building a strong and resilient frame that can support the high levels of force experienced during ground contact.

Similarly, as shown in figure 10.4, plyometrics are an effective way to develop the stretch–shortening cycle and associated stiffness properties, which in turn improve the manner in which youth interact with the ground when sprinting (Meyers et al., in press). For example, research has shown that when early-pubertal boys followed a 12-week program involving three sessions per week of combined resistance and plyometric training, they made significant improvements in 40-meter sprint times as compared with age-matched controls (Ingle, Sleap, & Tolfrey, 2006). Similarly, research examining the individual response of male youth to various forms of resistance training found that a high proportion of school-age boys exhibited worthwhile improvements in sprint performance when plyometric training was included in their 6-week training programs (Radnor et al., 2017).

DO YOU KNOW?

Due to the high ground reaction forces experienced during sprinting, developing relative strength levels should be seen as an important foundation for sprint performance.

Despite being acknowledged as an important quality for youth to possess, mobility and its associations with sprint performance in youth have received very little attention in the literature (Lloyd & Oliver, 2012). Although joints do not all undergo the same angular displacement during sprinting (the hip and knee extend and flex to a much greater extent than the ankle), children and adolescents require sufficient ranges of motion to enable efficient running technique. The relative importance of mobility for performance depends on the nature of the sport and the characteristics of the inherent movement patterns (Sands & McNeal, 2013). Although sprinting does not require extreme ranges of motion such as those displayed in acrobatic sports (e.g., gymnastics, figure skating), it does require multiple joints to transition sequentially and optimally from highly flexed to extended positions at high speed and often under large forces in order to produce high mechanical impulses (McNeal & Sands, 2006). In addition, though mobility development is an important feature in the dynamic warm-up phase of training sessions, little benefit is gained from developing extreme range of motion in a joint if the child or adolescent is unable to demonstrate sufficient stability and control throughout that range.

Since training prescription guidelines for strength and power are examined in chapter 9, the following sections examine prescription specifically for free, resisted, and assisted sprint training.

Volume and Intensity

Pediatric researchers have yet to examine the dose–response relationship for free, resisted, and assisted

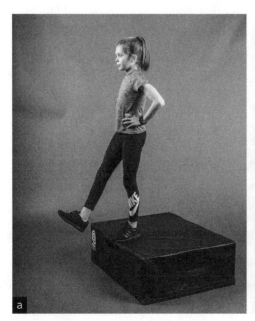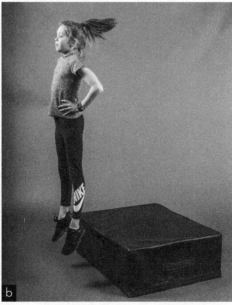

FIGURE 10.4   Pogo hopping is a form of plyometric exercise that targets rapid ground contact times and high amounts of stiffness.

sprint training. When quantifying the volume of sprint training, youth fitness specialists are best advised to measure the total distance covered during a training session by multiplying total repetitions by distance per repetition for each exercise. Intensity, on the other hand, is typically considered as a percentage of maximal speed but can also be viewed as a percentage of maximal effort (as measured by ratings of perceived exertion); if incorporating resisted or assisted sprint training into a session, practitioners must also consider the externally applied forces. When working to develop sprint ability, practitioners should prescribe drills that are performed at maximal intensity and allow youth sufficient time to recover between repetitions.

Various sprint distances are used to target specific qualities (e.g., acceleration, maximal velocity), and longer efforts call for more recovery time. Irrespective of the training drill, youth fitness specialists should always emphasize maintenance of correct technical execution and therefore may use different intensities when working on different elements of sprint training. For example, technical drills may be performed at low intensity to emphasize motor control and postural integrity; submaximal sprinting, or tempo running, may be performed at moderate to high intensity (60%-70% of maximal speed); and exercises targeting acceleration or maximal running velocity should be performed at high intensity (100% of maximal speed).

Due to the high-intensity nature of sprint training, and the fact that sprint training may feature as a component of an integrated neuromuscular training session (see chapter 12), the overall session volume is likely to be low. Rumpf and colleagues (2012) showed that the majority of youth-based sprint training studies have used training volumes of 240 to 480 meters per session, typically consisting of 8 to 15 repetitions of 10 to 30 meters per repetition. More recently, researchers have suggested a similar prescription (about 320 m) based on meta-analytical data and advocated up to 16 sprints of about 20 meters each per session (Moran et al., 2016). However, the optimal dosage for speed development has yet to be empirically examined and thus remains unclear. It is clear, however, that given the high neural requirements of sprinting, speed development sessions should *not* involve repeated bouts of submaximal-intensity repetitions with minimal rest if the end goal is to develop sprint performance. In addition, if youth fitness specialists observe that performance is deteriorating (e.g., decrements appear in sprint speed), then the session should be adapted or stopped altogether.

DO YOU KNOW?

When developing sprinting ability in children or adolescents, it is always better to undertrain than to overtrain to avoid fatiguing the central nervous system.

In-Session Recovery

In-session recovery depends on the nature of the training stimulus. For example, if the focus is on maximal acceleration or maximal running velocity, then full recovery should be encouraged; however, if the focus is on technical drills or tempo running, then shorter recovery periods can probably be used. Although there is a dearth of research examining the optimal rest period for speed development in youth, practitioners should acknowledge that the physiology of children allows them to recover more quickly than either adolescents or adults (Dotan et al., 2012). Therefore, whereas adults may be allowed more than 5 minutes for recovery after a 60-meter sprint (which would take anywhere from 6 to 8 sec), the rest time adopted by children and adolescents could be much less (e.g., 1-3 min). These notions are supported by meta-analytical data showing that a work-to-rest ratio of 1:25, or the adoption of rest intervals of greater than 90 seconds, is most beneficial for developing sprint performance (Moran et al., 2016).

Teaching Tip

USING YOUR SENSES TO MONITOR SPRINT PERFORMANCE

Although various digital tools are available for use in assessing and monitoring sprint performance, youth fitness specialists should not rely on them for coaching. When technology is used appropriately, it can enable valuable insights into the technical aspects of sprinting, but practitioners should initially rely on their eyes and ears to judge performance. Visually, performance decrements may be evident in a tenser running action, increased "sinking" of the hips on ground contact, or slower stride turnover. From an auditory perspective, reduced technical efficiency may manifest in the form of heavier and louder ground contact. In either case, the youth fitness specialist would need to make a judgment as to whether more rest is required before the next repetition, alternative technical cues are necessary, or the session should be terminated.

Training Frequency

Systematic review data have shown that most youth-based training studies have adopted a prescription of two or three sessions per week on nonconsecutive days (Moran et al., 2016; Rumpf et al., 2012). Training frequency ultimately depends on the individual participant's experience, technical competence, maturity status, and psychological development, as well as the training goal of the program. For example, a less mature, inexperienced, and technically incompetent young child may initially be exposed to sprint training once or twice per week in the form of "speed training" completed within the remit of a physical education class or integrated exercise session. In contrast, a mature, experienced, technically proficient adolescent sprinter who is in the speed and power development phase of training might engage in three or four sessions per week. Naturally, the frequency of sprint training sessions would need to be prescribed with an eye toward other requirements in the individual's overall training program.

Sample Speed Training Programs

The following tables provide sample training sessions focused on acceleration (tables 10.1 and 10.2) and maximal running velocity (tables 10.3 and 10.4) for beginners with low technical competence and for more advanced youth with higher technical competence. Notwithstanding the focus of the training session or the participant's technical ability, the sessions adopt a standard format that involves (a) an initial RAMP warm-up (not provided in the table below, but see chapter 7 for examples) designed to prepare the individual for the subsequent exercise and develop or retain athletic motor skill competencies; (b) a technique phase geared toward targeted technical development; and (c) the main phase, which provides youth with the opportunity to sprint for predetermined distances in order to develop specific aspects of sprint performance (e.g., acceleration, maximal running velocity). This systematic progression from warm-up through maximal effort sprinting should provide a logical and progressive approach to the session. However, as with other training modes, youth

TABLE 10.1   SAMPLE BEGINNER SESSION FOR ACCELERATION TRAINING IN YOUTH

Phase	Exercise	Volume (sets × reps)	Intensity (load)	Interset rest (sec)
Technique	Wall drive (single drive)	2 × 10 cycles	Body weight	30
	Harness march	3 × 10 m	Body weight	30
	"Tall and fall"	3 × 10 m	Body weight	30
	"Resist and release"	3 × 10 m	Body weight	30
Main	10 m acceleration sprint	3 × 10 m	Body weight	30
	10 m resisted sled sprint	3 × 10 m	Body weight + 30%	45
	20 m acceleration sprint	3 × 20 m	Body weight	60

TABLE 10.2   SAMPLE ADVANCED SESSION FOR ACCELERATION TRAINING IN YOUTH

Phase	Exercise	Volume (sets × reps)	Intensity (load)	Interset rest (sec)
Technique	Wall drive (switching)	2 × 10 cycles	Body weight	30
	Med ball dive pass	2 × 4 throws	1-8 kg med ball	15
	15 m kneeling start	3 × 15 m	Body weight	30
Main	15 m resisted sled sprint	4 × 15 m	Body weight + 30%	60
	20 m acceleration sprint	2 × 20 m	Body weight	60-120
	30 m acceleration sprint	2 × 30 m	Body weight	60-120
	Hollow sprinting (accelerating, decelerating, reaccelerating, decelerating)	4 × 40 m	Body weight	60-120

TABLE 10.3   SAMPLE BEGINNER SESSION FOR MAXIMAL VELOCITY TRAINING IN YOUTH

Phase	Exercise	Volume (sets × reps)	Intensity (load)	Interset rest (sec)
Technique	A-march	2 × 10 m	Body weight	30-60
	B-march	2 × 10 m	Body weight	30-60
	Pogo hop	3 × 10 m	Body weight	30-60
	High-knee	2 × 10 m	Body weight	30-60
Main	Flying 20 m sprint	4 × 20 m	Body weight	≥120
	30 m sprint	3 × 30 m	Body weight	≥120
	40 m sprint	2 × 40 m	Body weight	≥120

TABLE 10.4   SAMPLE ADVANCED SESSION FOR MAXIMAL VELOCITY TRAINING IN YOUTH

Phase	Exercise	Volume (sets × reps)	Intensity (load)	Interset rest (sec)
Technique	A-skip	2 × 15 m	Body weight	30-60
	B-skip	2 × 15 m	Body weight	30-60
	Pogo hop with dowel overhead	2 × 15 m	Body weight	30-60
	High-knee into run	2 × 20 m	Body weight	30-60
Main	Flying 20 m sprint	2 × 20 m	Body weight	≥120
	30 m sprint	2 × 30 m	Body weight	≥120
	40 m sprint	2 × 40 m	Body weight	≥120
	60 m sprint	2 × 60 m	Body weight	≥120

fitness specialists must be ready and able to progress or regress the exercises depending on the participant's technical competence. In some cases, if fatigue leads to noticeable deterioration in technique, the practitioner may even stop the session completely.

Agility

At one point, **agility** was defined as the ability to change direction rapidly (Bloomfield, Ackland, & Elliot, 1994); however, this definition appears to be simplistic when we look more closely at the manner in which agility-based movements are performed. As a result, researchers have since provided a more comprehensive definition of agility that encompasses rapid, whole-body movements requiring changes in direction, velocity, or both in response to a stimulus (Sheppard & Young, 2006). Figure 10.5 depicts the subcomponents of agility, which include both change-of-direction speed and perceptual and decision-making processes (Nimphius, 2014; Sheppard & Young, 2006).

Change-of-direction speed, which involves the ability to change direction rapidly, is typically displayed in closed, preplanned activities. For example, a group of young children may be participating in a sprint relay that requires them to accelerate from a start line to a cone 10 meters away, quickly decelerate, turn 180 degrees, and reaccelerate while returning to the start line. In this case, children are aware of the demands of the task before they start moving.

In contrast, free-play scenarios, recreational physical activity, and sport activity put a premium on **perceptual and decision-making processes** that enable the individual to respond to an external stimulus in open and reactive tasks. Although some of the anthropometric subcomponents (e.g., height, limb length) are largely unmodifiable, straight-line sprinting, technique, and leg muscle qualities are certainly modifiable, and thus they are prioritized when seeking to develop agility performance in youth. Emerging evidence also suggests that aspects of perceptual and decision-making

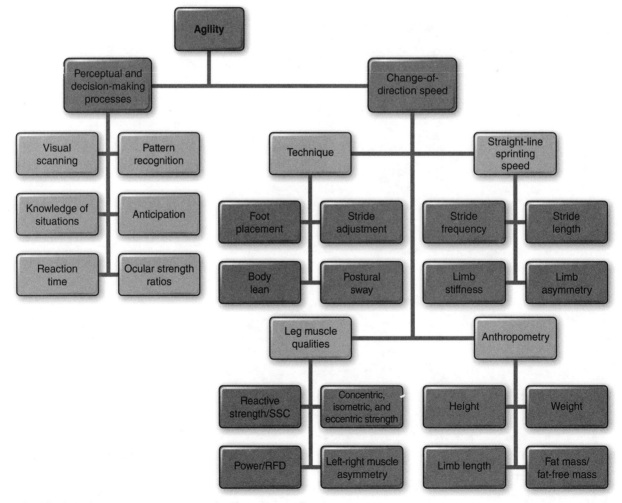

FIGURE 10.5   Determinants associated with agility performance.

Adapted from Nimphius (2014) and Sheppard and Young (2006).

factors are trainable and therefore that youth fitness specialists should try to develop such qualities as part of an overall training program.

Given our understanding of a constraints-led approach to motor skill performance (see chapter 8), it should be evident that agility technique will naturally be marked by large amounts of inter- and intra-individual variation as it is routinely modified based on interaction between task, individual, and environmental constraints (Gallahue, Ozmun, & Goodway, 2012). For example, when performing a closed and preplanned 45-degree cutting maneuver to the left, a child will be able to use anticipation and depth perception to predetermine an optimal footwork pattern and thereby maximize force application through the planted right foot. However, if the child is performing the same drill in an open and unplanned fashion with the option of cutting to either the right or the left in response to the movement or positioning of an opposing player, then the child's body positioning and the resulting application of force will be affected by a number of task and environmental constraints.

Due to the range of individual, task, and environmental constraints, no universal technique exists for change-of-direction speed. Even so, our understanding of biomechanics suggests that movement can be optimized by means of certain kinetic variables (e.g., force, rate of force development, torque) and kinematic variables (e.g., joint angular velocities, acceleration). The series of movement stages for performing an agility cutting maneuver are acceleration, then rapid deceleration, transition, and finally reacceleration. All of these stages feature different kinetic and kinematic characteristics. Specifically, acceleration requires high amounts of concentric force production, positive shin angles, forward body lean, and large changes in joint angles at the hip, knee, and ankle. In contrast, deceleration requires the individual to apply large braking forces, use a slight rearward lean, and adopt a negative shin angle. The force profile is also affected by task and environmental constraints; for instance, greater severity of cut (e.g., 90-degree versus 45-degree cutting angle) and later timing of the opponent's movement will likely result in increased eccentric force absorption and greater concentric force application.

Testing Agility in Youth

The definition of agility provided by Sheppard and Young (2006), which includes both change-of-direction speed and perceptual and decision-making skills, carries implications for our understanding of developmental changes in agility across childhood and adolescence; it also affects the manner in which we seek to assess and develop agility in youth (Lloyd et al., 2013). For example, a number of purported agility-testing protocols fail to expose individuals to a reactive stimulus, thus negating the need to use perceptual or decision-making abilities and therefore assessing only change-of-direction speed rather than true reactive agility.

Examples of protocols used in pediatric research include the repeated-change-of-direction test and sprint-with-180-degree-turns test (Hammami, Negra, Billaut, et al., 2017; Hammami, Negra, Shephard, & Chelly, 2017), the Illinois agility test (Negra et al., 2017), the eight-figure test (Vanttinen et al., 2011), the quadrant jump test (Eisenmann & Malina, 2003), Harre's circuit (Chiodera et al., 2008), the 5 × 10-meter sprint test (Philippaerts et al., 2006; Verschuren, Bloemen, Kruitwagen, & Takken, 2010), the zigzag test and 4 × 15-meter agility test (Jakovljevic, Karalejic, Pajic, Macura, & Erculj, 2012), the 4 × 10-meter shuttle run test (Roriz De Oliveira, Seabra, Freitas, Eisenmann, & Maia, 2014), the compass drill (Stojanovic et al., in press), the Balsom agility test (Garcia-Pinillos, Martinez-Amat, Hita-Con-

---

Teaching Tip

CHANGING DIRECTION AT SPEED: IMPORTANCE OF STRENGTH

The kinetic and kinematic demands of change-of-direction tasks highlight the importance of muscular strength. Performers need high amounts of concentric strength in order to accelerate, eccentric strength in order to decelerate, isometric strength in order to transition between deceleration and reacceleration, and concentric strength in order to reaccelerate. Although youth fitness specialists must of course teach sound movement technique (e.g., body lean, footwork, hip orientation), improvements in changing direction can often be achieved by helping an individual get stronger and therefore develop increased ability to produce and absorb force. In fact, research has highlighted the importance of strength characteristics for effective change-of-direction performance (Spiteri et al., 2015; Spiteri et al., 2014), especially when strength is expressed relative to body mass (Delaney et al., 2015).

treras, Martinez-Lopez, & Latorre-Roman, 2014), the 10 × 5-meter test (Figueiredo, Goncalves, Coelho, & Malina, 2009; Hirose & Seki, 2015; Valente-dos-Santos et al., 2014), the line drill (Vanderford, Meyers, Skelly, Stewart, & Hamilton, 2004), the T-test (Lovell et al., 2015; Negra et al., 2017), and the 505 agility test protocol (Faigenbaum et al., 2007; Thomas, French, & Hayes, 2009). In light of the limitations of these protocols, it is apparent that the existing evidence base has examined only change-of-direction speed in youth, which leaves our understanding of agility development in youth incomplete.

Natural Development of Agility in Youth

Due to the inherent limitations of previous testing protocols and the lack of longitudinal research examining agility development in youth, it remains unclear exactly how growth, maturation, and training interact with cognitive functioning and change-of-direction speed. Consequently, existing frameworks for long-term agility development have been forced to base their theoretical underpinnings on a combined understanding of the manner in which change-of-direction speed and cognitive functioning develop independently (Lloyd & Oliver, 2012; Lloyd et al., 2013).

Natural Development of Change-of-Direction Speed

In addition to a small amount of longitudinal data, cross-sectional studies show that change-of-direction speed develops naturally, albeit nonlinearly, in boys and girls as a consequence of growth and maturation (Chiodera et al., 2008; Eisenmann & Malina, 2003; Vanttinen et al., 2011). More recently, researchers have shown that within a group of boys, change-of-direction speed increased significantly from 12 to 14 years of age (Jakovljevic et al., 2012), an age range that typically coincides with the adolescent growth spurt. Eisenmann and Malina (2003) examined age- and sex-associated variation in a range of neuromuscular qualities, including change-of-direction speed, over a period of four to five years. Their study showed that boys and girls performed similarly in terms of change-of-direction speed prior to puberty; however, clear sex-associated differences were established during the adolescent growth spurt. The sex-associated variation during adolescence was attributable to continued neuromuscular adaptation in males (i.e., natural increases in strength and power) and a relative plateau in females, especially those who are untrained.

Age-related trends around the adolescent growth spurt in males are corroborated by research examining changes in physical fitness, including change-of-direction speed, in youth soccer players (Philippaerts et al., 2006; Vanttinen et al., 2011). Research by Vanttinen and colleagues (2011) showed that the greatest relative improvement in change-of-direction speed occurred in a group of youth male soccer players who transitioned from 13 to 14 years of age. These changes appeared to coincide with transient spikes in testosterone, height, and weight, which are reflective of typical changes associated with the adolescent growth spurt. Similarly, Philippaerts and colleagues (2006) determined that peak velocity of change in change-of-direction speed in their cohort of young players occurred approximately around peak height velocity.

Closer inspection of the determinants highlighted in figure 10.5 identifies a number of variables that, when interacting with growth and maturation, likely mediate adaptations in change-of-direction speed. For example, from an anthropometric perspective, height and weight increase at different rates and in a nonlinear manner throughout childhood and adolescence. Due to these naturally occurring developments, youth may be required to perform change-of-direction speed tasks with a disadvantaged anthropometric profile, especially during the adolescent growth spurt. During this stage of development, adolescents experience increases in body mass and in height of center of mass without concomitant increases in lower-limb strength, all of which can lead to performance decrements and increased risk of injury (Myer et al., 2009). Moreover, the anthropometric determinants displayed in figure 10.5 are largely unmodifiable. Therefore, practitioners are invariably more interested in the subcomponents that are modifiable, such as technical factors (e.g., body lean, foot placement, stride adjustment) and neuromuscular factors (e.g., various expressions of strength, stretch–shortening cycle function, rate of force development).

Natural Development of Cognitive Functioning

There is a dearth of research examining the effect of growth and maturation on cognitive functioning and agility performance. However, available literature in the fields of neuroscience and pediatric motor control suggests that repeated exposure to a given stimulus (or to related stimuli) results in faster response times and enhanced overall cognitive capacity due to synaptic pathway strengthening (Casey, Giedd, & Thomas, 2000), ongoing neural myelination (Paus et al., 1999), and synaptic pruning (Casey, Tottenham, Liston, & Durston, 2005). It also suggests that neural plasticity is heightened during childhood (Gogtay et al., 2004; Myer et al., 2015). Our understanding of cerebral development during childhood and adolescence (see chapters 2 and 8) can be applied to motor skill theory, which advocates exposing children to a depth and breadth of exercises and movement patterns in order to develop decision-making processes (Baker, Cote, & Abernethy, 2003). Further research has suggested that collective exposure to a range of sporting experiences may result in selective transfer of pattern-recall skills and may facilitate skilled task performance (Abernethy, Baker, & Cote, 2005). Given the highly variable nature of agility-based movements—whether in free play, recreational physical activity, or competitive sport—we must ensure that youth are able to execute agility-based movements when faced with a range of individual, environmental, and task constraints.

Trainability of Agility in Youth

As with designing programs for speed training, youth fitness specialists need to consider variables such as exercise selection, volume and intensity, recovery, and frequency when designing and implementing agility training programs for children and adolescents.

Trainability of Change-of-Direction Speed

The available literature has established that gains in change-of-direction speed in youth can be promoted through various training interventions, including change-of-direction sprints (Chaouachi, Chtara, et al., 2014), strength training (Hammami, Negra, Billaut, et al., 2017; Hammami, Negra, Shephard, et al., 2017; Jullien et al., 2008; Keiner, Sander, Wirth, & Schmidtbleicher, 2014), plyometrics (Asadi, Arazi, Ramirez-Campillo, Moran, & Izquierdo, 2017; Bedoya, Miltenberger, & Lopez, 2015; Meylan & Malatesta, 2009; Sohnlein, Muller, & Stoggl, 2014; Thomas et al., 2009), combined strength training and plyometrics (Faigenbaum et al., 2007; Garcia-Pinillos et al., 2014; Hammami, Negra, Shephard, et al., 2017), and small-sided games (Chaouachi, Chtara, et al., 2014; Young & Rogers, 2014). The effectiveness of strength training for change-of-direction speed was also shown in research in which 16-year-old soccer players used resistance training loads of up to 90 percent of 1RM over an eight-week training period (Hammami, Negra, Billaut, et al., 2017). The data showed that participants significantly improved in a range of tests for change-of-direction speed and that, although muscle volumes remained unchanged, significant increases were exhibited in muscle activity during vertical jumps. Altogether, these findings suggest that heavy strength training led to improvements in change-of-direction speed mainly through neuromuscular adaptations rather than through changes in muscle architecture.

Despite the scarcity of longitudinal studies examining the effects of long-term training on change-of-direction speed, a study by Keiner and colleagues (2014) showed that under-15, under-17, and under-19 soccer players all exhibited significant improvements in change-of-direction speed following a two-year strength training intervention. The study reported moderate to strong correlations between changes in relative strength levels and concomitant changes in change-of-direction speed for all age groups, thus highlighting the importance of efficient force production for successful change-of-direction speed performance.

In another study, meta-analytical data were analyzed to examine the influence of maturity stage on improvements in change-of-direction speed following exposure to plyometric training (Asadi et al., 2017). The analysis, which included 16 studies, found that plyometric training was effective for all youth but that older youth (ages 16 to 18 years) made more meaningful changes in performance, as evidenced by larger effect sizes. The study also indicated a positive relationship between training intensity and magnitude of improvement in change-of-direction speed. The benefits of higher-intensity training (presuming that technique remains competent) are echoed elsewhere in the pediatric literature, namely for improvements in strength and power in response to resistance training (Lesinski, Prieske, & Granacher, 2016) and for improvements in maximal aerobic capacity following endurance training (Baquet, van Praagh, & Berthoin, 2003).

Cumulatively, the existing evidence base highlights the effectiveness of neuromuscular-oriented training for change-of-direction speed, the relative trainability of strength in children and adolescents (Behringer, Vom Heede, Yue, & Mester, 2010), and the associations between change-of-direction speed and strength and power capacities (Delaney et al., 2015; Hammami, Negra, Billaut, et al., 2017; Jones, Bampouras, & Marrin, 2009; Keiner et al., 2014; Nimphius, McGuigan, & Newton, 2010; Spiteri et al., 2015). Therefore, it would seem prudent for youth fitness specialists to focus strongly on developing neuromuscular qualities (e.g., relative strength, power, stiffness properties) as part of any youth-based training program, irrespective of participants' training history or maturity status.

Trainability of Cognitive Functioning

The trainability of cognitive functioning for agility performance has been examined only minimally, but one study has attempted to determine the effectiveness of a short-term (three-week) reactive agility training intervention on perceptual and decision-making components of agility in a group of 18- to 20-year-olds

(Serpell, Young, & Ford, 2011). Participants took part in tests for reactive agility and change-of-direction speed using a previously validated protocol (Serpell, Ford, & Young, 2010) before being placed in either an experimental training group or a control group equivalent. Whereas the control group showed no significant performance changes over the intervention period, members of the experimental group improved their reactive agility test performance. Change-of-direction speed remained unchanged, but reactive agility perception and response time were significantly reduced, thus suggesting that improvements in reactive agility performance were attributable to adaptation in cognitive functioning. Although this study presents some novel insights into the potential trainability of cognitive functioning for agility performance, questions remain about how children and adolescents would respond to similar training interventions during different stages of maturation.

Training Prescription for Agility Development

Given that methods for developing strength and power are covered in chapter 9, the remainder of this section focuses on training prescription that targets the derivatives of agility, including **fundamental motor skill training**, **change-of-direction speed training**, and **reactive agility training**.

Fundamental motor skill training is needed in order to develop movement patterns inherent in successful execution of agility-related tasks, such as acceleration and deceleration mechanics, step patterns (e.g., jab, pivot, crossover, and gravity steps), cutting technique, backpedaling, and side-shuffling. Each pattern requires coordination of unilateral lower- and upper-body actions, as well as core bracing for force transmission along the kinetic chain. Therefore, in addition to training specific agility movement patterns, practitioners may also prescribe, in the same session, certain exercises that stress general movement patterns (e.g., single-leg stability tasks, core-bracing exercises).

Although correct technique will often be reinforced, change-of-direction speed training is designed primarily to enhance the participant's ability to apply forces during acceleration, deceleration, and reacceleration. These qualities can be developed through closed and preplanned exercises, such as the three-cone L-drill and the 5-0-5 drill.

Reactive agility training requires the child or adolescent to perform agility-based tasks in response to an external stimulus. The youth fitness specialist might use a variety of external stimuli, including auditory signals (e.g., verbal command, clap, whistle) and visual signals (e.g., light stimulus, video stimulus, opposition player). Sample exercises for reactive agility training could include partner mirroring (see figure 10.6), partner truck and trailer, or various versions of tag.

Researchers have suggested that while youth of all ages and abilities should be exposed to training in fundamental motor skills, change-of-direction speed, and reactive agility, the percentage of time devoted to each element should depend on the participant's technical competence and degree of maturation (Lloyd et al., 2013). Figure 10.7 provides a theoretical breakdown of how technical competence and stage of development can influence time devoted to various derivatives of agility training.

For beginners and less mature children, a large proportion of time should be spent on mastering fundamental motor skills, which serve as the foundations on which more complex movements can be developed in more reactive tasks and open-skill environments (Lubans et al., 2010; Oliver, Lloyd, & Meyers, 2011). This strategy not only aids long-term development of agility for performance but also, and perhaps of greater significance, helps with injury prevention through a structured and patient approach to agility

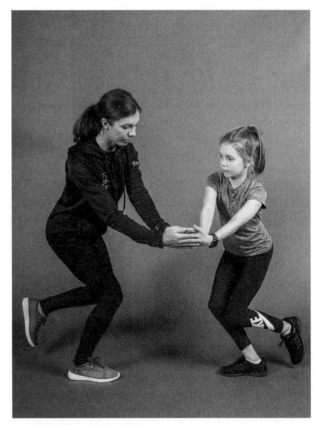

FIGURE 10.6   Partner mirroring.

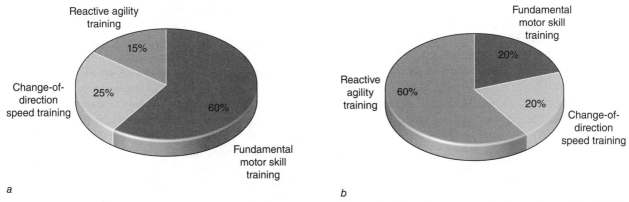

a   b

FIGURE 10.7   Sample distribution of percentage training time devoted to the derivatives of agility training for *(a)* a less mature and technically incompetent child and *(b)* a mature and technically competent adolescent.

training (Lloyd et al., 2013). For example, research has shown that unanticipated cutting maneuvers involve greater ligament loading at the knee joint than does straight-line sprinting, thus predisposing the anterior cruciate ligament to an increased risk of injury (Besier, Lloyd, Cochrane, & Ackland, 2001). By concentrating initial agility training on fundamental motor skill mastery (e.g., knee, hip, and ankle stability; single-leg movements; core bracing; step patterns), the child or adolescent should develop a more resilient and technically robust system with which to execute reactive and unanticipated movements. Once these fundamental motor skills have been mastered, the youth fitness specialist should be able to prescribe a higher proportion of more advanced, reactive drills while feeling confident that the child or adolescent has a strong, robust, and technically proficient system that is prepared to tolerate higher internal and external forces during free play and sporting activities.

Exercise Selection

Irrespective of which subcomponent is prioritized during a given session—fundamental motor skills, change-of-direction speed, or reactive agility—practitioners must select exercises that are developmentally appropriate for the child. Although children need to be physically and cognitively challenged for the purpose of ongoing development, they must also be prescribed exercises that they can perform safely with appropriate technique in order to maintain competent movement patterns. For example, an experienced adolescent might devote the majority of training time to reactive agility, but the warm-up could still incorporate exercises targeting fundamental motor skills and basic change-of-direction skills in order to reinforce correct movement mechanics that prepare the individual for the technical demands of the session. Prioritizing movement mechanics (e.g., acceleration and deceleration techniques; specific step patterns)

Teaching Tip

LEARNING TO SLAM ON THE BRAKES: DECELERATION TRAINING

Many studies have investigated the mechanics of effective acceleration during sprint performance, but the mechanics of effective deceleration have received considerably less attention. Decelerating effectively is critical both to one's ability to stop, either gradually or immediately, and to one's ability to decrease the velocity of movement before reaccelerating in another direction. From a purely physical standpoint, then, effective deceleration enhances performance in tasks that require sudden stoppages or rapid changes of direction (e.g., in preparation for, and during recovery from, tennis ground strokes) and should enable greater force transmission into subsequent movements (e.g., reaccelerating to evade an opposing player). However, the exceptionally high forces applied to the body over a very short time period during deceleration place children and adolescents at potential risk of injury if they are unable to decelerate competently. Therefore, youth fitness specialists should devote time to developing deceleration techniques at some point during an integrated fitness program.

at the start of a session—before engaging in more dynamic movements or small-sided games—has been proven to reduce the incidence of injury in young male and female athletes in both training and competitive environments (Junge, Rosch, Peterson, Graf-Baumann, & Dvorak, 2002; Mandelbaum et al., 2005; Richmond, Kang, Doyle-Baker, Nettel-Aguirre, & Emery, 2016; Rossler, Donath, Bizzini, & Faude, 2015).

Given that agility-based exercises are expressions of motor skill function, youth fitness specialists could adopt a constraints-led approach to agility training (as highlighted in chapter 8). When working with an inexperienced and technically incompetent child, the practitioner should initially look to use exercises that stress technical skill development (e.g., basic acceleration and deceleration mechanics; lateral hop and hold) with low degrees of freedom. In contrast, for an experienced young athlete who is technically proficient, the practitioner could manipulate multiple task constraints by prescribing exercises (e.g., reactive evasion drills) with a larger range of perceptual degrees of freedom and greater physical challenge in order to foster continued skill acquisition.

If the execution of closed, preplanned fundamental motor skills is viewed as the most simplistic and least demanding derivative of agility training, then small-sided games can be viewed as the more advanced end of the agility training continuum. Small-sided games would seem to offer the opportunity to simultaneously develop physical attributes, cognitive functioning, and technical and tactical qualities (Hill-Haas, Dawson, Impellizzeri, & Coutts, 2011). However, despite the apparent logic of this assumption, valid research remains somewhat scarce (Paul, Gabbett, & Nassis, 2016), and the amount of fatigue experienced by the child during such activities may prevent them from providing an optimal training stimulus for the development of agility. Of the available evidence, one study showed that six weeks of small-sided games and change-of-direction training were effective at improving linear sprinting, change-of-direction speed, and vertical jumping ability; however, small-sided games were more effective than change-of-direction drills in improving agility tests involving ball control (Chaouachi, Chtara, et al., 2014). Another study examined the effectiveness of small-sided games versus change-of-direction training on measures of agility and change-of-direction speed in a group of under-18 Australian Rules football players (Young & Rogers, 2014). The study showed that small-sided games improved agility performance mainly through very large improvements in speed of decision making but that change-of-direction training produced only small or even trivial changes in the same test variables.

Volume and Intensity

As suggested by the brief, intermittent nature of agility-based tasks, performance of these movements relies heavily on anaerobic metabolism. Therefore, in order to maintain the quality of agility training, work bouts should be brief and interspersed with sufficient recovery to facilitate full recovery. As with training for speed development, there is an inverse relationship between the volume and intensity of agility training, where *volume* refers to total repetitions × distance per repetition per exercise, and *intensity* reflects a percentage of maximal speed or maximal effort. The volume of training time devoted to agility development depends primarily on the following factors:

- Individual characteristics of the child or adolescent (e.g., training history, technical competence)
- Key training priorities for the individual
- Amount of time available in the training block or session (e.g., entire session or part of a session)

The dose–response relationship for agility training remains unclear; however, as with speed training, overall session volume is likely to remain low in order to maintain performance quality. Chaouachi and colleagues (2014) provide an example of training

Teaching Tip

EXECUTING MOVEMENTS CORRECTLY UNDER PRESSURE

If youth fitness specialists understand the technical model and the constraints-led approach to motor skill development, they can use relevant exercises and associated cues to develop sound fundamental agility-related movement patterns. In addition, youth should be taught how to perform such movements in a variety of tasks and environments. Thus, in many ways, the end goal for youth fitness specialists should be to develop robust and resilient movement patterns that youth can modify and use in the dynamic and unpredictable positions encountered in sport, recreational physical activity, and free play.

prescription for small-sided games, wherein total session volumes of up to 14 minutes (three exercises, 4 sets per exercise, and work bouts of 30 to 120 sec) were used to train 14-year-old soccer players. The training prescription for change-of-direction sessions involved up to 16 work sets spread over four exercises, for which the total distance increased from 360 to 520 meters and the total number of directional changes increased from 48 to 78 during the six-week training intervention. Similarly, a change-of-direction training study involving under-18 Australian Rules football players involved brief maximal-effort sprints over 2 to 5 meters with 1 to 5 changes of direction or speed for four activities per session (Young & Rogers, 2014). Overall, the study increased the total number of directional changes per session from 36 to 48 by the end of the program. Although research examining the trainability of perceptual and decision-making components of agility did not report specific training prescriptions (sets, reps, intensity, directional changes), total session duration lasted just 15 minutes (Serpell et al., 2011), which underlines the notion that agility training should focus on quality rather than quantity.

In-Session Recovery

As with sprint training, youth fitness specialists should try to ensure that youth are afforded sufficient time for full recovery. Researchers have used rest periods of about two minutes when prescribing brief activities for change-of-direction speed and noted work-to-rest ratios of 1:10 to 1:20 (Chaouachi, Chtara, et al., 2014). In contrast, studies involving small-sided games have used work-to-rest ratios of 1:1 (Young & Rogers, 2014) or ranging from 1:1 to 1:4 (Chaouachi, Chtara, et al., 2014); of course, the nature of small-sided games means that they are likely to include a higher proportion of subintervals within a given work set. Although many in-session recovery options are available, youth fitness specialists should make it a key objective to ensure full, or nearly full, recovery in order to aid maximal efforts in subsequent work bouts.

Training Frequency

Much like the optimal dosage (volume and intensity) for agility training remains unknown, the optimal training frequency is also yet to be established. Agility-based training interventions for youth (e.g., small-sided games and training for reactive agility and change-of-direction speed) have typically used two or three sessions per week for training periods of three to seven weeks (Chaouachi, Chtara, et al., 2014; Serpell et al., 2011; Young & Rogers, 2014). The optimal frequency of agility training requires further examination, but in the meantime youth fitness specialists should appreciate that change-of-direction speed and reactive agility can be developed as components of a training session in an integrated neuromuscular training program (Faigenbaum et al., 2011; Faigenbaum et al., 2007; Myer et al., 2011). Due to the fact that practitioners often have limited amounts of time to train youth, it is usually deemed appropriate to expose youth to some form of agility training two times per week.

Sample Agility Training Programs

Agility-based training programs should be based primarily on technical competence and secondarily on other variables, including stage of maturation, training experience, sex of the participant, and priority of the training block. To illustrate how agility training might differ when working with youth of differing abilities, tables 10.5 and 10.6 present sample training sessions for beginners with low technical competence and for more advanced youth with high technical competence. Although the sample sessions relate to a child and an adolescent, youth fitness specialists should remember

Teaching Tip

MONITORING DIRECTIONAL CHANGES IN A SESSION

At all levels, youth fitness specialists should visually observe and monitor each participant's movement technique while performing agility-based tasks in order to ensure correct dosage of training stimulus and reduce the risk of injury. Practitioners can also make use of subjective assessments, such as RPE scales, to monitor a participant's level of physical exertion during a session. They may also wish to measure the number of changes of direction completed per session, because these movements impose increased strain on the body, especially when they are performed at higher velocities (Hatamoto et al., 2014). Although empirical data are lacking, the eccentric trauma placed on the musculotendon unit when changing direction (e.g., during a 180-degree turn) is likely to be magnified as the volume of directional changes increases; in addition, more eccentric loading is experienced during reactive movements than during preplanned ones.

TABLE 10.5 SAMPLE BEGINNER SESSION FOR AGILITY DEVELOPMENT TRAINING IN YOUTH

Focus of training	Exercise	Volume (sets × reps)	Intensity (% effort)	Rest (sec)	Changes of direction
Fundamental motor skills	Hip mobility complex	2 × 10 (each drill)	Low	30-60	N/A
	Mini-band clam shell	2 × 8 (each leg)	Low	30-60	N/A
	Mini-band glute bridge	2 × 8 (each leg)	Low	30-60	N/A
	Single-leg balance with reach	2 × 30 seconds (each leg)	Low	30-60	N/A
	Single-leg partner mirroring	2 × 30 seconds (each leg)	Low	30-60	N/A

Focus of training	Exercise	Volume (sets × reps)	Intensity (% effort)	Rest (sec)	Changes of direction
Fundamental motor skills *(continued)*	Jump to low box	3 × 6	Low	30-60	N/A
	Countermovement jump and stick	2 × 4	Low	30-60	N/A
	Lateral squat jump and stick	2 × 4 (each side)	Low	30-60	N/A
Change-of-direction speed	Preplanned step pattern (drop, jab, pivot)	6 × each pattern	Moderate	30-60	~18
	Preplanned six-point grid court drill (2 m × 2 m)	4 × 10 sec	Moderate	30-60	~20
	Multidirectional preplanned relay (5 m)	4 × 10 sec	Moderate	30-60	~20
Reactive agility training	Randomized multidirectional ball throw with hold	4 × 6	High	60	~24
	Service box "piggy in the middle"	4 × 20 sec	High	60	~40

TABLE 10.6 SAMPLE ADVANCED SESSION FOR AGILITY DEVELOPMENT TRAINING IN YOUTH

Focus of training	Exercise	Volume (sets × reps)	Intensity (% effort)	Rest (sec)	Changes of direction
Fundamental motor skills	Hip mobility complex	2 × 10 (each drill)	Low	30-60	N/A
	Mini-band monster walk	2 × 8 (each leg)	Low	30-60	N/A
	Single-leg box squat	3 × 8 (each leg)	Low	30-60	N/A
	Lateral zigzag bound	4 × 4	Low	30-60	N/A

Focus of training	Exercise	Volume (sets × reps)	Intensity (% effort)	Rest (sec)	Changes of direction
Fundamental motor skills *(continued)*	Low-level multidirectional drop jump and stick	4 × 4	Low	30-60	N/A
Change-of-direction speed	Preplanned ball catch	6 × 10 sec	Moderate	60	~18
	Preplanned multidirectional ball pickup	6 × 10 sec	Moderate	60	~18
Reactive agility training	Randomized multidirectional ball throw	6 × 4	High	90	~24
	Lateral cone shuffle and react to catch ball	6 × 4	High	90	~16
	Half-court team tag	4 × 15 sec	High	90	~20
	Ball exchange competition	First to 7 points	High	90	~20

that training prescription is ultimately driven by technical competence. It is not surprising for practitioners to come across a naturally gifted child who displays high levels of athleticism or an adolescent who is technically very poor. Therefore, practitioners should never underestimate the value of direct observation to help them coach what they see in front of them. The sample sessions presented here are designed for a one-hour duration, but it is possible that strength and conditioning coaches may be required to tailor session contents to fit the available time; for example, 15 minutes of agility training could be integrated into the warm-up phase of a session focused on generic skills.

In comparing tables 10.5 and 10.6, it is evident that greater emphasis is placed on fundamental motor skills for youth with low technical competence, whereas reactive agility training becomes more of a focus for youth who are more technically competent. That said, due to the neural plasticity associated with the prepubertal years (Casey et al., 2000; Rabinowickz, 1986), practitioners should provide participants with some exposure to agility exercises that stress fundamental motor skills in sport-specific contexts and develop change-of-direction speed and reactive agility.

Summary

Research clearly shows that speed and agility are fundamental motor skills that combine to form the basis of many physical activities, including those typically witnessed in recreational free play and competitive sport. Although research indicates that maturation influences the training response in children and adolescents, randomized controlled trials examining the interaction between growth, maturation, and training are limited. Crucially, for practitioners, the available evidence for both speed and agility development shows that both children and adolescents can make worthwhile improvements in response to a range of training stimuli, provided that exercise prescription is commensurate with the needs of the individual. Certainly, for speed development, key training modes appear to be sensitive to maturation. More research is needed in order to examine the interaction of sex, maturity, and training, and the development of well-controlled longer-term interventions is crucial in order to further our understanding of the effect of long-term adaptations in speed and agility.

CHAPTER 11

Aerobic and Anaerobic Training

CHAPTER OBJECTIVES

- Discuss the determinants of aerobic and anaerobic fitness
- Examine how aerobic and anaerobic fitness develop naturally as a result of growth and maturation
- Critically review the trainability of aerobic and anaerobic fitness in children and adolescents
- Discuss relevant training strategies for aerobic and anaerobic development, as well as the process of manipulating training variables for long-term adaptation

KEY TERMS

Introduction

Exercise requires the support of **aerobic** and **anaerobic** metabolism to provide the energy required for contracting muscles and initiating force production and movement. The aerobic energy system is associated with endurance exercise because it can provide energy to sustain lower-intensity, prolonged exercise; it also enables metabolic recovery after bouts of higher-intensity exercise. The anaerobic system, on the other hand, is associated with high-intensity exercise of limited duration, which is characteristic of children's play. In the broad sense, anaerobic exercise can encompass speed, agility, strength, and power; however, because these specific components of fitness are discussed elsewhere in the book (see chapters 9 and 10), discussion of the anaerobic system in this chapter focuses on metabolism.

Aerobic and anaerobic energy can contribute simultaneously to a given type of exercise, and their relative contributions are determined by exercise intensity and duration as well as individual growth, maturation, and training history. Younger, more immature children rely less on **anaerobic glycolysis** and more on aerobic metabolism than do older, more mature adolescents (Boisseau & Delamarche, 2000). Consequently, a prepubertal child is likely to fatigue less and recover more quickly than an adolescent. Aerobic metabolism and anaerobic metabolism both develop naturally with maturation, though at different rates (Armstrong et al., 2015), and both systems can be positively influenced by training (Armstrong & Barker, 2011; Eriksson et al., 1973; Fournier et al., 1982). Youth fitness specialists should be aware of the influence of maturation on metabolic responses to exercise because they influence both acute responses and potential long-term adaptations to training.

In the course of daily life, active youth naturally engage in intermittent bouts of free play that are often characterized by explosive efforts of jumping, leaping, dodging, sprinting, throwing, and kicking interspersed with brief recovery periods as required. The ability to repeatedly perform explosive actions over long duration also characterizes fitness training and many other exercise activities, as well as many sports (e.g., team, invasion, and racket sports). Therefore, providing youth with opportunities to engage in free play, structured exercise activities, and sport helps to promote the development of both the aerobic and the anaerobic systems, which in turn provides children and adolescents with the capabilities to engage in exercise with energy and vigor. Improvements in aerobic and anaerobic fitness are also associated with health benefits and reduced risk of disease (Bangsbo et al., 2016; Costigan et al., 2015; Ortega et al., 2008).

Natural Development of Aerobic and Anaerobic Fitness

Youth who lead a healthy and active lifestyle will improve both their aerobic and their anaerobic fitness as a result of growth and maturation. These changes will result from both quantitative increases in size (e.g., increased muscle mass and internal organ size) and qualitative changes in function (e.g., alterations in muscle metabolism). Youth fitness specialists should be aware of how aerobic and anaerobic fitness develop naturally throughout childhood and adolescence and how these changes are driven by physiological processes. This knowledge will help practitioners design exercise programming and determine where training has improved fitness beyond what is expected as a result of growth and maturation.

Aerobic Fitness

As discussed in chapter 2, children are considered to be more reliant on aerobic metabolism and less reliant on anaerobic metabolism as compared with adults. This difference may derive partly from a greater proportion of type I muscle fibers in children, some of which may be converted to type II with maturation (Lexell et al., 1992); however, debate exists as to whether fiber type differentiation occurs during childhood and adolescence (Armstrong & Fawkner, 2008; Malina et al., 2004). In addition, glycolytic enzyme activity is lower in children and increases with maturation, as does muscle mass (Rowland, 2005). Thus, as children mature, they can produce greater power but also become subject to more rapid fatigue during high-intensity exercise. Given their substantial potential to improve anaerobic metabolism, children improve this quality faster than they improve aerobic metabolism during maturation (Ratel & Williams, 2008). Youth fitness specialists should be aware of the effects of these developmental changes; specifically, maturity brings greater ability to achieve high-intensity efforts but at the cost of greater fatigue and a need for more recovery time.

Aerobic metabolism is associated with endurance performance because it can provide energy over a long period of time. The primary physiological determinants of endurance include the following:

- **Peak oxygen uptake** ($\dot{V}O_2$peak), or the maximal rate at which energy can be supplied by aerobic metabolism
- **Lactate threshold**, or the highest exercise intensity that can be sustained for a prolonged period of time

Teaching Tip

ARE AEROBIC AND ANAEROBIC TRAINING WORTHWHILE FOR CHILDREN?

Researchers have debated whether immature children are responsive to anaerobic and aerobic training (Boisseau & Delamarche, 2000; Katch, 1983; Naughton et al., 2000), as well as when to initiate training. Recent evidence suggests that all youth can benefit from **metabolic conditioning** (Baquet et al., 2003, 2010; McManus et al., 2005; Sperlich, De Marees, Koehler, Linville, Holmberg, & Mester, 2011; Sperlich, Zinner, Heilemann, Kjendlie, Holmberg, & Mester, 2010) and that there is no need to align training with specific stages of maturation (Harrison et al., 2015). These findings mean that training gains can be made starting at a young age, and youth fitness specialists should encourage activities that promote the development of the aerobic and anaerobic systems in both children and adolescents.

- **Efficiency (economy)**, or the amount of metabolic energy required to perform work or exercise at a given intensity

The primary determinant is peak oxygen uptake, which is the product of cardiac output and the muscle's ability to extract and use oxygen. With growth and maturation, cardiac output increases as a function of increasing body size, heart size, and blood volume, all of which drive large absolute increases in $\dot{V}O_2$peak and endurance performance. These gains are greater in boys than in girls; specifically, between the ages of 8 and 16 years, absolute $\dot{V}O_2$peak increases by about 150 percent in boys and 80 percent in girls (Armstrong & Welsman, 2000).

Peak oxygen uptake can also be expressed relative to body size to provide a description of oxygen consumption per unit of body size. Traditionally, this expression has been rendered by means of ratio scaling, wherein $\dot{V}O_2$peak is divided by body mass to describe oxygen consumption in mL $\cdot$ kg^{-1} $\cdot$ min^{-1}. Viewed in this way, $\dot{V}O_2$peak tends to plateau with age in boys and decrease with age in girls, who are disadvantaged by the added fat mass that accompanies maturation (Armstrong & Welsman, 2000). Expressing $\dot{V}O_2$peak in terms of **ratio scaling** may be informative for activities in which youth must carry their own body weight, such as running (Armstrong et al., 2015). However, even though it remains popular, the use of ratio scaling to understand the relationship between physiological qualities and size has been criticized, particularly with regard to $\dot{V}O_2$peak (Welsman et al., 1996).

As an alternative, **allometric scaling** provides a more appropriate method for understanding the relationship between size and physiological function. Allometric scaling adjusts for changes in size and proportion in order to accurately examine the influence of growth and maturation on physiology. When $\dot{V}O_2$peak is allometrically scaled for both body mass and compo-

sition, it increases with age and maturity for both boys and girls, though boys still experience greater gains (Welsman et al., 1996). This finding suggests that some of the increase observed in $\dot{V}O_2$peak with growth and maturation is independent of increases in body size. However, given the ease of ratio scaling and reporting of $\dot{V}O_2$peak in terms of mL $\cdot$ kg^{-1} $\cdot$ min^{-1} this method should be considered acceptable for the youth fitness specialist. Peak oxygen uptake expressed with ratio scaling has been suggested to be useful in terms of helping to understand changes in aerobic function in relation to body size and it provides a variable that can be readily compared with healthy fitness standards (Ruiz et al., 2016).

The ability to maintain a high relative work rate, expressed as a percentage of $\dot{V}O_2$peak, is greater in children than in adolescents, and it declines with age and maturation. The lactate threshold is the point where, with increasing exercise intensity, lactate begins to accumulate rapidly, which leads indirectly to fatigue. With lower glycolytic activity and less muscle mass, children are less able to produce lactate and associated by-products; consequently, they suffer less fatigue. As a result, the lactate threshold is higher in children but decreases with maturation. This higher threshold allows children to sustain relatively higher exercise intensity when the threshold is expressed as a percentage of $\dot{V}O_2$peak. For instance, Tolfrey and Armstrong (1995) reported that the relative intensity at which a lactate threshold of 4 millimoles per liter was achieved decreased from 94 percent of $\dot{V}O_2$peak in prepubertal boys to 92 percent in teenage boys and 87 percent in adults.

The reduction in the relative exercise intensity at which the lactate threshold occurs has been attributed to increasing glycolytic enzyme activity with maturation (Fellman & Coudert, 1994; Reybrouck et al., 1985). Although the percentage of $\dot{V}O_2$peak at which the threshold occurs decreases slightly with matura-

Teaching Tip

MAXIMAL OR PEAK OXYGEN UPTAKE?

The terms *maximal oxygen uptake* ($\dot{V}O_2max$) and *peak oxygen uptake* ($\dot{V}O_2peak$) both refer to primary determinants of endurance and are often used interchangeably. They are not, however, the same. The term $\dot{V}O_2max$ should be used when a plateau in oxygen consumption is observed during a progressive exhaustive test as exercise intensity increases, thus indicating that oxygen consumption has reached its maximal rate. This plateau is displayed by only 20 percent to 40 percent of children during a progressive test (Armstrong et al., 1995; Rowland 1993). For most children, as exercise intensity increases, oxygen consumption continues to increase until the point of exhaustion. Therefore, we do not know if a true maximum for oxygen consumption has been achieved, and we use the term $\dot{V}O_2peak$ instead. Given the low proportion of children who can attain a true maximum, it is more appropriate to use $\dot{V}O_2peak$ with children.

tion, the large absolute increase in $\dot{V}O_2peak$ means that actual oxygen consumption at the threshold is higher in adolescents than in children. For instance, an 8-year-old boy with a $\dot{V}O_2peak$ of 1.5 liters per minute and a lactate threshold of 90 percent of $\dot{V}O_2peak$ would consume oxygen at a rate of 1.35 liters per minute at threshold. In contrast, a 16-year-old boy with a $\dot{V}O_2peak$ of 3.5 liters per minute and a lactate threshold of 85 percent of $\dot{V}O_2peak$ would consume oxygen at a rate of 3.0 liters per minute at threshold.

Running economy involves the oxygen cost required to run at a given steady-state speed and is typically expressed in terms of $mL \cdot kg^{-1} \cdot min^{-1}$. It has been suggested that running economy improves steadily with advancing age in children and adolescents (Krahenbuhl & Williams, 1992; Sallis et al., 1991). Improvements in running economy with increasing maturation have been confirmed when oxygen consumption is expressed in terms of both ratio and allometric scaling (Ariens et al., 1997). These findings suggest that as children mature, the oxygen cost of running at a given speed is lowered, thus providing a performance advantage. Data from Astrand (1952, presented in Morgan, 2008) show that between the ages of 5 to 6 and 16 to 18 years, the oxygen cost of running at 10 kilometers per hour decreased from 47 to 38 $mL \cdot kg^{-1} \cdot min^{-1}$ in boys and from 45 to 37 $mL \cdot kg^{-1} \cdot min^{-1}$ in girls. It has been suggested that girls may be more economical than boys (Bar-Or & Rowland, 2004), but the balance of evidence regarding a possible sex difference remains unclear (Morgan, 2008). Possible reasons for the impaired running economy observed in children are presented in figure 11.1; these factors would all improve with age, maturity, and training.

Perhaps more relevant are the performance gains observed in endurance with increasing age and maturation. For instance, one-mile run times have been shown to improve across all percentiles of girls and boys aged 9 to 17 years, although the gains seen in boys roughly double those seen in girls (Catley & Tomkinson, 2013). The sex-related difference in rate of improvement derives from the fact that growth and maturation improve absolute gains in oxygen consumption more in boys than in girls (at $\dot{V}O_2peak$ and at the lactate threshold), though both sexes improve

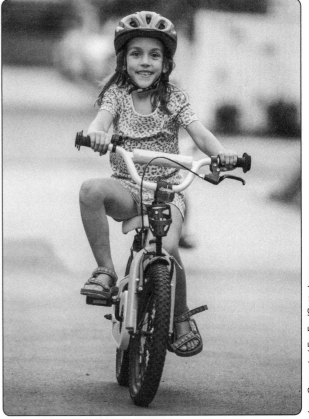

Getting children to take part in aerobic exercise can provide a multitude of fitness and health benefits.

Jure Gasparic / EyeEm/Getty Images

their economy. The developmental improvements are underpinned by physiological determinants, which are shown in figure 11.2. Improvements with age show what should be expected with a healthy lifestyle. However, youth fitness specialists must avoid being complacent—structured training is needed in order to ensure that aerobic fitness develops to its potential. Although aerobic fitness improves naturally, research indicates that, on average, modern-day children and adolescents complete a one-mile run approximately 90 seconds slower than the youth of 50 years ago (Tomkinson et al., 2013). Given the association between increases in size and function, it is not surprising that gains in both $\dot{V}O_2$peak and aerobic fitness have been reported to occur fastest around the time of the adolescent growth spurt (Malina et al., 2004; Philippaerts et al., 2006; Viru et al., 1999) due to rapid increases in muscle mass, heart volume, and blood volume.

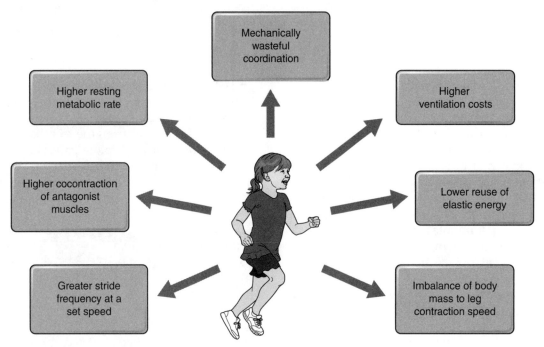

FIGURE 11.1   Possible reasons for the lower running economy observed in children as compared with adolescents and adults.
Data from Bar-Or and Rowland (2004) and Morgan (2008).

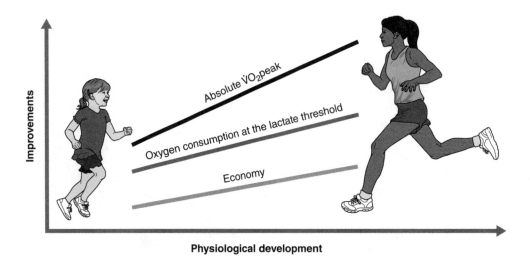

FIGURE 11.2   Changes in the key physiological determinants of endurance with advancing maturation (improvements for absolute oxygen consumption at the lactate threshold—not relative oxygen consumption).

Teaching Tip

NATURAL GAINS IN ENDURANCE PERFORMANCE

As compared with adults, children can sustain exercise at a relatively higher percentage of their peak oxygen uptake before they begin to fatigue. This difference occurs because children rely less on contributions from anaerobic glycolysis as exercise intensity increases, thus avoiding the fatiguing effects associated with lactate production. However, because children are also less coordinated and less economical, they convert less of their physiological energy to mechanical work. Most important, children are smaller, and increases in endurance performance are driven largely by increases in body size, cardiac dimensions, and blood volume. Therefore, as children mature, and particularly as they go through the growth spurt, their endurance performance naturally improves. However, youth fitness specialists should appreciate that a healthy lifestyle and structured training are needed in order to ensure that these developmental gains are realized.

Anaerobic Fitness

Energy for intense exercise lasting up to about 10 seconds is provided by the **ATP-PC system**, the abbreviated name of which refers to two phosphates: adenosine triphosphate and phosphocreatine. Whether storage levels of phosphocreatine increase with maturation is unclear (Armstrong et al., 2015), and this system has been suggested to be active at similar levels in children, adolescents, and adults (Berg et al., 1986). In contrast, the enzymes that catalyze anaerobic glycolysis are less active in children than in adolescents and adults (Berg et al., 1986; Haralambie, 1982). This difference means that children are less able to achieve sustained high work rates; instead, they are more reliant on aerobic metabolism even during prolonged bouts of intense exercise (e.g., 30 to 60 sec) and therefore produce less lactate and suffer less fatigue. Anaerobic performance is often considered in terms of power output during brief all-out exercise, or during performance in track events up to 400 meters in distance. Regardless of how maximal-intensity exercise is measured and standardized for body size, children always score significantly lower than adolescents, who in turn score lower than adults (Williams, 2008). In other words, anaerobic performance improves with age and maturation whether it is expressed in absolute or relative terms, though the latter is not necessarily the case for aerobic development.

Development of anaerobic capabilities throughout childhood and adolescence has been attributed to three potential factors: increasing muscle mass, increasing glycolytic activity, and improving neuromuscular coordination (Bar-Or & Rowland, 2004). The ratio between **peak anaerobic power** and **peak aerobic power**, known as the **power ratio**, changes from a factor of two at the age of 8 to a factor of three by age 14 (Bar-Or & Rowland, 2004), thus indicating that **anaerobic power** is developing faster than aerobic power.

In active play and in many sporting scenarios, youth are unlikely to engage in a single intense bout of exercise; nor are most youth likely to engage in long-duration, continuous bouts of exercise. Instead, most children naturally engage in intermittent activity characterized by periods of high-intensity and explosive actions interspersed with periods of lower intensity. As children mature, they grow larger and relatively more able to use anaerobic glycolysis, which means that they are able to achieve greater initial speed and power but with the consequences of greater fatigue and a slower rate of recovery. In fact, a large body of evidence now confirms that adults experience greater fatigue than children do during intermittent exercise (Ratel et al., 2006). Figure 11.3 shows some of the physiological factors that could explain why children experience less fatigue than adults and adolescents during high-intensity intermittent exercise.

In sport, repeated sprint ability involves the ability to perform a series of brief sprints with limited recovery between efforts (Spencer et al., 2004). This ability is a distinguishing characteristic of success in both youth and senior team sports (Abrantes et al., 2004; Reilly et al., 2000; Spencer et al., 2004). In a field-based repeated-sprint test involving a change of direction, mean sprint times decreased by 12 percent from under-12 to under-14 soccer players, by an additional 8 percent in the under-16 age group, and by yet another 6 percent to 12 percent at the senior professional level (Abrantes et al., 2004). Although maturity brings greater fatigue during all-out intermittent exercise, gains in the ability to sprint faster and produce more force and power mean that, overall, repeated sprint and intermittent exercise ability improve with maturation.

Aerobic and Anaerobic Trainability

Youth who have an active lifestyle will naturally improve their aerobic and anaerobic fitness, but these qualities can be further developed in both children and adolescents through appropriate training. When designing a training program, youth fitness specialists should consider the child's maturation and physiological capacity (e.g., ability to recover during intermittent work), as well as current fitness levels, previous exposure to training, and individual goals. Most important, practitioners must consider how to make training enjoyable and engaging when working with diverse populations that may range from sedentary youth who need to improve their health-related fitness to dedicated young athletes who want to improve their sport-specific fitness.

Aerobic Trainability

Much of the research on youth responsiveness to endurance training has examined $\dot{V}O_2$peak, which is recognized as the best single indicator of aerobic fitness (Armstrong & Barker, 2011). Research consistently demonstrates considerably higher $\dot{V}O_2$peak values for youth who are regularly involved in an endurance sport (e.g., swimming, cycling, distance running) than for untrained youth (Mahon, 2008). It is assumed that regular training causes positive adaptations in $\dot{V}O_2$peak in youth who participate in endurance activities, although some caution must be exercised when interpreting cross-sectional comparisons of different populations because findings may reflect a selection bias (toward those with naturally high levels of endurance) rather than a training effect.

Well-controlled intervention studies provide more robust evidence of the responsiveness of $\dot{V}O_2$peak to training. In a review of aerobic training in young people, Baquet and colleagues (2003) identified 22 studies that, taken cumulatively, suggest that gains of 5 percent to 6 percent in $\dot{V}O_2$peak can be achieved in children and adolescents through a training intervention. It is worth noting, however, that the vast majority of the studies involved prepubertal participants. Baquet and colleagues (2003) also examined the influence of program design on the training response and found that training-induced gains were increased when the following were true:

- Training frequency was three or more times per week.
- Session duration was more than 30 minutes.
- Exercise intensity was "all-out."

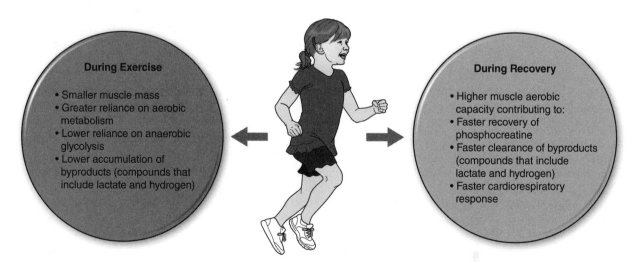

FIGURE 11.3 Physiological mechanisms that could explain the greater fatigue resistance of children as compared with adolescents and adults.

Adapted from Ratel, Duché, and Williams (2006).

Teaching Tip

FATIGUE RESISTANCE

In a study that included 10 repeated 10-second cycle sprints separated by either 30 seconds, one minute, or five minutes of recovery, Ratel and colleagues (2002) reported that prepubescent boys could maintain peak power with only 30 seconds of recovery, whereas pubescent boys and men needed five minutes of recovery to prevent fatigue. Specifically, with 30 seconds of recovery, peak power was reduced by 19 percent in pubescent boys and 29 percent in men; in addition, with all recovery intervals, blood lactate accumulation was always lower for prepubescent boys than for the other groups. Similar findings have been reported when comparing fatigue during a knee-extension muscle-endurance task in young, teenage, and adult males and females, although the differences plateaued by the teenage years in females (Dipla et al., 2009). From a practical perspective, these findings suggest that during brief, all-out exercise children require less recovery than adolescents and adults. Youth fitness specialists should not shy away from using brief bouts of recovery with immature children, because it will likely be necessary in order to provide an adequate training stimulus during intermittent exercise.

In a later review, Armstrong and Barker (2011) reported that the majority of training studies demonstrated that $\dot{V}O_2$peak was responsive to training in youth both under and over 11 years old. When training was successful, gains in $\dot{V}O_2$peak averaged 8 percent across studies, and training responses were not related to sex. This review evidence from Baquet and colleagues (2003) and Armstrong and Barker (2011) suggests that gains in $\dot{V}O_2$peak in the region of 5 percent to 8 percent can be expected in immature and mature boys and girls following short-term interventions (typically lasting 13 weeks or less).

Armstrong and Barker (2011) also observed that training responses were influenced by several factors, suggesting:

- Responsiveness to training is influenced by genetics.
- Training response is moderately influenced by baseline fitness level; those with lower initial fitness respond the most to training.
- $\dot{V}O_2$peak can be improved by any exercise that uses large muscle groups.
- $\dot{V}O_2$peak can be improved by either continuous or interval training, but training that combines both is most successful.
- Sessions that last 40 to 60 minutes are generally the most successful.
- Intensity is crucial; an intensity level of at least 85 percent of HRmax is recommended.

Harrison and colleagues (2015) performed a systematic review to examine the responsiveness of V.O$_2$peak and similar field-based measures (e.g., progressive shuttle running to exhaustion) to training in youth team-sport athletes. The authors reported that both interval training and sport-specific training (usually involving small-sided games) could improve endurance performance in 11- to 18-year-old players. As in previous reviews, the authors stated that periods of high-intensity effort are crucial in promoting gains in $\dot{V}O_2$peak. The mechanistic adaptations that underpin observed training gains in $\dot{V}O_2$peak in children and adolescents have been examined only in limited research. The available evidence suggests that gains can be attributed to increases in stroke volume and cardiac output, probably due to morphological and functional changes in the myocardium (e.g., increased heart volume and contractility) (Mahon, 2008). However, the majority of training studies have included male populations, and the lack of data from female participants, particularly team-sport players, is striking (Armstrong, 2016).

Few studies have examined the responsiveness of aerobic fitness to long-term systematic training. In one study involving prepubertal swimmers who trained at high volumes (10 sessions per week) over a one-year period, the findings indicated impressive gains of 29 percent in $\dot{V}O_2$peak (Obert et al., 1996). Another study reported that over a period of three years, academy soccer players aged 12 to 18 years old nearly doubled their yo-yo intermittent recovery distance (a test similar to a PACER) by more than 1,100 meters versus gains of only 315 meters in a control group (Wrigley et al., 2014). These players were likely exposed to high volumes of field-based training, such as full- and

Teaching Tip

DEBUNKING THE TRIGGER HYPOTHESIS

It has been suggested that children will not be responsive to training prior to the trigger of puberty and the associated increases in circulating androgenic hormones (Katch, 1983). However, accumulated evidence now suggests that children and adolescents are responsive to aerobic training throughout childhood and adolescence (Armstrong & Barker, 2011; Baxter-Jones & Maffulli, 2003; Harrison et al., 2015; McNarry et al., 2014). The previous belief that children had a blunted response to endurance training likely reflected the fact that children are naturally more reliant on aerobic metabolism compared to adults and thus need to train at higher relative intensities in order to experience adaptations (Armstrong & Barker, 2011). Therefore, youth should engage in well-designed programs that include bouts of vigorous, high-intensity exercise to support the development of aerobic fitness.

small-sided soccer games. Therefore, it seems likely that both children and adolescents can make sustained improvements in aerobic fitness with long-term, specific training programs.

Youth fitness specialists should be aware of the possible negative consequences of excessive training volumes in youth athletes. In fact, **nonfunctional overreaching**, the precursor to **overtraining**, was reported in 35 percent of adolescent swimmers from the United States, Japan, Greece, and Sweden (Raglin et al., 2000). Similarly, 27 percent of elite youth soccer players in Spain and the United Kingdom recalled experiencing nonfunctional overreaching, and 60 percent of those reported experiencing multiple bouts (Williams et al., 2017). Moreover, rates of both non-functional overreaching and overtraining itself have been reported to be greater in youth who specialize in an individual sport that is likely to include a high volume of aerobic training than in youth who focus on team sports (Kentta et al., 2001; Matos et al., 2011). Therefore, youth fitness specialists should prescribe sensible training loads that include adequate rest and recovery; they should not pursue training gains at the expense of potentially exposing young athletes to overtraining. The negative effects of overtraining are discussed further in chapter 12.

Although many studies have examined changes in $\dot{V}O_2$peak in response to training in youth, fewer have considered changes in the lactate threshold or in exercise economy. When comparing trained and untrained populations, evidence consistently demonstrates that trained young athletes accumulate less lactate than untrained youth when working at the same relative intensity (Armstrong & Welsman, 2008). It also seems possible that the lactate threshold occurs at a higher percentage of $\dot{V}O_2$peak in trained youth (Armstrong & Barker, 2011). For instance, Rotstein and colleagues (1986) reported that nine weeks of interval training performed three times per week enabled prepubertal

boys to increase their running velocity at the lactate threshold from 10 to 10.5 kilometers per hour.

An alternative measure is the **ventilatory threshold**, which requires measurement only of respiratory gases. This threshold represents the point at which ventilation begins to increase at a faster rate than oxygen consumption during a progressive exercise test, where the disproportionate increase in ventilation reflects increased production and buffering of lactic acid. Mahon and Vaccaro (1989) found that an eight-week intervention involving two sessions per week of continuous running and two sessions per week of interval running improved the ventilatory threshold of 10- to 14-year-old boys by 19 percent. McManus and colleagues (2005) reported that an eight-week training program involving interval sessions of repeated 30-second bouts of exercise increased oxygen consumption at the ventilatory threshold of 10-year-old boys by 18 percent, whereas a dose-matched continuous-exercise group had no training response. Thus it appears that youth can make gains in their lactate and ventilatory thresholds through short-term training programs. Improvements in either threshold in children and adolescents appear to depend on training at a relatively high intensity (Armstrong & Barker, 2011).

DO YOU KNOW?

The ventilatory threshold may be more sensitive to training than $\dot{V}O_2$peak in children and adolescents (Mahon, 2008).

The efficacy of short-term training programs intended to improve running economy in youth remains unclear. Both Pertray and Krahenbuhl (1985) and Lussier and Buskirk (1977) found that 11- to 12-week interventions involving technical training, running training, or a combination of the two did not improve running economy in 10-year-old boys and girls. Similarly, 10 weeks of high-intensity soccer training was shown not to improve running economy in 16-year-old players, although $\dot{V}O_2$peak did improve significantly (McMillan et al., 2005). In contrast, Larsen and colleagues (2005) reported that 12 weeks of run training at altitude improved running economy in 16-year-old Kenyan boys.

It may be that longer-term training is needed in order to achieve consistent gains in economy. Daniels and colleagues (1978) longitudinally observed middle-distance runners initially aged 10 to 13 years for a period of two to five years. The authors reported no change in $\dot{V}O_2$peak relative to body mass but concluded that improvements in running economy over time contributed greatly to improvements in race performance. However, longitudinal changes in economy may simply reflect an effect of growth and maturation rather than a training effect. Sjodin and Svedenhag (1992) found running economy to be better in 12-year-old runners than in controls, but the rate of improvement in economy over an eight-year period was similar for both groups. Based on available evidence, it remains unclear to what extent running economy is responsive to endurance training in children and adolescents. Research has demonstrated that strength training (Millet et al., 2002; Storen et al., 2008) and plyometric training (Spurrs et al., 2003) can improve running economy in adults; speculation has been offered that this type of training helped improve the economy of the women's marathon world-record holder (Jones, 2006). Strength and plyometric training may also be useful for enhancing economy in children and adolescents, but this possibility needs to be addressed by research.

Based on the available evidence, the likely gains in the primary determinants of aerobic fitness that can be expected with well-designed short-term training interventions in youth are shown in figure 11.4. Economy appears to be the component of fitness that is least responsive to short-term training, although research is needed to show whether short-term gains in economy can be achieved through strength and plyometric training programs. The greatest gains are seen in oxygen consumption at the lactate threshold, which should increase the upper limit of exercise intensity that a child can sustain for a prolonged period. Unfortunately, only limited evidence is available regarding long-term gains in the various determinants of endurance in well-controlled training studies.

Anaerobic Trainability

A wealth of studies and reviews have demonstrated that appropriate training and instruction can enable children and adolescents to sprint faster, become stronger, and jump higher and farther (e.g., Bedoya et al., 2015; Behringer, Vom Heede, Matthews, & Mester, 2011; Behringer, Vom Heede, Yue, & Mester, 2010; Rumpf et al., 2012). These training-induced gains in brief, explosive performance are underpinned by adaptations that are often attributed to positive changes in the neural system in youth. However, only limited research has directly examined the responsiveness of anaerobic metabolism to training in youth, and indirect measures of power output have often been used instead. Rotstein and colleagues (1986) subjected 10- and 11-year-old boys to intermittent running of 150 to 600 meters three times per week for three months. While the control group made no gains in performance, the training group increased both anaerobic power and **anaerobic capacity**, as represented by the peak and mean power achieved in a 30-second **Wingate anaerobic test**. In addition, McManus and colleagues (1997) reported significant improvements in the anaerobic power of 9-year-old girls following an eight-week training program during which participants completed three 10-second sprints and three 30-second sprints in each session. The improvements observed in cycling power output suggest some positive adaptation to anaerobic metabolism with training.

In classic earlier research, Eriksson and colleagues (1973) put 11-year-old boys through sprint training

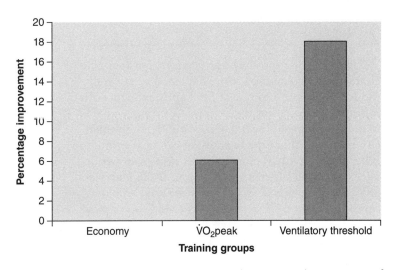

FIGURE 11.4   Expected improvements in the primary determinants of aerobic fitness with well-designed training interventions of short duration (13 weeks or less) in children and adolescents.

and used muscle biopsy analysis to determine that the training led to increases in the amount of anaerobic substrates (phosphocreatine and glycogen) stored in muscle. Fournier and colleagues (1982) submitted 16- and 17-year-old boys to three months of either continuous endurance training or interval sprint training at distances of 50 to 250 meters. The authors reported that endurance training resulted in increased oxidative enzyme concentration, whereas interval training resulted in increased glycolytic enzyme concentration. In both instances, enzyme activity returned to baseline after six months of detraining. In a longer training study, which lasted one year, Cadefau and colleagues (1990) subjected 15- and 16-year-old track athletes to training that focused on brief explosive efforts performed at maximal intensity, such as sprints up to 80 meters and jumps, as well as prolonged high-intensity interval runs of 100 to 500 meters together with some continuous running. The authors found that the training improved 60-meter and 300-meter sprint performance while also increasing muscle glycogen stores, concentration of rate-limiting glycolytic enzymes, and aerobic enzyme concentration. In contrast, the enzyme creatine kinase, which catalyzes the phosphocreatine reaction, was not increased with training. Collectively, these pioneering studies suggest that metabolic adaptations to training in youth are specific to the training stimulus, that anaerobic substrates and enzyme concentrations can adapt with training, and that training gains are lost with detraining.

DO YOU KNOW?

Training can improve anaerobic metabolism in youth, but these improvements are lost if the training stimulus is removed.

The ability to reproduce sprint efforts is a desirable characteristic in many sports. Repeated sprint training requires youth to repeat brief sprint efforts with minimal recovery between efforts. A primary goal is to improve repeated sprint ability, but the high-intensity nature of this type of training can also promote other training adaptations such as improved endurance capabilities (Ferrari Bravo et al., 2008; Harrison et al., 2015). Buchheit and colleagues (2010) employed repeated sprint training with 14-year-old soccer players once per week for ten weeks. The authors reported significant improvements in repeated shuttle sprint ability as well as significant improvements in 30-meter sprint time and jump performance. Tonnessen and colleagues (2011) also found that 16-year-old elite soccer players who completed repeated sprint training alongside their normal training once a week for 10 weeks

improved their repeated sprint ability as well as their maximal sprint speed. Ferrari Bravo and colleagues (2008) put 17-year-old soccer players through repeated sprint training twice a week for seven weeks. With training, mean time for a repeated sprint test improved by 2.1 percent while performance on an intermittent endurance test increased by 28 percent, gains that were greater when compared to a group training in intervals of 4 x 4 minutes of running at 90-95 percent HRmax. While there is limited research that has examined repeated sprint training in prepubertal children, the limited evidence available suggests that adolescents can improve their repeated sprint ability, and this type of training may also confer additional performance benefits. The youth fitness specialist may find repeated sprint training a useful supplement to normal sports training as it requires limited time and has been shown to provide meaningful training gains.

Aerobic and Anaerobic Training

Aerobic and anaerobic metabolism are often viewed as distinct qualities, contributing to either prolonged endurance exercise or briefer, more intense exercise, respectively. This view often leads to an approach wherein each metabolic system is targeted for training in isolation. However, it is clear that both aerobic and anaerobic metabolism contribute to any type of exercise and that these qualities need to be developed in all youth. Training programs that facilitate both aerobic and anaerobic development can provide practitioners with a time-efficient approach that confers both health and performance gains for children and adolescents. Whereas prolonged continuous training can promote improvements in aerobic performance (Armstrong & Barker, 2011), youth are more likely to enjoy and engage in intermittent types of exercise that are more representative of the activity they naturally take part in (Oliver et al., 2011). Furthermore, it has been shown that appropriately designed programs for high-intensity intermittent training are as good as, if not better than, continuous training at improving aerobic performance (Baquet, Berthoin, Dupont, Blondel, Fabre, & van Praagh, 2002; Baquet, Gamelin, Mucci, Thevenet, Van Praagh, & Berthoin, 2010; McManus et al., 2005) while also providing youth with health benefits (Costigan et al., 2015; Logan et al., 2014). Incorporating games and a skill element to exercise can also provide an effective training stimulus; the use of intermittent small-sided games has been shown to improve both aerobic and anaerobic fitness while also allowing for some technical development (Harrison et al., 2015; McMillan et al., 2005). Therefore, practitioners can employ a number of approaches to simultaneously target aerobic and anaerobic gains by using games and well-designed exercises that physiologically stimulate and psychosocially engage all participants.

General Principles of Aerobic and Anaerobic Training

Table 11.1 provides an overview of some general principles of training programs designed to promote improvements in aerobic and anaerobic function in children and adolescents. These principles are based on evidence presented earlier in this chapter and on extensive reviews of the trainability of aerobic and anaerobic qualities in youth (e.g., Armstrong & Barker, 2011, Baquet et al., 2003; Gamble, 2014; Harrison et al., 2015; Logan et al., 2014). The table reinforces the fact that aerobic and anaerobic qualities can be developed simultaneously, that common principles apply regardless of maturation, and that this type of training can benefit both children and adolescents.

The training principles provided in table 11.1 are designed to help maximize gains in performance. From this perspective, youth fitness specialists are advised to use a training frequency of at least three times per week, which is consistent with the available evidence (Baquet et al., 2003; Harrison et al., 2015). However, there may be times in a periodized program when the goal is simply to maintain (rather than improve) aerobic and anaerobic fitness, and at such times a lower training frequency may suffice. The mixed-intermittent approach is advocated for most youth because it ensures exercise of sufficient intensity to stimulate positive adaptations while also providing a medium for variable training that reflects the fact that youth are naturally active in an intermittent manner. In contrast, continuous exercise (covered later in this chapter) may provide some additional benefits, but it may be more appropriate for more mature youth endurance athletes.

Although a duration of at least 30 minutes has been suggested in order to increase gains in $\dot{V}O_2$peak in youth (Armstrong & Barker, 2011; Baquet et al., 2003), health benefits from high-intensity intermittent training have been reported in adolescents with training sessions as short as five minutes (Logan et al., 2014). Shorter-duration programs that succeed often do so through the use of particularly demanding high-intensity interventions. For example, Buchan and colleagues (2013) reported improvements in aerobic fitness and systolic blood pressure after adolescent boys and girls completed a training program consisting of four to six maximal 30-second sprints separated by 30-second recovery periods three times per week for seven weeks. Thus, although youth fitness specialists should not rely solely on the use of short exercise sessions, it is clear that short sessions can offer positive benefits when time is limited. Practitioners should also be cognizant of the duration and training load that can be imposed on youth who are involved in competitive sports. Even at a young age, team sports are often played for at least 60 minutes and at high intensity; as a result, they can contribute a substantial training load, as has been observed in youth soccer players (Wrigley et al., 2012). For instance, in some sports, it may not be unusual for an adolescent team-sport athlete to play in two competitive matches per week. Therefore, youth fitness specialists must balance both frequency and duration in order to ensure that youth athletes do not become overtrained.

By definition, anaerobic work is performed at high intensity, and all-out efforts are needed when the goal is to stimulate the largest, most powerful, most anaerobic muscle fibers. Even for aerobic training, the consensus view holds that exercise needs to be completed at high physiological intensity, which for children means working at a minimum of 85 percent of HRmax (Armstrong & Barker, 2011; Baquet et al., 2003; Harrison et al., 2015). When HR cannot be monitored, practitioners can use a **rating of perceived exertion** (RPE) to indicate exercise intensity. Based on data collected on boys and girls during running, an RPE rating of at least 7 on a scale of 10 equates to an intensity of at least 85 percent of HRmax, whereas an RPE of at least 8 equates to at

TABLE 11.1   GENERAL PRINCIPLES FOR MAXIMIZING AEROBIC AND ANAEROBIC GAINS IN CHILDREN AND ADOLESCENTS

Program variable	Program design
Frequency	3+ sessions per week
Session duration	5-60 min
Work intensity	≥85% HRmax effort
Mode of exercise	Whole-body or large-muscle-group
Format	Mixed-intermittent, ranging from <10 sec to 4 min and from structured interval work to relatively unstructured games

least 90 percent of HRmax (Utter et al., 2002). Metabolically, short work bouts (e.g., 5 sec) predominantly stress the ATP-PC system, moderate-duration bouts (e.g., 30 sec) predominantly stress the glycolytic system, and longer bouts (e.g., over 2 min) shift the emphasis to the aerobic system. Similarly, manipulation of recovery bouts from longer to shorter durations shifts reliance more from the ATP-PC system to anaerobic glycolysis and aerobic metabolism. In all instances, the aerobic and the anaerobic systems are both taxed, but manipulating the intensity and duration of work bouts and the amount of recovery determines which systems are stressed the most. Overall, the key principle for practitioners is simple: Youth should work at high intensity in order to promote aerobic and anaerobic adaptions.

The mixed-intermittent approach referred to in table 11.1 reflects the fact that intermittent exercise may be more engaging to youth than continuous exercise while providing considerable training gains; it also acknowledges that a mix of many types of intermittent exercise could and should be used. The literature supports the view that a variety of high-intensity intermittent training programs can provide youth with benefits for aerobic fitness (Harrison et al., 2015), anaerobic fitness (Buchheit et al., 2010; Cadefau et al., 1990), and health (Logan et al., 2014).

Figure 11.5 shows some of the options for prescribing intermittent exercise. The available formats can all be varied in terms of work and recovery duration, intensity and training design, and choice of activities ranging from games to more structured exercise drills. This flexibility means that youth fitness specialists have a variety of ways to keep youth interested and engaged in training.

Approaches to Mixed-Intermittent Exercise

When using a range of modes and types of intermittent exercise, youth fitness specialists should be mindful of how maturity, training history, and ability can influence the response to exercise. For example, matu-

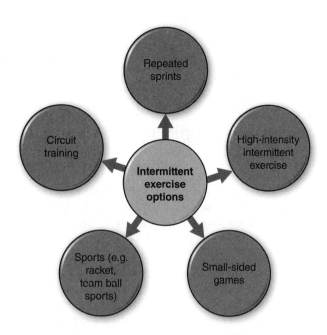

FIGURE 11.5   Various formats of intermittent exercise, which can be used to take a mixed-intermittent approach with youth.

rity influences metabolic processes related to energy provision during exercise, as prepubertal children rely more on aerobic metabolism but have less ability to use anaerobic glycolysis or produce lactic acid. In adolescence, however, they become more glycolytic and therefore able to produce more lactic acid but also require more recovery between exercise bouts (though this challenge can be reduced with training). These differences means that practitioners may need to adjust work and rest durations to match task demands with participants' maturity and training history—for instance, by providing more recovery time for youth who are advanced in maturity or by reducing recovery time for youth who are well trained. It has been suggested that allowing youth to self-limit their work and rest bouts could provide a practical method for implementing intermittent training and may also help prevent overtraining in immature participants

Teaching Tip

MIX IT UP

The mixed-intermittent approach shows that aerobic and anaerobic conditioning can be achieved through many forms of training, such as traditional exercise (e.g., running, rowing, cycling), conditioning, small-sided games (e.g., soccer, basketball, bucketball), and circuit training. Practitioners are encouraged to adopt a mixed approach not only to help promote aerobic and anaerobic gains but also to help achieve the bigger goal of exposing children and adolescents to a variety of exercise experiences throughout their development.

(Gamble, 2014). However, it remains undetermined whether children generally possess the cognitive ability to effectively self-regulate intensity and recovery in intermittent exercise.

Youth fitness specialists should take responsibility for ensuring that the demands of any session are appropriate for the needs of each individual. In this regard, the primary considerations should be individual ability and training history. Youth who are highly skilled may be able to perform complex tasks at high intensity, wherein they execute skills while tolerating high levels of physiological stress, thus allowing metabolic conditioning to be combined with technical training. In contrast, youth with lower technical ability are likely to compensate by lowering the intensity of work when an exercise becomes too technically demanding, thus removing the stimulus for aerobic and anaerobic adaptation. In such cases, practitioners should provide those participants with less technically demanding tasks and continued encouragement to maintain a high intensity of effort. In all scenarios, practitioners should provide training that considers both maturity and technical ability in order to ensure that each session is metabolically stressful.

Repeated Sprint Training

Repeated sprint training is brief and reflects the demands of many team sports, in which players are required to perform a series of sprints with minimal recovery between efforts during demanding periods of play. Repeated sprint training has been shown to be a useful mode of training in adolescent soccer players (Buchheit et al., 2010; Ferarri Bravo et al., 2008), and it may offer benefits for all youth. Sprint efforts are performed maximally, typically over a distance of 20 to 40 meters, and repeated 5 to 10 times with recovery durations of 30 seconds or less between sprints and a longer recovery (e.g., 3 min) between sets; participants complete two or three sets. If space is limited, sprints can be completed as shuttle sprints with a change of direction in the middle. As children mature and move faster, the sprint distance will need to be increased in order to maintain work duration; recovery time may also need to be increased in order to allow recovery from greater levels of fatigue. With training experience, the task can be progressed by increasing the sprint distance, including more sprints per set, increasing the number of sets, or reducing the recovery time between sprints or sets. Youth fitness specialists should be able to adapt these elements to introduce repeated sprint games that keep youth engaged and motivated—for example, prompting children to work in relay teams or repeatedly chase a partner.

High-Intensity Interval Training

High-intensity interval training (HIIT) differs from repeated sprint exercise in that it uses longer bouts of exercise. At the same time, it resembles sprint exercise in being a generic form of training that does not incorporate technical skills required in sports (e.g., working with a ball). Most often HIIT involves bouts of running at a high-intensity interspersed with periods of passive or active recovery. Review work has consistently identified the importance of exercise intensity in promoting $\dot{V}O_2$peak gains in children and adolescents (Armstrong & Barker, 2011; Baquet et al., 2003; Harrison et al., 2015)—a finding that is influenced by the popularity of HIIT studies in youth. The appeal of this type of training lies in the fact that participants maintain physiologically high work rates by alternating bouts of high-intensity exercise with bouts of recovery. As compared with continuous exercise of the same duration, this type of work induces greater overall heart rate response and involves more time spent with heart rate at a high level (e.g., >90% HRmax).

In one popular model of high-intensity intermittent training, adolescents complete four bouts of running for 4 minutes at 90 percent to 95 percent of HRmax separated by 3 minutes of active recovery (Ferrari Bravo et al., 2008; Impellizzeri et al., 2006). This approach has been shown to improve $\dot{V}O_2$peak, lactate threshold, running economy, and match performance in 18-year-old soccer players (Helgerud et al., 2001). More generally, among the many variations of HIIT, research has demonstrated success with training programs for adolescents using work and recovery bouts of 10 seconds each (Baquet et al., 2002), 15 seconds each (Buchheit et al., 2009), 30 seconds each (Buchan et al., 2013; Racil et al., 2013), and 30 seconds to 4 minutes of work with 30 seconds to 3 minutes of recovery (Sperlich et al., 2011). Programs can be as brief as four to six reps of 30-second maximal work alternating with 30 seconds of recovery (Buchan et al., 2013); they can also include longer efforts and recovery durations or multiple sets to extend total session time to 30 minutes (e.g., Ferrari Bravo et al., 2008; Sperlich et al., 2011). In all of these programs, work is completed at high intensity, ranging from close to maximal aerobic speed (the speed achieved in a $\dot{V}O_2$peak test) to all-out effort.

Youth fitness specialists can vary programs by manipulating session variables such as duration of work, duration of recovery, number of repetitions, and number of sets. For instance, in a HIIT program with 14-year-old soccer players, Sperlich and colleagues (2011) used repeated running efforts ranging in duration from 30 seconds to four minutes and separated by recovery durations lasting from 30 seconds to three minutes with the aim of achieving an intensity of 90 percent to 95 percent of HRmax in all sessions. The highly structured nature of HIIT means that this type of training is likely to be most appropriate for more mature youth who are inherently motivated to exercise and have accumulated a reasonable training history. This view is supported by the work of Harrison and colleagues (2015), who suggested that HIIT could be introduced when youth team-sport athletes begin to specialize (typically at 13 to 15 years old) and should form a main focus of training only after youth reach the investment stage in their chosen sport (typically from age 16 onward). Alternatively, HIIT may be a useful tool to use with special populations who need to perform low-skill exercise (e.g., using an exercise bike) in order to maintain a high level of exercise intensity. Adapted versions of HIIT are likely to be more beneficial for younger children and those who choose not to specialize in sport, with whom more emphasis can be placed on fun and enjoyment (see the next section).

Small-Sided Games

Children and adolescents often find it difficult to adhere to traditional training methods (e.g., continuous exercise, repeated high-intensity efforts) simply because they do not enjoy these types of exercise (Wall and Côt, 2007). Small-sided games can provide an alternative method for engaging youth of all abilities in a form of training that is similar to HIIT but more stimulating, fun, and enjoyable. During small-sided games, participants work as part of a team, complete work of varying intensities (including repeated sprint efforts), develop technical skills (e.g., catching, throwing, kicking), and move in multiple directions. Players in small-sided games are also called on to self-regulate

their work and rest periods, and such an approach may be a safe and effective way to prescribe HIIT-type exercise for youth (Gamble, 2014).

To maintain high work intensity, small-sided games are played in intermittent bouts—for example, repeated games lasting four minutes and separated by three-minute recovery bouts—that are similar in structure to a traditional HIIT session. In fact, small-sided games have been shown to be as effective as HIIT for improving aerobic fitness in youth (Harrison et al., 2014). Depending on the available time and space, the group size, and individual variables (e.g., skill level, maturation, training experience), practitioners can manipulate variables including work and recovery durations, size of the activity area, number of members per team, type of game, rules of the game, and technical difficulty. Small-sided games are typically played in limited space with team sizes ranging from two to six members. Youth fitness specialists should aim to adapt the demands of the game to suit the ability levels of participants and to meet the goal of promoting high work intensity during game periods.

Small-sided games have become a popular mode of training for youth sport because they allow coaches to train for physiological properties and technical abilities simultaneously. Research demonstrating the efficacy of small-sided games in youth sport are available for rugby league (Foster et al., 2010), handball (Buchheit et al., 2009), and soccer (Hill-Haas, Coutts, Dawson, & Rowsell, 2010; Hill-Haas, Coutts, Rowsell, & Dawson, 2009; Hill-Haas, Dawson, Coutts, & Rowsell, 2009). In many cases, simplified rules of the sport are used, as players complete four to six bouts of work lasting 2.5 to 4 minutes with recovery bouts of 3 minutes; players are encouraged to maintain a high intensity of effort.

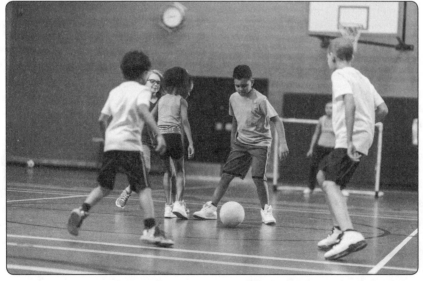

© Getty Images/FatCamera

Small-sided games can provide a fun and enjoyable format for getting youth to partake in high-intensity exercise.

Teaching Tip

SMALL-SIDED GAMES NEED NOT ALWAYS BE SPORT-SPECIFIC

Coaches often like to use small-sided games to mirror the demands of a sport and provide specificity of training. However, small-sided games should not be used to promote early specialization. Instead, all youth should get the opportunity to experience various games. All variations of small-sided games can provide physiological benefits that can then be transferred into a specific sport, should the child choose to participate in sport. More important, exposure to different small-sided games confers social and motor-skill benefits that allow for more holistic development opportunities.

In soccer, relative pitch size is often set at about 150 square yards or meters per player—for example, a pitch measuring 25 by 35 yards for a 3v3 game or 30 by 40 yards for a 4v4 game (Harrison et al., 2013; Hill-Haas et al., 2009).

Hill-Hass and colleagues (2010) demonstrated that work intensity can be increased during small-sided soccer games by introducing a rule to improve the chance of scoring, which, they speculated, may increase participants' motivation. Thus youth fitness specialists should be able to manipulate game rules to promote work intensity and variety in small-sided games—for example, requiring players to flood forward beyond a certain point before a shot is allowed, requiring players to run back to baseline each time a goal is scored, or introducing more than one ball or more than two goals.

DO YOU KNOW?

In small-sided games, reducing the number of players on each team can positively influence work intensity, whereas altering the pitch size has only a limited effect.

The use of small-sided games to develop aerobic and anaerobic fitness does not need to be limited to youth who are involved in sport. However, practitioners do need to consider the technical demands of the game; if a game is too technically demanding, then exercise intensity and enjoyment are likely to be reduced. Harrison and colleagues (2014) examined the responses of 13-year-old soccer players to small-sided games of soccer and a non-sport-specific game called bucketball. The authors found that players traveled farther, experienced higher physiological workloads, and performed more successful technical actions during bucketball than in soccer. In bucketball, a team can score a goal in the opponent's bucket only if all attacking players are in the opponent's half of the playing space and the shooter is positioned outside of a marked circle with a 2-meter radius around the bucket. Players can run with the ball and pass in any

direction, and control is swapped when a possession is lost or a bucket is scored; spare balls are placed around the perimeter to minimize stoppages. As with earlier studies of sport-specific small-sided games, Harrison and colleagues (2013) found that reducing team size positively influenced work intensity, particularly with regard to time spent at or above 90 percent of HRmax. Having fewer players also led each player to complete more technical actions.

It has been suggested that exercise intensity is reduced during small-sided games when a competitive environment is lacking—for instance, when one team dominates the other (Spittle et al., 2017). To avoid this pitfall, youth fitness specialists should match players and teams in terms of both technical and physical ability. This process should also avoid mismatches in maturation, because a team full of early-maturing youth may find it quite easy to dominant a team of late-maturing ones, in which case both sides may fail to work at a sufficiently high intensity.

Circuit Training

Circuit training can be a time- and space-efficient option for delivering a session with lots of variety to a large group; it can also benefit multiple components of fitness. Consequently, the positive benefits of circuit training have often been considered in relation to the delivery of physical education (Dorgo et al., 2009; Faigenbaum et al., 2011; Faigenbaum et al., 2015; Granacher et al., 2011; Mayorga-Vega et al., 2013) and with clinical populations (Verschuren et al., 2007; Wong et al., 2008). In this chapter, it is considered only briefly, from the perspective of aerobic and anaerobic development.

Circuit training that is intended to promote aerobic and anaerobic development should follow the general principles identified in table 11.1. Circuits should be designed to include exercises that target either the whole body or large muscle groups, and the intensity level should range from high to all-out effort in order to achieve physiological loads of at least 85 percent of HRmax. Dorgo and colleagues (2009) designed a circuit training program for 15- and 16-year-olds. Participants completed 10 to 14 reps of six or seven partner-resisted exercises in two mini-circuits (three or four exercises per circuit) with 20 to 30 seconds of rest between stations; the total number of sets progressed from 12 to 28 over a period of 18 weeks. Schoolchildren who combined the circuit training with additional aerobic training made extremely large improvements in one-mile run time.

In other studies, explosive anaerobic movements in primary and secondary PE students have been improved by circuit training interventions lasting six to eight weeks and including resistance and medicine ball exercises (Faigenbaum et al., 2011; Faigenbaum & Mediate, 2008; Granacher et al., 2011). Mayorga-Vega and colleagues (2013) delivered circuit training to 10- to 12-year-olds as part of their physical education classes. A circuit consisting of eight stations was repeated twice per session and twice per week over an eight-week period. Children worked for 15 to 35 seconds per station and rested for 25 to 45 seconds per station (for a combined one minute of work and rest per station). Although some exercises did not target large muscle groups, the authors still reported significant improvements in endurance performance, and these gains were maintained even when circuits were completed only once per week during a four-week follow-up period. Figure 11.6 shows a sample circuit designed to stimulate whole-body exercise and high work intensity in order to focus on aerobic and anaerobic training.

Continuous Exercise and Prolonged Intermittent Exercise

So far, the chapter has focused on intermittent exercise, which allows the high work intensities that are needed in order to promote both aerobic and anaerobic development. Whereas intermittent exercise can stimulate both the aerobic and anaerobic systems, continuous exercise does little to stress the anaerobic system. Even so, it can be a useful stimulus. In fact, Armstrong and Barker (2011) advise using a combination of intermittent and continuous exercise to elicit gains in $\dot{V}O_2$peak in elite young athletes, likely because they have both the training history and the motivation to complete long-duration continuous exercise at relatively high exercise intensities. The addition of continuous training may spice up an already-busy training schedule, and of course it is simply necessary for those who compete in continuous endurance events (e.g., cycling, swimming, rowing, running). Continuous exercise can also be useful for the general population. For instance, bike rides can be an enjoyable way for parents

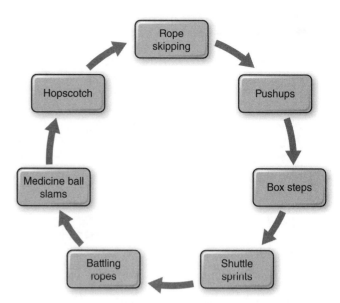

FIGURE 11.6 Sample circuit to target the aerobic and anaerobic systems.

to introduce children to a potential lifelong recreational activity. It is unlikely, however, that relatively untrained youth will complete continuous exercise for a duration or at an intensity that is sufficient to cause improvements in $\dot{V}O_2$peak, lactate threshold, or economy. Therefore, continuous exercise in the form of walking to school and taking a short bike ride may act more as a tool for helping youth to meet physical activity guidelines and maintain health and fitness, rather than stimulating further gains in aerobic or anaerobic fitness.

Sports, and in particular team ball sports, may offer an alternative and more appealing way for youth to take part in prolonged exercise. Sports such as basketball, hockey, and soccer are characterized by bouts of high-intensity effort interspersed with periods of lower-intensity exercise to allow for recovery. This mix can create a scenario in which participants maintain a high overall workload for a prolonged period of time. In a comprehensive review of HR responses in youth soccer, Alexandre and colleagues (2012) concluded that the average work intensity was about 85 percent of HRmax, which was consistent between competitive and friendly matches, from under-11 to under-17 age groups, between elite and non-elite youth, and between boys and girls. Furthermore, Billows and colleagues (2005) reported that elite male adolescent soccer players spend 66 percent of match time at 85 percent of HRmax or higher. Given that matches may be played over a period of 40 to 90 minutes, players spend a substantial amount of time working at high intensity. This workload may explain why the endurance of academy soccer players has been shown to develop at a much greater rate than that of controls (Wrigley et al., 2014).

Thus, organized competitive sport may motivate some youth and provide a good opportunity for exposure to high-intensity exercise. However, youth fitness specialists should remain mindful of the fact that the concept of competitive sport can be very unappealing to some youth, who may simply disengage from physical activity. Therefore, when introducing a sport, it may be most effective for many students if practitioners create a noncompetitive environment that ignores the score and focuses on physical effort.

Sample Training Programs

Tables 11.2 and 11.3 present two sample training programs—one for beginners (table 11.2) and the other for youth who are at an advanced stage of training (table 11.3). Each sample provides examples of different types of exercise. Beginner youth should aim for two or three 5- to 40-minute sessions per week at high to all-out intensity (at least 85% of HRmax or an RPE of 7), whereas advanced youth should aim for three or more 10- to 60-minute sessions per week at high to all-out intensity. Note that the terms *beginner* and *advanced* are not synonymous with *immature* and *mature*. For instance, practitioners often work with adolescents who have little experience of being active.

In addition, training for endurance should not be aligned to specific periods of maturation (Harrison et al., 2015). Instead, the need to get both children and adolescents to work at high exercise intensities is a fundamental principle of both aerobic and anaerobic training. As children mature, they become more anaerobic, which may mean that prepubertal children can recover very quickly while more mature youth may require more recovery time between bouts of exercise. However, chronic adaptation to training over time should include improved ability to work hard and recover quickly. In this regard, when prescribing training, youth fitness specialists should consider both maturity and training experience, as well as technical competence. Practitioners should also provide beginners with sessions that have low technical requirements in order to allow for high exercise intensity.

As shown in tables 11.2 and 11.3, various training modes are available to stimulate aerobic and anaerobic development. The mixed-intermittent approach is advocated to promote both high work intensity and variety in the training program. The available types of training should also allow youth fitness specialists to choose options that are most appropriate for each child, ranging from those who are highly competitive to those who have low skill and are often disengaged. In this way, meaningful work can be done in short bouts, and aerobic and anaerobic training can be easily incorporated into holistic training programs to promote athletic development.

TABLE 11.2   SAMPLE BEGINNER PROGRAM FOR AEROBIC AND ANAEROBIC TRAINING

Repeated sprints	Repeated sprint games (e.g., shuttle relays): • 3 sets of 6 × 10 m shuttle sprints • Relay teams of four (1:3 work-to-rest ratio) • 3 min rest between sets
High-intensity interval training	HIIT games: • 3 sets of 6 × 15 sec of work in a game format • 15 sec recovery between efforts • 3 min rest between sets
Small-sided games	Low-skill non-sport-specific game: • 3v3 • 3 sets of 3 min games • 3 min rest between sets
Circuit training	Low-skill exercises (whole body or large muscle group): • 2 sets of 7 exercises • 20 sec of work, 40 sec of rest • 3 min rest between sets
Continuous exercise	Short duration exercise (e.g., running, cycling, swimming): • 5-10 min • Likely intensity <85% of HRmax
Prolonged intermittent activity	Noncompetitive team-sport games (e.g., basketball, hockey, soccer): • 15+ min • High intensity interspersed with low intensity

TABLE 11.3   SAMPLE ADVANCED PROGRAM FOR AEROBIC AND ANAEROBIC TRAINING

Repeated sprints	Repeated sprints: • 4 sets of 6-8 sprints of 30-40 m • 15-30 sec recovery between sprints • 2 min rest between sets
High-intensity interval training	Traditional HIIT: • 4-6 bouts of 4 min of running • 3 min rest between sets
Small-sided games	High-skill sport-specific game (e.g., adapted soccer): • 3v3 • 6 sets of 4 min games • 3 min rest between sets
Circuit training	Low to high skill exercises (whole body or large muscle group): • 4 sets of 10 exercises • 30 sec of work, 30 sec of rest • 3 min rest between sets
Continuous exercise	Prolonged exercise (e.g., running, cycling, swimming): • 20-60 min • Intensity ≤85% of HRmax
Prolonged intermittent activity	Competitive team-sport games (e.g., basketball, hockey, soccer): • High intensity interspersed with low intensity • Up to 90 min

Summary

Both aerobic and anaerobic fitness develop naturally throughout childhood and adolescence. Children are more reliant on aerobic metabolism, but as they mature they develop more capacity to use anaerobic glycolysis. This sequence means that young children are fatigue-resistant and can recover more quickly during intermittent work, whereas adolescents are more explosive but experience more fatigue and recover more slowly, although this can improve with training. Despite these differences in physiology, a large body of evidence shows that both children and adolescents can make gains in aerobic and anaerobic performance with training. The intensity of exercise is particularly important in this endeavor, and youth fitness specialists should regularly expose healthy children and adolescents to metabolically stressful exercise. The target should be for youth to work at 85 percent of HRmax or higher, and all-out efforts are encouraged.

A mixed-intermittent approach is advocated to provide as much variety as possible with training prescription. A demanding stimulus can be provided by repeated work bouts ranging from brief sprints (e.g., 5 sec) to prolonged high-intensity efforts (e.g., 4 min) interspersed with recovery periods. This type of training can be packaged as games, circuits, and activities that keep youth motivated and engaged. Small-sided games provide a particularly good format for training because they allow many variables to be manipulated in order to meet the needs of different populations. When designing and progressing training programs, practitioners should consider the influence of maturation, as well as the interests of the participants, their technical abilities, and their training histories. More formalized and structured HIIT programs, as well as continuous training, can provide a good training stimulus but may be appropriate only for youth who are more mature, who are active in a sport system, and who have already accumulated a substantial training history.

CHAPTER 12

Integrative Program Design

CHAPTER OBJECTIVES

- Understand periodization and programming for youth
- Recognize the relationship between stress and adaptation
- Distinguish the hierarchical order of multilevel programming
- Understand how to incorporate multiple fitness components into youth training programs
- Appreciate how integrated training can be tailored to the needs and abilities of individual children and adolescents

KEY TERMS

Introduction

So far, this book has explored the importance of understanding pediatric exercise science and the fundamentals of training prescription for various fitness components in youth. This chapter brings all of the concepts together to illustrate how youth fitness specialists can design programs that facilitate long-term athletic development for all youth. Designing training programs for youth populations can be challenging, but the emergence of long-term athletic development models over the last 20 years has moved us toward a more coherent and structured approach for youth populations. Integrative program design for youth requires a unique blend of science (understanding the scientific principles of growth, maturation, and training) and art (designing and coaching training programs that are realistic and effective). Youth fitness specialists should adopt a methodical approach to program design in order to promote health and well-being, enhance physical fitness, and reduce the risk of injury (American College of Sports Medicine, 2009; Lloyd, Cronin, et al., 2016).

Periodization Versus Programming

The term **periodization** has been discussed and defined in a multitude of ways. Some of the earliest works on periodization defined it as systematic programming to promote physiological and performance-related adaptations commensurate with the needs of the individual (Matveyev, 1965; Nádori, 1962). More recent literature has described it as manipulation of training variables in a logical, sequential, and integrative manner in order to optimize training outcomes at predetermined time points (Haff & Haff, 2012). This approach stands in stark contrast to nonperiodized programming, which would involve random and less structured approaches to training. Meta-analytical data have shown that periodized training is more effective than nonperiodized training irrespective of

sex, training background, and age (Rhea & Alderman, 2004; Williams, Tolusso, Fedewa, & Esco, 2017) and that systematically programmed resistance training can lead to improvements in physical fitness (Lesinski, Prieske, & Granacher, 2016) and motor performance (Harries, Lubans, & Callister, 2012) in youth.

If periodization is viewed as the youth fitness specialist's overall philosophy of training that leads to subdivision of the training process into specific periods and phases, then **programming** refers to the process of actually constructing the training programs called for in the overall plan (American College of Sports Medicine, 2009). Regardless of the sporting involvement of the child or adolescent, the youth fitness specialist should view periodized programming as a means to enhance athleticism, reduce boredom, keep youth engaged in the training process, and spark ongoing interest in exercise and sport.

Although research examining the effects of long-term periodized training on children and adolescents remains scarce, youth fitness specialists should adopt a periodized approach to program design in order to promote athletic development, health, and well-being, and reduce injury risk (Lloyd, Cronin, et al., 2016). Meta-analytical data examining the effectiveness of resistance training in children showed that the mean intervention period across 42 studies was just 6 to 14 weeks (Behringer, Vom Heede, Yue, & Mester, 2010). However, more recent research has shown beneficial effects in athletes aged 11 to 19 years in response to longer training programs on measures of strength (Keiner et al., 2013), power (Sander, Keiner, Wirth, & Schmidtbleicher, 2013), and change-of-direction speed (Keiner, Sander, Wirth, & Schmidtbleicher, 2014). Regarding the potential long-term trainability of strength in young athletes, the data showed that trained 16- to 19-year-old soccer players expressed relative strength levels of two times body weight in the squat exercise following a two-year periodized training program (Keiner et al., 2013).

Research also shows that trained youth exhibit superior markers of athleticism over untrained youth for

Teaching Tip

PROGRAM DESIGN: PIECES OF A PUZZLE

Multiple strategies have been developed for program design, and there is no blanket model that can be applied to all individuals. Therefore, youth fitness specialists need to apply the information garnered from all chapters of this book in order to design and implement training programs that match the specific needs, goals, and abilities of the individuals with whom they work. The various components of a training program need to be arranged and aligned to be as relevant as possible and to be modifiable over time in order to maintain the effectiveness of the training stimulus.

measures such as aerobic fitness (Armstrong & Barker, 2011; Nikolic & Ilic, 1992), anaerobic fitness (Matos & Winsley, 2007), and muscle strength (Lesinski et al., 2016; Lloyd, Radnor, De Ste Croix, Cronin, & Oliver, 2016; Radnor, Lloyd, & Oliver, in press). However, the case for adopting a periodized approach to integrative program design is not limited to the enhancement of physical fitness. Periodized approaches should also help youth fitness specialists reduce injury risk while promoting physical and psychosocial health and well-being (Inoue et al., 2015; Lloyd, Cronin, et al., 2016). Practitioners should never sacrifice long-term success for short-term gains in fitness; indeed, such attempts will inevitably be built on poor foundations of movement. In addition, research has shown that injury risk can be increased by acute spikes in workload in both female adolescents (Watson, Brickson, Brooks, & Dunn, 2016) and male adolescents (Bowen, Gross, Gimpel, & Li, 2016) and by high workloads in the absence of preparatory conditioning (DiFiori et al., 2014; Fleisig et al., 2011; Jayanthi, LaBella, Fischer, Pasulka, & Dugas, 2015). Therefore, it is advisable to adopt a more progressive and systematic approach to the accumulation of training over time and to allow for adequate rest and recovery. By programming for long-term gains in athletic development and incorporating relevant testing and monitoring, practitioners better position themselves to prescribe appropriate workloads, assess injury risk factors, develop robust levels of fitness, and prepare youth for a lifetime of exercise and sport.

Although current long-term athletic development models offer generic guidelines for training, the process of designing, implementing, and modifying an integrative training program should be aligned with the needs of the individual and the demands of the chosen sport or physical activity. Youth fitness specialists should also be cognizant of external factors that may affect the training process for youth, such as the time available, facilities and resources, lifestyle behaviors, pressures of academic work, and the need for social interaction. For example, research has confirmed relationships between chronic lack of sleep and increased risk of injury (Milewski et al., 2014); in addition, external pressure from parents, coaches, or significant others can often place unrealistic expectations on youth (Bergeron et al., 2015). Both of these factors—lack of sleep and external pressure—can affect an individual's level of engagement in a training program. Practitioners also face challenges when young athletes are involved in multiple sports that are organized and delivered by different coaches. In these cases, it is essential to promote positive lines of communication between all personnel involved, including parents, coaches, and the athletes themselves. Cumulatively, youth fitness specialists should realize that designing and implementing integrative training is a multifaceted process that involves far more than a simple prescription of sets and reps for a particular exercise.

Balancing Training Stress and Recovery for Optimal Adaptation

Integrative program design requires effective sequencing of training blocks in order to maximize overall training response. The desired adaptation could involve improvements in one fitness component or a number of components, such as motor skill competence, muscle strength, aerobic fitness, speed, or agility. Irrespective of the desired fitness goal, the **training stress** must be balanced with sufficient time for rest, recovery, and growth in order for **adaptation** to occur (Lloyd, Cronin, et al., 2016). Although youth need sufficient exposure to exercise to prepare them for the physical demands of sport or recreational physical activity, their unique physiology also requires time for rest,

Teaching Tip

STARTING WITH THE END IN MIND

A periodized approach to programming remains relevant regardless of whether a practitioner is working with an overweight prepubertal boy who does not engage in physical activity or a prodigiously talented 17-year-old female with 10 years of high-quality training. Both individuals require training programs that help them work toward a predetermined goal, whether that goal is focused on health and well-being or on performance. With relevant goals in place, the youth fitness specialist can then "reverse engineer" the overall plan by programming sequential blocks of training that maximize the individual's chance of reaching the intended outcome. Although the level of detail and complexity will vary, and youth fitness specialists will always contend with individual differences, adopting a structured approach to the training process should result in a more favorable outcome.

Teaching Tip

ALLOWING FOR ADJUSTMENTS WHEN CREATING PROGRAMS

Due to the individual variation in the response to training and the dynamic and nonlinear nature of growth and maturation, youth fitness specialists must appreciate that any training program is subject to change. Certainly, they may have a preferred approach to integrative program design, but they must also be sensitive and willing to manipulate the training program in response to the individuals with whom they are working.

less intensive training, and growth processes (Oliver, Lloyd, & Meyers, 2011). Although children are able to recover from an acute bout of exercise (especially high-intensity exercise) at a faster rate than adults (Falk & Dotan, 2006), a child who gets insufficient rest during a training cycle or sporting season will experience accumulated fatigue, which can lead to nonfunctional overreaching or even overtraining, injury, or burnout (Meeusen et al., 2013). Thus, it could be argued that adopting a periodized approach to training is even more important for youth than for adults.

The interrelationship of training stress and recovery bouts in promoting adaptation has been explained in the literature. The earliest proposed hypothesis was that of the **general adaptation syndrome**, which characterized the way in which the body responds to a given training stress (Selye, 1956). This model posits three key phases, which can be applied to the concept of periodization of training (figure 12.1): the *alarm phase*, in which the individual is exposed to a training stress that causes an accumulation of fatigue and a decrement in baseline fitness (e.g., completes a training session); the *resistance phase*, wherein, with appropriate rest and recovery, adaptation enables the individual's fitness to return to baseline levels or greater; and the *exhaustion phase*, in which the individual is exposed to additional or prolonged training stress that does not enable recovery but further suppresses the body and in extreme cases can lead to a state of overtraining. Attaining a heightened level of baseline fitness after a bout of relatively intense training followed by sufficient recovery constitutes what is referred to as **supercompensation** (DeWeese, Hornsby, Stone, & Stone, 2015; Zatsiorsky & Kraemer, 2006).

Although the general adaptation syndrome model offers a logical theory for the process of the training response, it is somewhat simplistic. In reality, the training response is highly individualistic, and the task of achieving supercompensation across a large group of individuals is extremely challenging (Kiely, 2012). In addition, youth fitness specialists should realize that the training stress placed on the body can be magnified by the effects of other stressors, including growth and maturation, psychosocial factors, lifestyle behaviors, nutrition and sleeping habits, and work pressures (Bompa & Haff, 2009; Haff, 2013; Lloyd, Cronin, et al., 2016).

An alternative theory for the training response can be found in the **fitness-fatigue model** (Banister, Calvert, Savage, & Bach, 1975; Calvert, Banister, Savage, & Bach, 1976). This construct proposes that following exposure to training, preparedness (i.e., the state of readiness) is influenced by dynamic and fluid interaction between the positive effects of fitness and the negative effects of fatigue (see figure 12.2). The model uses the same premise as the general adaptation syndrome—that is, that supercompensation can manifest following exposure to training if the system is allowed an opportunity to recover. However, the fitness-fatigue model presents a more intuitive consideration of the interaction between the training stimulus and the response.

The original fitness-fatigue model displays single curves for fitness and fatigue, but exposure to training is likely to affect multiple components of fitness (e.g., maximal strength, endurance, speed) and of fatigue (e.g., central nervous system, endocrine system, structural tissue) (Chiu & Barnes, 2003). In addition, the interplay between fitness and fatigue is also influenced by factors such as training volume and intensity and the individual's training history, nutritional intake, and growth and maturation. For example, if a child is experiencing a growth spurt, then the negative effects of fatigue may be exacerbated by growth processes, which may call for the prescription of additional opportunities for rest and recovery. Youth fitness specialists should also be mindful that while all fitness and fatigue aftereffects are independent, they are also cumulative (Chiu & Barnes, 2003). As a result, if stressful training and a demanding competition schedule prevent a child or adolescent from getting sufficient rest and recovery, acute fatiguing aftereffects may accumulate to the point of chronic fatigue.

Despite the subtle differences between the general adaptation syndrome model and the fitness-fatigue model, some consistent hypotheses help explain the relationship between training stress and adaptive response. In summary, youth fitness specialists should remember the following realities:

- Regular training is required in order to enhance baseline fitness and develop physically robust youth.
- Training induces fatigue, which needs to be managed carefully in order to maximize preparedness for training, physical activity, or competition.

- Acute spikes in training workload should be avoided (especially after periods of inactivity); instead, fitness should be developed in a progressive and long-term fashion.
- Growth and maturation processes are likely to affect the interplay between fitness and fatigue following exposure to training.

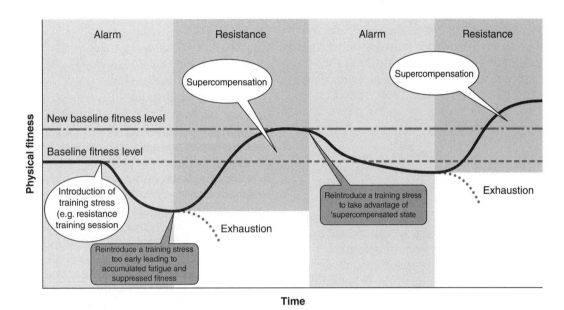

FIGURE 12.1   The general adaptation syndrome model. Note: The black curved line represents preparedness of the individual.

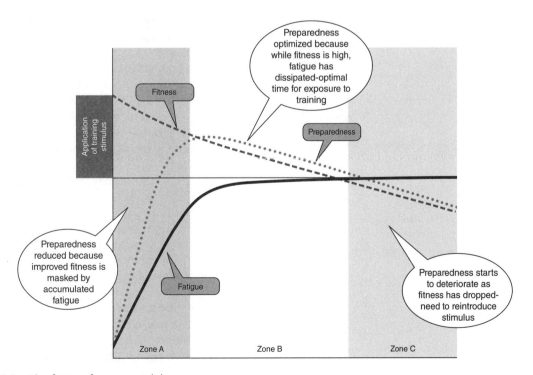

FIGURE 12.2   The fitness-fatigue model.

The Five Pillars of Training

When embarking on the process of integrative program design, practitioners should adhere to five key principles of training in order to maximize the adaptive response. These principles, referred to as the five pillars of training, include **individualization of training, training variation, progressive overload of training, reversibility of training,** and **training relevance.** The five pillars should be considered by youth fitness specialists at all stages of the programming process, irrespective of whether they are delivering integrative training to a group of children in a physical education class or to adolescents in a competitive after-school sport team. Failure to adhere to these pillars may reduce the likelihood that the training program will maximize the adaptive response.

Individualization of Training

The first pillar refers to the fact that individuals differ in a number of ways—for example, physical size and fitness, training experience, and technical competence—and therefore will differ as well in their ability to tolerate and respond to an exercise stimulus. For example, two children could cover the same distance during an anaerobic-capacity running session but experience different levels of fatigue and recover at different rates. Therefore, in order to optimize adaptations in children and adolescents, practitioners should use the available range of exercise modes, exercise variants, and exercise prescription variables (e.g., volume, intensity, frequency) to provide individualized training prescriptions.

DO YOU KNOW?

No two individuals will respond to training in the same manner; therefore, training needs to be individualized wherever it is feasible.

Training Variation

In order to design an effective integrated training program, youth fitness specialists need to manage the balance between training consistency and training variation. Although there is a need for some training consistency and ongoing instruction when programming for youth in order to facilitate learning, variation is also required in order to enable the development and mastery of skills (Farrow & Robertson, 2016). The concept of a constraints-led approach to skill development is discussed in chapter 8, and it is worth recalling the importance of variability in practice for ongoing adaptation (Farrow & Robertson, 2016; Shea & Wulf, 2005).

The need for variation should not, however, lead youth fitness specialists to assume that they cannot program the same exercise more than once without causing tedium. For one thing, participants need some form of consistent exposure to a given exercise, especially in the early stages of development; in addition, variation in programming can be elicited at a multitude of levels. For example, the squat pattern could be used as a common exercise in an integrated program, yet the youth fitness specialist could still achieve variation in terms of load (heavy or light), volume (low or high numbers of sets and repetitions), exercise variants (front squat, back squat, or overhead squat), tempo (fast and explosive, or slow and controlled), or range of motion (partial or full). In this example, resistance training skill competence in the squat pattern would be developed without monotonously exposing the child or adolescent to the same exercise with identical prescription variables. Similarly, in a large-group setting, comparable training sessions could be prescribed in terms of exercise selection, but differentiated variation could be applied through manipulation of one of the other prescription variables.

The balance between consistency and variation can be explained with the following examples. If the youth fitness specialist opts for high amounts of consistency in training with no variation (e.g., always keeps the same training modes, exercises, volumes, and intensities), then the training is likely to become monotonous, ultimately leading to a demotivated child who may even drop out of the program. From a physiological standpoint, failure to program variation into training leads to the manifestation of **accommodation,** in which the response of the biological system to a continued stimulus is decreased (Zatsiorsky & Kraemer, 2006). However, if the youth fitness specialist opts for high amounts of variation with no consistency, then the child is unlikely to stabilize the development of new skills and techniques. The optimal balance between variation and consistency remains unclear, but it undoubtedly depends on a multitude of factors related to the individual. In practical terms, when a youth fitness specialist works with an individual child or adolescent, it is relatively easy to react quickly to the performance at hand and adjust the exercise prescription where necessary. If, however, the practitioner is delivering an integrative training program to a large group (e.g., physical education class), then differentiated training (i.e., different levels of challenge for a particular exercise) should enable the training to meet the needs of many children, even with less favorable coach-to-child ratios.

Progressive Overload of Training

Youth fitness specialists need to manipulate prescription variables in an integrated training program in order to adequately disrupt the individual's current state of readiness (homeostasis) and elicit adaptation in the system (DeWeese et al., 2015). Unless homeostasis is disturbed by overload, adaptation will not occur. Moreover, the degree of challenge (overload) should increase as the child or adolescent becomes increasingly experienced, athletic, and technically competent.

However, the process of providing an overload to the system should be performed in a logical and progressive manner, in order to avoid an excessive stimulus that could lead to disproportionate degrees of challenge, breakdown in technique, injury or illness, loss of enjoyment, or demotivation. An example of progressive overload can be found in the external loads used for resistance training. Current guidelines advocate a load increase of 2 percent to 10 percent once the individual can complete the prescribed volume (sets × reps) in two consecutive training sessions (American College of Sports Medicine, 2009). Similarly, when prescribing motor skill training, youth fitness specialists can achieve overload by increasing the complexity of the movement task. If the practitioner is unsure how much or when to progressively overload a child or adolescent for any type of training modality, it is worth remembering that conservative progression with a long-term developmental perspective is preferred. Moreover, progression should never be prescribed at the expense of technical competence; in fact, when teaching youth, there is often a need to regress the training stimulus in order to reinforce desired technique and allow recovery from more intensive training.

Reversibility of Training

The adage "use it or lose it" characterizes the reversibility of training. This notion has also been addressed in terms of the training residual effect, which refers to the retention of adaptations acquired from systematic training once training ceases (Issurin, 2008b; Issurin, 2010). Although youth fitness specialists should identify key training objectives for an individual child or adolescent, the primary training focus should not cause other fitness qualities to be ignored. For example, if a child needs to develop motor skill competence and aerobic capacity, then training time may be biased toward those fitness qualities; this does not mean, however, that the practitioner can afford to overlook training intended to develop, or at least maintain, other important fitness qualities (e.g., strength, speed, power). Failure to expose youth to training modalities that develop particular fitness qualities is likely to lead to a detraining effect, in which any fitness gains revert back to baseline values or deteriorate even further (Faigenbaum et al., 2013). For example, research in children has shown that in a mere eight weeks after the cessation of resistance training, training-induced gains in lower-limb power and balance returned to pretraining values (Faigenbaum et al., 2013); in addition, detraining periods (e.g., long school holidays) have been suggested as potentially limiting performance gains in peak $\dot{V}O_2$ in children in school-based training interventions (Baquet, van Praagh, & Berthoin, 2003).

Meta-analytical data from adult athletes has shown that strength gains induced by resistance training can be maintained for up to three weeks of detraining, after which attained levels of strength begin to significantly diminish (McMaster, Gill, Cronin, & McGuigan, 2013). The detraining effect has also been examined in boys of different maturity stages following an eight-week strength training intervention (Meylan, Cronin, Oliver, Hopkins, & Contreras, 2014). Over the course of a detraining period of the same length, boys who were pre-peak height velocity (PHV) showed the greatest loss of strength and power, and those who were post-PHV showed some loss in sprint performance (both

Teaching Tip

TRAINING BALANCE: KEEPING THE PLATES SPINNING

The art of balancing training demands for different components of fitness can be likened to the act of spinning plates on poles, where the plates represent the fitness components. The youth fitness specialist should try to identify the primary fitness components that the individual needs to develop (no more than three at a time) and spin those plates very quickly. However, if the program ignores the other plates (i.e., fitness components), then the practitioner will see them fall to the ground; in other words, detraining will occur. Therefore, the art of programming is to provide concentrated doses of training for the most important fitness components while providing sufficient doses to at least maintain other components.

groups maintained or improved horizontal power performance). These data highlight the fact that youth fitness specialists need to provide regular exposure to multifaceted exercise interventions due to the transient nature of fitness components (Meylan, Cronin, Oliver, Hopkins, et al., 2014; Myer, Faigenbaum, et al., 2015).

Physical fitness can often be maintained with a lower training dosage than was required in order to cause the initial adaptation. However, although the lower dosage would represent a reduced volume or frequency of training, the training intensity would remain high. For example, in resistance training, the number of sets and repetitions might be reduced, but the percentage of 1RM would need to remain high.

Training Relevance

Specificity has been defined as the extent to which training resembles the demands experienced in the competitive task (Farrow & Robertson, 2016). This notion can lead coaches to prescribe exercises that simply mirror the movements of their sport. However, that approach fails to develop youth with well-rounded, adaptable movement vocabularies. In the case of youth athletes, it can also lead to consistent overloading of a very narrow band of movement competencies, which can eventually blunt motor skill development and increase the risk of overuse injury (Myer, Jayanthi, et al., 2015). Therefore, when designing integrative training programs, instead of focusing on *training specificity,* youth fitness specialists should concentrate on *training relevance* and consider whether the exercise prescription (e.g., training mode, exercise selection) is relevant to the goal of the program. Integrated training programs should be designed not simply to echo the movements seen in a sport but to elicit a desired training adaptation (Lloyd, Cronin, et al., 2016). Moreover, exercise should be prescribed to develop both the relevant kinetics (i.e., the types of force produced to cause motion) and the relevant kinematics (i.e., the way in which the body moves) and to elicit a transfer of training effect.

Steps to Successful Integrative Programming

It is well established that training programs need to be flexible in order to meet the needs, goals, and aspirations of children and adolescents and to be responsive to unpredictable events such as scheduling changes, injuries, and illness. At the same time, youth fitness specialists must approach the process of program design in a logical and systematic manner. It is far easier (and more effective) to manipulate a well-designed and logically structured training program than to randomly prescribe training sessions without any awareness of the long-term goals of the individual. The program design process outlined in the following sections begins with a needs analysis, then moves along the hierarchical order of programming, which begins with broader long-term planning and ends with the more intricately detailed design of training sessions.

Needs Analysis

The objective of any long-term integrative training program is to ensure that the details for any of the hierarchical levels of programming are aligned with the goals, needs, and abilities of the individual participant. To this end, the **needs analysis** involves systematically gathering information about the demands of the sport or physical activity and the characteristics and goals of the individual (Sheppard & Triplett, 2016). The breadth and depth of the analysis are likely to depend on the situation and the environment. For example, in an educational setting, it may refer to global factors related to a child's physical needs (e.g., fundamental motor skill competence) and developmental needs (e.g., motivation, confidence) in terms of recreational physical activity. In contrast, when working with young athletes in a sport academy, a practitioner is likely to produce a more intricate and detailed needs analysis in which the training priorities are based on more comprehensive testing modalities.

Needs Analysis of the Sport

Traditionally, the needs analysis process involves gathering information about the chosen sport or physical activity, such as the following:

- Physical demands (e.g., energy system requirements, force production characteristics, typical demands for specific components of fitness)
- Movement characteristics (e.g., common movement patterns and the kinetics and kinematics underpinning them)
- Injuries (e.g., common injuries, mechanisms of injury)

Needs Analysis of the Individual

It is equally important for practitioners to gather information about the characteristics and aspirations of the individual child or adolescent.

Informal initial conversations can be conducted to gain insight into the individual's physical activity history (e.g., sport or exercise participation), lifestyle behaviors (e.g., sleep patterns, nutritional intake), and medical conditions (e.g., hereditary conditions, previous or current injuries).

From a physical perspective, youth fitness specialists should then complete a fitness assessment (see chapter 6) to collect objective data and determine the child's levels of physical fitness, stage of maturation, and movement competence. This process should use valid and reliable testing methods that provide meaningful insights into the individual's fitness levels and help identify relevant fitness qualities to address in the training program.

From a psychosocial viewpoint, in addition to talking with and observing the child or adolescent, the youth fitness specialist can collate information about variables such as the individual's mood, anxiety, confidence, motivation, and self-perception by means of validated, child-friendly questionnaires, such as the Profile of Mood States—Adolescents (Terry, Lane, Lane, & Keohane, 1999), the Competitive State Anxiety Inventory-2 for Children (Stadulis, MacCracken, Eidson, & Sevrance, 2002), the Sport Motivation Scale (Pelletier, Rocchi, Vallerand, Deci, & Ryan, 2013), or the Pictorial Scale of Perceived Movement Skill Competence (Barnett, Ridgers, Zask, & Salmon, 2015). This information is extremely valuable for identifying psychosocial characteristics that youth fitness specialists can account for in the training program.

Designing appropriate training programs for youth is not a simple process. To the contrary, it requires careful consideration of a number of interrelated elements—for instance, training history, technical competence, biological maturation, and psychosocial maturity—that are likely to affect the decision-making process (see figure 12.3). However, although periodized programming can provide clear direction for the training process, practitioners must also be willing and able to adjust training sessions dynamically in order to provide an appropriate training stimulus to the individual in front of them rather than being blindly wedded to a predetermined program.

Hierarchical Order of Programming

In order to develop a long-term periodized plan, youth fitness specialists should recognize that a hierarchy of programming enables them to align the elements of the program all the way from global themes spanning multiple years to the details of specific training sessions (Haff, 2013; Haff & Haff, 2012). The process includes eight hierarchical levels, which offer multiple opportunities for practitioners to tailor programs to the specific needs of youth (see figure 12.4). These levels

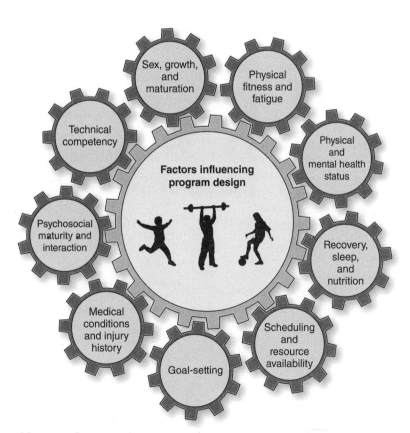

FIGURE 12.3   Range of factors influencing the program design process.

involve programming more broadly on a longitudinal perspective (**long-term plan** and **multiyear plan**); on the yearly and seasonal levels (**annual plan, macrocycle, periods,** and **phases**); and on the detailed levels of monthly (**mesocycle**), weekly (**microcycle**), and daily (**training day** and **training session**) planning. The process of building an integrative program can be viewed as an ascending funnel, wherein the detail of a given level of programming depends on the preceding level and is used to direct the content of the subsequent level. For example, the specific objectives of a macrocycle influence the design at the mesocycle level, which in turn dictates the programming of a given microcycle.

Level 1: Long-Term Athletic Development Plan

The first step in the programming process requires youth fitness specialists to establish a philosophy of long-term athletic development. When practitioners work with youth, they should have a view of the types of athletic qualities that a child or adolescent will need later in life in order to participate in sport or recreational physical activity. Recent literature has proposed a variety of models intended to help with the long-term physical development of youth (Balyi & Hamilton, 2004; Granacher et al., 2016; Harrison, Gill, Kinugasa, & Kilding, 2015; Lloyd & Oliver, 2012; Lloyd et al., 2015; Meylan, Cronin, Oliver, Hughes, & Manson, 2014; Pichardo et al., 2018). Although these models provide only generic frameworks for the programming process, they can offer global training objectives for youth to target based on their stage of development and technical ability. Of course, training goals will invariably change at the lower levels of hierarchical programming, but establishing a long-term training plan provides the youth fitness specialist with specific aims at key reference points in a child's or adolescent's development. For example, according to the youth physical development model (figure 4.6 in chapter 4), training foci during early and middle childhood should revolve around the development of motor skills, muscle strength, speed, power, and agility (Lloyd & Oliver, 2012). Thus, youth fitness specialists should identify these neuromuscular training qualities as key themes to ensure that they are emphasized at the level of annual programming.

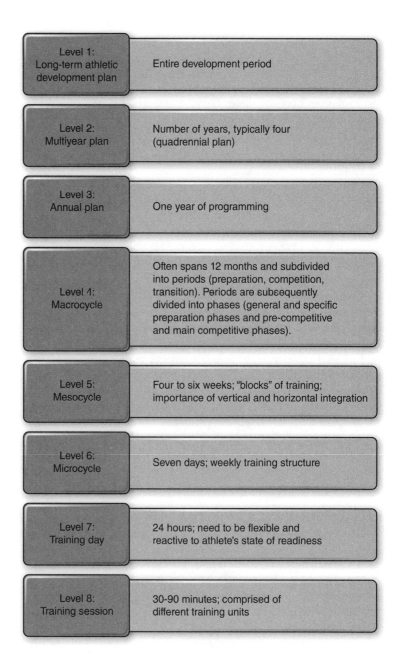

FIGURE 12.4 Hierarchical levels of planning.

Level 1: Long-term athletic development plan — Entire development period

Level 2: Multiyear plan — Number of years, typically four (quadrennial plan)

Level 3: Annual plan — One year of programming

Level 4: Macrocycle — Often spans 12 months and subdivided into periods (preparation, competition, transition). Periods are subsequently divided into phases (general and specific preparation phases and pre-competitive and main competitive phases).

Level 5: Mesocycle — Four to six weeks; "blocks" of training; importance of vertical and horizontal integration

Level 6: Microcycle — Seven days; weekly training structure

Level 7: Training day — 24 hours; need to be flexible and reactive to athlete's state of readiness

Level 8: Training session — 30-90 minutes; comprised of different training units

Level 2: Multiyear Plan

The next step involves creating a broad framework for the multiyear plan, which in turn incorporates a series of annual plans. Traditionally, the multiyear plan is quadrennial, which aligns with the time period between consecutive Olympic Games (Bompa & Haff, 2009). However, the multiyear plan philosophy should also be adopted by youth fitness specialists to systematically coordinate training over consecutive years in a sport system or educational setting. For example, a sport club could develop an athletic development program that spans its junior system, whereas a school could use the multiyear plan to program training over consecutive school years. Using school structures from the United States and the United Kingdom as examples, the educational sector offers opportunities for the following consecutive multiyear plans:

1. Preschool (U.S. and UK), ages 3-5
2. Kindergarten (U.S.), ages 5-6; or Infant School (UK) ages 4-7
3. Elementary School (U.S.), ages 6-11; or Junior School (UK), ages 7-11
4. Junior High School through High School Sophomore (U.S.) or Secondary School (UK), ages 11-16
5. High School Junior and Senior (U.S.) or 6th Form College (UK), ages 16-18

Table 12.1 provides an example of how a multiyear plan could be designed for the early years of childhood.

Viewing the long-term plan in terms of a series of multiyear plans enables the youth fitness specialist to become more systematic and selective in their programming. It also enables them to monitor youth in terms of athletic development. For example, individuals could be assessed for motor skill competence and for measures of health- and skill-related components of fitness at the end of each school year, and the results could be compared with predetermined, individualized improvement targets derived from a fitness testing battery. This approach helps practitioners track progression or regression and determine training goals for subsequent annual plans. Within these programs, however, wide variation will occur in individual development due to differing magnitudes, timings, and tempos of maturation (Lloyd, Oliver, Faigenbaum, Myer, & De Ste Croix, 2014). Thus, children should progress through integrative programs on the basis of their technical ability, not merely because

they are passing through a given school year. As in the academic educational system, where children who are underperforming in certain subjects are given supplementary learning support, youth should be afforded similar opportunities to target neuromuscular deficiencies and develop physical fitness by means of additional integrative neuromuscular training sessions in a bid to maintain progress in their athletic development.

Level 3: Annual Plan

With the global levels of programming in place (long-term and multiyear), the youth fitness specialist can now design the annual plan, which reflects 12 months of programming and is dictated by the overarching goals of the multiyear plan (Haff, 2013). The annual plan is still a higher-order level of programming and contains overarching training goals, but these goals will also help in designing and detailing subsequent levels of programming. For very young children or youth who do not participate in competitive sports, the annual plan often reflects the same length of time as the macrocycle. However, for youth who are involved in competitive seasonal sports, the annual plan may contain multiple macrocycles—for instance, one for a winter sport season and another for a summer sport season.

For practitioners who work with large groups, it is unlikely that a detailed annual plan will be made for each individual. Intuitively, however, youth may fall into integrative programs with specifics such as those aimed at improving motor skill competence, developing strength and power, or enhancing cardiorespiratory fitness. Therefore, when working with large groups, youth fitness specialists can design three to five annual plans and assign each child to the most appropriate one. This approach does not marginalize the individualization of training principles, because practitioners can still individualize training at a number of programming levels. Thus, while a group of children may be

TABLE 12.1   SAMPLE MULTIYEAR SCHOOL PLAN FOR EARLY YEARS

Year 1 (age 3)	• Large emphasis on exploratory play and fun • Balance, coordination, introduction to body-weight management exercises, and basic gymnastics
Year 2 (age 4)	• Large emphasis on exploratory play and fun • Increased exposure to body-weight management exercises and basic gymnastics
Year 3 (age 5)	• More focus on athletic motor skill competencies • Exploratory play still a priority but now with more instruction • More emphasis on body-weight management exercises and basic gymnastics
Year 4 (age 6)	• More emphasis on athletic motor skill competencies • Linking of multiple athletic motor skills for fun-based challenges • Body-weight management exercises and gymnastics of increased difficulty

▌ Teaching Tip ▌

MANAGING TRANSITIONS IN PHYSICAL EDUCATION AND SPORT

In addition to developing insight into physical fitness and growth and maturation processes, youth fitness specialists should also contemplate psychosocial development when progressing youth through multiyear plans. Among other psychosocial factors, practitioners should consider how to manage "transitions," or adjustments that go beyond the ongoing changes of everyday life (Sharf, 2009). Predictable transitions include moving from primary school to junior school or from youth sport to a more senior level (Morris, Tod, & Eubank, 2016). Unpredictable transitions, on the other hand, might involve serious injury or being deselected from a sport team (Stambulova, Alfermann, Statler, & Cote, 2009). Practitioners need to help children and adolescents navigate both predictable and unpredictable transitions; they should also be sensitive to such events when deciding on progression within a multiyear plan.

assigned to a particular annual plan, training can be differentiated at any or all of the subsequent levels of planning: mesocycle, microcycle, and training session. Similarly, training goals may change throughout the year, and an individual should be allowed to transfer to an alternative annual plan with different training priorities if appropriate. This approach provides a realistic strategy for practitioners who work with large ratios of children in an integrated program.

Level 4: Macrocycle

The macrocycle is the level of programming that spans a season (Haff, 2013; Viru, 1988), and each macrocycle is traditionally divided into three distinct periods: preparation period, competition period, and transition period. Whether an annual training program contains one or multiple macrocycles depends on the individual participant's needs, abilities, experiences, and degree of maturation. For example, a youth fitness specialist might need to build one macrocycle per year for a very young and inexperienced child who does not engage in competitive sport but two macrocycles per year for an adolescent who plays multiple seasonal sports.

The length of time that the child spends in each period depends on a number of factors, including training history, technical competence, stage of maturation, psychosocial development, and (for those involved in competitive sport) event schedules (refer back to figure 12.3 on page 247). Those responsible for a child's overall development, including the youth fitness specialist, should realize that apportioning the macrocycle into preparation or competition periods should be dictated not by the desire to win in competition but by the physical and psychosocial needs of the child. Indeed, for most young children, irrespective of whether they are involved in competitive sport or solely in recreational physical activity, they should be given more time in the preparation period. This is true

because youth typically make worthwhile gains in athleticism simply by developing their general motor skill competence, accompanying levels of muscle strength, and basic levels of fitness without the need for intricate and highly detailed programming (Haff, 2013; Lloyd, Cronin, et al., 2016).

Some training periods can be further subdivided into phases. For instance, the preparation period is separated into the general preparation phase and the specific preparation phase, whereas the competition period is divided into the precompetitive phase and the main competitive phase; the transition period is not typically subdivided. The process of subdividing a macrocycle into periods and phases lends itself more intuitively to youth who are participating in competitive sports and have clearly defined competition schedules, which make it easier to delineate preparation and competition periods and their subsidiary phases. However, youth fitness specialists can also apply the principles and processes of designing structured, integrative programs with youth who are not engaged in sport. For young athletes, the competition period is based on scheduled competitive events; for youth who are not engaged in sport, it might include an end-of-year fitness assessment (see chapter 6) toward which the child builds throughout the preceding preparation period.

Preparation Period   Classic periodization literature suggests that the general preparation phase (GPP) should focus on using a variety of training means to develop the foundations of an individual's training base across a range of fitness components and movement skills in order to prepare for training in the specific preparation phase (SPP) (Issurin, 2009). During the GPP, youth fitness specialists should try to develop a breadth and depth of athletic motor skills in children and adolescents while addressing both the quality of movement and the ability to produce and absorb forces. Current research on youth in general populations shows a high prevalence of physical inactivity (Tremblay et al., 2016) and low levels of motor skill and fitness (Moliner-Urdiales et al., 2010; Runhaar et al., 2010). Even young athletes who are entering sport pathways often show deficiencies in key athletic movement patterns (Parsonage, Williams, Rainer, McKeown, & Williams, 2014; Woods, McKeown, Haff, & Robertson, 2016). Therefore, regardless of involvement in sport, youth fitness specialists should recognize the value in programming for youth to spend longer periods of time in the GPP in order to develop basic levels of athleticism rather than progressing them to the SPP in the absence of the athletic qualities required for more advanced forms of training.

Arguably, in fact, annual plans for most children could simply involve 12 months of GPP. Indeed, only when youth have acquired a comprehensive training history and high levels of technical competence do these plans need to become more specific. Moreover, for children who are not engaged in competitive sport, the annual plan could consist of an entire year of preparation in which the integrated training is designed to prepare them for the demands of noncompetitive sport or recreational physical activity. This approach remains valid even for young athletes who have distinct competitive seasons, because they will likely continue to show physical adaptations simply from improving their base levels of athleticism within the confines of the GPP.

The SPP takes on a more sport-specific training emphasis and is ultimately intended to capitalize on the adaptations realized in the GPP (Bompa & Haff, 2009). When youth have been engaged in a long-term integrative program—and when training history and technical competence permit—youth fitness specialists will invariably need to be more systematic and intricate in their programming, and it is reasonable to devote more time to the SPP in order to build on already-developed athletic qualities. For example, recent evidence (albeit with small sample sizes) shows that increases in strength and power slow as training experience increases and that worthwhile changes in both qualities may take longer in athletes who are closer to their ceiling of potential (Baker, 2013). Therefore, as training experience increases, practitioners will likely need to develop more sophisticated arrangements of mesocycles (typically, blocks of four to six weeks) and more refined microcycles (typically seven days).

Competition Period

The precompetitive phase is designed to bridge the preparation and competition periods and to provide exposure to more gamelike training environments (Haff, 2013; Haff & Haff, 2012). During this phase, the volume of training should be reduced to avoid high levels of accumulated fatigue and encourage supercompensation; training intensity, however, should be maintained or slightly increased to retain high levels of neuromuscular performance. When working with young athletes, this phase of training can involve intra-squad games or warm-up games against outside opposition. In educational settings, the precompetitive phase can be used to focus on game-based activities with emphasis on motor skill development. For example, a group of children might follow an integrative training program with a major emphasis on developing fundamental motor skills and basic muscle strength. During the precompetitive phase, the program might devote a higher proportion of training time to participation in games that stress fundamental motor skills in a challenging and reactive environment.

The notion of a main competitive phase is unlikely to feature in integrated programs used with inexperienced youth, for whom general preparatory training typically provides a suitable training stimulus.

Teaching Tip

TAPERING: THE KEY TO OPTIMIZING PERFORMANCE

If a youth fitness specialist is responsible for the integrated program of a talented and athletic adolescent with an advanced training history, then the main competitive phase might include a **tapering** period in the lead-up to a major competition. The tapering process is highly individualized, and very little research has been conducted on it in youth populations; however, meta-analytical data in adults suggest that the optimal time frame for a taper is 7 to 14 days, during which training volume is reduced by 41 percent to 60 percent but intensity is maintained (Bosquet, Montpetit, Arvisais, & Mujika, 2007). For practitioners who work with elite sport performers, it is wise to identify the best tapering strategy prior to adopting it for an important competitive event, in light of the influence of both physiological and psychosocial factors.

This is especially true for very young children and for youth who are not engaged in competitive sport. However, for youth who are involved in sport and will participate in organized events within a sport season, practitioners will need to consider the overall stress placed on the child during the main competitive phase. Because competitive sport participation typically provides the largest form of physical stress on a child or adolescent, it is critical to program for sufficient rest and recovery during the main competitive phase.

Transition Period   Irrespective of training history, youth need to be afforded transition periods that enable recovery and regeneration within an integrated training program. These periods not only facilitate recovery from bouts of exercise but also allow growth-related processes to occur (Lloyd, Cronin, et al., 2016). Transition phases are also important for youth who are engaged in sports, because they help safeguard against the negative effects of accumulated fatigue and reduce the risk of overuse injury by giving youth an opportunity to take a break from the repetitive rigors of sport. In baseball, for example, guidelines have been introduced to restrict young pitchers to no more than eight months of pitching during a 12-month period in order to reduce the risk of overuse injury in the upper arm (Rice, Congeni, & Council on Sports Medicine and Fitness, 2012). In such cases, the time spent not pitching offers the child an opportunity to devote more time to the integrative training program, wherein they have the opportunity to improve fitness, target muscle imbalances, and address any injuries.

DO YOU KNOW?

Depending on the needs of the individual, youth fitness specialists can use the scheduled breaks in school terms (e.g., summer holidays) as convenient transition periods when programming for school-aged youth.

Using transition periods can be a challenging process, because many youth are involved in multiple sports during their childhood and adolescent years. In addition, some youth are encouraged to participate in certain activities or to specialize in a single activity year-round by the ambitions of their parents or coaches (Tofler, Knapp, & Larden, 2005). For children or adolescents who find themselves in either of these situations, a clear transition period may not exist; that is, multisport athletes may experience sport seasons that trail one another or even overlap, as in the case of winter and summer sports. This situation should be avoided because it will prevent youth from having a clear break from sport practice and competition throughout the year and will also reduce their opportunities for general preparatory conditioning. This prospect underlines the need for a holistic and well-rounded approach to integrative program design that prioritizes communication between parents, youth fitness specialists, coaches, athletic directors, and medical personnel (Lloyd, Cronin, et al., 2016).

Figure 12.6 presents examples of how annual plans could be outlined for youth of varying abilities and experiences. Specifically, figure 12.6a shows how an annual plan can be divided into the macrocycle and its constituent periods and phases for an inexperienced young child who is not involved in competitive sport, whereas figure 12.6b shows planning for an experienced and technically competent late adolescent who is involved in rugby. The figure also provides examples of how training goals can be aligned with key training phases.

Level 5: Mesocycle

The next step in the programming process requires youth fitness specialists to design the mesocycle, which typically consists of a four- to six-week period and is often referred to as a "block" of training (Issurin,

---

Teaching Tip

WRITING DOWN YOUR GOALS TO STAY ON TRACK

Once the macrocycles, periods, and phases have been created as part of an annual plan, it is good practice for youth fitness specialists to outline the training goals for each phase. The purpose here is to ensure that when planning the lower levels of the hierarchical order (i.e., mesocycles, microcycles, and training sessions), youth fitness specialists can align specific exercise prescriptions (e.g., volume, intensity, exercise mode) with the established goals of the higher levels of programming. For example, when detailing training session content for a particular week in a preparation period, practitioners can align their prescription with the overarching goals of the phase in which the session is positioned. Establishing clear goals and including them in the annual plan should help practitioners visualize the programming process by providing clear reference points for logical progression in the integrative program.

2008a). The proposed duration is designed to enable the desired biochemical, morphological, and neuromuscular adaptations to occur without excessive accumulation of fatigue (Issurin, 2010), thereby reducing the chance of involution (DeWeese et al., 2015; Viru, 1995; Zatsiorsky & Kraemer, 2006), or reduction in preparedness (Haff & Haff, 2012), which may lead to decrements in performance, increased injury risk, or burnout. The key training priorities for a given training block are ultimately determined by the training goals identified in the preceding macrocycle phase; for instance, the main training objectives for the general preparation phase should be outlined before deciding the details of a mesocycle within that phase. Coincidentally, for

(a) Annual plan

Month	September	October	November	December	January	February	March	April	May	June	July	August
Week start	09/04/2017–09/25/2017	10/02/2017–10/30/2017	11/06/2017–11/27/2017	12/04/2017–12/25/2017	01/01/2018–01/29/2018	02/05/2018–02/26/2018	03/05/2018–03/26/2018	04/02/2018–04/30/2018	05/07/2018–05/28/2018	06/04/2018–06/25/2018	07/02/2018–07/30/2018	08/06/2018–08/27/2018
Week no.	1–4	5–9	10–13	14–17	18–22	23–26	27–30	31–35	36–39	40–43	44–48	49–52
School terms	Autumn term 1	(Half term) Autumn term 2		Christmas holiday	Spring term 1	(Half term) Spring term 2		Easter holiday / Summer term 1		Summer term 2		Summer holiday
MACRO	MACROCYCLE 1											
Periods	PREPARATION			TRANSITION	PREPARATION			TRANSITION	PREPARATION			TRANSITION
Phases	GPP			TRANS	GPP			TRANS	GPP		SPP	TRANSITION

Goals (a):

PREPARATION / GPP (Sept–Dec):
- Fun warm-up activities (e.g., animal shapes)
- Introduced to a range of motor skills
- Increase basic levels of muscular strength
- Opportunities for deliberate play and sampling
- Game-based activities for development of multiple qualities (strength, balance, speed, and agility)

TRANSITION (Christmas): Active recovery

PREPARATION / GPP (Jan–Mar):
- More emphasis on bodyweight management training
- Develop competency in motor skills
- Enhance levels of muscular strength
- Ongoing opportunities for deliberate play and sampling
- Game-based activities for development of multiple qualities (strength, balance, speed, and agility)

TRANSITION (Easter): Active recovery

PREPARATION / GPP (April–May):
- Further enhancement of motor skill competency and muscular strength
- Focus on more advanced bodyweight management training
- Game-based activities for development of multiple qualities (strength, balance, speed, and agility)

SPP (June–July):
- More challenging tasks for development of motor skill competency and muscular strength
- Additional focus on developing muscular power
- Game-based activities for greater skill challenge

TRANSITION (August): Active recovery

(b) Annual plan

Month	September	October	November	December	January	February	March	April	May	June	July	August
Week start	09/04/2017–09/25/2017	10/02/2017–10/30/2017	11/06/2017–11/27/2017	12/04/2017–12/25/2017	01/01/2018–01/29/2018	02/05/2018–02/26/2018	03/05/2018–03/26/2018	04/02/2018–04/30/2018	05/07/2018–05/28/2018	06/04/2018–06/25/2018	07/02/2018–07/30/2018	08/06/2018–08/27/2018
Week no.	1–4	5–9	10–13	14–17	18–22	23–26	27–30	31–35	36–39	40–43	44–48	49–52
Competition schedule		Friendly, Friendly	Away, Home, Home, Away, Away, Home	Home, Home, Home, Away, Away		Home, Away, Home, Away	Cup semifinal		Cup final			
School terms	Autumn term 1	(Half term) Autumn term 2		Christmas holiday	Spring term 1	(Half term) Spring term 2		Easter holiday / Summer term 1		Summer term 2		Summer holiday
MACRO	MACROCYCLE 1											
Periods	PREPARATION	COMPETITION PERIOD						TRANSITION		PREPARATION		
Phases	SPP	PCP / MCP		TRANS	MCP			TRANS		GPP		

Goals (b):

SPP (Sept):
- Major focus on strength and power development
- Speed and acceleration
- Motor skill maintenance

PCP (Oct): Warm-up fixtures for game sharpness

MCP (Oct–Nov):
- Develop high force and rate-of-force development, emphasis on weightlifting and more complex movements
- Ongoing development of acceleration/max speed
- Sport-specific conditioning

TRANS (Dec): Active rest and recovery

MCP (Jan–Mar):
- Develop high force and rate-of-force development, emphasis on weightlifting and more complex movements
- Ongoing development of acceleration/max speed
- Sport-specific conditioning
- Peaking strategies employed close to cup final

TRANS (April–May):
- Active rest and recovery
- Address individual imbalances/injuries

GPP (June–Aug):
- Maintain competency across range of athletic motor skill competencies
- Correct/enhance technical deficiencies
- Increase levels of muscular hypertrophy and muscular strength
- Small-sided games for specific conditioning
- Acceleration/deceleration technical development

FIGURE 12.6 Sample annual plans for (a) an inexperienced young child who is not involved in competitive sport and (b) an experienced and technically competent late adolescent who is involved in rugby.

integrative programs in the education sector, the four- to six-week duration of a mesocycle often aligns with school-term arrangements (Pichardo et al., 2018). For example, a six-week half-term could incorporate a six-week mesocycle, and an eight-week half-term could be divided into two four-week mesocycles. By adopting this structured approach, practitioners can set themes for mesocycles in each term in order to ensure that youth are following a training program that facilitates long-term athletic development.

When programming at the mesocycle level, youth fitness specialists should be cognizant of both **vertical integration** and **horizontal integration** (Bompa & Haff, 2009; Haff & Nimphius, 2012). Vertical integration reflects the notion that a number of fitness qualities need to be trained in order to maintain or improve existing levels; however, the fitness quality that most needs improvement should be prioritized. For example, a young and inexperienced child with a low training age may need to apportion training time to improve running speed and agility, muscle strength, motor skill competence, and endurance capacity; however, more training time should be devoted to developing the most important quality at that time (e.g., motor skill competence). Horizontal integration, on the other hand, involves sequencing priorities so that, ideally, training progresses in a logical sequence in which

one block lays the foundation for the next (Zamparo, Minetti, & di Prampero, 2002). For instance, in order to develop muscle strength in an adolescent boy, a 16-week training period could be separated into an initial 4-week block of training focused on resistance training technical competence, followed by four-week blocks focused on muscle hypertrophy, basic strength development, and, finally, maximum strength.

Figure 12.7 provides a conceptual framework for prioritizing training foci and arranging them in sequential training blocks (i.e., implementing horizontal integration) in order to develop key fitness components. For example, if looking to develop speed in youth, a logical starting point could be to focus on developing running technique, followed by blocks where speed training priorities are based on improving acceleration and deceleration, then maximal speed, and finally speed endurance. In simple terms, this approach would attempt first to develop the ability to run with technical proficiency, second to enhance the ability to use those techniques over short distances, third to develop the ability to sprint over longer distances, and finally to improve the ability to perform repeated bouts of sprinting. This sequence is merely one example, and youth fitness specialists should horizontally integrate sequential training blocks according to the needs of the indi-

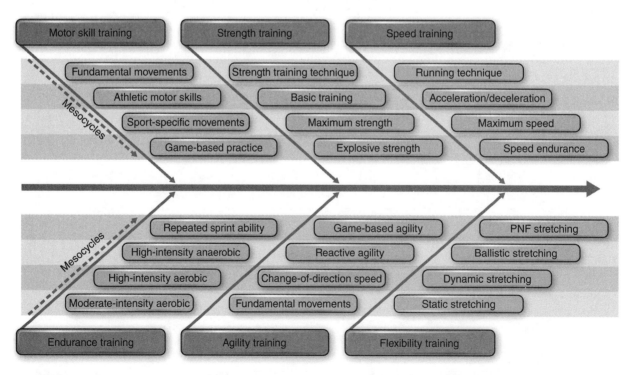

FIGURE 12.7   Sample progression showing how primary training emphases can be progressed systematically (i.e., horizontally integrated) to develop individual components of fitness.

vidual and the adaptation sought at any given time in an annual plan.

Developmental trajectories through horizontally integrated blocks of training are likely to be nonuniform. Individuals should be allowed to progress at different rates, and the duration of mesocycles should be designed to elicit the desired adaptation. Accordingly, the blocks shown in figure 12.7 do not necessarily represent equal amounts of time, and they need not be followed strictly at all times. For example, consecutive blocks of basic strength training could be prescribed if the child or adolescent is particularly weak; similarly, if a young athlete is in-season, then the practitioner might focus endurance training purely on repeated sprint ability and high-intensity anaerobic training in order to mirror the energy demands of the chosen sport. Ultimately, the horizontal integration of training blocks is up to the discretion of the practitioner and should be arranged to optimize the desired training adaptation.

Concurrent training refers to the combination of resistance training and endurance training, which can lead to an interference effect because these two types of training trigger different cellular signaling pathways (Fyfe, Bishop, & Stepto, 2014; Wilson et al., 2012). Research (albeit based on adult data) indicates that when combined with resistance training, the endurance training stimulus leads to compromises in the development of muscle mass, strength, and power as compared with resistance-only interventions (Hawley, 2009; Wilson et al., 2012). The interference effect has led to debate about the optimal arrangement of resistance and endurance training to alleviate the blunting response of concurrent training on neuromuscular qualities (especially if the goal is to develop high levels of strength and power). The interference effect has yet to be fully explained on a mechanistic level in children or adolescents, but pediatric research has shown that concurrent training does not appear to negatively affect development of explosive strength and $\dot{V}O_2$max in prepubescent boys and girls (Alves, Marta, Neiva, Izquierdo, & Marques, 2016; Marta, Marinho, Barbosa, Izquierdo, & Marques, 2013) or in adolescent boys (Santos, Marinho, Costa, Izquierdo, & Marques, 2012). Nor does it detrimentally affect improvements in body composition or metabolic profiles in obese youth as compared with either training mode in isolation (Garcia-Hermoso, Ramirez-Velez, Ramirez-Campillo, Peterson, & Martinez-Vizcaino, 2016).

Overall, research suggests that when the situation so dictates (e.g., when contact time is limited), youth fitness specialists can program resistance and endurance training concurrently, although care should be taken to ensure that the endurance training stimulus is of high intensity (Wilson et al., 2012). If the schedule permits, it may be prudent to keep the training modes separate or at least to sequence training in order to maximize the chance of eliciting a positive training adaptation (Fernandez-Fernandez et al., 2018). This separation of training exposures could range from a number of hours to training on different days (Baar, 2014; Robineau, Babault, Piscione, Lacome, & Bigard, 2016); ultimately, it depends on the demands of the overall schedule (e.g., school and social commitments, sport training, availability of facilities).

One important goal of periodization is to meet the demands of the requisite exercise stimulus while managing fatigue to avoid overtraining (DeWeese et al., 2015). In order to achieve supercompensation, youth fitness specialists need to manipulate the training program to provide a dose of training, but they must also enable periods of rest, recovery, and growth. Depending on the length of the mesocycle (four to six weeks), practitioners can choose from a myriad of possible loading structures. The one that is most commonly used (and arguably most appropriate for youth) is the 3:1 layout (Bompa & Haff, 2009; Matveyev & Zdornyj, 1981), wherein the child or adolescent is exposed to three consecutive weeks of incremental workload, followed by one week of reduced workload (often termed a "deload week"). The purpose of this loading strategy is to provide an incremental training stimulus in the first three weeks, then use the reduced workload in the final week of the block to facilitate rest and recovery and, hopefully, to achieve supercompensation. When working with youth, the deload week also offers a subtle change in the training stimulus, which may help maintain interest and motivation. Figure 12.8 provides a representation of how the 3:1 mesocycle structure is designed in accordance with the theory of supercompensation.

In this context, the term *workload* refers to the total stress placed on the individual during the week. In other words, the youth fitness specialist needs to consider the total physical stress placed on the child or adolescent—from various modes of training, physical education lessons, and competition—rather than focusing on only one factor (e.g., how many kilograms are lifted in a resistance training session). Each of these stressors will have its own unit of measurement to quantify absolute external training load; for instance, volume loads could be used for resistance training, whereas distance or time could be used for endurance training. Practitioners can also use a session rating of perceived exertion (sRPE) measure (Borresen & Lambert, 2009; Foster, Daines, Hector, Snyder, & Welsh, 1996), which, in combination with external load metrics (e.g., distance, load), provides a better indication of

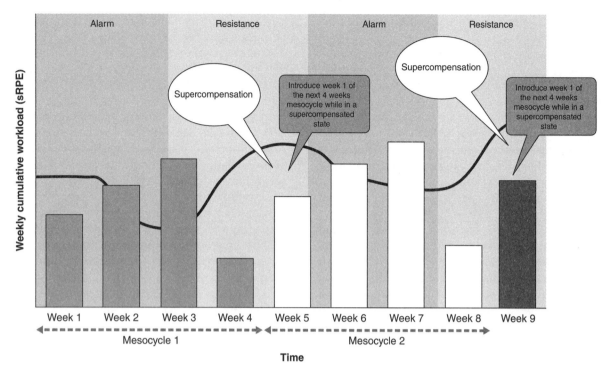

FIGURE 12.8   3:1 mesocycle arrangement applied to successive blocks of training in order to promote supercompensation. Note: The black curved line represents preparedness of the individual.

internal training stress. The sRPE has been validated in youth populations for a range of training modes (Eston, Lambrick, & Rowlands, 2009; Robertson et al., 2008; Robertson et al., 2005; Robertson et al., 2000). For more detailed examinations of suitable monitoring and assessment tools for youth, see chapters 6 and 13.

Level 6: Microcycle

Now, with blocks of training outlined, the youth fitness specialist should design the microcycle level of programming. This level typically covers a seven-day period (Haff & Haff, 2012; Issurin, 2010), which is often referred to as the "training week." The content and prescription assigned to this level of programming are dictated by the goals and objectives of higher-order levels (e.g., annual plan, macrocycle, mesocycle), but this level is the most important one in terms of balancing the many demands placed on the child or adolescent in order to optimize adaptation. The objective of the microcycle is to program the training week so as to stimulate adaptation and promote recovery. In order to do so, practitioners can program for youth to accumulate training in ratios of training and recovery days (e.g., 1:1 or 3:1). However, recovery days in these ratios should not consist of inactivity, which would violate accepted recommendations for daily physical activity (WHO, 2010). Instead, these days should enable recovery from formalized training (e.g., speed or resistance training). Therefore, youth should still

be encouraged to engage in physical activity through less-intensive training aimed at facilitating recovery, improving motor control, and enhancing joint stability and functional range of motion (Faigenbaum & McFarland, 2006). Alternatively, for very young children, recovery days might simply be reserved for the child to accumulate 60 minutes of moderate to vigorous physical activity through free-play options.

Youth fitness specialists should try to arrange training within the week in accordance with likely recovery rates for various subsystems. For example, international consensus guidelines advocate that youth participate in two or three resistance training sessions per week separated by at least 24 hours for recovery (Lloyd, Faigenbaum, et al., 2014); similar guidelines are reported in the literature for speed training in youth (Moran, Sandercock, Rumpf, & Parry, 2016; Rumpf, Cronin, Pinder, Oliver, & Hughes, 2012). However, it is highly unlikely that youth fitness specialists will have total autonomy over a youth athletic development program; inevitably, other commitments or scheduled activities will make the ideal scenario unachievable. For example, if a youth fitness specialist is delivering integrative training within a school curriculum, then time-tabled lessons will ultimately dictate the frequency and sequencing of training. Similarly, the realities of youth sport often require sport training and competition to be scheduled prior to integrative training sessions. In either of these instances, practitioners must apply their understanding of training theory and pediatric exercise science to make the most informed decisions possible regarding the structure of the microcycle. Figure 12.9 provides examples of how microcycle design might differ for an inexperienced young child who is not involved in competitive sport (12.9a) and

an experienced and technically competent late adolescent who is involved in rugby (12.9b).

Level 7: Training Day

The penultimate step in the programming process involves planning the training day, which consists of daily activity dictated by the goals and objectives of the

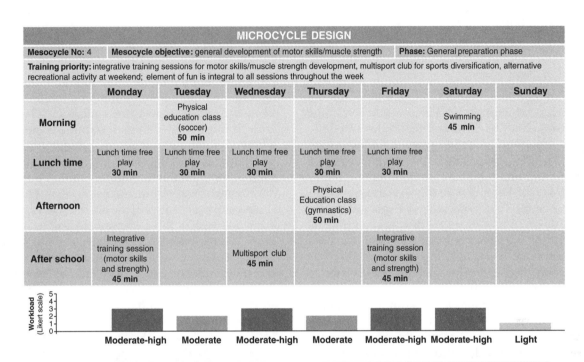

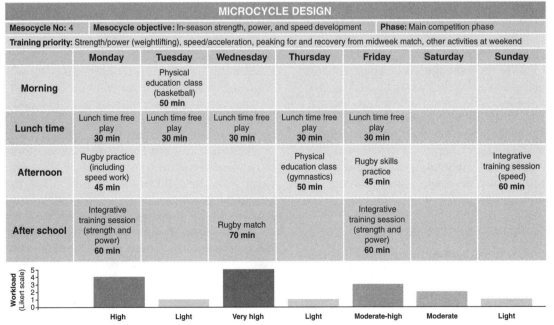

FIGURE 12.9   Sample microcycles for (a) an inexperienced young child who is not involved in competitive sport and (b) an experienced and technically competent late adolescent who is involved in rugby.

Teaching Tip

LIMITED OPPORTUNITY TO TRAIN?

For a multitude of reasons, there may be only one or two dedicated training opportunities per week to deliver integrative training to youth. In such cases, youth fitness specialists should remember that while a training session may address a series of components (e.g., mobility, speed, strength), the most important training goals should always be prioritized and given the greatest amount of training time. Practitioners should always ask what type of training stimulus will most benefit the child or adolescent. More often than not, neuromuscular qualities (e.g., coordination, strength, speed, power) should be prioritized due to the fact that youth will generally accumulate a reasonable degree of endurance-related activity during free play and sport training but often have limited (if any) exposure to the targeted neuromuscular training that can be delivered by qualified professionals.

microcycle in which it resides. For most youth, training days are likely to be governed by school schedules and holiday periods. Unfortunately, opportunities for exposure to appropriately designed integrative training programs may be limited to time slots before and after school. Exceptions to this scenario may occur when the youth fitness specialist delivers integrative training during curriculum time or when youth are on a holiday break from school, both of which can offer greater flexibility for scheduling training.

One area of concern for practitioners relates to the schedule conflicts that can arise when youth are involved in multiple bouts of sport training, competition, or recreational physical activity on the same day. Unless they are managed carefully, these situations can lead to very high workloads in a condensed period of time, which can cause high amounts of accumulated fatigue and potentially place youth at increased risk of injury or nonfunctional overreaching (Williams et al., 2017). Research indicates that youth should be given sufficient time for recovery between repeated bouts of exercise in the same day (Bergeron, Laird, Marinik, Brenner, & Waller, 2009; Jayanthi, Dechert, Durazo, Dugas, & Luke, 2011), and practitioners should use such guidelines when constructing their microcycles and training day schedules. Chapter 13 provides a more detailed overview of the potential risks and warning signs of nonfunctional overreaching, overtraining, and associated injury risk.

Level 8: Training Sessions

The final step in the programming process involves creating the individual training sessions, which typically consist of a series of training components (e.g., warm-up, motor skills, speed and agility, strength and power). This level of programming includes the greatest level of detail as the youth fitness specialist stipulates the variables of exercise prescription (e.g.,

intensity, volume, density, rest intervals). The content and the time devoted to each training component in a given session depend on the goals and objectives laid down in the preceding levels of programming (e.g., mesocycles, microcycles), as well as the stage of development and training experience of the child or adolescent. For example, if the practitioner is programming one, two, or three 30-minute sessions in a week for an inexperienced child (as depicted in figure 12.9a) and is seeking to develop both neuromuscular and endurance qualities, then the plan may need to integrate training modes in a concurrent fashion (Alves et al., 2016; Marta et al., 2013; Santos et al., 2012). However, if programming two or three 60-minute sessions for an experienced adolescent who has specialized in a given sport (as depicted in figure 12.9b), then training modes might be isolated to specific training sessions; for instance, weekly training might be divided into two neuromuscular training sessions and one speed-based session.

Although youth fitness specialists should plan training sessions in advance, they also need to be flexible, responsive, and willing to adapt based on the state of readiness and technical competence shown by the individual both before and during the session (Verkhoshansky, 2009). For example, although a session may have been planned to include a loaded squatting exercise, if the child has injured an ankle, then the practitioner will need to resort to a contingency plan that avoids stressing the injured body part. Similarly, if an athlete shows greater than expected signs of fatigue, then the session may need to be altered to reduce the volume and intensity of work and promote recovery.

DO YOU KNOW?

Practitioners should observe youth as they walk through the door, because their mood and appearance will say a lot about their readiness to train.

Summary

The process of designing integrative training programs requires practitioners to blend scientific principles with the practical realities of coaching and teaching youth. The meeting of these two elements should result in a developmentally appropriate training program that facilitates long-term adaptation based on the needs, abilities, and aspirations of the individual child or adolescent. Through the programming process, youth fitness specialists should balance training stress with suitable recovery bouts to promote rest and regeneration. The programming process should employ hierarchical ordering, and practitioners are encouraged to adopt a systematic, long-term approach to designing integrative programs with strong emphasis on general preparatory conditioning.

At the same time, youth fitness specialists should be acutely aware that due to the dynamics of working with youth, what is initially written in the annual plan is not cast in stone. To the contrary, successful programming for long-term athletic development requires practitioners to be responsive and willing to modify training programs in accordance with the unpredictable nature of youth. Ideally, decision making about program design should be based on sound principles of pediatric exercise science and informed by insights from relevant coaching experience. Designing integrative training is only the first step—the program will truly come alive only if it is delivered by a youth fitness specialist who possesses a sound understanding of pedagogy and high-level coaching skills.

PART III

CONTEMPORARY ISSUES

CHAPTER 13

Young Athletes and Sport Participation

CHAPTER OBJECTIVES

- Understand the role of the relative age effect in youth sport
- Understand the risks associated with excessive training in young athletes
- Distinguish between various tools for monitoring and assessing physical fitness, health, and well-being in young athletes
- Be aware of common injuries experienced by young athletes as well as strategies for reducing injury risk
- Recognize strategies for fostering positive relationships with parents of young athletes

KEY TERMS

Introduction

Published data from the United States indicate that some 27 million 6- to 17-year-olds participate in team sports (Sporting Goods Manufacturers Association, 2011). Additional U.S. survey data show that roughly 60 million 6- to 18-year-olds engage in organized athletics, and three-quarters of them participate in more than one sport (National Council of Youth Sports, 2008). On a global scale, despite some inconsistencies in reporting methods, recent data indicate that about 50 percent of youth participate in some form of organized sport (Tremblay et al., 2016), though the proportion is lower among females than among males (Eime et al., 2016; Zimmermann-Sloutskis, Wanner, Zimmermann, & Martin, 2010). Global data have also shown higher participation rates reported in the United States than in European countries in children aged 5 to 12 years (59% versus 38%, respectively) and in adolescents aged 13 to 17 years (57% versus 31%) (Hulteen et al., 2017).

Organized sport has the potential to offer children and adolescents a number of physical, psychological, and social benefits (Brenner & Council on Sports Medicine & Fitness, 2016). Although sport alone is not always enough to ensure that youth accrue all of the available health benefits (Leek et al., 2011; Vella et al., 2016), long-term exposure to sport can help young athletes develop greater levels of physical fitness than age-matched nonathletes (Armstrong & Welsman, 2005). For example, young athletes in training are typically stronger (Dotan et al., 2013; Halin, Germain, Buttelli, & Kapitaniak, 2002), more powerful (Wrigley, Drust, Stratton, Atkinson, & Gregson, 2014), and both more aerobically fit (Ballester, Huertas, Yuste, Llorens, & Sanabria, 2015) and more anaerobically fit (Ara et al., 2004). Sport also offers youth a platform for enhancing self-esteem (Eime, Young, Harvey, Charity, & Payne, 2013) and self-perception (Wiersma, 2000) and provides opportunities to foster life skills (Gould & Carson, 2008; Wright & Cote, 2003) and develop friendships (Schaefer, Simpkins, Vest, & Price, 2011; Weiss & Smith, 2002).

Although success in sport is often measured in terms of the competitive result (i.e., winning or losing), youth participate in sport largely to have fun, learn new skills, and make friends (Allender, Cowburn, & Foster, 2006; Hardie Murphy, Rowe, & Woods, 2017; Smoll, Cumming, & Smith, 2011). When organized appropriately, sport can lead to positive youth development by promoting enjoyment, challenge, and the mastering of fundamental skills (Merkel, 2013). However, if youth find training to be boring, feel that a sport takes too much time, suffer an injury, or experience low self-perceived competence, they may drop out (Hardie Murphy et al., 2017). In addition, although the literature shows many benefits of participating in youth sport, a growing body of evidence also shows that young athletes may be subject to increased risk of injury and disengagement from sport unless their development is managed carefully (DiFiori et al., 2014). In that light, this chapter addresses the challenges of working with youth who are involved in sport. More specifically, it highlights contemporary issues that, if appropriately managed, can positively influence the developmental process for young athletes.

Previous chapters have emphasized the need for all youth to develop athleticism—that is, the ability to repeatedly perform a variety of movements with precision and confidence in a variety of environments, which requires competence in a range of health- and skill-related components of fitness (Lloyd et al., 2016). Still, it can be challenging to define what a **young athlete** is because the term encompasses diverse levels of skill (e.g., low versus high technical skill) and competition (e.g., school, regional, national, or international level) (Beunen & Malina, 2008; Malina, Bar-Or, 2004). For the purposes of this chapter, the term *young athlete* refers to children and adolescents who are selected for, and routinely participate in, organized competitive sports.

Understanding the Relative Age Effect in Youth Sport

The manner in which growth and maturation influence the development of physical fitness is clearly outlined in chapter 3. Despite the large interindividual variation observed in the timing, tempo, and magnitude of maturation, youth sport participants are nearly always grouped according to chronological age (Lloyd, Oliver, Faigenbaum, Myer, & De Ste Croix, 2014). These groupings typically result in the use of consecutive age groups (e.g., under-12s, under-13s, under-14s), and January 1 is often used as a cutoff date for each selection year (Cobley, Baker, Wattie, & McKenna, 2009). This approach can lead to two children participating in the same competition category despite being born almost 12 months apart (Helsen et al., 2012). As a result, this method of grouping often leads to the **relative age effect** phenomenon due to unequal distribution of birthdates within an age-grouped cohort. For example, if January 1 is used as the cutoff date, a child born between January and March is much more likely to be selected than a child born between October and December of the same year because the first child has had more time for growth and development, thus favoring advanced maturation (Schorer, Cobley, Busch, Brautigam, & Baker, 2009). That child has also had an extra year to be physically active, participate in sport training, and learn new skills.

Research has shown that the relative age effect varies according to age group, type of sport, sex, and level of performance (Delorme, Boiche, & Raspaud, 2010a, 2010b; Williams & Reilly, 2000). It is most apparent in younger age groups (e.g., under-10s), in which children selected for sport teams are typically born in the first or second quarter of the year. In fact, the distribution of young athletes in representative sport teams who were born in the first quarter has been reported to be as high as 50 percent and as low as 10 percent for those born in the last quarter (Del Campo, Vicedo, Villora, & Jordan, 2010; Till et al., 2010). Retrospectively analyzed data from the Olympics and the Youth Olympic Games (Hoffman, Wulff, Busch, & Sandner, 2012; O'Neill & Cotton, 2012) indicate that the relative age effect appears to remain present in older populations; however, it is most prevalent in the youngest age groups.

Data show that the relative age effect is prominent in a range of sports, including alpine skiing (Muller, Muller, Hildebrandt, & Raschner, 2016), soccer (Helsen et al., 2012), ice hockey (Sherar, Baxter-Jones, Faulkner, & Russell, 2007), tennis (Ulbricht, Fernandez-Fernandez, Mendez-Villanueva, & Ferrauti, 2015), track and field (Brazo-Sayavera, Martinez-Valencia, Muller, Andronikos, & Martindale, 2016), baseball (Thompson, Barnsley, & Stebelsky, 1991), and rugby league (Till et al., 2010). Most of the evidence addresses only boys and shows a biased representation of selected young players from the first and second quarters of the year. For some sports (e.g., tennis), greater stature confers an obvious advantage in terms of greater biomechanical leverage; however, an inverse relative age effect may be present in some other sports, such as gymnastics, in which relatively short stature and lower fat mass are advantageous for meeting the sport's rotational demands.

Research indicates that the extent and determinants of relative age effects differ between males and females (Nakata & Sakamoto, 2012; Schorer et al., 2009; Vincent & Glamser, 2006). For example, research from the United States has shown that the relative age effect is more prevalent in males than in females in the Olympic soccer development program (Vincent & Glamser, 2006). More specifically, the data indicated a strong relative age effect at all levels of competition in the male program; however, in the female program, a moderate relative age effect was present in the higher levels of competition (regional and national teams) but not at the lower level (state teams). Similar findings were reported in youth handball, where male teams at all levels of play included more overrepresentation than female teams of athletes born in the first quarter of the year (Schorer et al., 2009). However, whereas the relative age effect appeared to decrease with increases in competition level in male teams, the opposite was true for females, thus suggesting that as competition for selection intensifies in female athletes (especially at higher levels of play), a greater relative age effect emerges.

In addition to physical contributions, the relative age effect can be explained in part by psychosocial maturity. Relatively older youth tend to have an initial performance advantage and to experience greater success, which can lead to greater motivation based on their self-perception of athletic competence and recognition from significant others, such as coaches, teachers, and parents. In addition, youth who are selected for sport teams as a consequence of the relative age effect are typically then exposed to more training opportunities and thus acquire greater depth of experience. Cumulatively, these factors predicate the potential "snowball effect" of the relative age effect in youth sport, wherein selection of relatively older athletes for sport teams during childhood can result in relatively younger and less mature peers being lost from the sport system despite being extremely talented.

Teaching Tip

WHAT A DIFFERENCE A YEAR MAKES

It is becoming increasingly popular for sport organizers to try to identify "talent" at an early age in order to maximize their chances of developing athletes with the potential to excel (Goncalves, Rama, & Figueiredo, 2012). A child born at the beginning of a season has had almost a year longer to grow and mature and to learn and refine skills than a child born at the end of the season. Relatively speaking, this difference in learning time and training age looms largest in the youngest age groups. In order to minimize the chance of deselecting youth simply because they are "young for their year," sport organizers must consider not only physical size and athleticism but also technical competence and skill level.

Emerging data show that the relative age effect can also lead to biases in position allocation in youth sport (Romann & Fuchslocher, 2013; Towlson et al., 2017). One of the disadvantages of biasing youth toward particular positions on a team from an early age is that they are likely to develop a blunted portfolio of athletic motor skills due to being repeatedly exposed to a narrow band of position-specific skills (Lloyd et al., 2016). In addition, the relative age effect has been associated with sport-related injury risk in both pre- and postpubescent youth (Stracciolini et al., 2016). Specifically, in the prepubescent cohort, children born within six months before the age cutoff displayed a higher risk of injury, likely because relatively younger children succumb to injury more readily due to smaller body size. In contrast, in the postpubescent group, adolescents born in the five months after the age cutoff were most at risk of injury, which may be explained by their spending more time participating in sport and physical activity (Stracciolini et al., 2016).

Potential solutions proposed for the relative age effect in youth sport include annually rotating cutoff dates for year groups and adopting a greater range of age categories (Helsen, van Winckel, & Williams, 2005). Indeed, one can hope that sport teams and associations adopt a long-term view of talent and athletic development that prioritizes **process goals** (e.g., development of technique, well-rounded athleticism, and psychosocial characteristics) over **outcome goals** (e.g., winning championships, securing professional contracts). In the meantime, however, the relative age effect remains a robust phenomenon in youth sport (Helsen et al., 2012).

In order to reduce the influence of maturation on competitive inequity, reduce the risk of injury, and improve the process of talent identification (Cumming, Lloyd, Oliver, Eisenmann, & Malina, 2017; Malina, 2009), some sport governing bodies have turned to the practice of **bio-banding**, which groups youth according to physical size or maturation rather than chronological age. Although classification can be based on size (e.g., weight, height), it would be more prudent to group young athletes according to maturity status. Among the many methods for estimating maturity (see chapter 3), youth fitness specialists are often best advised to assess somatic maturity through the use of growth rates (Lloyd, Oliver, et al., 2014), maturity offsets (Mirwald, Baxter-Jones, Bailey, & Beunen, 2002), or percentage of predicted adult stature (Khamis & Roche, 1994). Using these tools, practitioners can cluster younger athletes into groups based on their proximity to peak height velocity (pre, circa, or post) or into bands of predicted adult height (PAH) (e.g., PAH <85%, PAH 85%-90%, PAH 90%-95%, PAH 95%-100%).

These groupings can then be used to assign players to maturity-based teams or groups for the purposes of competitive matches, sport training practices, and strength and conditioning sessions (Cumming et al., 2018; Cumming et al., 2017).

Grouping according to size or maturity should not preclude youth fitness specialists from considering technical competence and psychosocial development in their decision making. In addition, research has shown that selection bias in talent scouts can be eliminated when junior soccer players wear shirts with numbers on reflecting their relative age (Mann & van Ginneken, 2017). Such strategies can enable better understanding of young athletes as individuals and therefore aid the holistic development of sporting talent to encourage ongoing participation in exercise and sport. Therefore, youth fitness specialists should not view bio-banding as a total substitute for age-grade groupings. Instead, bio-banding should be used periodically as part of a hybrid development model in which young athletes are challenged in different performance environments, ultimately providing a more diverse and holistic learning experience.

Monitoring Training in Young Athletes

The programming process requires the intricate balancing of volume and intensity of training on both the acute and the chronic levels to promote athletic development and augment sport performance. The need to monitor **training load** in young athletes is heightened by the advent of early specialization and its associated high volumes of sport-specific practice and competition (Brenner & Council on Sports Medicine & Fitness, 2016). Another challenge in programming for young athletes involves the complex interaction between training, growth, and maturation, which makes it especially important to routinely assess the efficacy of the training program in promoting adaptation.

Monitoring refers to the routine evaluation of various physiological or perceptual metrics in order to determine the effectiveness of a training intervention, maximize performance, and minimize the risks of overtraining, injury, and illness. Monitoring typically involves asking athletes to complete frequent, short-duration protocols at a lower-order level of planning (e.g., microcycle, training day, training session). Monitoring data should help the youth fitness specialist respond to weekly or daily fluctuations in athlete preparedness and should directly influence training prescription, recovery, and nutritional strategies. Monitoring is different from **assessment** (covered in detail in chapter 6), which involves less frequent measurement (one to three times per year) of a range of physical, physiological, and psychosocial indices and can be costlier and time-intensive. Data obtained from assessments are used to provide benchmarks and identify training objectives for young athletes on a higher-order level of planning (e.g., macrocycle, mesocycle).

Quantifying Training Loads for Young Athletes

The training loads experienced by young athletes can be divided into **internal loads** and **external loads**. A recent consensus statement on the monitoring of training loads in athletes defined internal loads as consisting of the relative physiological and psychological stressors experienced by an athlete, whereas external loads were defined as objective measures of work performed by the athlete (Bourdon et al., 2017). As opposed to relying solely on either internal or external load metrics, youth fitness specialists should use a combined approach to determine the overall degree of stress related to competition or training.

This approach is especially needed due to the fact that the training response is highly variable, both within and between individuals (Hecksteden et al., 2015; Mann, Lamberts, & Lambert, 2014). For example, two young soccer players could have identical external training loads (e.g., cover the same distance; complete the same number of accelerations, decelerations, and changes of direction; and spend equal percentages of game time in high-velocity running) yet respond very differently from an internal perspective (e.g., in terms of heart rate, oxygen consumption, or hormonal response). Therefore, if external data were used in isolation to quantify the players' training loads, the data would fail to portray the actual stress placed on the athletes during the competition or training session. This failure would be even more concerning in light of previous research examining the variability of internal and external load metrics in young soccer players, which showed external load metrics to be more variable than internal load metrics (e.g., rating of perceived exertion, heart rate) (Hill-Haas, Coutts, Rowsell, & Dawson, 2008). Figure 13.1 presents typical tools used to quantify internal and external loads.

External Load Metrics

While a number of metrics could be used to monitor external training load in young athletes, the measures typically align with either resistance training (e.g., strength training, plyometrics) or locomotive activities (e.g., running/sprinting, sport-specific movements).

Resistance Training   The most basic way to monitor resistance training is to record the number of repetitions completed. However, due to intra- and interindividual variation in the absolute loads lifted across sets and exercises, this method is unlikely to yield insight into physical stress. Absolute volume load can be calculated by multiplying volume and intensity (sets × repetitions × external load in kg), and the result can be used to quantify the total load lifted for a given exercise, session, or training week. Even though absolute volume load is probably the most commonly used monitoring metric for resistance training, it does not account for interindividual differences in strength. In fact, two young athletes could perform the same number of repetitions using the same external load, but due to differing strength levels or anthropometric differences they could be exposed to vastly different levels of physical stress.

For example, if two young basketball players each complete three sets of five repetitions of a back squat using 80 kilograms, then the absolute volume load

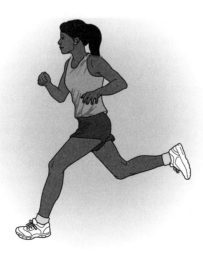

Internal loads

- Heart rate
- Rating of perceived exertion (RPE)
- Blood lactate
- Oxygen consumption
- Hormonal analysis
- Muscle damage
- Wellness and well-being questionnaires
- Psychological analyses
- Training impulse (TRIMP)

External loads

- Power output
- Volume loads
- Speed
- Acceleration
- Changes of direction
- Distance or time
- Notational analysis
- Global positioning system (GPS)
- Accelerometer-derived parameters

FIGURE 13.1   Monitoring tools used to quantify internal and external training loads in young athletes.

Teaching Tip

ENGAGING YOUNG ATHLETES IN THE MONITORING PROCESS

The collection and recording of monitoring data can be time-consuming, and youth fitness specialists should encourage young athletes to be proactive about data collection. This process may take some time, and it needs to be grounded in mutual trust to ensure that accurate data are recorded; however, following a period of instruction, familiarization, and relationship building, young athletes should be encouraged to record data themselves. Ideally, the data are entered immediately into a spreadsheet on a laptop or tablet to facilitate data analysis and subsequent feedback. In addition to reducing time pressure on the practitioner, actively encouraging young athletes (especially adolescents) to move toward self-sufficiency empowers them to become responsible for their own personal development.

would be 1,200 kilograms for each athlete. However, if maximal strength is 100 kilograms for athlete A and 120 kilograms for athlete B, then athlete A is working at a higher relative level of maximal strength. As an alternative to absolute volume load, the youth fitness specialist might instead quantify the relative volume load (sets × repetitions × %1RM), which accounts for interindividual differences in strength (Scott, Duthie, Thornton, & Dascombe, 2016). In the same example, then athletes A and B would be working at 80 percent and 67 percent of their 1RM loads, respectively, thus resulting in a relative volume load of 1,200 arbitrary units (AU) for athlete A and 1,005 AU for athlete B.

Other metrics for monitoring resistance training in young athletes exist—for example, calculating mechanical work (McBride et al., 2009) or using repetition velocities (Gonzalez-Badillo & Sanchez-Medina, 2010; Sanchez-Medina & Gonzalez-Badillo, 2011). Calculating mechanical work requires simultaneous measurement of force and displacement of the center of the barbell, and the associated time and financial costs are likely to render this method impractical for youth fitness specialists. Similarly, quantifying repetition velocities from accelerometers and linear position transducers (McMaster, Gill, Cronin, & McGuigan, 2014) involves significant financial cost and raises questions of feasibility in large-group environments. In addition, it remains unclear how reliable and valid these approaches are for monitoring resistance training performance in young athletes.

Plyometrics are often used as a resistance training mode in the training programs of young athletes (Lesinski, Prieske, & Granacher, 2016; Moran et al., 2017), but the monitoring of external plyometric training loads remains poorly understood. Previous guidelines have suggested that the number of foot contacts can be used to assign various plyometric volume thresholds (Potach & Chu, 2016). However, as with repetition count for resistance training, the use of foot contacts in isolation fails to account for differences in intensity.

Although laboratory-based studies have attempted to quantify plyometric intensity by means of kinetic or electromyographic analysis (Ebben, Fauth, Garceau, & Petushek, 2011; Ebben, Simenz, & Jensen, 2008; Jarvis, Graham-Smith, & Comfort, 2016), these approaches may not be suitable for training programs that simultaneously cater to the need of multiple young athletes. Thus the quantification of plyometric training intensity in young athletes requires further research to facilitate plyometric prescription by youth fitness specialists.

Locomotive Activities   As with resistance training, various tools are available for quantifying external training loads in locomotive activities (e.g., acceleration, maximal velocity sprinting, endurance training). For example, power output can be tracked during cycling by means of bike-mounted mobile power meters (e.g., SRM) or air-braked ergometers (e.g., Wattbike) in field-based or laboratory environments, respectively (Nimmerichter & Williams, 2015). Some of the most commonly used tools for measuring external load metrics during locomotive-based activities are global positioning system (GPS) devices and accelerometers, which have been used to investigate training and competition demands in young athletes (Castagna, Manzi, Impellizzeri, Weston, & Barbero Alvarez, 2010; Hartwig, Naughton, & Searl, 2011; Hoppe et al., 2014). Typically, external load metrics obtained from GPS analysis include total distance, high-speed running distance, average running velocity, and distance or number of repetitions completed within a range of speed or acceleration thresholds (Bourdon et al., 2017; Malone, Lovell, Varley, & Coutts, 2017; Vanrenterghem, Nedergaard, Robinson, & Drust, 2017).

The simplest option for youth fitness specialists is to record distance covered during a session, but this approach only indicates the volume of training while failing to provide insight into intensity. In contrast, akin to the means of quantifying volumes and intensities of workload in resistance training, GPS technology can be used to measure volume (i.e., total distance covered) while intensity can be represented by the percentage of maximum speed. Volume loads can then be calculated in terms of total distance covered multiplied by mean percentage of maximum speed. Alternatively, total distances can be banded into specific individualized speed thresholds, such as high-speed running, jogging, and walking (Halson, 2014).

Due to the volume of data captured, youth fitness specialists must possess sound understanding of the application of GPS metrics and be aware of certain limitations. Notably, variances occur in the filtering processes used by different systems (Bourdon et al., 2017); higher sampling frequencies are necessary in order to optimize reliability and validity of the captured data (Varley, Fairweather, & Aughey, 2012); and the accuracy of velocity measurements is reduced during acceleration, deceleration, and change-of-direction activities (Akenhead, French, Thompson, & Hayes, 2014). Recently, accelerometers have been integrated with GPS technology to estimate external forces placed on the body (Vanrenterghem et al., 2017), and some recent research has used the technological approach to determine the work output of young soccer players (Barron, Atkins, Edmundson, & Fewtrell, 2014).

Internal Load Metrics

Similar to monitoring external training loads in young athletes, a number of options are available to the youth fitness specialist to monitor internal training loads. Invariably, these tools fall into one of two categories; *physiological* or *psychological*.

Physiological   As indicated earlier, internal training loads reflect the relative physiological and psychological stressors experienced by an athlete during practice or competition (Bourdon et al., 2017; Halson, 2014). From a physiological perspective, two internal load metrics that practitioners can monitor are heart rate and blood lactate.

Heart rate is often used in place of maximal oxygen consumption ($\dot{V}O_2max$) due to the strong linear relationship between the two (Hui & Chan, 2006), and percentage of maximum heart rate is often used to prescribe and monitor aerobic or anaerobic exercise intensity (Halson, 2014). By using a heart rate monitor

Assessment of Strength, Power, and Locomotive Performance in Youth

Although the assessment of fitness is discussed in chapter 6, youth fitness specialists should be aware of more advanced testing protocols that can be used to derive greater insight into strength and power qualities in young athletes. For example, neuromuscular function can be assessed by means of a range of jump protocols (e.g., squat jump, countermovement jump, drop jump) that use either contact mats (Lloyd, Oliver, Hughes, & Williams, 2009) or force plates (Read, Oliver, Croix, Myer, & Lloyd, 2016). Common variables used by practitioners and researchers include contact time, flight time, jump height, peak force, peak velocity, impulse, reactive strength index, and rate of force development (Halson, 2014; McMaster et al., 2014). These variables can be used to assess the effectiveness of training interventions (e.g., whether the training program results improve maximal force production, or peak force) or to determine the state of neuromuscular readiness in response to fatigue (e.g., whether the reactive strength index returns to baseline levels before starting a new training session). Other types of equipment used for assessing neuromuscular function in young athletes include linear position transducers (Dayne et al., 2011; Ford, Myer, Brent, & Hewett, 2009), motion analysis systems (Leard et al., 2007), and isokinetic dynamometers (Chaouachi et al., 2014). Irrespective of the testing equipment or protocol used, it is critical to use them correctly; youth require familiarization sessions, clear and child-friendly instructions, and child-sized equipment whenever possible.

Youth fitness specialists should also assess various aspects of locomotive performance in young athletes. For example, thanks to technology, practitioners can measure displacement (using electronic timing gates) or velocity (using radar guns) as a function of time (Haugen & Buchheit, 2016) in order to assess high-speed running or sprinting performance. Although these options can be costly and labor-intensive, technological advancements have led to the development of a commercially available mobile phone application that is reliable and valid for measuring sprint performance (Romero-Franco et al., 2017). Using this app, youth fitness specialists can quantify a range of sprint-related variables, including split times over 40 meters, maximal theoretical horizontal force, maximal theoretical velocity, maximal power, and mechanical effectiveness (Romero-Franco et al., 2017). With the proviso that reliability and validity must be determined, the ease of use of mobile applications for monitoring external loads makes them a potentially appealing option for practitioners.

with a high sampling frequency, youth fitness specialists can observe various indices, such as average heart rate, maximum heart rate, time spent in various heart rate zones, heart rate reserve, and heart rate recovery. Although heart rate is not a direct measure of physical activity in youth and can be influenced by a range of factors (e.g., stress, anxiety, fitness) (Armstrong & Welsman, 2006), it does indicate the relative stress placed on the cardiopulmonary system during exercise (Armstrong, 1998). Earlier research has shown that young male athletes typically display lower resting heart rates and increased stroke volumes than their nonathletic peers (Obert, Stecken, Courteix, Lecoq, & Guenon, 1998; Rowland, 2016; Rowland, Unnithan, Fernhall, Baynard, & Lange, 2002; Rowland, Wehnert, & Miller, 2000; Sundberg & Elovainio, 1982). As with external metrics, volume loads can be determined from heart rate data, in this case by multiplying the percentage of maximal heart rate (i.e., intensity of exercise) by the total time spent in activity (i.e., volume of exercise).

Blood lactate concentrations are sensitive to manipulations in exercise intensity and duration and can be collected by using various measuring instruments in either field- or laboratory-based environments. Using capillary blood samples enables researchers to determine internal loads from blood lactate responses during graded or all-out exercise (Goodwin, Harris, Hernandez, & Gladden, 2007). Research has shown that young athletes accumulate less lactate than untrained youth at the same relative exercise intensity (Pfitzinger & Freedson, 1997) and reach the lactate threshold at a higher percentage of peak $\dot{V}O_2$ (Fernhall, Kohrt, Burkett, & Walters, 1996). Any drawing of blood samples should be performed by a qualified phlebotomist, and full ethical processes should be strictly adhered to (e.g., informed parental consent and child assent).

Psychological
The metrics discussed so far involve the use of advanced equipment (and, in the case of blood lactate assessment, the collection of blood samples) to quantify the physiological internal loads, but practitioners can also use noninvasive, subjective assessment tools to distinguish the psychological internal loads experienced by young athletes.

One option is the rating of perceived exertion (RPE) scale, which is commonly used in practice and has appeared extensively in the pediatric literature as a valid means of quantifying the perception of physical effort. Multiple RPE scales have been developed for use with young children to facilitate the process of understanding the association between written terminology and exercise intensity. Examples include the Perceived Exertion Scale for Children (see figure 13.2), the Children's OMNI Scale of Perceived Exertion (see figure 13.3), and the facial RPE scale, all of which use a combination of a numerical Likert scale and pictorial descriptions.

For each of these measurement scales, the young athletes provide a numerical value representative of how hard they found the activity to be by pointing at the appropriate region of the scale either during or upon completion of the session. This value provides an indication of the intensity of the exercise, which when multiplied by the duration of the exercise provides an indication of the session volume load (i.e., session RPE), which is presented in arbitrary units. These arbitrary

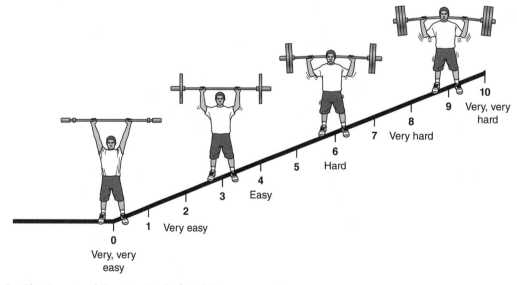

FIGURE 13.2   The Perceived Exertion Scale for Children.

Reprinted by permission from A.D. Faigenbaum, L.A. Milliken, G. Cloutier, et al., "Perceived Exertion During Resistance Exercise by Children," *Perceptual and Motor Skills* 98, no. 2 (2004): 627-637.

units can then be tracked over the course of the training program to provide insight into loading across the microcycle, mesocycle, and macrocycle levels of programming. RPE scales are also transferable across different forms of exercise. For example, RPE has been used to quantify workload in youth during resistance training (McGuigan et al., 2008), jump-rope training (Buchheit, Rabbani, & Beigi, 2014), small-sided games (Koklu, Alemdaroglu, Cihan, & Wong, 2017), and sport-specific training (Haddad et al., 2011). Although RPE is typically used to quantify training load during a session, more recent research has examined the validity of a weekly RPE measure in adolescent male athletes (Phibbs et al., 2017); however, the typical error of estimate associated with that approach was found to be substantial.

Additional methods of determining internal training loads in young athletes include the use of subjective wellness questionnaires. One example is the Profile of Mood States—Adolescents (POMS-A) questionnaire, which uses Likert-scale answers to 24 questions to detect mood state in adolescents (Terry, Lane, Lane, & Keohane, 1999). Other survey-based assessments for detecting changes in mood state include the Training Distress Scale (TDS), which has been shown to identify mood disturbances in stale young athletes (Kentta, Hassmen, & Raglin, 2001); the Recovery–Stress Questionnaire for Athletes (RESTQ-Sport), which is sensitive in detecting overreaching and neuromuscular readiness in young soccer players (Brink, Visscher, Coutts, & Lemmink, 2012); and a well-being questionnaire used to assess perceptual

fatigue in young rugby players (Oliver, Lloyd, & Whitney, 2015). In most cases, subjective questionnaires must strike a balance between asking enough questions to acquire relevant information but not including so many items as to burden the athlete.

Thus, a number of accessible subjective assessment questionnaires are available for youth fitness specialists to adopt in order to monitor internal training loads in their athletes. Be mindful, however, that not all of them were developed for use with all age groups and that cognitive ability may limit the effectiveness of using certain scales with certain groups of individuals. Moreover, given ongoing developments in modern technology, and considering that some of the published questionnaires are long and narrowly focused, practitioners may seek to develop their own monitoring questionnaires (Saw, Main, & Gastin, 2015). If so, they must establish the validity and reliability of the instrument to ensure that it provides useful information.

The Acute-Chronic Workload in Young Athletes

If training loads are not managed or active rest is overlooked, acute spikes or very high volumes of training can increase the risk of injury or illness (Brink et al., 2012; Dennis, Finch, & Farhart, 2005; Drew & Finch, 2016; Fleisig et al., 2011; Lovell, Galloway, Hopkins, & Harvey, 2006; Malisoux, Frisch, Urhausen, Seil, & Theisen, 2013; Olsen, Fleisig, Dun, Loftice, & Andrews, 2006), especially during the years surrounding and including the adolescent growth spurt (DiFiori et al.,

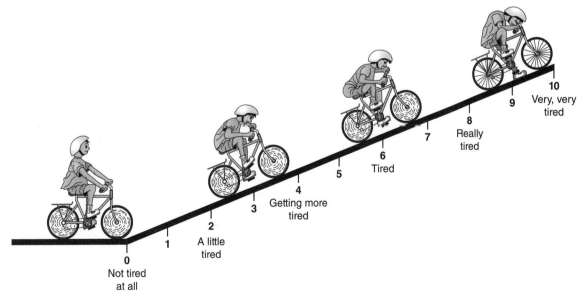

FIGURE 13.3   The Children's OMNI Scale of Perceived Exertion.

Reprinted by permission from R.J. Robertson, F.L. Goss, N.F. Boer, et al., "Children's OMNI Scale of Perceived Exertion: Mixed Gender and Race Validation," *Medicine & Science in Sports & Exercise* 32, no. 2 (2000): 452-458.

Teaching Tip

IMPORTANCE OF LOOKING AT AND LISTENING TO THE YOUNG ATHLETE

Youth fitness specialists should remember that while many subjective questionnaires are available for assessing mood state and general well-being, the process of evaluating the young athletes should begin from the moment they enter the training facility. Practitioners should observe athletes as they walk through the door in an attempt to identify whether they are demonstrating enthusiasm, energy, and general alertness, or, instead, whether they appear lethargic, confused, or demotivated. Quite often, visual observation and an informal conversation can provide insight into an athlete's state of mind, especially when the practitioner has established a good relationship with the individual over time. Simple questions (e.g., How are you feeling today? Are you ready to train?) will often prompt a discussion about an athlete's readiness to train; if the response is negative, then a more objective follow-up may be required.

2014; Huxley, O'Connor, & Healey, 2014). For example, a 10-year prospective analysis showed that 9- to 14-year-old pitchers were 3.5 times more likely to experience an injury leading to elbow or shoulder surgery or retirement when they pitched more than 100 innings per year (Fleisig et al., 2011). Similar data from youth baseball have shown that a high seasonal workload (more than 600 pitches) doubled the risk of elbow injury in young pitchers (Lyman et al., 2001). Comparable data have been reported in cricket, in which adolescent fast bowlers were three times more likely to experience overuse injury when they were given fewer days for recovery between bowling sessions (Dennis et al., 2005).

Although the monitoring of training loads in young athletes should help reduce the relative risk of injury, practitioners also need to ensure that their athletes receive sufficient training to prepare them for the demands of their sports. The evidence indicates unequivocally that developmentally appropriate training reduces the relative risk of injury in young athletes (Emery & Meeuwisse, 2010; LaBella et al., 2011; Lauersen, Bertelsen, & Andersen, 2014; Soligard et al., 2008). Therefore, youth fitness specialists need to monitor training loads and recovery intervals in order to ensure that the dosage of training is sufficient to enhance performance but not enough to lead to injury.

DO YOU KNOW?

About 50 percent of overuse injuries in young athletes could be prevented with appropriately designed preparatory strength and conditioning (Valovich McLeod et al., 2011).

Injury can also be caused by lack of fitness and the use of inadequate loads (Gabbett, 2016; Lovell et al., 2006). Recent literature, albeit primarily based on adult data, has illustrated this risk in terms of the acute-to-chronic workload ratio (Gabbett, 2016; Hulin et al., 2014; Hulin, Gabbett, Lawson, Caputi, & Sampson, 2016). This ratio considers training load by relating the athlete's recent acute training (e.g., during the past week) to the chronic load completed over a longer period (e.g., four weeks). When the acute training load is similar to or lower than the chronic training load, the acute-to-chronic ratio is less than 1.0 and fitness should prevail; however, when the acute load is much higher than the chronic load, the ratio is greater than 1.0 and fatigue is likely to predominate. Research from multiple sports shows that in adults an acute-to-chronic workload ratio of more than 1.5 appears to be a threshold above which injury risk increases (Ehrmann, Duncan, Sindhusake, Franzsen, & Greene, 2016; Hulin et al., 2014; Hulin et al., 2016; S. Malone, Roe, Doran, Gabbett, & Collins, 2017). It remains unclear whether the same thresholds apply to young athletes, but it seems prudent for youth fitness specialists to adopt the approach of helping participants gradually build a chronic training history in a systematic and progressive manner in order to acquire well-developed physical qualities and reduce injury risk. Therefore, training prescription for young athletes should avoid sudden spikes in training load, which appear to heighten the risk of injury (Malisoux et al., 2013).

Integrating Training Load Metrics for Young Athletes

By now it is clear that a range of measures are available to help youth fitness specialists determine the loads experienced by young athletes during competition and training. It is also evident that focusing solely on either internal or external training load does not provide adequate information to help practitioners make good decisions about training prescription or competitive involvement. Instead, the best insights are gained by

Teaching Tip

MAKE YOUR DATA COUNT

Any monitoring battery should be able to produce data that can inform practice. Certain protocols may be used to compile longitudinal data for the purpose of identifying workload trends in relation to physical performance and injury risk. In most cases, however, the battery should produce data that can be used immediately to help direct training prescription and identify athletes at risk of injury or overtraining.

taking an integrated approach using both types of load measures. When deciding which internal and external load metrics are most appropriate for their athletes, practitioners need to consider the financial costs and measurement error associated with the relevant equipment, the variables addressed by the selected protocols, the time required and feasibility of using the equipment, and the likely level of buy-in from athletes and technical coaches.

In the realm of youth sport, some practitioners (e.g., those at an elite soccer academy) have a sizeable budget with which to purchase monitoring tools. Of course, most practitioners do not work at the elite level and therefore are more likely to have only a small operating budget. Regardless of financial resources, youth fitness specialists should try to establish a monitoring battery that provides insight into both internal and external training loads, provides reliable and valid data to enable detection of worthwhile changes in performance, and produces data with sufficient timeliness to influence training prescription as needed.

Excessive Workloads in Young Athletes

Although youth sport offers multiple benefits to children and adolescents in terms of physical fitness, health, well-being, and psychosocial development, the common focus on competitive success and elite performance at an early age can lead to negative health outcomes (DiFiori et al., 2014). In fact, modern-day youth appear to be subject to increased pressure for high volumes of repetitive, intense, and specialized training, which has been shown to carry detrimental ramifications for both physical and psychosocial health (Brenner & Council on Sports Medicine & Fitness, 2016).

Of course, the promotion of physical or physiological adaptation requires disruption of the individual's homeostasis (i.e., internal environment), which causes some performance decrement due to **acute fatigue** (Selye, 1956). In contrast, **functional overreaching**, which also results from intentional training, leads to

performance decrements that are greater than those experienced from acute fatigue alone and can take several days to several weeks to fully restore (Meeusen et al., 2013). **Nonfunctional overreaching**, on the other hand, is characterized by unintentional decrements in performance as a result of an imbalance between the training dosage and opportunities for recovery. Restoration of performance capacity following nonfunctional overreaching is likely to take several weeks to several months. Finally, **overtraining** has been defined as a syndrome that induces prolonged impairments in performance accompanied by maladaptation of biological, neurochemical, and hormonal systems (Meeusen et al., 2013). It can be just as debilitating as an orthopedic injury, and recovery may take several months to years.

Thus, if workloads become excessive in the absence of adequate rest, excessive fatigue can accumulate and may ultimately lead to a nonfunctionally overreached or overtrained state (see figure 13.4). To safeguard young athletes, youth fitness specialists and other significant figures (e.g., coaches, parents) must collaboratively manage physical training and overall workloads to prevent nonfunctional overreaching and overtraining.

Young athletes face increased risk of nonfunctional overreaching or overtraining when they are exposed to long periods of high-volume physical training and competition, when they experience other sources of nontraining stress (e.g., pressure to win, time away from family), and when they get inadequate rest (Matos, Winsley, & Williams, 2011). As previous research has highlighted, nonfunctional overreaching and overtraining have been experienced by 30 percent to 40 percent of youth who are involved in sport (Birrer, Lienhard, Williams, Röthlin, & Morgan, 2013; Kentta et al., 2001; Matos et al., 2011; Raglin, Sawamura, Alexiou, Hassmen, & Kentta, 2000). Both of these conditions can lead to adverse medical consequences, and sport organizers should never allow them to manifest in young athletes (Oliver, Lloyd, & Meyers, 2011).

Research from youth soccer found a performance decrement lasting more than a month in 10 percent

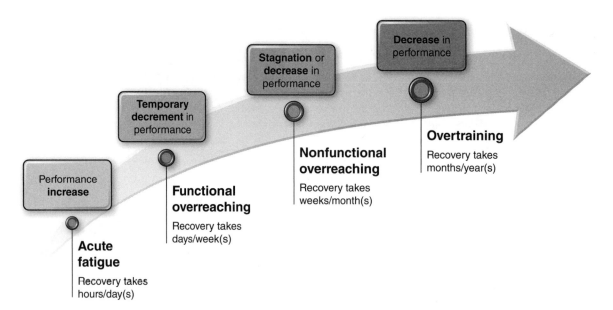

FIGURE 13.4   Representation of how an imbalance between training stressors and recovery can progress from intentionally eliciting acute fatigue to unintentionally promoting overtraining.

of male and female players who were followed over the course of a competitive season (Schmikli, Brink, de Vries, & Backx, 2011). The study showed that the underperforming soccer players presented with higher submaximal heart rates during an incremental shuttle run test, significantly higher scores for anger and depression on the Profile of Mood States inventory, and an indication of the uncoupling of adrenocorticotropic hormone (ACTH) and salivary cortisol levels, which can indicate adrenal insufficiency and chronic fatigue. Research in youth soccer players has also shown that those who became ill during a competitive season reported higher levels of general and sport-specific stress, lower levels of recovery, and more disturbed sleep before the illness appeared (Brink et al., 2012). Finally, more recent data have shown that about 30 percent of young male soccer players from elite English and Spanish clubs had experienced nonfunctional overreaching and that 60 percent of those players experienced multiple bouts (Williams et al., 2017). Cumulatively, the existing literature suggests that nearly one in three young athletes are likely to experience nonfunctional overreaching or overtraining and that these affected athletes are likely to experience reoccurring bouts. This reality highlights the importance of developing strategies to identify young athletes who are at risk for either condition before the negative health outcomes begin to manifest.

Additional challenges are faced by practitioners managing workloads for athletes who succeed in sport from a young age. Research shows that determinants of sport-related injury in young athletes included very high volumes of participation in a single sport (Fleisig et al., 2011; Jayanthi, LaBella, Fischer, Pasulka, & Dugas, 2015; Pasulka, Jayanthi, McCann, Dugas, & LaBella, 2017) and congested playing schedules (LaPrade et al., 2016; Luke et al., 2011). Although succeeding in sport can be a rewarding experience for children and adolescents, those who are responsible for the long-term development of young athletes must not place unrealistic or unmanageable burdens on them or on their parents. For example, it is not uncommon for a talented young soccer player to play for a school team, an age-based club team, and, due to their high ability, an older age-based team within the same club. If the player is then also selected for a representative team (e.g., age-based national or international team), the playing schedule is likely to become unsustainable.

Without careful planning, this scenario could prevent the individual from being exposed to integrative neuromuscular training, preclude getting enough rest and recovery, and reduce sleep quality and volume, all of which could result in nonfunctional overreaching or overtraining. Similarly, children who are deemed "talented" at a young age may find themselves playing for multiple teams across multiple sports. Although sport diversification and sampling are advocated, practitioners still must consider young athletes' overall workload—even if they are not deemed to have specialized—in order to appropriately manage their accumulated fatigue and reduce their relative risk of injury.

Teaching Tip

MONITORING FOR INDIVIDUAL RESPONSIVENESS TO TRAINING

Two athletes who appear very similar in technical ability, physical fitness, and biological maturation may cope very differently with training and nontraining stress. Therefore, youth fitness specialists need to be able to recognize when young athletes are working near their physical and psychological limits and prevent them from being exposed to excessive training with incomplete recovery. Early signs of nonfunctional overreaching or overtraining can include lethargy, loss of motivation, bad moods, increased anxiety, impaired sleep, suppressed appetite, and decreased performance (Meeusen et al., 2013). Practitioners can help prevent maladaptive responses to training by planning and monitoring young athletes' activity and by interacting with them on an individual basis.

Sport-Related Injuries in Young Athletes

Increased sport participation rates among youth have led to greater incidence of sport-related injuries (Emery, 2010; Kerssemakers, Fotiadou, de Jonge, Karantanas, & Maas, 2009). In the United States, more than 3.5 million youth sport injuries per year require a medical visit (American Academy of Orthopaedic Surgeons, 2012), and comparable data from Europe indicate that nearly 1.3 million sport-related injuries reported in 2009 required hospitalization for children under the age of 15 years (Bauer & Steiner, 2009). Similarly, Canadian data suggest that 30 percent to 40 percent of youth annually experience a sport-related injury requiring medical attention (Emery & Tyreman, 2009; Emery, Meeuwisse, & McAllister, 2006). In addition, emerging data suggest that young athletes who specialize in a single sport from an early age are more likely to experience sport-related injuries, especially overuse injuries of the lower limbs (Bell et al., 2016; Hall, Barber Foss, Hewett, & Myer, 2015; Jayanthi et al., 2015; McGuine et al., 2017).

Acute injuries occur during a single traumatic event and typically take the form of fractures, sprains, strains, and concussions. In contrast, **overuse injuries** are caused by repetitive submaximal microtrauma to the musculoskeletal system in the absence of sufficient time for recovery and subsequent adaptation (DiFiori et al., 2014; Stein & Micheli, 2010). Examples of overuse injuries include stress fractures, tendinopathies, osteochondritis dissecans, and patellofemoral pain (Shanmugam & Maffulli, 2008). Pediatric sport-related injuries vary according to age, sex, sport type, participation level, and playing position (Caine, Caine, & Maffulli, 2006; Schroeder et al., 2015). For example, data show that acute traumatic injuries are more likely to occur in children (particularly in the upper extremities), whereas overuse injuries are more probable in adolescents (especially in the hips and lower limbs) due to the growth spurt (Stracciolini, Casciano, Levey Friedman, Meehan, & Micheli, 2013).

When injuries are grouped by sex, females have been shown to experience a higher percentage of overuse injuries than traumatic injuries, whereas the opposite is seen in males (Stracciolini et al., 2014). Research has shown that 46 percent of the sex differences in overuse injuries could be attributed to the nature of the sports played by young males and young females (Stracciolini, Casciano, Friedman, Meehan, & Micheli, 2015). Specifically, Stracciolini and colleagues (2015) reported that a greater proportion of males participated in contact and collision sports (e.g., basketball, American football, rugby, soccer), which are more likely to result in acute traumatic injuries, whereas females were typically involved in high-overuse sports (e.g., dance, track and field, swimming, gymnastics), which of course are associated with a higher risk of overuse injuries. The authors suggested that the remaining sex differences in overuse injuries could be explained by biological differences associated with growth and maturation (Stracciolini et al., 2015), and the existing literature indicates that these biological differences include variations in femoral notch size, Q angle, hormonal profile, and lower-extremity strength and flexibility (Alentorn-Geli et al., 2009). These differences underline the unique challenges that practitioners face when working with young athletes.

It is beyond the scope of this chapter to critically discuss all types of acute and chronic injuries that young athletes might experience. However, certain injuries have been researched in the pediatric literature and have received notable media attention due to their prevalence, severity, and financial cost (Stein & Micheli, 2010). These injuries include **sport-related concussion**, **Little League shoulder** and **Little League elbow**, **lower-back pain**, **anterior cruciate ligament injury**, and **calcaneal apophysitis**.

Sport-Related Concussion

Sport-related concussion consists of the clinical syndrome of traumatic brain injury induced by an event such as a direct blow to the head or neck, which transmits an impulsive force to the head (McCrory et al., 2017). Sport-related concussions are common in competitive sport, and children and adolescents appear to be the most at risk (Fridman, Fraser-Thomas, McFaull, & Macpherson, 2013; Grady, 2010), perhaps due to their weaker neck muscles, their larger head-to-body ratio, and the vulnerability of the developing brain (Sim, Terryberry-Spohr, & Wilson, 2008). Youth also appear to experience symptoms of concussion for longer periods than adults (Field, Collins, Lovell, & Maroon, 2003; Howell, Osternig, & Chou, 2015) and to be at heightened risk of sustaining a sport-related concussion in collision sports such as American football, soccer, lacrosse, and ice hockey (Lincoln et al., 2011; Pfister, Pfister, Hagel, Ghali, & Ronksley, 2016). Certain sports indicate sex differences in concussion incidence, with boys showing higher incidence in American football, although participation rates are much higher among boys in that sport. However, in sports with more comparable participation rates, girls appear to be at greater risk of concussion when similar sports are considered (e.g., basketball, soccer, softball and baseball) (Gessel, Fields, Collins, Dick, & Comstock, 2007; Lincoln et al., 2011). The discrepancy may derive from biomechanical differences such as head size, neck strength, and neck girth (Covassin & Elbin, 2011; Covassin, Savage, Bretzin, & Fox, 2017; Dick, 2009). Data also show that females tend to experience greater severity and suffer more prolonged symptoms following a sport-related concussion (Berz et al., 2013).

Recent international consensus guidelines suggest that a diagnosis of sport-related concussion is likely to be established if one or more of the following clinical signs are present in the child or adolescent (McCrory et al., 2017):

- Somatic symptoms (e.g., headache)
- Cognitive symptoms (e.g., feeling "foggy")
- Emotional symptoms (e.g., mood swings)
- Physical signs (e.g., amnesia, loss of consciousness)
- Balance impairment (e.g., gait instability)
- Behavioral changes (e.g., irritability)
- Cognitive impairment (e.g., slowed reactions)
- Sleep disturbance (e.g., drowsiness)

The presentation of symptoms from sport-related concussion can be delayed; therefore, the preferred response is always to take a conservative and cautious approach. When concerns arise that a child or adolescent may have experienced a concussion, the individual should be immediately withdrawn from sport participation (McCrory et al., 2017), which reduces recovery time (Elbin et al., 2016). Similarly, under no circumstances should a child or adolescent be allowed to return to sport if symptoms are still present. Following a period of enforced active rest and symptom-limited resumption of physical activity, youth must pass a full and thorough neurophysiological assessment (e.g., the Child-SCAT3) by a trained physician before gradually returning to sport practice and competition (Gomez & Hergenroeder, 2013; McCrory et al., 2017).

Youth fitness specialists and youth coaches should *not* be responsible for making clinical diagnoses or judgments about whether a child or adolescent has experienced a concussion or when an individual can resume sport participation. Youth who have experienced a concussive event should be encouraged to obtain a baseline neurocognitive test (e.g., ImPACT test; Covassin, Elbin, Stiller-Ostrowski, & Kontos, 2009) performed by an appropriately trained medical professional (McCrory et al., 2017). Advanced technological strategies aimed at preventing sport-related concussion have shown promising results (Myer, Yuan, Barber Foss, Smith, et al., 2016; Myer, Yuan, Barber Foss, Thomas, et al., 2016). In addition, recent evidence has shown that concussion incidence was reduced in adolescent rugby players following exposure to a five-month training program focused on preactivity movement control that included a range of resistance, plyometric, balance, landing, and cutting exercises (Hislop et al., 2017).

Little League Shoulder and Little League Elbow

Young athletes can experience a range of acute sport-related injuries (e.g., dislocations, fractures, abrasions) in the shoulder, elbow, wrist, hand, and fingers (Brooks & Hammer, 2013), and they are most often accidental in nature. Whereas accidental injuries are difficult to avoid, youth fitness specialists are better able to manage and reduce the relative risk of overuse injuries. Young athletes who participate in throwing sports face heightened risk of shoulder and elbow injuries, largely due to the chronic, repetitive overhead motion of throwing. Although a number of sports involve overhead motions (e.g., tennis, gymnastics, cricket, track and field), the most common throwing-related overuse injuries are Little League shoulder and Little League elbow, so named for the prevalence of shoulder and elbow injuries in young baseball pitchers (Lyman et al., 2001; Matsuura et al., 2016).

Little League shoulder involves epiphysiolysis resulting from the high rotational stresses placed across the proximal humeral physis during overhead throwing (Leonard & Hutchinson, 2010; May & Bishop, 2013). Similarly, Little League elbow is caused by excessive traction, compression, and shear forces around the elbow during repetitive throwing (Hennrikus, 2006). Research has found that the incidence of shoulder pain in young baseball pitchers is about 30 percent and that key risk factors include arm fatigue and a pitch count of more than 75 per game (Lyman et al., 2001). Similarly, incidence data have indicated that roughly 30 percent of youth pitchers experience elbow pain (Matsuura et al., 2016; Matsuura, Suzue, Kashiwaguchi, Arisawa, & Yasui, 2013), and about 60 percent of those players exhibit radiographic abnormalities (Matsuura et al., 2013). More recently, a 10-year prospective study revealed that 25 of 481 young baseball pitchers (5%) required elbow surgery or shoulder surgery or were forced into premature retirement due to injury, thus highlighting the adverse effects of these injuries consequent to excessive training and competition (Fleisig et al., 2011).

Little League elbow most commonly occurs medially, and medial epicondylar apophysitis (irritation and inflammation of the tendon insertion site) is often caused by valgus stress and repetitive microtrauma in the medial collateral ligament and flexor pronator muscles (Hennrikus, 2006). Young athletes who suffer with this condition typically report a gradual onset of pain that intensifies with throwing, which can lead to medial elbow tenderness and mild swelling. Little League shoulder, in turn, is caused by rotational stress placed on the proximal humerus, which leads to separation of the epiphysis from the diaphysis (Leonard & Hutchinson, 2010). Young athletes who suffer from this condition typically present with diffuse shoulder pain that is aggravated by throwing. Although youth fitness specialists are not qualified to diagnose or treat injuries, they can play in a role in helping to reduce the risk faced by young athletes who experience these overuse conditions. Risk reduction strategies that have been validated by research and are available to youth fitness specialists include the following:

- Monitoring workloads to ensure that young athletes adhere to throwing guidelines (e.g., maximum pitch counts for games)
- Limiting young pitchers to no more than eight months of pitching within a year
- Ensuring the use of correct throwing biomechanics
- Enforcing the maintenance or correction of postural integrity

- Using a progressive warm-up before throwing with maximal effort
- Avoiding throwing when fatigued
- Implementing a well-rounded strength and conditioning program, including exercises that specifically strengthen the shoulder complex (e.g., rotator cuff and periscapular)

Lower-Back Pain

Research indicates that lower-back pain is prevalent in 10 percent to 15 percent of young athletes across a range of sports (d'Hemecourt, Gerbino, & Micheli, 2000; Mueller et al., 2016). The incidence appears to increase with age (higher rates of back pain are reported in adolescent athletes), and rates fluctuate according to the type of sport played (Haus & Micheli, 2012). Young athletes face heightened risk if they participate in sports that expose them to high amounts of axial loading in addition to flexion and torsional forces through the spine (Sward, 1992). Prevalence of back pain in adolescent athletes has ranged from 26 percent to 30 percent in female adolescent dancers (Steinberg et al., 2013) and young fast bowlers (Noorbhai, Essack, Thwala, Ellapen, & van Heerden, 2012) and from 85 percent to 89 percent in gymnasts (Hutchinson, 1999) and divers (Baranto, Hellstrom, Nyman, Lundin, & Sward, 2006). As with other regions of the body, the etiology of back pain may involve acute trauma or chronic overuse (Haus & Micheli, 2012); however overuse injuries appear to be more common (Purcell & Micheli, 2009). The most frequently reported back injuries in young athletes include spondylolysis, spondylolisthesis, apophyseal injury to the vertebral ring, disc degeneration or herniation, sacroiliac joint pain, and lumbar Scheuermann's disease (Kerssemakers et al., 2009; Purcell & Micheli, 2009; Young & d'Hemecourt, 2011).

The spine is more vulnerable in young athletes than in other athlete populations due to the disproportionate growth rates of skeletal and soft tissues, which can lead to muscle imbalances and reduce flexibility. In addition, the youth spine is skeletally immature, which leaves the epiphyseal growth plates, cartilaginous end plates, and ring apophyses at greater risk of herniation or avulsion fractures due to the repetitive loading experienced during sport participation (Purcell & Micheli, 2009). Thus, during the rapid growth associated with adolescence, these vertebral structures form the weakest portions of the spinal column and are at the greatest risk of injury during high force transmission (Haus & Micheli, 2012). It is likely that the risk of these injuries increases even further when young athletes specialize in a single sport from an early age and are exposed to excessively high volumes of repetitive loadings. We must remember, however, that mechanical loading is required in order to promote the bone remodeling process (see chapter 2). Therefore, it is recommended that a variety of loadings are required to alter the point of force application and promote ongoing skeletal development while minimizing the risk of overstressing specific regions of the musculoskeletal system (Lloyd et al., 2016).

Although physicians are of course responsible for diagnosing and treating lower-back pain in young athletes, youth fitness specialists can play a role in primordial prevention aimed at arresting the emergence of risk factors for overuse-related back injury. Specifically, they can help young athletes avoid excessive training loads and focus on the development and maintenance of correct posture and proper technique. Practitioners should also ensure that sufficient training time is devoted to strengthening the abdominals and the lumbar region of the back, mobilizing the thoracic spine and thoracolumbar fascia, and improving or at least retaining flexibility in the musculature surrounding the hips and lower limbs (Purcell, 2009). Young athletes should be exposed to this type of training at least two or three times per week, starting from an early age, in order to maximize their chances of maintaining a healthy spine throughout their sport career and into their later years.

Anterior Cruciate Ligament Injury

For multiple reasons, anterior cruciate ligament (ACL) injury is one of the most catastrophic injuries that a young athlete can sustain. The reasons include the considerable time spent unable to participate in sport, the financial burden of treatment (about $25,000 per injury), the negative effect on mental health, the increased risk of unfavorable weight gain, and the detrimental effect on academic performance (de Loes, Dahlstedt, & Thomee, 2000; LaBella et al., 2014; Myer et al., 2014). ACL injury occurs during **dynamic lower-extremity valgus** (see figure 13.5), which typically involves a combination of hip adduction and internal rotation, knee abduction, tibial external rotation and anterior translation, and ankle eversion (Hewett, Myer, & Ford, 2006). Even when athletes make a successful return to their sport, some 25 percent go on to sustain a second knee injury (Paterno, Rauh, Schmitt, Ford, & Hewett, 2012; Paterno et al., 2010; Wiggins et al., 2016), either in the ACL-reconstructed knee or in the contralateral normal knee (Shelbourne, Gray, & Haro, 2009). In addition, ACL injury dramatically increases the chance of suffering from radiographic osteoarthritis later in life (Parkkari, Pasanen, Mattila, Kannus, & Rimpela, 2008). As with initial ACL injury, major risk

factors for ACL re-injury appear to include reduced neuromuscular control and aberrant movement biomechanics, which are influenced by abnormal trunk and lower-extremity movement patterns and strength levels (Hewett, Di Stasi, & Myer, 2013).

Data show that ACL injuries can result from clear contact or collisions with another player or from noncontact situations such as cutting and pivoting movements (Hewett, Myer, et al., 2006). Noncontact ACL injuries appear to be more common in athletes than in nonathletes (Boden, Dean, Feagin, & Garrett, 2000) and are more preventable with appropriate preparatory conditioning. In fact, a large body of research has investigated the potential mechanisms of ACL injury, and various risk factors have been designated as either unmodifiable (e.g., anatomical, developmental, and hormonal factors) or modifiable (e.g., biomechanical and neuromuscular factors); an overview of these risk factors is presented in figure 13.6 (Alentorn-Geli et al., 2009; Hewett, Myer, Ford, Paterno, & Quatman, 2016). Although ACL injury invariably involves a multifactorial etiology, youth fitness specialists should be most concerned with the modifiable risk factors, especially neuromuscular qualities such as muscular strength

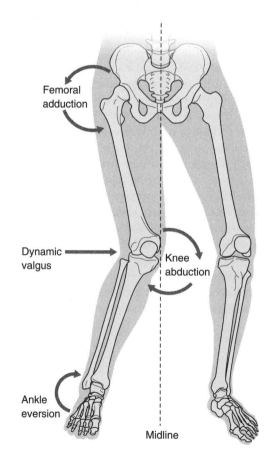

FIGURE 13.5 Joint actions leading to dynamic lower-extremity valgus.

and power, motor control, balance, and proprioception (Hewett, Myer, et al., 2006).

ACL injury rates increase with age in both males and females (LaBella et al., 2014), and there are no discernable sex-related differences in ACL injury rates during childhood (Shea, Pfeiffer, Wang, Curtin, & Apel, 2004). Research indicates that the risk of ACL injury rises markedly at or just after peak height velocity (Granan, Forssblad, Lind, & Engebretsen, 2009), at which point adolescent females exhibit a higher rate of ACL injury than their male counterparts (Hewett, Myer, & Ford, 2004; Voskanian, 2013). The increased risk at this stage of development results from the rapid increase in body mass and height of center of mass as a result of the growth spurt. Combined, these changes place greater torque on the knee, especially during tasks that involve landing, cutting, or pivoting (Hewett et al., 2004). These increased torques are somewhat mediated in males by their natural increases in neuromuscular capacities (e.g., strength, power, coordination), but the same neuromuscular spurt is not evident in females (Myer et al., 2009). These sex-related differences explain the greater attention that young female athletes have received in the academic literature and the heightened importance placed on female-focused programs to reduce the incidence of ACL injuries by targeting neuromuscular deficiencies (Noyes & Barber Westin, 2012; Sugimoto et al., 2015). These efforts also highlight the likely benefit of initiating integrative neuromuscular training early in life to lay the foundations for movement competence and basic strength qualities in order to minimize the deleterious effects of the growth spurt.

DO YOU KNOW?

Young athletes who experience an ACL injury are 10 times more likely to suffer from early-onset osteoarthritis.

Despite the devastating nature of ACL injury, youth fitness specialists should be encouraged by research that has examined the effectiveness of neuromuscular interventions aimed at preventing ACL injury and reported favorable outcomes for young athletes (Alentorn-Geli et al., 2014; Hewett, Ford, & Myer, 2006; Soligard et al., 2008). In general, the most effective neuromuscular interventions have adopted a range of training modalities, including strength training and plyometrics; balance, stretching, and coordination work; and technique development. Strength training in particular appears to be an integral component of intervention and has led to the most desirable outcomes (Lauersen et al., 2014; Sugimoto et al., 2016), although plyometrics appears to be the most commonly used training tool (LaBella et al., 2014).

Despite limited literature addressing young male populations, neuromuscular interventions have been shown to be effective in young female athletes (Sugimoto, Myer, McKeon, & Hewett, 2012). Meta-analytical data show that the greatest reduction in ACL injuries occurs in younger age groups (14 to 18 years)

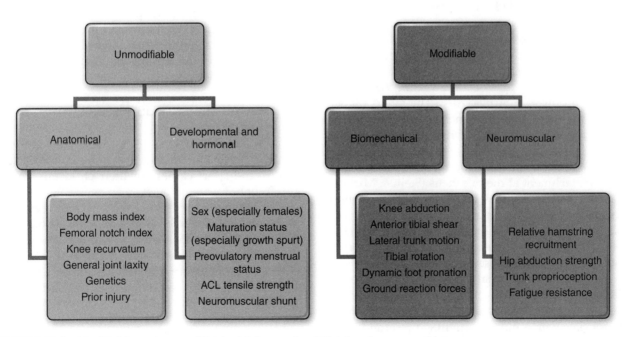

FIGURE 13.6   Modifiable and unmodifiable risk factors for ACL injury in young athletes.

Based on Alentorn-Geli, Myer, Silvers, et al. (2009), and Hewett, Myer, Ford, et al. (2016).

as compared with those in their late teens (18 to 20 years) or adulthood (over 20 years), which suggests an age-related association between neuromuscular interventions and reduction of ACL injury risk (Myer, Sugimoto, Thomas, & Hewett, 2013). Additional research has indicated increased effectiveness when adolescent females were exposed to a higher dosage of neuromuscular intervention (Sugimoto, Myer, Foss, & Hewett, 2014). Specifically, the data showed greater returns when youth were exposed to multiple sessions per week (two or more) lasting more than 20 minutes each. More recent data indicate similar optimal dosages of neuromuscular training for preventing overuse and acute injuries in young athletes; specifically, researchers suggested a total weekly training volume of up to 60 minutes spread over two or three training sessions (Steib, Rahlf, Pfeifer, & Zech, 2017).

Cumulatively, current data indicate that youth fitness specialists should try to expose youth to multifaceted neuromuscular interventions from the earliest age possible (Renstrom et al., 2008) and ensure ongoing exposure to developmentally appropriate activities that target neuromuscular deficits.

Calcaneal Apophysitis

Commonly referred to as Sever's disease, calcaneal apophysitis is an overuse-related injury in the heel that is typically experienced by youth (especially boys) aged 8 to 14 years; incidence is magnified around periods of growth and at the commencement of new sport seasons (Hendrix, 2005; Kennedy, Knowles, Dolan, & Bohne, 2005). Earlier data indicated that the incidence of calcaneal apophysitis falls between 2 percent and 16 percent (Scharfbillig, Jones, & Scutter, 2008), and more recent European data indicate 61 cases across 34 general practices, resulting in an incidence rate of about 4 per 1,000 patients over the course of three years (Wiegerinck, Yntema, Brouwer, & Struijs, 2014). The rate is higher in young athletes than young nonathletes due to their greater levels of repetitive activity (Micheli & Ireland, 1987). The etiology of calcaneal apophysitis involves repetitive, submaximal microtrauma in the Achilles tendon attachment at the calcaneus (Stein & Micheli, 2010). As is often the case with overuse injuries, young athletes may experience a gradual increase in pain, in this case around the heel, with the onset of exercise; about 60 percent of sufferers complain of discomfort in both heels (Cassas & Cassettari-Wayhs, 2006).

Here again, only qualified physicians should diagnose and treat this condition, but youth fitness specialists can help mediate the associated pain by appropriately manipulating training prescription. To

that end, practitioners should bear in mind that, in addition to structural differences in youth populations (i.e., heightened vulnerability in the apophysis), the risk of experiencing calcaneal apophysitis is increased by growth-related reductions in flexibility in the gastrocnemius and soleus muscles and in the Achilles tendon (Stein & Micheli, 2010). Therefore, practitioners should include stretching and strengthening of the relevant musculature of the lower limb in athletic development programs for young athletes (Micheli & Ireland, 1987), especially during periods of rapid growth.

Fostering Parental Support for Young Athletes

Parents play a significant role in cultivating a positive environment in which young athletes can develop both physically and psychosocially. From the practical, logistical, and financial perspectives, parents are typically responsible for transporting their children to and from sport practices and competitions, purchasing relevant sports equipment, paying for memberships in sport organizations, providing emotional support, and helping youth understand the sporting experience (Elliott & Drummond, 2017; Fraser-Thomas & Cote, 2009). Parents can also influence the development of young athletes by the roles they adopt and the behaviors they demonstrate before, during, and after sport practices and competitions (Harwood & Knight, 2015; Knight, Berrow, & Harwood, 2017). Due to parents' substantial influence on their children, youth fitness specialists need to develop positive relationships and build rapport with the parents of the young athletes with whom they work. Although practitioners should never try to instruct parents about how to parent, they can promote educational and supportive opportunities to foster effective parenting in and around the sport environment.

Supportive Versus Pressuring Parenting

It is not unusual for parents to assume a highly active role in the sport careers of their children. Unless carefully harnessed, however, an overzealous parent can exhibit behaviors and perform actions that serve as a source of stress for young athletes (Smoll et al., 2011). In the phenomenon known as achievement by proxy distortion, parents live vicariously through their children's sporting endeavors (Tofler, Knapp, & Larden, 2005; Wiersma, 2000), which can lead parents to make decisions on behalf of children rather than supporting and empowering them to make decisions of their own. This dynamic has been referred to as the **reverse-dependency phenomenon**, wherein parents define their own self-worth in terms of their child's sporting achievements (Smoll, 1998). In this situation, parents may pressure young athletes to participate in additional practices, play an excessive number of games, or even play when injured due to fear of failing to win, being deselected, or simply "missing out" in comparison with another child.

From the perspective of athletic development, this scenario could mean that a young athlete is encouraged to complete additional training sessions (potentially delivered by unqualified personnel) outside of the prescribed program when the athlete may need to rest and recover. Alternatively, an athlete may be encouraged to train despite injury for fear that the head coach might otherwise view the athlete as unavailable for the next competition. In such instances, youth fitness specialists must communicate appropriately with the young athlete, the parent, and the technical coach to ensure, wherever possible, that a logical and collaborative approach to training is adopted and that the health and well-being of the child remain central to the program.

Although parental involvement in youth sport can often be perceived in a negative light (e.g., the "pushy parent"), youth fitness specialists should remember that most parents are simply eager for their children to improve and enjoy their chosen sport. Efforts should always be made to foster a supportive environment for young athletes. When children perceive that their parents are positively involved and satisfied with their performance, they typically report enhanced enjoyment of sport (McCarthy & Jones, 2007). In contrast, research shows that when children deem their parents to be overinvolved, exerting too much pressure, or holding unrealistic expectations, they report increased levels of anxiety (Gould, Eklund, Petlichkoff, Peterson, & Bump, 1991). Therefore, although youth sport parenting is complex and dynamic—and though flexibility is required in managing the sport parenting environment—the goal should be to develop a motivational climate in which young athletes are empowered to develop self-esteem, self-worth, self-confidence, resilience, a growth mind-set, and a range of life skills (Lloyd et al., 2015; Visek, Harris, & Blom, 2013).

A recent position paper advocates that expertise in sport parenting is reflected by actions and behaviors that enhance the likelihood of children achieving their sporting potential, cultivate positive psychosocial experiences, and develop a range of positive developmental outcomes (Harwood & Knight, 2015). Furthermore, the authors propose a series of postulates that, if adhered to, should enable parents to develop an appropriate environment for their child:

1. Select appropriate sport opportunities for the child and provide necessary types of social support.
2. Understand and apply an authoritative or autonomy-supportive parenting style.
3. Manage the emotional demands of competition and serve as emotionally intelligent role models for children.
4. Foster and maintain healthy relationships with significant others in the youth sport environment.
5. Manage the organizational and developmental demands placed on them as stakeholders in youth sport.
6. Adapt their involvement and support to different stages of their child's athletic development and progression.

The Importance of Education

Although youth fitness specialists are unlikely to be called on to manage fallout over team selection or deselection, they may need to educate parents about the training, testing, and monitoring principles and methods used in the long-term athletic development program. They may also need to educate parents about rates of progression or regression in young athletes and clarify the arrangement of subgroups in team training sessions.

Research has indicated that even physical educators and coaches require education opportunities to improve their limited knowledge and understanding of the design and implementation of resistance training for youth (Froberg, Alricsson, & Ahnesjo, 2014; McGladrey, Hannon, Faigenbaum, Shultz, & Shaw, 2014). Given that parents are less likely to have a background in sport science or long-term athletic development, they may well have concerns about the safety of resistance training modalities (e.g., weightlifting, strength training, plyometrics) regardless of the strength of evidence now promoting its use among youth (Lloyd, Faigenbaum, et al., 2014). Similarly, due to the risks associated with early sport specialization, youth fitness specialists may prescribe activities in a training session that do not necessarily resemble the sport in which a young athlete is involved. Parents, however, may not understand the benefits of sport diversification or the principles of training variety for long-term athletic development. To reduce the risk of conflict with parents, practitioners may benefit from providing educational opportunities to clearly outline the central philosophy of the long-term athletic development program in which a child is involved.

Practical Strategies for Parents

Given the importance of promoting a supportive and educated culture among the parents of young athletes, youth fitness specialists should consider how best to interact with parents in order to communicate their philosophies and approaches to athletic development in a positive manner. Too often, parents of young athletes are told what *not* to do (e.g., "do not coach your child from the sidelines") rather than being encouraged in what *to* do (e.g., "please discuss your child's experience of today's session after practice has ended"). Parents do not like to be told how to parent their child, but adopting positive language helps practitioners to create a supportive and collaborative environment, which ultimately leads to greater buy-in from parents. Table 13.1 provides examples of communication strategies for interacting with various types of parents (Smoll et al., 2011). Table 13.2 provides a range of practical solutions for fostering an appropriate climate in any long-term athletic development program. Youth fitness specialists should not feel compelled to use all of these options but should select those that are most appropriate for the specific environment in which they work.

Summary

Well-organized youth sport offers a platform for children and adolescents to have fun, challenge themselves, learn new skills, enhance their physical fitness, gain confidence, and develop their social network of friends. However, given the increased emphasis on specialization in a single sport and the heightened training loads assigned at early ages, young athletes can be vulnerable to the negative aspects of youth sport. These facets include maturity-related selection or deselection, sport-related injury, loss of motivation and confidence, overtraining, and excessive expectations from significant others such as parents and coaches.

Fortunately, with an understanding of pediatric exercise science and an appreciation for the long-term athletic development process, youth fitness specialists can play an integral role in the development of young athletes as part of a holistic athletic development program. Youth sport programs should promote the development of healthy, proficient, and resilient young athletes who are able to flourish and succeed in a sustainable and enjoyable environment. Youth fitness specialists should seek to develop positive relationships with parents and other personnel involved in a young athlete's career. Irrespective of whether a young athlete will be highly successful at a senior level of sport, the athlete should be given the tools to remain active in sport or recreational physical activity throughout life.

TABLE 13.1 COMMUNICATION STRATEGIES FOR INTERACTING WITH PARENTS

Parental behavior	Sample scenario	Example of what to do	Example of what to say
Disinterested	Parent is absent from training sessions or competitions and not always responsible for transporting child to and from practice.	Do not assume that lack of presence means lack of caring or interest; absence could be due to other commitments (e.g., work). Make contact to find out why the parent is unable to attend.	"Dear Mrs. Shaw, I appreciate that parents are really busy, and I just wanted to touch base to make sure you were aware of how well your daughter is progressing at the moment. It would be great to see you at training because familial support is always welcomed. If it would be easier, maybe we can arrange to discuss her development over the phone?"
Hypercritical	Parent is dissatisfied or unnecessarily critical of child's performance during a training session involving competitive sprint drills.	Be diplomatic, reinforce the importance of praise and encouragement, and encourage parents to focus on process goals (e.g., technical execution) rather than outcome goals (e.g., comparing performance against that of other players).	"Hi Mr. Daniels. I know you're trying to help your son, but he really does seem to get nervous when he constantly hears critical feedback. It seems that he has more fun when he hears positive feedback, so maybe we can focus on that instead?"
Highly vocal	Parent is outwardly critical or abusive to coaches, players, or other parents during a warm-up session before a competitive activity.	Avoid entering into a heated argument with the parent; instead, try to speak privately to explain the pitfalls of shouting. Emphasize that it can be distracting and demotivating for young athletes and other observers.	"Hi Mrs. Taylor. I realize that it's easy to get excited about your son's performance and that you are coming from a good place, but the kids are just here to have fun and learn. We definitely need your support, but the kids don't need to take things too seriously."
Coaching from the sideline	Parent gives young athletes strategy and coaching feedback from the sideline during a conditioning-based, small-sided game.	Unless the sideline coaching puts young athletes at risk of injury (e.g., bad technical advice), avoid instant engagement or confrontation. Instead, opt for private discussion with the parent to outline the effects of multiple coaching inputs for young athletes.	"Mr. Wilmore, I really appreciate your concerns and passion for the children, but it's really confusing for your daughter and the rest of the team when you're coaching from the sidelines. I'd really appreciate it if we could save any discussions about training for after the sessions."
Overprotective	Parent appears worried and threatens to remove the child from a resistance training session due to fears of harm.	Try to allay fears by educating the parent in basic terms about the program's philosophy and the safety of various training modes. Emphasize that the athletic development program is grounded in technical competence and that youth are not progressed unless they can demonstrate appropriate form in relevant exercises.	"Hi Mrs. Lewis. I understand your concerns about your daughter doing resistance training. Please be reassured that this is a safe and effective thing for her to do. We won't ask your daughter to do any exercises unless she is absolutely ready for them. I can provide you with all of the information you need to help you understand that it is okay for your daughter to take part in this resistance training session."

Adapted from Smoll, Cumming, and Smith (2011).

TABLE 13.2   PRACTICAL STRATEGIES FOR ENGAGING WITH PARENTS OF YOUNG ATHLETES

Strategy	Overview	Advantages	Disadvantages
Coach–parent meeting	The purpose of the meeting is to discuss the progress or personal situations of individual athletes.	The meeting creates an opportunity to provide detail on a case-by-case basis and address specific questions from parents.	This strategy can be time-consuming.
Open house for parents	This type of meeting is designed to enhance parents' understanding of the athletic development program and gain their cooperation and support.	This meeting enables the practitioner to address a large number of parents simultaneously in a face-to-face forum. It may also foster communication and support among the parents.	This is not the place to discuss details or address questions that are specific to individual athletes.
Training diary and progress reports	These tools can be used daily or weekly to document factors such as training loads, progressions, regressions, and achievement of milestones.	This strategy enables ongoing communication between the youth fitness specialist and parents. It also facilitates a transparent and collaborative approach to monitoring progress and training loads.	This approach does not necessarily involve face-to-face communication, and it does require some level of understanding from parents with respect to the training diaries.
Information dissemination	This approach can distribute information in the form of flyers, fact sheets, tips, or infographics. It can be delivered via a team or program website, included in a program handbook, or displayed in poster format in the training facility.	This approach makes information available in a range of forms for parents to access as needed or desired. It can help dispel misunderstandings or concerns from parents—for instance, regarding the safety of resistance training, the trainability of children versus adolescents, or issues related to growth and maturation.	This strategy relies on parents to acquire the information. In addition, unless it is written in a parent-friendly manner, certain parents may find some of the content uninteresting or difficult to understand (and some parents may be unable to read).
Digital communication	The youth fitness specialist can use digital forums (e.g., website, e-mail, social media) to connect with parents on a regular basis.	Depending on the environment, these communications can be used to provide informal updates about the progression of the team as a whole or to convey more specific information about the progress of an individual athlete. Regular updates from social media sources can help parents feel like "part of the program."	By nature, this strategy lacks face-to-face contact. The practitioner needs to monitor usage to ensure that content is screened and uploaded only by the account holder. Some social media streams are limited to small pieces of information and therefore do not help provide parents with detailed insight.

CHAPTER 14

Exercise for Overweight and Obese Youth

CHAPTER OBJECTIVES

- Identify global trends in overweight and obesity among children and adolescents
- Examine comorbidities associated with overweight and obesity in youth
- Explore the influence of hypoactivity on body composition and lifestyle behaviors
- Describe the benefits of aerobic, resistance, and combined exercise training for youth who are overweight or obese

KEY TERMS

Introduction

In modern society, lack of daily physical activity and ease of access to lower-quality processed foods have contributed to high levels of overweight and obesity among children and adolescents (Dunford & Popkin, 2018; Hills, Andersen, & Byrne, 2011; Luger et al., 2017). Over the past few decades, the proportion of youth worldwide who are obese stands at about 20 percent (NCD Risk Factor Collaboration, 2017; Ng et al., 2014). In the United States, the prevalence of obesity in youth aged 2 to 19 years stands at about 19 percent (Hales, Fryar, Carroll, Freedman, & Ogden, 2018), and similar rates have been reported in Australia (Ho, Olds, Schranz, & Maher, 2017), Canada (Rao, Kropac, Do, Roberts, & Jayaraman, 2016), China (Zhao, Ma, Pan, Chen, & Sun, 2016), and Europe (Wijnhoven et al., 2013). In 2016, the prevalence of obesity among boys and girls was more than 30 percent in several countries, including Nauru, the Cook Islands, and Palau (NCD Risk Factor Collaboration, 2017). Notably, an increasing number of young children are severely obese and frequently have immediate health consequences due to their extreme adiposity (Skinner, Ravanbakht, Skeleton, Perrin & Armstrong, 2018; Spinelli, Buoncristiano, Kovacs et al., 2019). This phenomenon affects all socioeconomic groups, irrespective of age, sex, or ethnicity, and without targeted interventions it is estimated that a majority of today's children will be obese by age 35 (Ward et al., 2017).

These troubling trends hold significant ramifications for health care providers and youth fitness specialists because of the increasing prevalence of obesity-related comorbidities such as type 2 diabetes, hypertension, and asthma (Grant-Guimaraes, Feinstein, Laber, & Kosoy, 2016; McCrindle, 2015; Valaiyapathi, Gower, & Ashraf, 2018). A **comorbidity** is a disease or condition that occurs in the presence of another, primary disease or disorder. Management of overweight and obesity in clinical settings and fitness centers is needed in order to address these health care concerns before youth become more resistant to interventions later in life. A change in current attitudes and social behaviors is required because the long-term effects of overweight and obesity are not just pathophysiological processes, but rather phenomena that influence economic and political processes (Finkelstein, Graham, & Malhotra, 2014; B. Lee et al., 2017; Sonntag, Ali, & De Bock, 2016). Although ongoing participation in active play, exercise, and sport activities early in life can help prevent the onset of unwanted weight gain during childhood and adolescence (Henrique et al., 2018; Ortega et al., 2011; Rodrigues, Stodden, & Lopes, 2016), contemporary trends in overweight and obesity highlight the need

for multifaceted interventions because these conditions will not simply resolve themselves in due course. From a public health perspective, reducing the prevalence of overweight and obesity among children and adolescents has become a priority for the 21st century (Institute of Medicine, 2015; National Academies of the Sciences, 2016; NCD Risk Factor Collaboration, 2017).

Although it is important to consider the complex interaction between genetic, environmental, and socioeconomic influences (Heymsfield & Wadden, 2017), the root cause of overweight and obesity in most individuals is a positive energy balance characterized by excessive caloric intake, poor food quality, and limited caloric expenditure—all of which are fueled by modern-day lifestyles (De Miguel-Etayo, Bueno, Garagorri, & Moreno, 2013; Kumar & Kelly, 2017; Lustig et al., 2016; Pereira, Bobbio, Antonio, & Barros Filho Ade, 2013). Consequently, youth fitness specialists need to be aware of the challenges (both real and perceived) of treating overweight and obesity in children and adolescents due to the multitude of physical, psychosocial, and environmental factors that influence this condition. Important considerations include the age of the child, stage of maturity, diet quality, lifestyle activity, training experience, family engagement, cultural traditions, presence of comorbidities, and stigmatization of youth with obesity (Kelleher et al., 2017; Kumar & Kelly, 2017; H. Lu et al., 2015; Pont, Puhl, Cook, & Slusser, 2017).

As discussed in chapter 6, **body mass index** (BMI) is an accepted measure of body fatness in children and adolescents (a BMI calculator is available at www.cdc.gov). More accurate and expensive techniques are used in clinical and research settings (e.g., dual energy X-ray absorptiometry, or DEXA), but BMI provides a feasible and reasonable estimate of adiposity in children and adolescents (Freedman, Ogden, Blanck, Borrud, & Dietz, 2013; Martin-Calvo, Moreno-Galarraga, & Martinez-Gonzalez, 2016). At the same time, BMI may overestimate body fatness in youth with a high level of muscle mass and underestimate adiposity in sedentary youth with reduced muscle mass. Furthermore, it does not distinguish adipose type or fat distribution, which are important considerations (Gishti et al., 2015; Slyper et al., 2014). Youth fitness specialists should consider these limitations when assessing BMI in children and adolescents.

Due to normal growth and development processes, the classification of BMI scores into weight-status categories for children aged 2 years and older is age- and sex-specific. Pediatric reference standards define **overweight** as having a BMI at or above the 85th percentile but below the 95th percentile for children and adolescents of the same age and sex. **Obesity** is defined as having a BMI at or above the 95th percentile (Kuczmarski et al., 2000). Although the term severe obesity (or extreme obesity) has been previously defined as having a BMI >99th percentile (Barlow, 2007), a new classification system uses a relative BMI measure to better reflect adiposity among youth with obesity (Freedman & Berenson, 2017). As shown in table 14.1, three new subclasses of obesity are class I, class II, and class III with class II and III obesity associated with greater health risks (Skinner, Perrin, Moss, Skelton, 2015).

Comorbidities of Obesity During Childhood and Adolescence

Obesity can lead to adverse health consequences that affect almost every system in the body (Juonala et al., 2011; Kumar & Kelly, 2017; Michalsky et al., 2015; Rankin et al., 2016). If left untreated, these diseases and comorbidities worsen over time, and some experts predict that the epidemic of childhood obesity will likely shorten the lifespan of the current generation (Daniels, 2009; Hruby et al., 2016). The health- and fitness-related concerns that are linked to excess adiposity pose significant challenges to clinicians and youth fitness specialists who may not be accustomed to treating and managing obesity, hypertension, and type 2 diabetes in children and adolescents.

Increasingly, environmental "obesogenic" factors that drive physical inactivity and unhealthy food choices during the growing years are responsible for the emergence of chronic diseases and comorbidities that were once considered rare in youth (Fisberg, Maximino, Kain, & Kovalskys, 2016). Over the long term, increased food intake, poor food quality, and decreased physical activity lead to the accretion of lipids in many body compartments, which in turn can result in physical ailments and psychosocial disorders (Ebbeling, Pawlak, & Ludwig, 2002; Kelly et al., 2013; Schwimmer, Burwinkle, & Varni, 2003; Slyper et al.,

2014). Clearly, then, obesity is a multisystem disease that affects pathological processes as well as childhood experiences, peer relationships, and quality of life. Figure 14.1 provides descriptions of various obesity-related comorbidities and conditions that warrant special attention.

Cardiovascular Conditions

Obesity during childhood and adolescence is associated with risk factors for cardiovascular disease, including hypertension, dyslipidemia, impaired fasting glucose, and physical inactivity (Greco, Sood, Kwon, & Ariza, 2016; Juonala et al., 2010; Steinberger et al., 2016). Obese youth also tend to have lower levels of aerobic fitness than normal-weight peers, and the relationship between high body mass index and low cardiovascular endurance is stable throughout the growing years (Lang et al., 2018; Lopes et al., 2018). Furthermore, there is evidence that obese youth have impaired endothelial function and increased arterial stiffening, which are early signs of subclinical atherosclerosis (see figure 14.2 on page 289) (Hudson, Rapala, Khan, Williams, & Viner, 2015; Meyer, Kundt, Steiner, Schuff-Werner, & Kienast, 2006). The development of atherosclerotic plaque is a lifelong process that begins early in life, and obesity plays a critical role in the development of cardiovascular disease risk factors that mediate the evolution of early atherosclerosis (Falaschetti et al., 2010; Stoner et al., 2017).

Although each risk factor alone warrants consideration, obesity has been found to exert the greatest effect on carotid artery intima-media thickness (CIMT) in children (White et al., 2017). Increased CIMT is a hallmark of atherosclerosis and a potential harbinger of future cardiovascular disease events (Le, Zhang, Menees, Chen, & Raghuveer, 2010). In a very large cohort of more than 2 million male adolescents, an increase in BMI in late adolescence was strongly associated with cardiovascular mortality during 40 years of follow-up (Twig et al., 2016). Collectively, these findings highlight the importance of multifaceted interventions

TABLE 14.1 BODY MASS INDEX AND WEIGHT STATUS IN CHILDREN AND ADOLESCENTS

Category	Body mass index
Overweight	BMI ≥ 85th percentile < 95th percentile
Obese	BMI ≥ 95th percentile
Subcategory: class 1 obesity	BMI ≥ 95th percentile
Subcategory: class 2 obesity	BMI ≥ 120% of 95th percentile
Subcategory: class 3 obesity	BMI ≥ 140% of 95th percentile

Data from Kuczmarski, Ogden, Grummer-Strawn, et al. (2000), and Freedman and Berensen (2017).

Teaching Tip

YOUTH AT RISK

Although age- and sex-specific BMI thresholds have been established for overweight and obesity, we also need to identify youth who are at risk for developing these conditions. In a landmark study of some 2.3 million adolescents, a BMI in the 50th to 74th percentiles (currently within the normal range) was associated with increased risk for all-cause mortality in young adulthood and midlife (Twig et al., 2016). Although the specific level of BMI that warrants clinical attention is debatable, waiting until youth become overweight or obese is not in the best interest of their health and well-being. Simply being below the established BMI threshold for overweight or obesity does not necessarily mean that a child is healthy. We need to identify youth who are at risk for overweight and obesity before they decrease their time spent in physical activity, develop unhealthy eating habits, and become more resistant to intervention. School and community-based interventions that assess BMI can help to inform parents and caregivers about a healthy weight range.

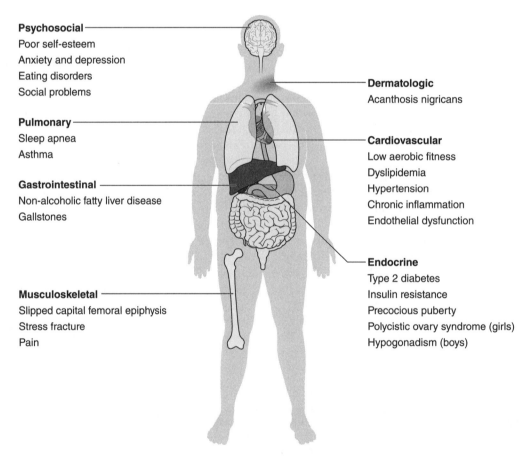

Psychosocial
Poor self-esteem
Anxiety and depression
Eating disorders
Social problems

Pulmonary
Sleep apnea
Asthma

Gastrointestinal
Non-alcoholic fatty liver disease
Gallstones

Musculoskeletal
Slipped capital femoral epiphysis
Stress fracture
Pain

Dermatologic
Acanthosis nigricans

Cardiovascular
Low aerobic fitness
Dyslipidemia
Hypertension
Chronic inflammation
Endothelial dysfunction

Endocrine
Type 2 diabetes
Insulin resistance
Precocious puberty
Polycistic ovary syndrome (girls)
Hypogonadism (boys)

FIGURE 14.1   Obesity-related comorbidities in children and adolescents.

Adapted from C.B. Ebbeling, D.B. Pawlak, and D.S. Ludwig, "Childhood Obesity: Public-Health Crisis, Common Sense Cure," *Lancet* 360, no. 9331 (2002): 473-482.

to increase physical activity, reduce sedentary time, and improve cardiovascular risk factor profiles in obese youth (Dumuid et al., 2018; García-Hermoso, Cerrillo-Urbina, et al., 2016; Saavedra, Escalante, & Garcia-Hermoso, 2011).

DO YOU KNOW?

In youth with obesity and other risk factors for cardiovascular disease, the vascular age of blood vessels is more like that of a 45-year-old than that of normal-weight peers (Le et al., 2010).

Endocrine Conditions

A troubling consequence of obesity during childhood and adolescence has been the increasing incidence of type 2 diabetes in school-age youth (Lobstein & Jackson-Leach, 2016). Although type 2 diabetes was once referred to as "adult-onset diabetes," an increasing number of children and adolescents now exhibit type 2 diabetes or other obesity-related cardiometabolic comorbidities (Lobstein & Jackson-Leach, 2016; Valaiyapathi et al., 2018). Type 2 diabetes is a polygenetic disorder arising from **insulin resistance**, which is a common manifestation of obesity in youth (Thota, Perez-Lopez, Benites-Zapata, Pasupuleti, & Hernandez, 2017). Under conditions of insulin resistance, cells fail to respond normally to the hormone insulin, and blood sugar levels rise. Because insulin resistance generally has no signs or symptoms, this prediabetic condition may go unrecognized and contribute to a formal diagnosis of type 2 diabetes (Lee, Fermin, Filipp, Gurka, & DeBoer, 2017). Youth who present with type 2 diabetes early in life appear to have a more rapid deterioration of glycemic control and progression of serious complications as compared with those who are diagnosed later in life (Levitt Katz et al., 2018; Nadeau et al., 2016).

Childhood obesity is also associated with earlier onset of puberty in girls (De Leonibus et al., 2014; Kaplowitz, 2008), which in turn is predictive of a higher BMI during adulthood and a greater risk of obesity (Prentice & Viner, 2013). **Precocious puberty**, defined as puberty that begins at an earlier age than expected, is influenced by complex interactions between genetic, ethnic, environmental, and lifestyle factors, including obesity (Cesario & Hughes, 2007). Although many factors may help explain the link between obesity and early puberty, the hormone leptin may play an important role due to its influence on regulating appetite and reproduction (Kaplowitz, 2008; Shalitin & Kiess, 2017). Because leptin is secreted from adipose tissue, obese youth have higher leptin levels, which may contribute to earlier onset of puberty.

Obese girls are also at greater risk of developing **polycystic ovary syndrome**, which is the single most common cause of infertility in young women (Rosenfield, 2015). This syndrome is characterized by hyperandrogenism (i.e., androgen excess) and persistent menstrual disorders; common signs include acne and hirsutism (excessive face and body hair) (Rosenfield, 2015). In addition, obese youth are at increased risk for **hypogonadism**, which is characterized by a reduction or absence of hormone secretions from the testes or ovaries (Viswanathan & Eugster, 2014). Hypogonadism can influence pubertal progression, as well as the development of primary and secondary sex characteristics. Testosterone concentrations of obese pubertal and postpubertal males (aged 14-20 yr) are reportedly 40 percent to 50 percent lower than those of age- and maturity-matched peers with a normal BMI (Mogri, Dhindsa, Quattrin, Ghanim, & Dandona, 2013).

Pulmonary Conditions

Obese youth are more likely than normal-weight children to suffer from **obstructive sleep apnea** (OSA) (Spilsbury, Storfer-Isser, Rosen, & Redline, 2015). OSA is caused by complete or partial obstruction of the upper airways during sleep, which leads to fragmented sleep and intermittent hypoxia or oxygen deficiency.

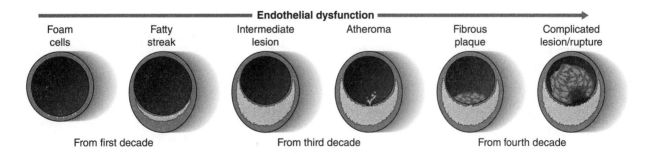

FIGURE 14.2   Endothelial dysfunction begins early in life and is a marker for atherosclerosis.

The condition appears to independently increase the risk of developing dyslipidemia, hypertension, and insulin resistance in youth, thus raising concerns about the development of serious conditions that can persist into adulthood (Bhushan, Ayub, Thompson, Abdullah, & Billings, 2017; Patinkin, Feinn, & Santos, 2017). Obesity during childhood and adolescence is also associated with **asthma,** which is characterized by reversible airflow obstruction and bronchospasm (K. Lu, Manoukian, Radom-Aizik, Cooper, & Galant, 2016; Mebrahtu, Feltbower, Greenwood, & Parslow, 2015). Whereas underweight is associated with reduced risk of asthma, obesity increases the likelihood of developing asthma symptomatology, including coughing, wheezing, shortness of breath, and chest tightness (Mebrahtu et al., 2015). The severity of asthma symptoms in overweight and obese youth can be improved through weight loss and physical activity (Leinaar, Alamian, & Wang, 2016; van Leeuwen, Hoogstrate, Duiverman, & Thio, 2014).

Gastrointestinal Conditions

The prevalence of **nonalcoholic fatty liver disease** (NAFLD) increases incrementally in youth with increases in BMI (Anderson et al., 2015). NAFLD is characterized by hepatic fat accumulation (steatosis) in the absence of excessive alcohol intake. Most youth with NAFLD are asymptomatic, although abdominal pain and fatigue are present in some young patients. During the early stage of NAFLD, fat accumulation in the liver results in insulin resistance and hyperinsulinemia. Without treatment, fat accumulation in the liver exacerbates insulin resistance and metabolic dysfunction, which can eventually lead to end-stage liver disease (Ciocca, Ramonet, & Álvarez, 2016). Early detection and lifestyle management are critical to preventing the progression of this condition and related comorbidities (Utz-Melere et al., 2018). Imaging techniques may confirm the presence of a fatty liver, but a liver biopsy is the gold standard for confirming an NAFLD diagnosis (Ciocca et al., 2016). Obesity is also associated with the increasing occurrence of **gallstones** in youth (Koebnick et al., 2012). Gallstones are formed inside the gallbladder and contain hard deposits of digestive fluid and cholesterol. Although small gallstones may be harmless, others can block the flow of digestive fluids and cause inflammation, infection, and pain.

Musculoskeletal Conditions

Excess adiposity during childhood and adolescence is associated with a higher prevalence of musculoskeletal disorders (Paulis, Silva, Koes, & van Middelkoop,

2014; Toomey et al., 2017). For instance, overweight and obesity place additional mechanical pressure on the growth plates of the tibia and can result in **Blount's disease** (tibia vara), which is characterized by lower-limb deformity resembling a bowleg. Overweight and obese youth are also more likely to experience musculoskeletal pain and lower-extremity stress fractures (Krul, van der Wouden, Schellevis, van Suijlekom-Smit, & Koes, 2009; Ryder et al., 2016). Musculoskeletal pain and consequent reduction in muscle strength and physical functioning may contribute to a cycle of weight gain and physical inactivity, which, in turn, affect capacity for daily functioning and quality of life (Tsiros et al., 2016). A high BMI is also a risk factor for **slipped capital femoral epiphysis** (SCFE) during the growing years, especially in youth with a BMI-for-age at or above the 95th percentile (Aversano, Moazzaz, Scaduto, & Otsuka, 2016). SCFE is a disorder of the proximal femur wherein the "slip" is a result of an abnormally high load across a normal physis or a normal load across a weak physis, or both (Witbreuk et al., 2013). This condition can cause pain, stiffness, and instability in the hip region; without treatment, it can lead to serious complications.

Dermatologic Conditions

One common skin condition observed in obese youth is **acanthosis nigricans**. This dermatosis is characterized by rough skin, irregular wrinkles, and hyperpigmentation and typically develops near the neck, armpits, and groin. Although its onset may be insidious, acanthosis nigricans is a notable marker of insulin resistance, which worsens with increasing severity of this condition (Koh, Lee, Kim, & Moon, 2016). Acanthosis nigricans is typically asymptomatic, although the unsightly appearance of coarse, thickened, and hyperpigmented skin may arouse psychological distress in some individuals.

Psychosocial Conditions

The psychosocial comorbidities of obesity during childhood and adolescence include anxiety, depression, poor self-esteem, social isolation, and decreased health-related quality of life (Pont et al., 2017; Rankin et al., 2016; Sutaria, Devakumar, Yasuda, Das, & Saxena, 2019). Obese youth may experience teasing and bullying related to their body size, and this abuse can carry serious consequences for their emotional health and well-being (Pont et al., 2017). Weight-related teasing has been found to be associated with social isolation, poor self-perceptions, preference for sedentary activities, disordered eating habits, and avoidance of health care services (Hayden-Wade et al., 2005; He, Cai, & Fan, 2017;

Pont et al., 2017). Over time, teasing can lead to depressive symptoms and suicidal ideations (Eisenberg, Neumark-Sztainer, & Story, 2003). In a cross-sectional study of children and adolescents who had been referred to a hospital for evaluation of obesity, researchers reported that severely obese youth had a similar health-related quality of life as those diagnosed with cancer (Schwimmer et al., 2003). Given that the causal pathways between obesity and psychosocial comorbidities may be bidirectional (Faith et al., 2011; Zhu et al., 2017), multifaceted interventions are needed to enhance peer relationships, support behavior change, and improve lifestyle behaviors in a welcoming and nonstigmatizing environment in order to optimize physical and mental health in youth with obesity.

DO YOU KNOW?

Several medications used to treat major depression and psychotic disorders in youth and adults can contribute to substantial weight gain due to an increase in appetite.

Lifestyle Hypoactivity and Obesity

Positive behaviors established early in life tend to track or carry over into adulthood; therefore, children who engage regularly in physical activity are more likely to be active later in life (Fraser et al., 2017; Meredith-Jones et al., 2018; Telama et al., 2014). The same can be said for negative behaviors, including physical inactivity and poor eating habits (Bugge, El-Naaman, McMurray, Froberg, & Andersen, 2013; Evensen, Wilsgaard, Furberg, & Skeie, 2016; Rääsk et al., 2015). Because adiposity in children is associated with lifestyle behaviors, interventions are needed early in life to increase physical activity, reduce sedentary time,

and inform parents and caregivers about the importance of healthy lifestyle choices. Heavier children are more likely to be classified as having low motor skill competence than normal-weight peers (Han, Fu, Cobley, & Sanders, 2017; Silva-Santos, Santos, Vale, & Mota, 2017), and motor coordination appears to track moderately during the growing years (Henrique et al., 2018; Lima, Bugge, Pfeiffer, & Andersen, 2017). Even during infancy, motor delay has been shown to be more likely in overweight infants who have higher subcutaneous fat as compared with non-overweight infants who have lower subcutaneous fat (Slining, Adair, Goldman, Borja, & Bentley, 2010).

In order to support physical development, we need to promote daily physical activity and provide regular opportunities to practice and reinforce fundamental movement skills. Because normal-weight children show better motor skill proficiency than those who are overweight or obese (Lima et al., 2017; Marmeleira, Veiga, Cansado, & Raimundo, 2017), it is appropriate to target neuromuscular deficiencies in youth who are overweight or obese in order to encourage active play and regular participation in exercise, games, and sport activities. Although obesity tends to persist throughout infancy and early childhood without targeted interventions (Nader et al., 2006; Roy et al., 2016), children with a BMI below the 50th percentile during the primary school years are less likely to reach overweight status by age 12 years than youth with a BMI above the 85th percentile (Nader et al., 2006). Indeed, efforts to alter BMI trajectories should begin early in life, ideally before the age of 6 years (Buscot et al., 2018). These findings underscore the need for public and health services to begin **primordial prevention** in order to prevent the appearance of risk factors in the first place (Tanrikulu, Agirbasli, & Berenson, 2017). Primordial prevention is intended to establish healthy communities, change the social environment, and maintain

Teaching Tip

PARENTS' PERCEPTIONS

Parents and caregivers often underestimate a child's overweight or obesity status (Hochdorn et al., 2018; Manios et al., 2015). Without knowledge of related comorbidities and the potential effect of healthy lifestyle behaviors on a child's physical, psychosocial, and cognitive well-being, it is unlikely that current trends in overweight and obesity will improve. Youth fitness specialists are uniquely positioned to educate parents and speak about the importance of establishing healthy lifestyle behaviors early in life, including healthy food choices, daily physical activity, and adequate sleep. Simply identifying a child as overweight or obese is not enough and may even contribute to additional weight gain across childhood (Robinson & Sutin, 2016). Instead, we need to deliver ongoing education in schools, fitness centers, and health clinics in an informative and nonjudgmental manner in order to reach parents and caregivers with the ultimate goal of helping youth to establish long-lasting healthy behaviors.

lifestyle behaviors that exert a positive influence on health and well-being. The stages of prevention are outlined in table 14.2.

Over time, the gap between youth with lower and higher levels of physical fitness tends to widen, and the evolution of these changes is strongly related to a child's weight status (D'Hondt et al., 2013; DAS Virgens Chagas, Carvalho, & Batista, 2016; Dowda, Taverno Ross, McIver, Dishman, & Pate, 2017; Lima et al., 2017). As youth transition from childhood to adolescence, those who maintain higher levels of moderate to vigorous physical activity (MVPA) tend to maintain more favorable levels of adiposity as compared with those who are less active (Dowda et al., 2017). Because time spent in MVPA is associated with decreases in body mass index during the growing years (Mitchell et al., 2013), concerted efforts are needed to provide all youth with opportunities to engage in daily MVPA as part of active transportation, free play, structured exercise, and organized sport activities at school and in the community. Notwithstanding the critical importance of healthy food choices at home and at school, the right dose of MVPA early in life may enhance a child's resilience with regard to excess adiposity.

Given the immediate and long-term consequences of overweight and obesity on the lifestyle behaviors of children and adolescents, youth fitness specialists need to be aware of the synergistic relationship between hypoactivity and excess adiposity. Behavioral factors such as increasing physical activity as well as limiting screen time (both television and electronic devices) and improving sleep hygiene seem to be the most amenable to change, and therefore lifestyle interventions at home and in school should be part of the solution (Dumuid et al., 2018; Li, Zhang, Huang, & Chen, 2017; Roman-Viñas et al., 2016). For example, digital media time for children aged 2 to 5 years should be limited to no more than 1 hour per day to allow ample time for other activities and to establish healthy habits associated with lower rates of obesity (American Academy of Pediatrics Council on Communications

and Media, 2016). In addition, due to the evidence linking short sleep duration with obesity in children, adequate amounts of sleep should be recommended for all youth (Li et al., 2017). Sleep recommendations (including naps) for children 3 to 5 years, 6 to 12 years, and 13 to 18 years are 10 to 13 hours, 9 to 12 hours, and 8 to 10 hours per day, respectively (Paruthi et al., 2016). Proper sleep hygiene practices include turning off all screens 30 minutes before bedtime and avoiding stimulants such as caffeine during the late afternoon and evening.

DO YOU KNOW?

The presence of a television in the bedroom is directly related to the risk of obesity in children and adolescents.

Exercise Interventions for Overweight and Obese Youth

As discussed throughout this text, regular participation in both structured and unstructured physical activities offers observable health and fitness value to boys and girls. Even though children are physically and psychosocially less mature than adults, the benefits of regular physical activity are attainable by all participants regardless of age, body size, or level of maturity. The key is to design exercise interventions that are developmentally appropriate and consistent with individual needs, goals, and abilities so that all participants can gain competence and confidence in their physical abilities while also experiencing the sheer enjoyment of games, exercise, and sport activities.

Regular participation in exercise training can exert a positive effect on health and is an important component of youth weight management programs (García-Hermoso, González-Ruiz, Triana-Reina, Olloquequi, & Ramírez-Vélez, 2017; Kelley, Kelley, &

TABLE 14.2   STAGES OF PREVENTION FOR REDUCING HEALTH RISKS

Stage	Goal	Example
Primordial	Prevent the appearance of risk factors themselves.	Establish and reinforce healthy eating habits and physical activity behaviors early in life.
Primary	Reduce the presence of risk factors to prevent disease and improve health.	Provide nutrition and exercise counseling for an overweight child.
Secondary	Intervene to slow or stop the progression of a disease.	Provide diabetes screening for an obese child.
Tertiary	Control negative consequences of an established disease.	Provide clinical rehabilitation for an obese child with diabetes.

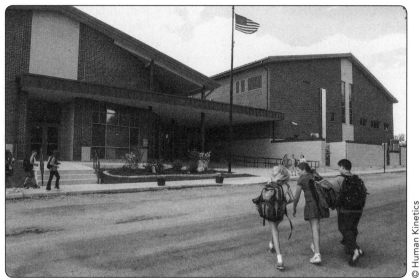

A walking school bus offers a healthy way for children to get to school.

Pate, 2017; Stoner et al., 2016). In addition to favorable changes in fat mass and lean body mass, regular exercise has been shown to lower elevated blood pressure, improve blood lipids, enhance metabolic health, and reduce carotid intima-media thickness in obese youth (Bea, Blew, Howe, Hetherington-Rauth, & Going, 2017; Dias, Green, Ingul, Pavey, & Coombes, 2015; García-Hermoso et al., 2019; Poitras et al., 2016). The potential psychosocial benefits of exercise for obese youth include improvements in mental functioning and health-related quality of life, and the greatest gains are observed in those with elevated symptoms (Davis et al., 2011; Eime, Young, Harvey, Charity, & Payne, 2013; Goldfield et al., 2015; Goldfield et al., 2017; Melnyk et al., 2015). The potential physical and psychosocial benefits of regular exercise for obese youth are shown in figure 14.3 (Bea et al., 2017; García-Hermoso, Ramírez-Vélez & Saavedra, 2019.; Goldfield et al., 2015; Han et al., 2017; Kelley et al., 2017; Zwolski, Quatman-Yates, & Paterno, 2017).

Youth fitness specialists are uniquely positioned to enhance the health and well-being of obese children and adolescents by helping them overcome barriers to physical activity and by preparing them for a lifetime of free play, exercise, and sport (see table 14.3). Traditional interventions include periods of aerobic exercise at a predetermined intensity, but overweight and obese youth are less willing and sometimes unable to participate in prolonged periods of endurance training. Obese youth tend to perceive physical activity negatively and may find sedentary activities more reinforcing than normal-weight youth (Salvy, Bowker, Germeroth, & Barkley, 2012). Moreover, excess body fat hinders the performance of weight-bearing physical

activity such as jogging and may increase the risk of musculoskeletal injury (McHugh, 2010). These observations underscore the importance of considering the type, intensity, frequency, and progression of exercise training when designing interventions for overweight and obese youth.

Although all youth should be physically active on all days of the week, obese youth often lack sufficient competence and confidence in their ability to engage in outdoor play and recreational games with energy and interest. Total physical activity is inversely associated with fat mass in youth, and the decline in MVPA tends to start early in life (Gillis, Kennedy, & Bar-Or, 2006; Schwarzfischer et al., 2018). Longitudinal findings indicate that higher levels of MVPA at age 6 or 7 years remain inversely associated with fat mass at age 11 years (Griffiths et al., 2016; Schwarzfischer et al., 2018). Given that overweight and obese children will not simply "outgrow" physical inactivity, inactive youth need exercise interventions that include neuromuscular training to "activate" them so that they can experience the physical and psychosocial benefits of regular exercise (Lloyd et al., 2015; Myer et al., 2011).

New insights into the design of pediatric weight management programs suggest that resistance training or combined aerobic and resistance training (e.g., circuit or interval training) can provide a safe, effective, and worthwhile method of conditioning for all youth, regardless of body size (Bharath et al., 2018; Dietz, Hoffmann, Lachtermann, & Simon, 2012; Jung et al., 2018; Marson et al., 2016; Sigal et al., 2014). Scientific reports and clinical observations support the contention that participation in multifaceted interventions that are engaging, challenging, and enjoyable provide overweight and obese youth with a chance to feel good about their accomplishments and experience the benefits of exercise training (Faigenbaum, 2009; Goldfield et al., 2015; Sigal et al., 2014). Obese youth tend to be relatively strong, because the excess body mass supported during daily activities seems to act as a chronic training stimulus. Consequently, the high adherence rates to interventions that include resistance training are not surprising, given that this type of exercise gives obese youth a chance to shine as they learn new exercises, experience success, and receive unsolicited feedback from their normal-weight peers, who are often impressed with the amount of weight they can lift.

Notwithstanding the potential benefits of aerobic training (e.g., walking, cycling, swimming) for health and fitness indicators in obese children and adolescents (Marson et al., 2016), youth fitness specialists should also recognize the unique benefits of resistance training for body composition and metabolic profiles in younger populations. Muscular strength has been found to be negatively associated with metabolic risk in youth (Gomes, Dos Santos, Katzmarzyk, & Maia, 2017; Steene-Johannessen, Anderssen, & Kolle, 2009), and longitudinal findings indicate that **phenotypes** of muscular fitness (i.e., muscular strength, power, and endurance) during childhood can be used to predict **metabolic syndrome** in adulthood (Fraser et al., 2016). The term *phenotype* refers to an individual's observable characteristics, which are influenced by one's genotype as well as environmental factors. Metabolic syndrome

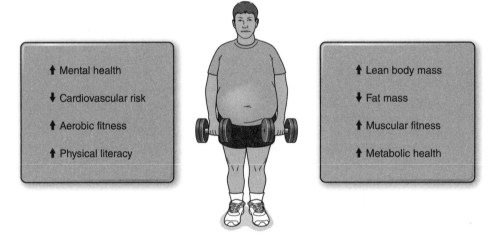

FIGURE 14.3   Potential benefits of regular exercise for overweight and obese youth.

TABLE 14.3   POTENTIAL BARRIERS TO EXERCISE IN OBESE YOUTH ALONG WITH ACTION STEPS

Potential barrier	Comment from child	Action step
Lack of energy	"I'm tired."	Schedule exercise when youth feel more energetic; perform shorter bouts; try outdoor activities.
Lack of motivation	"Exercise is boring."	Try an active game or challenging sport activity; add variety to the weekly exercise routine; identify personal goals.
Lack of skill	"I can't do it."	Develop basic movement skills and improve muscle strength; offer physical activity choices; emphasize enjoyable activities.
Lack of peer support	"My friends don't exercise."	Plan social events that involve physical activity; join a local recreation center; exercise with family members.
Weight bias	"People will tease me."	Increase socialization and shift the focus to healthy behaviors; try activities that highlight muscle strength.
Lack of time	"I'm too busy."	Add physical activity to daily routine; walk to school; play active games at recess; walk the dog; try exergaming instead of watching television.
Lack of parental involvement	"My parents don't exercise."	Inform parents about the importance of healthy lifestyle behaviors; encourage family fitness activities; infuse physical activity into the daily routine.

is a clustering of risk factors (including obesity, dyslipidemia, elevated blood pressure, and elevated fasting plasma glucose) that has been linked with cardiovascular disease and type 2 diabetes (Alberti et al., 2009). Because the benefits of resistance exercise for health and fitness markers in children and adolescents have been found to be independent of cardiorespiratory fitness (Smith et al., 2014), resistance exercise may be particularly beneficial during introductory programs to set the stage for more advanced exercise interventions as health and fitness improve.

These observations are clinically relevant because regular participation in exercise interventions that include resistance training have been shown to improve physical fitness, body composition, and metabolic health in overweight and obese youth (Alberga et al., 2015; Bea et al., 2017; Racil et al., 2016). Following 16 weeks of progressive resistance training that included loads greater than 85 percent of 1RM, researchers reported a significant decrease in body fat and a significant increase in insulin sensitivity along with a 96 percent adherence rate in overweight adolescents (Shaibi et al., 2006). Given that these metabolic adaptations remained significant after adjustment for changes in total fat mass and total lean mass, heavy resistance training likely resulted in qualitative changes in skeletal muscle that enhanced insulin action (Shaibi et al., 2006). In support of these findings, researchers have reported that 12 weeks of resistance training improved endothelial function, metabolic profiles, body composition, and physical fitness in obese adolescents (I. Dias et al., 2015). Indeed, the benefits of exclusive resistance training (without concurrent aerobic exercise) on overweight and obese youth extend beyond gains in muscular fitness and include favorable adaptations in cardiometabolic and musculoskeletal health (McGuigan, Tatasciore, Newton, & Pettigrew, 2009; Sothern et al., 2000; Yu et al., 2005).

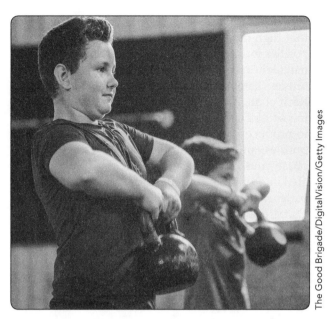

The Good Brigade/DigitalVision/Getty Images

Obese youth tend to enjoy resistance training because they are often the strongest participants in class.

Different types of exercise have been integrated into training programs for obese youth with the goal of enhancing metabolic health, improving body composition, and optimizing training-induced adaptations. Following 22 weeks of aerobic, resistance, or combined training, researchers reported reductions in percentage body fat following all types of training in obese adolescents, although combined training tended to be superior to aerobic training alone in more adherent youth (Sigal et al., 2014). Others found that the combination of aerobic and resistance training was more effective than aerobic training alone in improving visceral adiposity, metabolic profile, and inflammatory markers in obese adolescents following a one-year intervention (Dâmaso et al., 2014).

Teaching Tip

"THIN-FAT" KIDS

Although the benefits of exercise training for children and adolescents with a high BMI are well known, youth fitness specialists should not overlook the importance of daily MVPA for youth with an acceptable BMI but excess adiposity—the so-called "thin-fat phenotype" (Kurpad, Varadharajan, & Aeberli, 2011). Youth with this phenotype may look skinny, but they tend to have higher levels of fat, lower levels of physical fitness, and greater risk for cardiometabolic disease than children with normal body composition (Fairchild, Klakk, Heidemann, Andersen, & Wedderkopp, 2016). In addition, these youth may present with unhealthy lifestyle behaviors. Youth fitness specialists should recognize the clinical importance of enhancing cardiorespiratory and muscular fitness both in obese youth and in inactive boys and girls with an acceptable BMI.

In support of these findings, other researchers found that high-intensity interval training exerted a more positive influence on blood lipids, lean body mass, and metabolic measures in obese adolescent females than did less-intense training protocols (Racil et al., 2013; Racil et al., 2016). Collectively, interventions combining aerobic and resistance training have been found to produce favorable changes in fat mass, metabolic profiles, and inflammatory state in overweight and obese youth, and these changes tend to be accentuated in programs with higher exercise intensities and better exercise adherence (Costigan, Eather, Plotnikoff, Taaffe, & Lubans, 2015; Crisp, Fournier, Licari, Braham, & Guelfi, 2012; García-Hermoso, Ramírez-Vélez, et al., 2018; Jung et al., 2018).

Guidelines for Training Overweight and Obese Youth

Pediatric obesity is a challenging problem, and there is no single weight-management program with proven efficacy for all children and adolescents. The most effective treatment programs for obesity involve behavioral strategies aimed at increasing physical activity, enhancing food quality, improving sleep hygiene, and reducing screen time (Kumar & Kelly, 2017; Oude Luttikhuis et al., 2009; Poitras et al., 2016). Youth fitness specialists should recognize the value of multifaceted interventions that provide participants with an opportunity to develop healthy habits as an ongoing lifestyle choice. Exercise guidelines for overweight and obese youth are outlined in this section, and important concepts related to nutrition and healthy food choices are discussed in chapter 16.

Rather than focusing on "weight talk," pediatric weight management programs should emphasize establishing and maintaining healthy behaviors that reduce risk factors and promote a positive body image (Golden, Schneider, Wood, & AAP Committee on Nutrition, 2016; Shaibi, Ryder, Kim, & Barraza, 2015). With guidance and encouragement from parents, health care providers, and youth fitness specialists, participants in weight management programs can gain competence and confidence in a wide variety of physical abilities while improving their cardiometabolic and musculoskeletal health. In addition to improving overall body composition as a long-term goal, it is important in the short term to establish healthy lifestyle behaviors and reduce disease risk factors through habitual physical activity, including exercise training. In some cases, weight management (not weight loss) may be a desirable goal for overweight children because BMI will decrease as children grow (Barlow, 2007). Recommendations for weight loss and weight maintenance are outlined in table 14.4 (Barlow, 2007).

An integrated approach to pediatric weight management should include regular opportunities to participate in school- and community-based physical activities, including structured exercise training. However, obese youth often have low perceptions of their physical abilities and are less likely to participate actively in outdoor games, physical education, and fitness classes with energy and interest (Roura, Milà-Villarroel, Lucía Pareja, & Adot Caballero, 2016; Sampasa-Kanyinga, Hamilton, Willmore, & Chaput, 2017). In addition, weight-related teasing or struggling to complete an endurance run can understandably influence one's attitude toward and motivation to engage in exercise. Youth fitness specialists should be aware of these concerns and develop exercise interventions that are consistent with the physical and psychosocial needs of normal-weight youth as well as children and adolescents who are obese. In a fitness class or sport program, youth fitness specialists

TABLE 14.4　WEIGHT MAINTENANCE AND WEIGHT LOSS GOALS FOR OVERWEIGHT AND OBESE CHILDREN AND ADOLESCENTS

Age (yr)	BMI (percentile)	Weight goal
2-5	85-94	Weight maintenance or slow weight gain
	≥95	Weight maintenance (or weight loss up to 1 lb [0.45 kg]/mo if BMI >22)
6-11	85-94	Weight maintenance
	95-99	Gradual weight loss (1 lb/mo)
	>99	Weight loss (max 2 lb [0.9 kg]/wk)
12-18	85-94	Weight maintenance or gradual weight loss
	95-99	Weight loss (max 2 lb/wk)
	>99	Weight loss (max 2 lb/wk)

Adapted from Barlow (2007).

should address individual concerns, use appropriate language, and create a welcoming environment that accommodates youth of diverse body sizes.

In order to maximize the potential benefits of habitual physical activity for inactive children, practitioners should consider the type, intensity, tempo, and frequency of training when designing exercise interventions because these program variables can influence training outcomes and enjoyment of the exercise experience (Malik, Williams, Bond, Weston, & Barker, 2017; McMurray & Ondrak, 2013). According to research findings, exercise training that includes aerobic, resistance, or combined training can be safe and effective for overweight and obese youth (García-Hermoso, Cerrillo-Urbina, et al., 2018; Kelley et al., 2017; Marson et al., 2016). In addition, high-intensity interval training has been found to be effective for improving aerobic fitness, body composition, and cardiometabolic risk factors in obese youth (Thivel et al., 2019).

A variety of training modalities and combinations of exercises, sets, and repetitions have been shown to provide an adequate stimulus for favorable changes in body mass index, metabolic parameters, aerobic capacity, and muscle strength in overweight and obese youth (Bea et al., 2017; García-Hermoso, Cerrillo-Urbina, et al., 2016; Kelley et al., 2017; Schranz, Tomkinson, & Olds, 2013). Although low-intensity training is appropriate for beginners who need to learn safe training procedures while gaining confidence in their physical abilities, moderate to higher intensities may eventually be needed in order to optimize training adaptations in youth (Fiorilli et al., 2017; García-Hermoso, Cerrillo-Urbina, et al., 2016; Racil et al., 2016; Thivel et al., 2018). Notably, recreational football and high-intensity interval training elicited similar improvements in muscular and cardiovascular fitness measures in overweight and obese children (Cvetković et al., 2018). However,

all youth programs need to be carefully prescribed and sensibly progressed in order to reduce the risk of injury, maintain exercise adherence, and establish long-lasting behavior change.

Program Design Considerations for Youth Weight Management

When designing pediatric weight management programs, youth fitness specialists should consider the age of the child, maturity level, training experience, severity of obesity, related comorbidities, and parental support. Parents often provide the impetus for initiating a program, and they are often driven by concerns about their child's psychological health and well-being (Kelleher et al., 2017). Youth fitness specialists should speak with parents about their concerns because active engagement, modeling of desirable behaviors, and ongoing support are critical to the long-term success of any pediatric weight management program (Kelleher et al., 2017; Næss, Holmen, Langaas, Bjørngaard, & Kvaløy, 2016). Since parents may face barriers to managing their child's weight status, practitioners should show parents how to infuse physical activity into their lifestyles so that it becomes part of the family routine. Outdoor play, an afternoon at the playground, or small-sided games of basketball can provide an enjoyable activity that increases daily energy expenditure while providing an opportunity to practice and reinforce motor skills developed during structured exercise training.

Although habitual physical activity (e.g., walking to school, using the stairs) is beneficial and should be encouraged, it may be insufficient to bring about significant changes in cardiometabolic disease risk factors (McMurray & Ondrak, 2013). Therefore, we

Teaching Tip

CLINICAL SCREENING

Clinical evaluation of an obese child or adolescent is geared toward identifying the causes of obesity and related comorbidities (U.S. Preventive Services Task Force et al., 2017). The evaluation typically includes a medical history, physical examination, dietary history, and physical activity assessment. The clinician may also ask questions about participation in outdoor play, physical education, school recess, after-school activities, and organized sport as well as nonacademic screen time (e.g., with a television, tablet, or video game) in order to aid in designing exercise interventions consistent with individual interests and abilities. It may also be helpful to gain understanding of emotional comorbidities associated with obesity, including weight-based bullying and depression, in order to address damaging weight stigma (Pont et al., 2017).

Teaching Tip

WORDS MATTER

Exercise programs for youth who are obese should include ongoing guidance and encouragement from youth fitness specialists. Instead of negative comments and sarcastic remarks, practitioners should use language and strategies that educate, inspire, and empower. Accordingly, neutral terms such as *unhealthy body weight* and *unhealthy lifestyle* are preferred over more loaded terms such as *obese* and *fat* (Hirschfeld-Dicker, Samuel, Tiram Vakrat, Dubnov-Raz, 2019; Pont et al., 2017). In addition, motivational interviewing is a patient-centered technique that can help obese youth explore ambivalence, express their thoughts, and take responsibility for their own actions, all of which may promote healthy behavior changes (Resnicow et al., 2016; Wong & Cheng, 2013). By asking open-ended questions, providing affirmations, listening reflectively, and talking about the pros and cons of change, youth fitness specialists can help facilitate lifestyle modification. The manner in which practitioners talk with youth really does matter.

need to distinguish public health recommendations (e.g., accumulating ≥60 min of daily MVPA) from prescribed exercise programs that target specific fitness outcomes and clinical measures. Although there is no established minimum age for participation in pediatric weight management programs that include structured exercise, obese children as young as five years old have benefited from exercise training in supervised settings (Tan, Chen, Sui, Xue, & Wang, 2017). Regardless of age or program goals, exercise interventions should provide an opportunity for all participants to gain competence and confidence in their physical abilities so that they are able to perform more complex and intense bouts of exercise as the program is progressed over time.

Aerobic exercise such as walking and cycling has been found to be associated with improvements in cardiovascular health in obese children and adolescents (Corte de Araujo et al., 2012; Marson et al., 2016). In addition to reducing CIMT (García-Hermoso et al., 2017), regular aerobic training lasting four to 12 weeks is associated with improvements in cardiometabolic risk factors in obese youth (Marson et al., 2016; García-Hermoso et al., 2019). Yet some obese youth may be unable or less willing to participate in prolonged periods of moderate to vigorous aerobic exercise without rest. Therefore, interval-type games and exercise programs that include higher-intensity bouts of both aerobic and resistance training may be a worthwhile approach because it is characterized by short bouts of physical activity interspersed with brief rest periods, which is more consistent with how youth move and play (Bond, Weston, Williams, & Barker, 2017; Thivel et al., 2019). Youth may find high-intensity interval training to be more enjoyable than continuous aerobic exercise due to feelings of reward, excitement, and success (Malik, Williams, Weston, & Barker, 2018). Table 14.5 outlines sample beginner and advanced exercise programs for overweight and obese youth.

Many factors influence the willingness of an obese child to commence and continue an exercise program, including the opportunity to build strength, improve fitness, and experience pleasant social interaction with peers and youth fitness specialists (Pescud, Pettigrew, McGuigan, & Newton, 2010). The following steps for success provide a series of ideas for encouraging participation in physical activity as an ongoing lifestyle choice.

Step 1. Activate and Motivate

If youth fitness specialists underestimate the physical abilities of overweight and obese youth and gradually increase the intensity and volume of exercise training, participants are less likely to drop out or suffer an injury. The goals of youth fitness programming should extend beyond gains in physical fitness and include teaching participants about healthy behaviors, promoting safe training procedures, and sparking an ongoing interest in daily physical activity. Instead of employing a pass-fail mentality that may discourage youth from participating, practitioners should view the exercise session as a challenge in which all participants have an opportunity to feel good about their performance and get excited about their progress. Accordingly, emphasis on guaranteed outcomes should be limited, and the focus should be placed instead on intrinsic factors such as skill improvement, personal successes, and positive peer relationships. Youth fitness specialists should teach participants how to perform exercises correctly and should introduce the concept of a fitness workout that includes warm-up, conditioning, and cool-down phases. The first few weeks of the program are critical to forming meaningful connections with each participant in order to build a strong foundation for more advanced training in the future. In short, habitual physical activity does not guarantee favorable changes in health-

TABLE 14.5   SAMPLE BEGINNER AND ADVANCED EXERCISE PROGRAMS FOR OVERWEIGHT AND OBESE YOUTH

| Session phase | BEGINNER | | ADVANCED | | COACHING TIP |
	Time (min)	Sample exercises	Time (min)	Sample exercises	Create a welcoming and nonstigmatizing area.
Dynamic warm-up	5	Medicine ball (1-2 kg) movements	10	Body-weight and medicine ball (2-3 kg) movements	Observe mobility and skill level; set a positive tone.
Movement preparation	5	Demonstration and practice of proper exercise technique	5	Review and reinforcement of technique-driven progression	Identify session goals and exercise modifications.
Circuit training	15-20	6-10 exercise stations using body weight, medicine balls, elastic bands, and dumbbells; moderate intensity; 30 sec exercise to 30 sec rest	25-30	10-15 exercise stations using body weight, medicine balls, fitness ropes, and dumbbells; moderate to high intensity; 30-60 sec exercise to 30 sec rest	Monitor subjective exercise perceptions and any physical discomfort; modify exercise or rest interval if needed.
Games	5	Moderate-intensity skill-building activities with balls and balloons	10	Higher-intensity aerobic and sport activities	Foster inclusion with team-building activities.
Cool-down	5	Static and dynamic stretching	5	Static and dynamic stretching	Reflect on positive achievements; seek feedback; listen to concerns.

and fitness-related measures; rather, any adaptations that take place will be determined by individual effort combined with qualified instruction, realistic goals, enthusiastic leadership, and a well-designed training program.

Step 2. Be Strong and Fit

Exercise for obese youth should include resistance training to increase neuromuscular fitness, which may in turn lead to gains in motor skill performance, desirable changes in body composition, and improvements in health-related measures (Behringer, Vom Heede, Matthews, & Mester, 2011; Thivel et al., 2016; García-Hermoso et al., 2019). These training-induced adaptations are particularly important for obese youth, who typically have only limited experience with organized exercise programs. Although excess adiposity can hinder the performance of weight-bearing aerobic exercises and body-weight resistance exercises (e.g., pull-ups, push-ups), it does not hamper weight-machine exercises or selected free-weight and medicine ball exercises. The choice of exercise is an important consideration when designing programs for obese youth who have limited experience with resistance training. Instead of walking on a treadmill for 30

minutes, obese youth may enjoy and benefit from a circuit training session that includes shorter bouts of higher-intensity exercise interspersed with brief rest periods as needed (Thivel et al., 2019). This type of choice is where the art and science of designing pediatric weight management programs come into play, because the fundamental principles of exercise science must be balanced with the individual needs and physical abilities of overweight and obese youth in order to reduce boredom, enhance exercise adherence, and optimize training outcomes.

Step 3: Integrate, Don't Isolate

There is no single combination of aerobic and resistance training that will promote favorable adaptations in cardiometabolic parameters and body composition in all obese youth, but the integration of various exercise intensities and training modalities into youth programs will likely yield the most favorable changes (Buchan et al., 2011; Dâmaso et al., 2014; García-Hermoso, Cerrillo-Urbina, et al., 2018; Sigal et al., 2014). Aqua aerobics, resistance training, recreational sports, and outdoor games all offer health- and fitness-related benefits for obese youth. In one study, a 12-week recreational soccer intervention consisting of 60-minute sessions performed three times per week improved cardiometabolic and physical fitness markers in obese youth (Vasconcellos et al., 2016). By integrating whole-body exercises into a program and varying the intensity and volume of training over time, participants continue to be challenged, and the training stimulus continues to be effective.

Step 4: Foster Inclusion

All children and adolescents should be encouraged to adopt a healthy lifestyle and should be given multiple opportunities throughout the day to participate in games, exercise, and sport activities. It may be difficult, however, for obese youth to participate in these activities, due to weight stigma, teasing, and negative instructional experiences (Pont et al., 2017; Rukavina & Doolittle, 2016; Salvy et al., 2012). Indeed, obese youth may be asked to participate in exercise activities that are embarrassing or too difficult, which will likely lead to disinterest and dropping out. Consequently, youth fitness specialists need to foster inclusion for obese youth and facilitate positive peer relationships and experiences for all participants. To create an inclusive climate in the exercise area, practitioners can review rules and expectations, highlight the strengths and abilities of obese children, and publically recognize prosocial behavior. They can also allow an obese child to rest between activities and, when appropriate, provide choices among activities or exercises. It may also be worthwhile to talk with the class about different body sizes in various sports—for instance, American football, rugby, gymnastics, and soccer.

Although all participants should be held accountable for their actions and behaviors, youth fitness specialists should foster social inclusion by encouraging peer relationships that help obese youth feel worthwhile. Since obese youth tend to spend more time alone than normal-weight youth, the novelty of interacting with others in an exercise class has the potential to improve their exercise performance (Salvy et al., 2012). In some cases, private or small-group exercise training may provide an opportunity to address specific needs and concerns.

Step 5: Think Long-Term

Scientific evidence supports participation in structured exercise training for obese youth, although long-term adherence to lifestyle interventions remains challenging (Danielsson, Bohlin A., Bendito, Svensson, & Klaesson, 2016; Khalsa, Kharofa, Ollberding, Bishop, & Copeland, 2017; Theim et al., 2013). Degree of obesity is a predictor of treatment outcomes, and the longer a child is obese the less likely it is that treatments will work (Danielsson, Kowalski, Ekblom, & Marcus, 2012). Without a sustained commitment to healthy behaviors at home and at school, it is less likely that lifestyle-induced benefits will stick. Maintaining healthy habits throughout childhood and adolescence is likely to require effective long-term intervention strategies and ongoing support from parents, health care providers, school administrators, and fitness professionals. In addition, the importance of identifying and managing this disease early in life must be underscored because the age at start of treatment has been found to affect treatment efficacy (Danielsson et al., 2016).

Summary

The growing prevalence of obesity in youth is associated with serious physical and psychosocial comorbidities that directly affect the health and well-being of youth and their families. If left untreated, this disease may shorten the life span of the current generation. Managing it requires sustained, multifaceted interventions and ongoing support from families, school administrators, fitness professionals, and health care providers. In addition to encouraging habitual physical activity throughout the day, exercise programs should be prescribed to foster favorable changes in body composition, enhance cardiometabolic health, and promote improvements in psychosocial well-being. Although different types of MVPA can offer health-related benefits for obese youth, the performance of both aerobic and resistance exercise at moderate to high intensity has been found to result in favorable training outcomes. Youth fitness specialists are uniquely positioned to design, implement, and progress exercise training programs that are consistent with the needs, interests, and body size of youth who are overweight or obese.

CHAPTER 15

Exercise for Youth With Selected Clinical Conditions

CHAPTER OBJECTIVES

- Understand the physical and psychosocial benefits of exercise for youth with clinical conditions
- Identify barriers to and facilitators of participation in exercise programs for youth with clinical conditions
- Describe appropriate exercise training strategies for youth with clinical conditions
- Gain insights into designing exercise programs for youth with asthma, diabetes, and physical or intellectual disabilities

KEY TERMS

asthma (p. 303)

acetone (p. 307)

bronchoconstriction (p. 303)

diabetes mellitus (p. 306)

diabetic ketoacidosis (p. 307)

differentiation (p. 303)

exercise-induced bronchospasm (p. 304)

glycolated hemoglobin (p. 307)

hyperglycemia (p. 306)

hyperinsulinemia (p. 307)

hypoglycemia (p. 308)

insulin resistance (p. 307)

intellectual disability (p. 311)

ketoacidosis (p. 307)

metabolic syndrome (p. 307)

physical disability (p. 310)

polydipsia (p. 307)

polyuria (p. 307)

prediabetes (p. 307)

Introduction

Physical activity is important for all children and adolescents regardless of physical prowess or intellectual ability (Bar-Or & Rowland, 2004; Riner & Hunt Sellhorst, 2017). Regular participation in active play, structured exercise, and competitive sport is positively associated with favorable changes in physical fitness, cognitive development, and psychosocial well-being (de Greeff, Bosker, Oosterlaan, Visscher, & Hartman, 2018; Donnelly et al., 2016; Korczak, Madigan, & Colasanto, 2017; Poitras et al., 2016; Spruit, Assink, van Vugt, van der Put, & Stams, 2016). Yet most children and adolescents are not as active as they should be, and those with clinical conditions are less active, more sedentary, and at greater risk for obesity than their typically developing peers (Einarsson, Jóhannsson, Daly, & Arngrímsson, 2016; Papas, Trabulsi, Axe, & Rimmer, 2016; Rimmer & Marques, 2012; Shields & Synnot, 2016; Sit et al., 2017; Tremblay et al., 2016). Although broadly defined, clinical conditions include a variety of diseases, disabilities, and impairments that affect physical functioning, psychosocial well-being, and lifestyle behaviors.

In light of the increasing prevalence of clinical conditions among children and adolescents (Mayer-Davis, Lawrence, Dabelea, Divers, Isom, Dolan, et al., 2017; Pulcini, Zima, Kelleher, & Houtrow, 2017; Van Cleave, Gortmaker, & Perrin, 2010), targeted interventions are needed to enhance the health and well-being of all youth. Without opportunities to be physically active at school and in the community, youth with clinical conditions are more likely to suffer from negative health outcomes as the divergence between those with lower and higher levels of physical fitness will likely widen over time (Bloemen et al., 2015; Hands, 2008; Magnussen et al., 2012; McMurray, Harrell, Creighton, Wang, & Bangdiwala, 2008; Poitras et al., 2016). Daily physical activity that is consistent with individual needs and abilities can help reduce the physical, psychosocial, and economic burden associated with poor health (Lee, 2017; Poitras et al., 2016; Shields & Synnot, 2016). From a public health perspective, increasing physical activity among all children and adolescents, including those with clinical conditions, has become a top priority (U.S. Department of Health and Human Services, 2016; World Health Organization, 2018).

Although some clinical conditions, including physical and intellectual disabilities, are present from the developmental period of life, others, such as diabetes, can be subclinical for many years before surfacing as a recognizable clinical condition. Regardless of the disease or disorder, a primary goal for youth fitness specialists is to spark a lifelong interest in exercise and sport through daily participation in both less structured physical activities (e.g., outdoor play) and more structured ones (e.g., sport practice). Although general recommendations for increasing physical activity are appropriate for most children and adolescents, youth fitness specialists should be aware of the complexities and concerns associated with designing exercise interventions for youth with clinical conditions. Practitioners need to understand the diseases, disabilities, and impairments that are common in pediatric populations and develop awareness of the potential benefits of physical activity in order to optimize the safety, efficacy, and enjoyment of exercise and sport activities for all participants. Not only can youth with clinical conditions experience the physical and psychosocial benefits of regular exercise, but also a physically active lifestyle may help to manage their clinical conditions and improve their quality of life.

Some clinical conditions may limit participation in exercise and sport activities, and youth fitness specialists should approach such conditions as a challenge and develop strategies to overcome misperceptions, break down barriers, and forge pathways that encourage ongoing participation as youth gain competence and confidence in their physical abilities. Participation in physical activity can be facilitated by early interventions that develop fundamental movement skills, encourage socialization, promote inclusion, and educate families about the importance of daily physical activity (Jaarsma, Dijkstra, Geertzen, & Dekker, 2014; Shields & Synnot, 2016). Potential barriers, on the other hand, include dependence on others, poor instructor skills, lack of local opportunities, time constraints, and unwillingness to be inclusive (Shields & Synnot, 2016; Wright, Roberts, Bowman, & Crettenden, 2018). Another potential barrier reported by pediatricians is their own lack of knowledge about youth exercise guidelines (Carson, Barnes, LeBlanc, Moreau, & Tremblay, 2017). Strategies for overcoming barriers to physical activity are outlined in table 15.1.

Given the importance of promoting participation in exercise and sport activities, youth fitness specialists are well-suited to confer with health care providers to design and implement interventions for children and adolescents with clinical conditions. Indeed, youth fitness specialists are integral to the Exercise Is Medicine campaign spearheaded by the American College of Sports Medicine and are uniquely qualified to provide education and training related to pediatric exercise in order to promote active lifestyles early in life. In addition, by educating parents and caregivers about the critical importance of regular physical activity, and by identifying barriers to and facilitators of exercise and sport programs, youth fitness specialists can help

TABLE 15.1   OVERCOMING BARRIERS TO PHYSICAL ACTIVITY FOR INACTIVE YOUTH

Barrier	Action step
Lack of knowledge about the importance of physical activity	Educate youth, parents, and caregivers about potential benefits of physical activity and gain support from health care providers.
Fear of participating in exercise or sport activities	Screen youth for participation, seek qualified instruction, and modify activity as needed.
Lack of convenient access to fitness facilities	Find a local playground, go to a nearby park, and ask about after-school programs.
Perception that exercise is boring	Exercise with friends and family, play new games and activities, or try shorter bouts of active play at various times of day.
Lack of confidence in physical abilities	Take an exercise class, practice with a sport coach, or try activities such as walking or cycling.
Fear of injury	Follow safety rules, develop proper technique, and seek guidance when needed.
Weather	Play inside, dance with friends, or find a school or center that offers indoor activities.
Time constraints	Shorten exercise bouts to 10 or 15 minutes and incorporate daily physical activity such as walking and stair climbing into your routine.

provide equal access to activity-friendly programs in schools and the local community. Proactive teaching or coaching that gives participants with different needs the opportunity to learn, engage, and participate effectively regardless of ability or disability is referred to as **differentiation**.

Although the benefits of a physically active lifestyle are observable across clinical populations regardless of age or health condition, this chapter provides specific insights for designing exercise programs for youth with asthma, diabetes, or physical or intellectual disabilities (obesity is addressed in chapter 14). Children and adolescents with these clinical conditions respond favorably to exercise training, and youth fitness specialists often work in exercise, recreation, and sport centers in which youth may present with these conditions. Regular physical activity may also benefit youth with other clinical conditions—including cancer (Rustler et al., 2017; San Juan, Wolin, & Lucía, 2011), cerebral palsy (Kim, Kim, Yang, Lee, & Koh, 2017; Verschuren, Peterson, Balemans, & Hurvitz, 2016), and depression (Bailey, Hetrick, Rosenbaum, Purcell, & Parker, 2018; Korczak et al., 2017)—and youth fitness specialists are encouraged to seek additional information when designing and supervising exercise programs for children and adolescents with those conditions. In any case, the guidelines and recommendations presented in this chapter should be adopted with sound clinical judgment because responses and adaptations to exercise training are unique to each participant.

Asthma

Asthma is a chronic pulmonary condition that affects millions of children and adolescents worldwide (Akinbami, Simon, & Rossen, 2016; de Aguiar, Anzolin, & Zhang, 2018). This clinical condition is an inflammatory disorder characterized by periodic episodes of **bronchoconstriction** and airflow limitation that are often reversible (Philpott, Houghton, & Luke, 2010). Bronchoconstriction involves narrowing of the airways in the lungs caused by tightening of surrounding smooth muscle. Typical symptoms of asthma include wheezing, coughing, shortness of breath, and chest tightness (Moore, Durstein, & Painter, 2016; Philpott et al., 2010). Although there is no cure for asthma, it can be managed through pharmacological and nonpharmacological strategies including regular exercise. Without medical therapy and compliance with treatment plans, youth who suffer from severe asthma are at greater risk for respiratory distress and sudden death (Gullach et al., 2015; Nievas & Anand, 2013).

DO YOU KNOW?

Asthma is a common reason for missing school and can lead to poor academic performance and reduced quality of life (Hsu, Qin, Beavers, & Mirabelli, 2016).

Asthmatic events are typically triggered by allergens such as animal dander, mold, pollen, and smoke, although symptoms may also be associated with breathing cold or dry air (Moore et al., 2016). In some youth, asthma symptoms may be exacerbated by physical exertion, which results in a condition called **exercise-induced bronchospasm** (EIB). The phenomenon of EIB is characterized by a transient narrowing of the airways that occurs during or after exercise. Clinicians can diagnosis EIB by assessing changes in lung function provoked by an exercise challenge (Caggiano, Cutrera, Di Marco, & Turchetta, 2017). EIB can also occur in children with normal airways who do not appear to have asthma (Molis & Molis, 2010; Wanrooij, Willeboordse, Dompeling, & van de Kant, 2014), in which case it is referred to as EIB without apparent asthma (Moore et al., 2016).

Although we do not yet fully understand the pathophysiology by which exercise can cause an asthma attack or a sudden worsening of symptoms, the mechanisms likely relate to the heating and drying of the airways during exercise, which can lead to respiratory water loss (Molis & Molis, 2010). In turn, the water loss from the airway surface can cause a change in the concentration or osmolarity of the airway surface liquid, which can trigger a release of inflammatory mediators including histamines, cytokines, and leukotrienes (Anderson & Kippelen, 2008; Carlsen, Anderson, & Bjermer, 2008). This proinflammatory response, along with airway dehydration, can result in an early airway closure that reduces the forced expiratory volume in the first second (FEV_1). This type of obstructive limitation can trigger symptoms and limit exercise performance.

EIB may also be related to airway epithelial injury from breathing a high volume of irritant gases or particles (Anderson & Kippelen, 2008). For example, breathing air saturated with chlorine from pool water or ultrafine particles from ice resurfacing machines in ice rinks can lead to alterations in smooth muscle contractile properties and consequent bronchoconstriction (Anderson & Kippelen, 2008; Kanikowska, Napiórkowska-Baran, Graczyk, & Kucharski, 2018).

Managing Asthma in Youth

Once a child has been properly diagnosed with asthma, the key is to take the necessary steps to manage the condition in order to minimize the occurrence of asthmatic events. When asthma is well controlled, the child has minimal or no symptoms, makes minimal use of quick-relief inhalers (e.g., albuterol), and is subject to no limitations on physical activity. Allergy testing can identify environmental triggers and raise awareness about the importance of avoiding potential irritants, such as cat dander, dust mites, and seasonal allergens. In addition, most youth with asthma use medication either daily or prophylactically to reduce airway inflammation and provide bronchoprotection during physical activities. Inhaled corticosteroids (e.g., flunisolide) often serve as the first line of therapy for asthma because they can reduce inflammation, swelling, and mucus production in the airways. In some cases, additional medications may be needed as add-on therapies.

Because fear of an asthma attack can be a major barrier to exercise, educating youth and their parents about preventive inhalers and the differences between exercise-induced breathlessness and asthma symptoms may increase participation in exercise and sport programs (Jago R., Searle, Henderson, & Turner, 2017; Winn et al., 2018). It may also help to note that the World Anti-Doping Association permits the use of selected inhaled steroids, provided that the athlete has a therapeutic-use exemption certificate; however, all oral and injected B-adrenoceptor agonists are prohibited unless the athlete has a declaration-of-use certificate.

Youth who have asthma that is properly controlled should be encouraged to participate in exercise and sport programs due to the overall beneficial effects, which include more days free from asthma symptoms, which of course reduces the need for asthma medications (Andrade, Britto, Lucena-Silva, Gomes, & Figueroa, 2014; Basaran et al., 2006; Crosbie, 2012; Eichenberger, Diener, Kofmehl, & Spengler, 2013; Wanrooij et al., 2014). Although additional research is needed about the effects of exercise training on airway inflammation and bronchial hyperresponsiveness, aerobic exercise or a combination of aerobic exercise and resistance training have been found to decrease the severity of EIB by raising the threshold for triggering bronchospasm (Fanelli, Cabral, Neder, Martins, & Carvalho, 2007; Philpott et al., 2010). In another study, following 16 weeks of supervised aerobic exercise and resistance training performed twice per week, children with moderate to severe asthma made significant improvements in physical fitness and saw reductions in the severity of EIB and postexercise breathlessness (Fanelli et al., 2007). These findings are supported by others who reported significant improvements in aerobic fitness or quality of life following 16 weeks of aerobic games and strength building activities (Lu, Cooper, Haddad, & Randon-Aizik, 2018), 8 weeks of moderately intensive basketball training (Basaran et al., 2006) or 6 weeks of active play in children with asthma (Westergren et al., 2016). Although different types of physical activity have been explored as ancillary interventions for youth with asthma—for example, tai chi chuan (Lin et al., 2017) and breathing exercises (Macêdo, Freitas,

Teaching Tip

INCLUSIVE APPROACH

An inclusive approach to physical activity hinges on the overarching concept that all children and adolescents should have an opportunity to participate in developmentally appropriate physical activities while learning new skills, making friends, and experiencing the joy of active play and exercise (Hastie & Martin, 2006; National Association for Sport and Physical Education, 2011). Because youth with clinical conditions may lack confidence in their physical abilities and may have fewer social connections than their peers in the program, youth fitness specialists need to foster an inclusive environment in which all youth can participate safely and feel protected from social embarrassment and repeated failure. Practitioners should facilitate inclusion by addressing individual needs, modifying games and activities as appropriate, and collaborating with others because the benefits of learning from people who differ from ourselves can be meaningful and long-lasting.

Chaves, Holloway, & Mendonça, 2016)—exercise and sport training that enhance aerobic fitness have been the primary nonpharmacological approach for managing asthma in children and adolescents.

Exercise Guidelines for Youth With Asthma

Both asthma and obesity have become more prevalent over the past few decades, and it is not uncommon for children with persistent asthma to be physically inactive (Holderness et al., 2017; Lochte, Nielsen, Petersen, & Platts-Mills, 2016; Willeboordse, van de Kant, van der Velden, van Schayck, & Dompeling, 2016). In addition, some youth with asthma or EIB may become symptomatic during or after participating in exercise or sport and, understandably, may self-limit their participation in physical activity (Glazebrook et al., 2006; Winn et al., 2018). Because children with low levels of physical activity face an increased risk of new-onset asthma (Lochte et al., 2016), practitioners need to help youth adhere to exercise interventions by providing them with opportunities to gradually improve their physical fitness before engaging in prolonged periods of exercise training. High adherence to therapeutic interventions for managing asthma can lower a child's odds of experiencing an asthma event (Guarnaccia et al., 2016; Guarnaccia et al., 2017).

DO YOU KNOW?

Exercise-induced bronchospasm is the most common chronic condition among Olympic athletes (Couto et al., 2018).

When designing exercise interventions for youth with asthma, youth fitness specialists should limit exposure to environmental allergens, cold weather, and unaccustomed bouts of strenuous exercise.

Although children and adolescents with well-controlled asthma can participate in various types of physical activity, practitioners should consider a variety of exercise and sport activities based on the desired type of physical effort, ventilatory demands, and environmental factors. Most team sports (e.g., basketball, field hockey, soccer) are characterized by brief bouts of high-intensity effort and tend to be well tolerated. Although youth with stable asthma can benefit from participation in sports such as swimming (Beggs et al., 2013; Lahart & Metsios, 2018), long-distance events may be more challenging. Practitioners should consider the potential for problems related to chlorine-based irritants in pool water; in fact, some evidence links pool use with asthma development (Andersson et al., 2015; Bernard, Nickmilder, & Dumont, 2015).

The exercise guidelines discussed in parts I and II of this text are appropriate for most children and adolescents who have asthma that is properly controlled (National Institute for Health and Clinical Excellence, 2013). Notwithstanding the importance of aerobic exercise for youth with asthma, resistance training may also be beneficial as a way to counter the potential adverse effects of long-term corticosteroid use, which can include growth retardation and reduced bone mineral density (Aljebab, Choonara, & Conroy, 2017; Skoner, 2016). Regular participation in weight-bearing physical activities during the growing years has been found to build bone mass and enhance bone structure (Gómez-Bruton, Matute-Llorente, González-Agüero, Casajús, & Vicente-Rodríguez, 2017; Larsen et al., 2018), and these osteogenic effects may offset the adverse effects of selected asthma medications.

In addition, a variable-intensity (i.e., interval) warm-up that is well designed may reduce the likelihood of exercise-induced asthma symptoms in some individuals (Mtshali, Mokwena, & Oguntibeju, 2015; Stickland, Rowe, Spooner, Vandermeer, & Dryden, 2013). Therefore, it may be appropriate to gradually

Teaching Tip

ASTHMA ACTION PLAN

Youth fitness specialists should become familiar with each participant's asthma action plan in order to improve parent and child understanding of asthma management, enhance adherence to physical activity recommendations, optimize asthma-related outcomes, and plan for emergencies. An asthma action plan provides instructions for avoiding asthma triggers, taking medications, treating symptoms, and seeking medical care (National Heart, Lung, and Blood Institute & National Asthma Education and Prevention Program, 2007). The signs and symptoms of a severe asthma attack requiring emergency medical care include gasping for air, consistent wheezing, bluish lips, lack of improvement after using a rescue inhaler, and chest retractions (in which areas below the ribs appear "sucked in" during inhalation). An asthma action plan is recognized as an important component of high-quality asthma care, but adherence tends to be poor in primary care practice (Yawn, Rank, Cabana, Wollan, & Juhn, 2016). Youth fitness specialists should support health care efforts by teaching youth how to effectively manage their condition through healthy lifestyle choices that include regular physical activity. A sample asthma action plan is available from the Allergy and Asthma Foundation of America at www.aafa.org.

introduce bouts of higher-intensity exercise into the warm-up. It may also be worthwhile for young athletes with asthma to perform warm-up activities 45 to 60 minutes before the scheduled event because the lingering effects of warm-up exercises may reduce subsequent asthmatic symptoms (Philpott et al., 2010). Finally, efforts to sustain participation in exercise and sport through group activities and team games may be particularly important for youth with asthma because the physiological benefits of physical activity are most apparent following three months of training (Lu, Cooper, Haddad, & Radom-Aizik, 2018; Wanrooij et al., 2014; Winn et al., 2018).

Program design considerations for youth with asthma are outlined in figure 15.1.

Diabetes Mellitus

Diabetes mellitus (DM) refers to a group of metabolic disorders characterized by abnormally high blood glucose (blood sugar) levels—a condition referred to as **hyperglycemia**. There are four types of diabetes mellitus based on etiologic origin. Type 1 diabetes mellitus (T1DM) typically begins early in life and is most often caused by autoimmune destruction of the insulin-producing beta cells of the pancreas. Type 2 diabetes mellitus (T2DM) is the most common form and is characterized by an insulin secretory defect combined with insulin resistance in skeletal muscle, adipose tissue, and liver tissue. The third type is gestational diabetes mellitus, which is diagnosed during pregnancy, and the fourth type is caused by other specific origins such as genetics or medication (American College of Sports Medicine, 2018; American Diabetes Association, 2015). Some youth do not fit clearly into a T1DM or T2DM category, and disease progression

can vary considerably among individuals. This section focuses only on T1DM and T2DM.

The precursor to DM is **prediabetes**, which may go unrecognized for years because it lacks distinct symptoms despite elevated blood glucose values. Youth with prediabetes are at increased risk for developing T2DM and other serious health problems, including cardiovascular disease. Useful diagnostic tests are based on fasting plasma glucose levels and **glycolated hemoglobin** (HbA1C), which reflects average blood glucose control over the past two to three months (American Diabetes Association, 2015). Because a fasting plasma glucose test provides information about blood sugar levels only at a specific point in time, glycolated hemoglobin provides a better indication of glycemic control. Table 15.2 outlines diagnostic criteria for prediabetes and DM in youth and adults; it can also be important to consider possible effects of age, race, and ethnicity when screening for or diagnosing clinical conditions.

Although various mechanisms may be responsible for DM, the primary factors include defects in insulin secretion from the pancreas and deficits in the body's ability to use insulin. T1DM is caused by a near absolute insulin deficiency; therefore, an external source of insulin is required. Individuals with T1DM have a higher tendency to develop **diabetic ketoacidosis**, which is a serious complication arising from lack of insulin. If the cells in the body cannot receive glucose for energy, the body burns fat for energy and consequently produces high levels of ketones, which make blood more acidic. Typical symptoms of diabetic ketoacidosis include hyperglycemia, fatigue, **polyuria** (frequent urination), **polydipsia** (increased thirst), and **acetone** breath (fruity odor) (American College of Sports Medicine, 2018). Ketones include acetone (the same chemical used in nail

FIGURE 15.1   PROGRAM DESIGN CONSIDERATIONS FOR YOUTH WITH ASTHMA

- Try to avoid asthma triggers, such as cold weather and high allergen counts.
- If exercising in cold weather, place a scarf or face mask over the mouth and nose.
- Use medication before physical activity if instructed to do so by a health care provider.
- Warm up sufficiently before exercise and sport activities.
- Start exercising at a low or moderate intensity and progress gradually.
- Advance exercise intensity to the personalized ventilatory threshold (about 80% of maximum HR).
- Include at least two 60-minute training sessions per week.
- Monitor asthma symptoms and exposure to triggers.
- Reduce exercise intensity if asthma symptoms appear.
- Carry a rescue inhaler and know how to use it.
- If at an elite level, consult with a physician to review asthma medications.

polish remover) that can cause breath to smell sweet. Diabetic **ketoacidosis** is potentially life-threatening and requires immediate medical care.

Common features of T2DM, on the other hand, include excess adiposity and **insulin resistance**, which is a pathological condition characterized by the inability to achieve normal levels of blood glucose in response to insulin. Because insulin-resistant cells are less sensitive to insulin, which is required for glucose use, blood glucose levels eventually rise above the normal range as the beta-cells are unable to produce enough insulin. Youth with high insulin resistance have low insulin sensitivity, which means that they will require greater amounts of insulin in order to lower their blood glucose levels. Excess insulin circulating in the blood relative to the level of glucose, known as **hyperinsulinemia**, is seen in a number of metabolic conditions. For example, it is associated with **metabolic syndrome**, which is a collection of cardiovascular disease risk factors including hyperglycemia, high blood pressure, excess body fat, and dyslipidemia (Vanlancker et al., 2017). The growing prevalence of metabolic syndrome and DM in youth derive in part from modern lifestyles characterized by physical inactivity and poor choices about foods and beverages (Lee, Fermin, Filipp, Gurka, & DeBoer, 2017; Mayer-Davis, Lawrence, Dabelea, Divers, Isom, Dolan, et al., 2017).

DO YOU KNOW?

Puberty is associated with significant changes in physiology, including a transient reduction in insulin sensitivity. The sensitivity returns to normal at the completion of puberty in healthy youth but may continue in youth who are obese (Hannon, Janosky, & Arslanian, 2006; Kelsey & Zeitler, 2016).

Without sustained interventions beginning early in life, uncontrolled DM can increase the risk of developing both microvascular complications (e.g., neuropathy, retinopathy) and macrovascular complications (e.g., stroke, coronary artery disease) (Dabelea, Stafford JM2, & Mayer-Davis EJ3, 2017). Early-onset T2DM in youth appears to follow an aggressive disease course characterized by rapidly progressive beta-cell decline and accelerated development of diabetes complications (Amutha et al., 2017; Nadeau et al., 2016; Viner, White, & Christie, 2017). Findings from the multicenter Treatment Options for Type 2 Diabetes in Adolescents and Youth (TODAY) study found that loss of glycemic control in youth with T2DM is rapid and may be three to four times more severe than in adults with this disease (Nadeau et al., 2016; Narasimhan & Weinstock, 2014). Rapid progression of complications in youth with T2DM was also observed in the Canadian First Nations Report, which found that renal and neurological complications began within 5 years of diagnosis and that major complications (e.g., dialysis, blindness, amputation) began to manifest 10 years after diagnosis (Dart et al., 2014; Hannon & Arslanian, 2015). Consequently, comprehensive interventions that target lifestyle behaviors early in life are needed in order to manage DM in children and adolescents before they suffer from clinical complications and become more resistant to treatment options.

Managing Diabetes Mellitus in Youth

Clinical conditions such as DM affect the entire family; as a result, educational efforts that include parents and siblings are needed in order to create an environment and support network that keeps blood glucose

TABLE 15.2   DIAGNOSTIC CRITERIA FOR PREDIABETES AND DIABETES MELLITUS

Prediabetes	Diabetes
Fasting plasma glucose = 100-125 mg/dL (5.5-6.9 mmol/L)	Fasting plasma glucose ≥126 mg/dL (≥7.0 mmol/L)
2 hr plasma glucose = 140-199 mg/dL (7.8-11.0 mmol/L) during oral glucose tolerance test	2 hr plasma glucose = 140-199 mg/dL (7.8-11.0 mmol/L) during oral glucose tolerance test
Glycolated hemoglobin (HbA1C) = 5.7%-6.4%	Glycolated hemoglobin (HbA1C) ≥6.5%

Adapted from American Diabetes Association (2015).

levels as close to normal as possible and thereby avoid complications. Because a diagnosis of DM can feel overwhelming, youth fitness specialists should work with health care providers to dispel misperceptions, promote adherence, and educate families about lifestyle choices that can improve health and well-being. Lifestyle interventions can lead to profound health benefits for youth with DM, but the intervention should be tailored to the specific needs of the individual; in addition, youth fitness specialists should be aware of potential complications because blood glucose responses to physical activity are highly variable in youth with DM (Colberg et al., 2016).

Practitioners also need to address the common parental fear that increasing physical activity will increase the frequency of **hypoglycemia** in youth with DM (Michaud, Henderson, Legault, & Mathieu, 2017). Hypoglycemia is characterized by blood glucose levels below 70 milligram per deciliter (<3.9 mmol/L) and is a relative contraindication to exercise (Colberg et al., 2016). The early signs and symptoms of hypoglycemia include shakiness, dizziness, sweating, hunger, headache, and tingling of the mouth and fingers. Youth with DM (and their parents and youth fitness specialists) should be aware of these signs and symptoms and should monitor blood glucose levels before, occasionally during, and after exercise and, if needed, make appropriate dietary or medication changes in consultation with a health care provider (Colberg et al., 2016). Given that hypoglycemia can occur 12 hours or more after exercise (McMahon et al., 2007), frequent glucose monitoring is needed in order to detect and prevent later-onset hypoglycemia.

In order to improve clinical outcomes, youth fitness specialists need to provide children and adolescents with information about exercise that is understandable and reasonable to carry out. Living healthfully with DM requires the individual to exercise regularly, follow nutrition guidelines, and take medications as prescribed. Lifestyle behavior change is the cornerstone of therapy for youth with DM, because most interventions target diet, physical activity habits, or both (Brackney & Cutshall, 2015; Ho et al., 2013; Savoye et al., 2014). Although evidence for lifestyle intervention effects is limited after the diagnosis of T2DM (Kriska et al., 2018; Zeitler et al., 2012), an intensive 12-month lifestyle intervention demonstrated favorable treatment effects in obese youth without diabetes and in youth with prediabetes (Savoye et al., 2014). Youth fitness specialists should be aware of the challenges involved in changing lifestyle behaviors in youth who have DM due to the influence of various types of factors—social (e.g., family dynamics), mental (e.g., depression), and environmental (e.g., lack of access to healthy foods and physical activity). To overcome these challenges, practitioners need to design interventions that are feasible, sustainable, and meaningful for children and adolescents.

Exercise Guidelines for Youth with Diabetes Mellitus

Children and adolescents with DM should be encouraged to accumulate at least 60 min of moderate to vigorous physical activity per day to enhance cardiorespiratory and musculoskeletal fitness, although special precautions are needed in order to maximize benefits and safety (Colberg et al., 2016). Due to low initial levels of physical fitness in most youth with DM (de Lima et al., 2017; Pivovarov, Taplin, & Riddell, 2015), youth fitness specialists should begin with less intense activities before progressing to more intense bouts of aerobic exercise and sport. Exercise training that consists of aerobic exercise, resistance training, or both has been found to improve cardiovascular disease risk factors, reduce insulin resistance, and decrease HbA1C in youth with DM (Ishiguro et al., 2016; Marson, Delevatti, Prado, Netto, & Kruel, 2016; Quirk, Blake, Tennyson, Randell, & Glazebrook, 2014; Riddell et al., 2017; Roberts & Taplin, 2015; Stoner et al., 2016; Umpierre et al., 2011). A meta-analysis of 10 trials involving youth with T1DM found significant improvements in HbA1c following exercise training (at least three times per week for at least 60 minutes per session) and highlighted the potential benefits of doing supervised aerobic and resistance training (MacMillan et al., 2014).

Since aerobic exercise and resistance training have proven to be beneficial in individuals with T1DM and

Pump Therapy

Some youth with T1DM use continuous subcutaneous insulin infusion (i.e., an insulin pump) as an alternative to multiple daily insulin injections in order to maintain near-normal blood glucose levels (Karges et al., 2017). An insulin pump is a computer-driven device about the size of a cell phone that is worn outside the body on a belt or in a pocket (see figure 15.2). It delivers insulin into the body via a thin plastic tube ending in a small, flexible plastic cannula or a very thin needle inserted just below the skin and taped securely in place. Although insulin pumps can improve glucose control, youth fitness specialists should be aware of concerns related to pump therapy. Sweating and rapid movements during exercise can cause the pump infusion set to become loose or cause the skin to become irritated. Thus, it may be beneficial to insert the cannula or needle on the buttocks covered by a tight garment. If extra protection is needed, a variety of accessories are available, including spandex belts and pouches that hold the insulin pump in place.

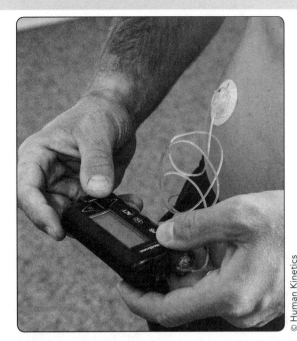

© Human Kinetics

FIGURE 15.2   Insulin pump on a young athlete.

T2DM (MacMillan et al., 2014; Yang, Scott, Mao, Tang, & Farmer, 2014), youth fitness specialists should ask about individual preferences and consider the potential benefits of integrating both types of training into the exercise program as described in other chapters. In addition, varying the training stimulus by alternating bouts of moderate and vigorous exercise can optimize cardiometabolic benefits for youth with DM (Cockcroft et al., 2015; Colberg et al., 2016).

In the absence of contraindications—including uncontrolled hypertension, severe proliferative retinopathy, and recent treatments using laser surgery (American College of Sports Medicine, 2018)—youth with DM can participate in well-designed resistance training programs. Following an introduction to resistance training with light to moderate loads, higher training intensities can be gradually introduced into the exercise program to enhance training-induced gains in muscular strength and metabolic health (Bea, Blew, Howe, Hetherington-Rauth, & Going, 2017; Gordon, Dolinsky, Mughal, Gordon, & McGavock, 2015). Although flexibility training is a recognized component of health-related physical fitness, this type of exercise should not replace aerobic and resistance training, because flexibility training does not exert a favorable effect on glycemic control, insulin action, or body composition. However, exercise sessions should begin with a well-designed dynamic warm-up in order

to prepare youth for the demands of the upcoming session while improving flexibility and mobility. Program design considerations for youth with DM are presented in figure 15.3.

Physical and Intellectual Disabilities

As with able-bodied children and adolescents, youth with physical or intellectual disabilities should be encouraged to engage in exercise and sport activities. From community-based events all the way to the Paralympic Games and Special Olympics, opportunities are available for youth with disabilities to participate in exercise and sport programs. However, special precautions are needed to prescreen youth with disabilities in order to identify factors that may predispose a child to injury (Murphy, Carbone, & American Academy of Pediatrics Council on Children With Disabilities, 2008). In addition, youth fitness specialists may need to modify game rules, use specialized equipment, and take special care to ensure a safe training environment. As a whole, it is important to raise awareness about the importance of daily physical activity while recognizing the unique abilities of youth with physical or intellectual disabilities.

The interaction between individuals with physical or intellectual impairments and attitudinal and

FIGURE 15.3   PROGRAM DESIGN CONSIDERATIONS FOR YOUTH WITH DIABETES MELLITUS

- Begin with short bouts (10 min) of aerobic exercise and moderate-intensity (e.g., <60% of 1RM) resistance exercise.
- Perform aerobic exercise on most days of the week and resistance exercise on two or three days per week.
- Accumulate at least 60 minutes of moderate- to vigorous-intensity physical activity per day.
- Allow no more than two consecutive days without exercise.
- Seek guidance and supervision on exercise training and progression from a youth fitness specialist.
- Encourage parent modeling and support of regular exercise.
- Carry a medical ID identifying DM, as well as glucose tablets or similar food items for hypoglycemia.
- Be aware that dehydration may contribute to a compromised thermoregulatory response and elevated blood glucose levels.

Adapted from American College of Sports Medicine (2018).

environmental barriers is complex and may limit participation in community- and school-based programs on an equal basis with others. Environmental factors can affect an individual's health and well-being, and efforts are needed to increase access to exercise and sport activities in order to avoid excluding people with disabilities. Youth fitness specialists should challenge negative attitudes and behaviors in order to increase visibility and participation in physical activities by youth with disabilities. Without concerted efforts to educate caregivers, recognize personal abilities, and address barriers to physical activity, youth with disabilities may not be able to experience the physical and psychosocial benefits of exercise and sport.

Disability is a complex term that includes impairments (e.g., paralysis), activity limitations (e.g., difficulty with walking), and participation restrictions (e.g., discrimination) (World Health Organization, 2001). Although each child with a disability has unique needs, this section focuses on youth with physical and intellectual disabilities. **Physical disabilities,** such as cerebral palsy and spinal cord injuries, can impair mobility and physical functioning. Cerebral palsy results from a defect or lesion in the developing brain and causes mobility limitations due to motor impairments, spasticity, and muscle weakness (Bax, Flodmark, & Tydeman, 2007; Verschuren et al., 2016). Other physical disabilities include hearing loss or visual impairment. Although some youth with a physical disability are ambulatory, others require the use of a wheelchair or assistive device.

Intellectual disabilities are neurodevelopmental disorders that become apparent before 18 years of age and are characterized by deficits in both intellectual functioning and adaptive behaviors, including phys-

ical functioning, social interactions, and communication skills (Schalock et al., 2010). Down syndrome is the most common chromosomal anomaly among newborns with intellectual disabilities; it occurs when an extra chromosome 21 is present through nondisjunction or translocation (van den Driessen Mareeuw, Hollegien, Coppus, Delnoij, & de Vries, 2017). Youth with mild intellectual disabilities can learn self-care and practical skills, although others need considerable support due to additional physical and emotional problems. Common elements of physical and intellectual disabilities are outlined in table 15.3.

Establishing Healthy Lifestyles for Youth With Physical or Intellectual Disabilities

Due to the increasing prevalence of physical inactivity, obesity, and low physical fitness in youth with disabilities (Hinckson & Curtis, 2013; Papas et al., 2016; Segal et al., 2016; Wouters, Evenhuis, & Hilgenkamp, 2019), it is crucial to help them establish healthy lifestyles early in life in order to reduce the risk of cardiometabolic disease later in life. Lack of regular physical activity, increased screen time, and unhealthy weight gain are associated with a higher disease burden in youth with disabilities (Bertapelli, Pitetti, Agiovlasitis, & Guerra-Junior, 2016; Grover et al., 2015; Papas et al., 2016). Similarly, adults with disabilities tend to be less active, eat poorer diets, and exhibit higher rates of diabetes and heart disease than the general population (Carroll et al., 2014; Leser, Pirie, Ferketich, Havercamp, & Wewers, 2017). By establishing healthy behaviors early in life, youth with disabilities may be more active later in life and thereby reduce their

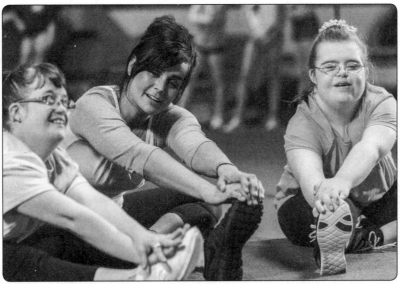

kali9/E+/Getty Images

Activity-based interventions offer health and fitness benefits for youth with clinical conditions.

risk of cardiometabolic disease (Cairney, Veldhuizen, King-Dowling, Faught, & Hay, 2017; Hartman, Smith, Westendorp, & Visscher, 2015).

The health- and fitness-related benefits of physical activity for youth with disabilities include favorable changes in aerobic fitness, muscle strength, motor skills, and body composition (Ash, Bowling, Davison, & Garcia, 2017; Bloemen et al., 2015; Johnson, 2009; Wu et al., 2017). Through regular participation in exercise and sport activities, youth with disabilities can enhance their physical fitness while learning new skills and socializing with others (Ash et al., 2017; O'Brien et al., 2016; Zwinkels et al., 2019). Furthermore, the psychosocial benefits of exercise and sport can favorably influence a child's overall health and well-being (Murphy et al., 2008). Youth with disabilities may feel isolated from their peers and may be particularly vulnerable to teasing and marginalization, which can adversely affect their self-esteem and health-related quality of life (Jemtå, Fugl-Meyer, Oberg, & Dahl, 2009; Uzark et al., 2012). Therefore, exercise and sport programs should be characterized by qualified instruction and team-building activities so that participants have an opportunity to socialize with others while learning new skills and improving their physical abilities. Youth fitness specialists should create a safe, welcoming, and supportive environment while focusing on individual needs and concerns. In addition to the importance

TABLE 15.3   COMMON ATTRIBUTES OF SELECTED INTELLECTUAL AND PHYSICAL DISABILITIES

Disability	Attributes
Cerebral palsy	Movement difficulties, muscle weakness, muscle spasms, poor balance, poor coordination
Cystic fibrosis	Persistent cough, frequent lung infections, exercise limitations, problems with digestion
Muscular dystrophy	Progressive muscle weakness, difficulty standing, unsteady gait
Spina bifida	Muscle weakness, numbness in limbs, paralysis, incontinence
Hearing impairment	Delayed speech, inability to locate or respond to sounds, withdrawal from social interaction
Visual impairment	Hazy or blurred vision, repeated blinking, sensitivity to light, poor eye–hand coordination
Down syndrome	Cognitive impairments, low muscle tone, slow physical development
Prader-Willi syndrome	Constant sense of hunger, weight gain, poor muscle tone, cognitive impairments
Fragile X syndrome	Delayed speech, learning problems, hyperactivity, social anxiety

Data from Moore, Durstein, and Painter (2016); Bloemen, Backx, Takken, et al. (2015); Hodge, Lieberman, and Murata (2012); and Philpott, Houghton, and Luke (2010).

of enhancing both health- and skill-related fitness measures, parents of youth with disabilities value the social benefits of exercise programs for their children (Wiart, Darrah, Kelly, & Legg, 2015).

Exercise Guidelines for Youth With Physical or Intellectual Disabilities

Youth with clinical conditions, including physical or intellectual disabilities, should be screened by their health care provider before participating in an exercise or sport program. For example, children with Down syndrome should be screened radiographically for atlantoaxial instability, which can lead to dislocation and spinal cord compression (Bull & Committee on Genetics, 2011; Hankinson & Anderson, 2010). The goal of prescreening is not to exclude youth with disabilities from exercise or sport but to recommend appropriate physical activities and sport options in the least restrictive environment (Murphy et al., 2008). Consequently, health care providers and youth fitness specialists need to work together to enhance the safety and efficacy of exercise and sport programs for youth who are increasingly vulnerable to a lifestyle of sedentary behaviors.

Youth fitness specialists should beware of preconceived notions about the physical abilities of youth with disabilities, who are often able to do more than many people think. Most youth with disabilities can learn new skills and participate in a variety of exercise and sport activities that are consistent with individual strengths and abilities. At the same, youth with disabilities generally do have lower levels of cardiorespiratory fitness and are less active than children without disabilities (Hinckson & Curtis, 2013; Oppewal, Hilgenkamp, van Wijck, & Evenhuis, 2013; Sit et al., 2017). Fatigue is also an important consideration, and youth fitness specialists should be mindful that high levels of fatigue may affect participation and adherence to exercise programs (Maher et al., 2015).

The best approach for beginners may be to participate in exercise sessions characterized by brief bouts of low- to moderate-intensity physical activity interspersed with rest periods as needed. Over time, the program can be progressed by gradually increasing the exercise intensity. High-intensity interval training has been found to promote improvements in a wide range of health-related outcomes in healthy children and adolescents (Bond, Weston, Williams, & Barker, 2017), and similar findings have been observed in youth with physical disabilities (Zwinkels et al., 2019). Notably, six months of sport training that included soccer, basketball, hockey, and running games such as tag improved anaerobic performance and decreased fat mass in youth with physical disabilities (Zwinkels et al., 2018). Since most outdoor play and sport activities include short bouts of vigorous physical activity, it seems practical to integrate this type of training into exercise programs for youth with physical and intellectual disabilities.

DO YOU KNOW?

Junior Paralympic athletes with different types of disabilities have competed in a variety of sports and performed a number of impressive feats, including a 448-pound (203 kg) bench press.

In addition to aerobic games and activities, exercise programs for youth with disabilities should include exercises that target strength, flexibility, and skill-related fitness (Fragala-Pinkham, Haley, & O'Neil, 2008; Gupta, Rao, & Kumaran, 2011; Hartman, Smith, Houwen, & Visscher, 2017; Kachouri et al., 2016; Sugimoto, Bowen, Meehan, & Stracciolini, 2016). Through improvements in muscular strength, cardiorespiratory endurance, and skill-related fitness, youth with disabilities can gain confidence in their physical abilities, improve their exercise performance, enhance their independence, and boost their cognitive functioning—all while experiencing the enjoyment of exercise and sport (Hartman et al., 2017;

Teaching Tip

RISKS AND REWARDS

Misperceptions about the risks of physical activity, combined with insufficient counseling about the benefits of exercise and sport for children and adolescents with disabilities, appear to be at least partly responsible for the increasing prevalence of physical inactivity and sedentary behaviors in this young population (Murphy et al., 2008; Shields & Synnot, 2016). To address these issues, youth fitness specialists should provide reassurance that regular participation in exercise and sport activities can be safe, effective, and enjoyable for children and adolescents with disabilities, provided that the program is properly designed, sensibly progressed, and supervised by qualified professionals. The relative risks associated with physical activity should be balanced with the relative risks of physical inactivity and associated comorbidities.

FIGURE 15.4   PROGRAM DESIGN CONSIDERATIONS FOR YOUTH WITH DISABILITIES

- Prescreen youth for medical conditions in order to minimize the risk of illness or injury.
- Begin with less intense activities interspersed with rest periods as needed.
- Gradually increase exercise intensity and training volume.
- Integrate aerobic and resistance exercises into exercise sessions.
- Encourage socialization in group activities.
- Recognize the warning signs of hyperthermia.
- Encourage participation in sport activities when appropriate.
- Emphasize variety and enjoyment to sustain participation.

Teaching Tip

EYE TO EYE

It is important for youth fitness specialists to interact appropriately with children and adolescents who have disabilities. Look at and speak directly to the child rather than to a caregiver. At times, it may be necessary to sit, kneel, or move to the side in order to establish eye contact. Ask if the child needs help and seek to understand what the child can or cannot do. Convey your thoughts in an easily understandable form and allow extra time for the child to answer questions. Help all participants feel welcome in the program by respecting and communicating with each child at the same eye level. Do not assume that a child with a disability has low intelligence.

Johnson, 2009; Murphy et al., 2008). Because health and fitness benefits can be gained from different types of physical activity, youth fitness specialists should consider a child's preferences when designing interventions (Baksjøberget, Nyquist, Moser, & Jahnsen, 2017; Shields, Synnot, & Kearns, 2015). Practitioners should identify local exercise or sport programs that meet the needs of youth with clinical conditions so that participants can find something they really enjoy. Program design considerations for youth with physical and intellectual disabilities are outlined in figure 15.4.

Group exercise and sport activities may be particularly beneficial for youth with physical and intellectual disabilities because they can enhance physical fitness while promoting a social interaction and a sense of inclusion and achievement (Crawford, Burns, & Fernie, 2015; Murphy et al., 2008). Programs such as the Special Olympics offer exercise and sport activities for youth and adults with intellectual disabilities. The Special Olympics offers year-round training and competitions in more than 30 Olympic-style summer and winter sports for individuals aged eight years and older, as well as a young athletes program for children aged two to seven years (Special Olympics, 2019). Researchers

and practitioners involved with the Special Olympics continue to provide evidence and inspiration that individuals with disabilities can, and should, participate in exercise and sport activities (Baran et al., 2013; Crawford et al., 2015; Myśliwiec & Damentko, 2015). In addition to improving physical skills, involvement in programs such as the Special Olympics provides an opportunity for personal growth, social interaction, and lasting friendships.

Summary

The physical and psychosocial benefits of regular physical activity for children and adolescents, especially those with clinical conditions, are observable and long-lasting. In light of current trends of physical inactivity, health care providers should ask youth and their parents about their physical activity habits and should refer their inactive patients to qualified fitness professionals. Health care providers and youth fitness specialists have a responsibility to inform families about the inevitable consequences of physical inactivity and to facilitate participation in exercise and sport programs that are developmentally appropriate and consistent with each individual's physical and intellectual abilities.

CHAPTER 16

Nutrition for Youth

CHAPTER OBJECTIVES

- Understand the roles of nutrition and energy balance in supporting growth, maturation, and a healthy lifestyle
- Understand how macronutrients can contribute to a healthy diet for youth
- Understand how micronutrients can contribute to a healthy diet for youth
- Identify practical ways to provide youth with healthy and nutritious meals, snacks, and drinks

KEY TERMS

Introduction

A healthy diet and an active lifestyle should be viewed as fundamental rights for all youth. These two factors support physical and psychological development and help to minimize the risk of disease. Adequate nutrition is required in order to support the processes of growth and maturation, thus providing lifelong health benefits. For instance, rapid growth and development of the brain in the early years of life requires a plentiful supply of **macronutrients** and **micronutrients** (Bourre, 2006a, 2006b). In contrast, malnutrition during adolescence can impair growth and weaken the bones (Rogol et al., 2000), and nutritional status can influence the timing of sexual maturation (Malina et al., 2004). It has also been shown that nutrition and dietary habits influence psychosocial well-being (Alaimo et al., 2001), cognitive function (Cohen et al., 2016), and academic performance of children (Florence et al., 2008). Healthy eating can also help protect children, directly or indirectly, from maladies including cardiovascular disease, diabetes, metabolic syndrome, and cancer (Centers for Disease Control and Prevention, 2011).

It is important for youth to establish a good diet early in life because eating behaviors tend to track from childhood into adolescence and adulthood (Movassagh et al., 2017). Although youth fitness specialists are not called on to plan diets for youth, they can act as good nutritional role models; provide youth with access to good food and beverage choices; educate children, parents, caregivers, and coaches about the benefits of a healthy diet; and provide practical tips eating healthily. To help practitioners advocate healthy eating, this chapter addresses current nutritional guidelines.

DO YOU KNOW?

Children should eat a diet that includes a variety of nutrient-dense foods and beverages while limiting the intake of solid fats, salt, added sugars, and refined grains (Morgan, 2017).

Youth health fitness specialists should consider both the quantity and the quality of food in children's diets (quality of food is discussed in more detail later in this chapter). **Energy balance** consists of the difference between the amount of energy consumed and the amount of energy expended. Consuming too much energy through a poor diet and expending too little energy through an inactive lifestyle leads to a positive energy balance, meaning that more calories are taken in than expended; over the long term, this dynamic causes excessive weight gain, as is the case in overweight and obese youth. In contrast, a diet that is too low in energy to meet the demands of an active lifestyle leads to a negative energy balance; over time, this pattern leads to weight loss and potentially negative health outcomes, which in turn can impair growth and delay maturation (Rogol et al., 2000). Negative energy balance may be found in children living in poverty (Kurpad et al., 2005), but it can also be observed in young athletes (e.g., Gibson et al., 2011). To achieve a healthy lifestyle, youth should be physically active and consume a diet that meets their energy needs, thus maintaining an energy balance that supports growth, maturation, and physical activity.

It is especially difficult for sedentary youth to avoid a positive energy balance when contemporary society normalizes excessive calorie intake and creates obesogenic environments (Gidding et al., 2005; Lipek et al., 2015). Given the high prevalence of overweight and obese children, it is likely that, in addition to providing physical activity opportunities, youth fitness specialists will need to develop nutritional interventions to reduce energy intake and improve food quality. For example, frequent or excessive consumption of high-calorie "energy" or "sport" drinks has been linked to a range of adverse outcomes, including increasing levels of overweight and obesity in youth (American Academy of Pediatrics, 2011; Visram et al., 2016). Practitioners can encourage healthier replacements, such as no- and low-sugar drinks, as part of an integrated approach to help youth achieve a healthy energy balance and improve their overall health (U.S. Department of Agriculture, 2015).

The estimated energy needs of boys and girls are presented in tables 16.1 and 16.2, respectively. As these tables indicate, energy requirements depend on age and physical activity level. All children should be active, but some are not, and sedentary children require fewer daily calories to meet their energy needs. Based on the information presented in the tables, sedentary boys and girls require 35 percent to 40 percent less energy than their very active peers, and this difference needs to be taken into account in their diet. The energy requirements shown in tables 16.1 and 16.2 are based on boys and girls of average size. Of course, energy requirements increase during puberty to support rapid growth and increased body size, which means that the nutritional needs of two same-age children may vary considerably. Youth fitness specialists should be aware of the individual energy needs of each child based on a variety of factors. To facilitate this process, the Institute of Medicine (IOM; 2005) has produced equations for estimating the energy requirements of boys and girls based on age, weight, and physical activity (table 16.3 on page 317).

In the IOM predictive equations, physical activity levels are defined as sedentary if the child is never

TABLE 16.1   ESTIMATED TOTAL ENERGY EXPENDITURE* FOR AVERAGE-SIZE BOYS WITH DIFFERING ACTIVITY LEVELS

Age (yr)	Mass (kg)	Height (m)	Sedentary (kcal/day)	Low-active (kcal/day)	Active (kcal/day)	Very active (kcal/day)
3	14.3	0.95	1,150	1,300	1,450	1,650
4	16.2	1.02	1,200	1,350	1,450	1,750
5	18.4	1.09	1,250	1,450	1,650	1,850
6	20.7	1.15	1,300	1,500	1,700	2,000
7	23.1	1.22	1,400	1,600	1,800	2,100
8	25.6	1.28	1,450	1,650	1,900	2,200
9	28.6	1.34	1,500	1,750	2,000	2,350
10	31.9	1.39	1,600	1,850	2,100	2,450
11	35.9	1.44	1,700	1,950	2,250	2,600
12	40.5	1.49	1,800	2,100	2,400	2,800
13	45.6	1.56	1,900	2,250	2,600	3,000
14	51.0	1.64	2,050	2,450	2,800	3,250
15	56.3	1.70	2,200	2,600	3,000	3,450
16	60.9	1.74	2,300	2,700	3,150	3,650
17	64.6	1.75	2,350	2,750	3,200	3,750
18	67.2	1.76	2,350	2,800	3,250	3,800

*Values rounded to the nearest 50 kcal/day.

Adapted from Institute of Medicine (2005).

TABLE 16.2   ESTIMATED TOTAL ENERGY EXPENDITURE* FOR AVERAGE-SIZE GIRLS WITH DIFFERING ACTIVITY LEVELS

Age (y)	Mass (kg)	Height (m)	Sedentary (kcal/day)	Low active (kcal/day)	Active (kcal/day)	Very active (kcal/day)
3	13.9	0.94	1,050	1,200	1,400	1,650
4	15.8	1.01	1,100	1,300	1,450	1,730
5	17.9	1.08	1,150	1,350	1,550	1,850
6	20.2	1.15	1,250	1,450	1,600	1,950
7	22.8	1.21	1,300	1,500	1,700	2,050
8	25.6	1.28	1,350	1,550	1,800	2,150
9	29.0	1.33	1,400	1,650	1,850	2,250
10	32.9	1.38	1,450	1,700	1,950	2,350
11	37.2	1.44	1,500	1,800	2,050	2,500
12	41.6	1.51	1,600	1,900	2,150	2,600
13	45.8	1.57	1,650	1,950	2,250	2,750
14	49.4	1.60	1,700	2,000	2,300	2,800
15	52.0	1.62	1,700	2,050	2,350	2,850
16	53.9	1.63	1,700	2,050	2,350	2,850
17	55.1	1.63	1,700	2,000	2,350	2,850
18	56.2	1.63	1,650	2,000	2,300	2,850

*Values rounded to the nearest 50 kcal/day.

Adapted from Institute of Medicine (2005).

active, low if active for less than one hour pay day, moderate if active for about one hour per day, and very active if active for more than one hour per day. Given the subjective nature of applying physical activity levels in predictive equations—as well as the influence of maturation and the metabolic variability in energy requirements between individuals—these equations should be used only as a guide (Desbrow et al., 2014). Greater insight can be gained through longitudinal monitoring of youth, which allows youth fitness specialists to measure markers of growth and development. When these markers are combined with knowledge of an individual's diet and physical activity habits, they help indicate whether energy balance is being achieved or whether targeted intervention is needed.

As discussed in chapter 14, childhood obesity is a critical contemporary issue because it is associated with a number of negative outcomes. Since the late 1980s, the prevalence of obesity in youth has almost doubled in the United States (Ogden et al., 2016). This increase in obesity was preceded by a 20-year period during which the proportion of food that children consumed from fast food restaurants increased by 300 percent and the calorie intake from soft drinks also increased (St-Onge et al., 2003). The "empty calorie" foods consumed by youth are obtained in roughly equal proportions from fast food restaurants, convenience stores, and schools (Poti et al., 2014). Regularly consuming more energy than is necessary for healthy functioning, growth, and physical activity leads to a positive energy balance and weight gain (Hill et al., 2012) as the excess energy is stored as excess body fat. The imbalance between energy intake and energy expenditure has contributed to the high rates of childhood obesity observed around the globe (Hill et al., 2012, Swinburn et al., 2011).

Although youth athletes tend to eat better diets than their nonathlete counterparts (Croll et al., 2006), their diets are still likely to be suboptimal. Highly active youth athletes may underestimate their energy requirements due to the large amount of energy needed to support both growth and high levels of physical activity. Negative energy balance, which results from expending more energy than one consumes, may lead to impaired growth, delayed puberty, menstrual dysfunction, loss of muscle mass, and increased susceptibility to injury and illness (Purcell & Canadian Paediatric Society Paediatric Sports and Exercise Medicine Section, 2013). Reduced growth during the competitive season has been reported in young wrestlers and attributed to the high energy demands of training and the restriction of food intake in order to make weight classifications (Roemmich & Sinning, 1997). However, when the negative energy balance is reversed during the off-season, youth wrestlers have been shown to accelerate and catch up on their growth (Roemmich & Sinning, 1997; Tipton & Tcheng, 1970). Youth fitness specialists should be aware of the energy needs of young athletes and help make nutrient-rich foods and drinks accessible before, during, and after training as required.

Components of Diet and Recommended Daily Intakes

As shown in figure 16.1, the diet is comprised of six essential nutrients, each of which can be classified as either a macronutrient or a micronutrient. Three key

TABLE 16.3   EQUATIONS FOR ESTIMATING ENERGY REQUIREMENTS OF BOYS AND GIRLS BASED ON AGE, PHYSICAL ACTIVITY (PA) LEVEL, WEIGHT, AND HEIGHT

Group (yr)	Estimated energy requirements (kcal/day)*	PHYSICAL ACTIVITY (PA) COEFFICIENT**			
		Sedentary	Low active	Active	Very active
Boys 3-8	88.5 − (61.9 × age) + PA × (26.7 × weight + 903 × height) + 20	1.00	1.13	1.26	1.42
Boys 9-18	88.5 − (61.9 × age) + PA × (26.7 × weight + 903 × height) + 25	1.00	1.13	1.26	1.42
Girls 3-8	135.3 − (30.8 × age) + PA × (10.0 × weight + 934 × height) + 20	1.00	1.16	1.31	1.56
Girls 9-18	135.3 − (30.8 × age) + PA × (10.0 × weight + 934 × height) + 25	1.00	1.16	1.31	1.56

*Age is in years, weight is in kilograms, and height is in meters.

**Apply a physical activity (PA) coefficient based on the physical activity level of the child.

Data from Institute of Medicine (2005).

Teaching Tip

EMPTY CALORIES

Imbalance between energy (calories) consumed and energy expended (activity performed) can lead youth to become overweight and obese. In addition, overweight and obese youth are less likely to eat fruits, vegetables, and whole grains and more likely to routinely consume fast food, ready meals, refined grains, sweets, and other foods and drinks containing added sugar. These types of food tend to be calorie dense and nutrient low and therefore have been labeled as "empty calories" (Caballero, 2007). Not only does the excessive calorie intake contribute to weight gain but also the lack of nutrients can carry negative health consequences. Youth fitness specialists should recognize that a healthy diet involves more than simply achieving energy balance; indeed, what children eat is equally as important as how much they eat.

macronutrients are carbohydrate, protein, and fat, all of which provide energy and are needed in large amounts; in addition to carbohydrate for energy, dietary fiber is a type of carbohydrate that aids digestion. Another macronutrient, water, does not provide energy but is still needed in large amounts in order to support body function. Micronutrients include vitamins and minerals, affect numerous body functions, such as bone health, immune function, metabolism, oxygen transport, and antioxidant activity (Fox & Kerksick, 2016).

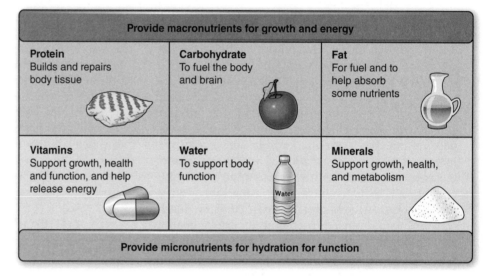

FIGURE 16.1   The six essential nutrients of the diet.

All six essential nutrients are needed in order to support growth and development, promote and maintain good health, and support an active lifestyle. Under- or overconsumption of essential nutrients can lead to negative health outcomes in youth, and nutrient requirements change with growth and development. The Centers for Disease Control and Prevention (2011) identify that physical activity and a healthy diet provide a multitude of benefits, helping to protect children against obesity, cardiovascular disease, metabolic syndrome and type 2 diabetes. The same guidelines also suggest that a lack of micronutrients in the diet can contribute to poor bone health, fatigue, attention deficits, impaired psychomotor development and increased susceptibility to infections in children. Youth fitness specialists should be aware of the nutrient requirements of growing children and well informed about how to meet these needs.

The Institute of Medicine (2005) provided the following definitions of commonly used terms for describing nutritional needs:

- Recommended daily allowance (RDA): average daily dietary nutrient intake level sufficient to meet the requirements of nearly all healthy individuals

- Adequate intake (AI): estimation or approximation of adequate average daily intake for apparently healthy individuals; used when RDA cannot be determined

- Tolerable upper intake level (UL): highest average daily nutrient intake likely to pose no risk and cause no adverse health effects in almost all individuals in the general population

- Estimated average requirement (EAR): average daily nutrient intake estimated to meet the requirement of half of healthy individuals

Collectively, the nutrient reference values covered by RDA, AI, UL, and EAR are referred to as **recommended daily intakes** (RDI) (Institute of Medicine, 2005). Although RDAs exist for the carbohydrate and protein, they are not adjusted for size or physical activity levels. Rather, they are provided as set values for all of the population based on sex and age. No RDA or AI is provided for fat, because there is insufficient information to determine a level of fat intake at which risk of inadequacy or prevention of chronic disease occurs (Institute of Medicine, 2005). From 1 to 18 years of age (and into adulthood), the RDA for carbohydrate is set at 130 grams per day for both males and females, whereas the protein requirement increases from 19 grams per day for a 3-year-old to 46 and 52 grams per day for 14- to 18-year-old girls and boys, respectively (Institute of Medicine, 2005). As the RDA, those quantities are deemed sufficient to meet the health needs of most individuals. The RDA of 130 grams per day of carbohydrate is based on the average minimum amount of glucose used by the brain, but it is expected that the total consumption of this macronutrient would exceed that amount in order to meet the overall energy needs of an individual. For instance, where guidelines include the amount of carbohydrate required for support of all energy needs, it is recommended that from age 11 years onward girls consume at least 267 grams per day and boys at least 333 grams per day (Public Health England, 2016).

A more useful approach for establishing the macronutrient needs of youth may be the **acceptable macronutrient distribution range (AMDR)**, which provides a range of intakes for a particular energy source that are associated with reduced risk of chronic disease and provide adequate intake of essential nutrients (Institute of Medicine, 2005). AMDR provides a percentage range within which the calories from a given macronutrient should contribute to the total energy intake. Globally, AMDR is the subject of good agreement; for instance, recommendations from North America (Institute of Medicine, 2005) and the Nordic countries (Nordic Council of Ministers, 2014) are similar, albeit with slightly different upper ranges for carbohydrate and fat. Figure 16.2 shows AMDR along with the target macronutrient contribution to energy to be used in dietary planning. If based on the estimated energy requirements of a child, AMDR can be used to calculate macronutrient requirements while accounting for sex, size, and activity level (Zakrewski & Tolfrey, 2016).

To calculate macronutrient needs in absolute amounts (grams), energy requirements for each macronutrient should be converted based on its **energy density**. Consider a very active American 13-year-old boy of average height and weight. As shown in table 16.1, this individual would have an estimated energy requirement of 3,000 kilocalories per day. Using AMDR and the target contribution in figure 16.2, the boy would require about 1,575 kilocalories from carbohydrate, 975 from fat, and 450 from protein. These amounts equate to 394 grams of carbohydrate, 108 of fat, and 113 of protein in the daily diet.

DO YOU KNOW?

Both carbohydrate and protein provide four kilocalories of energy per gram, whereas fat has more than double the energy density at 9 kilocalories per gram.

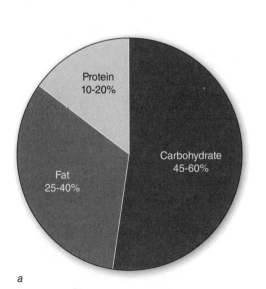
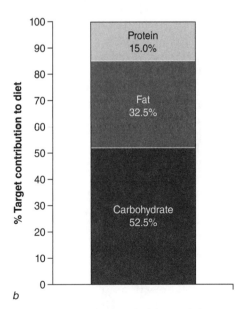

FIGURE 16.2 *(a)* Acceptable macronutrient distribution range for children aged 2 years and older and *(b)* macronutrient target contribution to diet based on ADMR midpoint.

Based on recommendations from Nordic Council of Ministers (2014).

Nutritional goals for selected micronutrients are provided by the RDIs given in table 16.4; the type of RDI (e.g., RDA, AI, UL) provided for each micronutrient depends on what information is available. Table 16.5 shows food sources of selected vitamins and minerals and demonstrates that youth need a varied diet in order to meet micronutrient needs. It is important to meet the recommended intakes of micronutrients because they support metabolism and tissue function; in fact, micronutrient deficiencies are associated with disease and other negative health outcomes. Vitamins and minerals often work synergistically to support function and development, as in the combined role played by vitamin D and calcium in promoting healthy bone growth.

In contrast to macronutrients, micronutrient needs do not differ across physical activity levels, but the consequences of failing to reach recommended intakes may be more acute in athletic youth (Mangieri, 2017). Youth athletes need adequate intake of micronutrients to help support performance and recovery; for instance, Geiker and colleagues (2017) show that adolescent swimmers with higher levels of vitamin D also had greater muscle strength. In summarizing available evidence, Story and Stang (2005) reported that American adolescents routinely consumed suboptimal levels of vitamins A, B$_9$ (folate), and E and of the minerals iron, zinc, magnesium, and calcium (they also had excessive levels of salt intake). Deficits notwithstanding, the use of supplements to provide excess levels of micronutrients may be harmful, and concerns have been raised that initial use of over-the-counter supplements may be associated with other risk-taking behaviors (Shenkin, 2006). Nutrient needs should normally be met through the diet (Desbrow et al., 2014), and prolonged supplementation is not associated with reduced disease risk or additional health benefits in individuals who eat a balanced healthy diet (Nordic Council of Ministers, 2014). If supplementation is truly needed for health reasons, it should be prescribed by a medical professional.

DO YOU KNOW?

There is no scientific justification for using supplements to adjust an unbalanced diet (Nordic Council of Ministers, 2014).

Vitamins can be divided into two classifications; water soluble and fat soluble. Water-soluble vitamins, which include the B vitamins and vitamin C, help catalyze metabolic reactions that break down and synthesize macronutrients. These vitamins have a high turnover rate because they are absorbed into the blood and do not remain in the system for long periods (Schoenfeld & Aragon, 2016). Fat-soluble vitamins include A, D, E, and K and are stored in adipose tissue; they contribute to processes including bone formation and antioxidation. Like vitamins, minerals can be divided into two categories: major minerals (also referred to as *macrominerals*) and trace minerals. Major minerals are required in amounts of at least 100 milligrams per day, whereas trace minerals are required in smaller amounts. With regard to growth, development, physical activity, and health, particularly important vitamins and minerals include iron, vitamin D, calcium, zinc, and sodium.

Macronutrients and Dietary Fiber

Appropriate intake of macronutrients and dietary fiber is needed in order to support growth and development, fuel active living, and maintain good health. The distribution of macronutrients in the diet determines the overall energy intake, but it is equally important to consider the type and quality of each macronutrient. Youth fitness specialists and others who are responsible for guiding youth should consider the food and beverage choices available for meeting macronutrient needs, as well as the potential consequences for youth who consume diets consisting of either desirable or undesirable sources of carbohydrate, fat, and protein.

Carbohydrate: Starch and Sugar

Carbohydrate, in the form of starch and sugar, provides energy for the cells of the body and the brain, the latter of which is the only carbohydrate-dependent organ in the body (Institute of Medicine, 2005). AMDR suggests that carbohydrate should contribute 45 percent to 65 percent of needed daily energy (Institute of Medicine, 2005); a value of 52 percent or 53 percent has been suggested as a suitable target for the general population (Nordic Council of Ministers, 2014), and a minimum target of 50 percent has been suggested for youth athletes (Petrie et al., 2004). Thus carbohydrate serves as the major source of energy in the diet, providing energy to support growth and daily functioning and to fuel exercise, particularly high-intensity exercise. Youth have limited internal stores of carbohydrate, and they begin to deplete during physical activity. During heavy exercise, youth can use carbohydrate stores at a rate of 1.0 to 1.5 gram per kilogram of body mass per hour, which means that a 50-kilogram child could deplete 50 to 75 grams of carbohydrate per hour of exercise (Fox & Kerksick, 2016). Therefore, it is important to provide youth with a diet that includes regular intake of carbohydrate throughout the day; moreover, active youth may require considerable additional carbohy-

TABLE 16.4   MICRONUTRIENT KEY FUNCTIONS AND DIETARY REFERENCE INTAKES FOR CHILDREN AND ADOLESCENTS

	Key functions	RDI*	CHILD 1-3	FEMALE 4-8	FEMALE 9-13	FEMALE 14-18	MALE 4-8	MALE 9-13	MALE 14-18
Vitamins									
A (mg)	Vision, wound healing, growth, immune function	RDA	300	400	600	700	400	600	900
B₁ (thiamin) (mg)	Metabolism of macronutrients, growth, appetite, digestion, healthy nerves	RDA	0.5	0.6	0.9	1.0	0.6	0.9	1.2
B₂ (riboflavin) (mg)	Tissue respiration, growth	RDA	0.5	0.6	0.9	1.0	0.6	0.9	1.3
B₃ (niacin) (mg)	Oxidation, synthesis of glycogen and fatty acids	RDA	6	8	12	14	8	12	16
B₆ (mg)	Growth, synthesis and breakdown of proteins and fatty acids	RDA	0.5	0.6	1	1.2	0.6	1	1.3
B₉ (folate) (mcg)	Synthesis of nucleic acids, maturation of blood cells	RDA	150	200	300	400	200	300	400
B₁₂ (mcg)	Folate (B₉) metabolism and central nervous system metabolism	RDA	0.9	1.2	1.8	2.4	1.2	1.8	2.4
C (mg)	Collagen synthesis, iron absorption and transport, antioxidant action	RDA	15	25	45	65	25	45	75
D (IU)	Bone formation, absorption of calcium and phosphorus in the intestines	RDA	600	600	600	600	600	600	600
E (mg)	Antioxidant action	RDA	6	7	11	15	7	11	16
K (mcg)	Blood clotting, synthesis of intestinal bacteria	RDA	150	200	300	400	200	300	400
Minerals									
Calcium (mg)	Bone and tooth formation, blood clotting, nerve transmission	RDA	700	1,000	1,300	1,300	1,000	1,300	1,300
Copper (mcg)	Support of iron and many enzymes	RDA	340	440	700	890	440	700	890
Iron (mg)	Formation of hemoglobin, resistance to infection	RDA	7	10	8	15	10	8	11
Magnesium (mg)	Oxidation, nerve transmission, muscle contraction	RDA	80	130	240	360	130	240	410
Manganese (mg)	Support of enzymes involved in protein synthesis and energy metabolism	AI	1.2	1.5	1.6	1.6	1.5	1.9	2.2
Potassium (mg)	Acid–base balance, muscle activity (including cardiac)	AI	3,000	3,800	4,500	4,700	3,800	4,500	4,700
Selenium (mcg)	Tissue respiration, fat metabolism, antioxidant action	RDA	20	30	40	55	30	40	55
Sodium	Acid–base balance, muscle contraction	UL	1,500	1,900	2,200	2,300	1,900	2,200	2,300
Zinc	Support of enzyme systems and insulin	RDA	3	5	8	9	5	8	11

*RDA = Recommended Daily Allowance, AI = Adequate Intake, UL = Tolerable Upper Intake Level

Adapted from Schoenfeld and Aragon (2016) and USDA (2015).

drate before, during, and after competition or training.

When eaten, digestible carbohydrate is broken down into the simple sugar glucose, which enters the blood and causes blood glucose levels to rise. Blood glucose can then be used to help supply immediate energy; if energy release is not required, it can be converted to glycogen and stored in skeletal muscle and in the liver. To aid this process, rises in blood glucose stimulate the release of the hormone insulin, which prompts muscle and liver cells to absorb glucose from the blood. If blood glucose levels then begin to fall (i.e., later in the day or with continued exercise), the stored glycogen can be converted back to glucose in order to help fuel muscles and the brain. This ability to maintain stable blood glucose levels is important for health and enables the body to avoid **hyperglycemia** and **hypoglycemia**, both of which can carry serious health implications.

Consumption of carbohydrate, particularly sugar, is implicated in the development of metabolic syndrome and type 2 diabetes, the latter of which is characterized by high levels of blood glucose and absence of or resistance to insulin. Acute and chronic complications of type 2 diabetes can lead to many negative and often severe outcomes for youth (Pinhas-Hamiel & Zeitler, 2007). In 2000, the American Diabetes Association referred to an emerging problem of type 2 diabetes in children, suggesting that if the trend was not reversed it could lead to major challenges to society. Unfortunately, between 2001 and 2009 the prevalence of type 2 diabetes in U.S. children and adolescents increased by 31 percent (Dabelea et al., 2014), a trend which has been observed around the world (Reinehr, 2013). The rise in adolescent diabetes is creating a major clinical challenge and health care burden (Viner et al., 2017), and preventing this disease should be a priority. As part of this effort, youth fitness specialists should be aware of the link between type 2 diabetes and sugar-sweetened beverages, artificially sweetened beverages, and fruit juice (Imamura et al., 2016).

TABLE 16.5   FOOD SOURCES OF SELECTED VITAMINS AND MINERALS

Micronutrient	Food sources
Vitamins	
A	Milk, eggs, liver, fortified cereals, orange fruits and vegetables, dark green vegetables
B	Fish, red meat, poultry, milk, cheese, eggs
B_1	Fortified breads, cereals, and pastas; lean meats; dried beans; soy foods; peas; whole grains
B_2	Meat, dairy products, legumes, nuts, green leafy vegetables, broccoli, asparagus, fortified cereals
B_3	Red meat, poultry, fish, peanuts, fortified cereals
B_6	Potatoes, bananas, beans, seeds, nuts, red meat, poultry, fish, eggs, spinach, fortified cereals
B_9	Liver, dried beans and legumes, green leafy vegetables, oranges, fortified bread, rice, cereals
C	Citrus fruits, strawberries, kiwi, guava, peppers, tomatoes, broccoli, spinach
D	Egg yolks, oily fish, fortified milk and juices
E	Vegetable oils, nuts, green leafy vegetables, avocados, whole grains
K	Green vegetables (leafy and nonleafy), meat, liver, fish, eggs
Minerals	
Calcium	Milk, cheese, yogurt, sardines, salmon, fortified foods (e.g., juice, tofu)
Copper	Shellfish, liver, kidney, whole grains, beans, nuts, dark leafy greens, dried prunes
Iron	Meat, fish, poultry, liver, heart, firm tofu, beans and legumes, nuts, seeds, fortified foods (e.g., flour, bread, pastas, cereal)
Magnesium	Spinach, Swiss chard, bran cereals, wheat germs, dried beans and legumes, nuts, seeds
Manganese	Whole grains, beans, nuts, leafy vegetables, bran cereals, tea
Potassium	Bananas, papaya, sweet potato, dark leafy greens, avocado, milk, yogurt, dried beans, meat, nuts, seeds
Selenium	Brazil nuts, mixed nuts, oysters, fish, meat, liver, poultry, eggs,
Sodium	Salt
Zinc	Yogurt, milk, cheese, dried beans, seeds, meat, liver, poultry, fish, seafood

Carbohydrate is often divided into two categories—simple and complex—depending on the number of sugar units present. Simple carbohydrates, such as glucose and fructose, contain only one or two sugars. They are easy to break down and when consumed cause blood glucose and insulin secretion to rise rapidly. Forms of carbohydrate containing more than two sugars, known as oligosaccharides and polysaccharides, are classified as complex. These carbohydrates tend to be found in foods that also contain fiber, vitamins, and minerals and they take longer to digest. They can cause blood sugar and insulin to rise more slowly. The polysaccharides known as glycogen and starch serve as the storage forms of carbohydrate in plants and in animals, respectively (Institute of Medicine, 2005). Another source of carbohydrate is found in sugar alcohols, which should not feature in a youth diet.

Consuming simple carbohydrates such as glucose and fructose can cause blood glucose and insulin levels to increase rapidly. If simple sugars are consumed routinely, the repeated and long-term stress can lead to **insulin resistance** as body cells become unresponsive to increased insulin. As a result, blood sugar remains high, which can lead to a state of hyperglycemia, symptoms of which can include headaches, lethargy, inability to concentrate, and increased thirst. In response to insulin resistance, insulin-producing cells work harder to produce more of this hormone, but over time this adjustment can cause damage and ultimately lead to reduced insulin production and inability to regulate blood glucose. This process describes the development of type 2 diabetes.

DO YOU KNOW?

Refined starches, such as white bread and white pasta, provide carbohydrate that contains little fiber or other nutrients.

Therefore, youth fitness specialists must consider not only the quantity of carbohydrate consumed but also the quality of that carbohydrate. For example, Lustig and colleagues (2016) replaced a substantial amount of dietary sugar intake by obese youth with starch while maintaining overall energy consumption. In just nine days, in comparison with a control group, obese youth on a low-sugar but calorie-equivalent diet, significantly improved their markers of metabolic health; specifically, they exhibited reductions in blood pressure and low-density lipid cholesterol, improvements in glucose tolerance, and enhanced **insulin sensitivity**.

The glycemic index (GI) provides a method for classifying carbohydrate-rich foods according to their effect on postprandial blood glucose (Zakrewski & Tolfrey, 2016). Glycemic index is measured by monitoring the blood glucose response following ingestion of 50 grams of a particular type of carbohydrate; it is expressed relative to a standard reference of either glucose or white bread, which are given a score of 100. A lower glycemic index indicates a source of carbohydrate that causes a lower but more prolonged release of sugar into the blood, thus causing less stress on the body and providing a steadier supply of energy.

Compelling evidence supports the use of low-glycemic-index diets for disease prevention in adults (Barclay et al., 2008), and similar evidence is emerging in regard to youth (Fajcsak et al., 2008; Rouhani et al., 2013). Table 16.6 identifies sources of carbohydrate with a low, medium, or high glycemic index. Youth fitness specialists can use this information to help plan meals and snacks for youth in their care—for example, by opting for unrefined grains, cereals, and legumes over refined cereals and snacks. However, practitioners should also consider the overall nutritional value of any food or drink and how it might fit with the overall needs of the child. The preference is for carbohydrate to be derived from sources that are lower in GI and higher in fiber and micronutrient density; this goal can be accomplished by replacing refined grains with whole grains and cereals and by consuming more fresh fruit, vegetables, and pulses (e.g., beans, peas, chickpeas, lentils).

Given the health benefits of a diet that includes carbohydrate from nutrient-rich foods, as well as the potential negative effects of consuming too much sugar, the consensus view holds that consumption of **added sugar** should be limited (Vos et al., 2017). Added sugar is defined as any sugar or syrup added to a food or beverage during processing or preparation. Major sources of added sugar include soft drinks, fruit drinks, energy drinks, cakes and doughnuts, sweet pies, cookies, pastries, ice cream and other frozen desserts, and jams (U.S. Department of Agriculture, 2015). Many countries and food agencies have adopted the WHO recommendation that added sugar should not account for more than 10 percent of the calories consumed in one's diet (World Health Organization, 2015). It is further recommended that added sugar eventually be limited to 5 percent of total energy consumed (World Health Organization, 2015). The American Heart Association has extended the recommendation, noting that youth aged 2 to 18 years should consume no more than 25 grams of added sugar per day (Vos et al., 2017). As a point of reference, a 12-ounce (350 mL) can of soda generally contains about 40 grams of added sugar.

Evidence shows that people in countries that generally follow a Western diet consume added sugar in excess of the recommended 10 percent limit (Nordic

PUBERTY AND OBESITY IN THE DEVELOPMENT OF TYPE 2 DIABETES

Insulin resistance is the greatest risk factor for development of type 2 diabetes and is perhaps the greatest current health threat to children (Keskin et al., 2005). Insulin sensitivity declines naturally by about 30 percent during puberty, and this reduction affects the body's ability to regulate blood glucose, but sensitivity should recover after puberty (Amiel et al., 1986; Goran & Gower, 2001). High-sugar diets have also been implicated in the process of childhood and adolescent obesity, and obese youth are likely to be insulin resistant and to exhibit impaired insulin production (Keskin et al., 2005; Luger et al., 2017). Consequently, pubertal and obese youth are more at risk of developing type 2 diabetes. In response, youth fitness specialists should educate pubertal, overweight, and obese youth and encourage them to move toward a diet that replaces simple, refined sugars with nutritious foods containing complex carbohydrates, as well as good sources of protein and healthful fat.

TABLE 16.6   LOW-, MEDIUM-, AND HIGH-GLYCEMIC-INDEX FOODS

	Low GI (0-55)	Medium GI (56-70)	High GI (>70)
Cereal	Wheat bran (42) Whole grain (48) Rolled-oat porridge (55)	Muesli (57) Raisin bran (61) Wheat biscuits (69)	Toasted oats (74) Whole-wheat pieces (75) Puffed rice, chocolate (77) Instant porridge (79) Toasted corn (81) Crisped rice (87)
Bread	Corn tortilla (46) Buckwheat bread (47) Rye Bread (50) Chapati (52)	White pita (57) Hamburger bun (61) Rice bread (67) Croissant (69)	White bagel (72) Wholemeal bread (74) White bread (75) English muffin (77) White baguette (95)
Fruit	Apple (36) Orange (43) Grapes (46) Banana (51) Kiwi (53)	Apricot (57) Pineapple (59) Papaya (59) Raisins (64)	Watermelon (76) Dried dates (103)
Vegetables	Raw carrots (16) Yam (37) Carrots (39) Green pea (48) Sweet corn (54)	Sweet potato (63) Beetroot (64)	Rutabaga (72) Pumpkin (95) Parsnip (97)
Staples	Soybeans (16) Chickpeas (28) Lentils (32) Baked beans (48) Spaghetti (49) Noodles (55)	Basmati rice (58) Couscous (65) Brown rice (68) Cornmeal (69)	White rice (73) Potato (78) French fries (75) Tapioca (81) Instant mashed potatoes (87)
Snacks and sweet foods	Hummus (6) Custard (38) Fruit yogurt (41) Apple muffin (44) Banana cake (47)	Potato chips (56) Cream cracker (56) Blueberry muffin (59) Ice cream (61) Popcorn (65) Pancakes (67) Crumpet (69)	Cupcakes (73) Doughnut (76) Waffles (76) Rice crackers (87)
Drinks	Fruit smoothie (32) Soy milk (34) Tomato juice (38) Full-fat milk (39) Apple juice (40) Orange juice (50)	Soda (59)	Sport drink (78) Rice milk (86) Energy drink (95)

Based on information from Atkinson, Foster-Power, and Brand-Miller (2008) and Foster-Powell, Holt, and Brand-Miller (2002).

Council of Ministers, 2014). Moreover, intake of added sugar is particularly high among children and adolescents (U.S. Department of Agriculture, 2015); in fact, added sugar accounts for about 17 percent of calories consumed by the average 9- to 18-year-olds in the United States. Almost half of that intake comes in the form of sugary beverages (U.S. Department of Agriculture, 2015), which are linked to overweight and obesity in youth (American Academy of Pediatrics, 2011) and increase the risk of type 2 diabetes (Nordic Council of Ministers, 2014).

Carbohydrate: Dietary Fiber

Dietary fiber is a form of carbohydrate that is resistant to human enzymes and consequently nondigestible. Fiber normally contains a mix of polysaccharides and is found in edible plant foods, including grains, cereals, fruits, and vegetables; as a result, sources of dietary fiber typically contain other digestible macro- and micronutrients as well. When consumed, fiber delays gastric emptying, thus providing a sensation of fullness that may help with weight management; it may also reduce postprandial blood glucose concentrations and exert a beneficial effect on insulin sensitivity. Other benefits may include reducing blood cholesterol concentrations and preventing constipation (Institute of Medicine, 2005).

Fibers are categorized as either soluble or insoluble. Soluble fibers are found in some grains, fruits, pulses, and root vegetables; when consumed, these fiber dissolve and form a gel in the gut. Insoluble fibers, on the other hand, are found in cereals, whole grains, some vegetables, and seeds and nuts. Both soluble and insoluble fibers aid digestion and are considered good for gut health. The long-term benefits of a diet high in fiber include reduction in risk of developing type 2 diabetes (Fung et al., 2002; Schulze et al. 2004) and reduction in coronary heart disease (Pereira et al., 2004).

Analysis of the National Health and Nutrition Examination Survey revealed that U.S. children and adolescents consume an average of 14 grams of fiber per day; although consumption increased over a 10-year-period, the levels achieved still fell below recommended guidelines (McGill et al., 2015). RDAs for dietary fiber are widely available, and the U.S. Department of Agriculture (2015) recommends that children aged 1 to 3 years consume 14 grams per day and that 14- to 18-year-old girls and boys consume 25 and 31 grams, respectively. These values are based on the needs of children of average size with average levels of physical activity. Fiber needs are considered to be the same in children and adults, and consumption of 14 grams per 1,000 kilocalories of dietary intake per day is viewed as an adequate to reduce coronary heart disease (Institute of Medicine, 2005).

As with macronutrient needs, the fiber needs of youth should be based on their estimated energy requirements. On this basis, a very active 13-year-old boy of average size would have an estimated daily energy requirement of 3,000 kilocalories (table 16.1) and a dietary fiber need of 42 grams per day. Youth can increase fiber intake by replacing refined grains with whole grains (e.g., whole-grain cereal, bread, pasta) and increasing consumption of beans, legumes, fruits, vegetables, seeds, and nuts.

Fat

Fat is an essential macronutrient that provides energy and contributes to many other functions in the body, including the absorption of vitamins A, D, E, and K; the building of cell membranes; the production of sex hormones; and the development of the brain and eyes. Although fat plays an important role in the body, dietary fat is often associated with overweight and obesity in youth and linked to increased risk of

Teaching Tip

SHOULD YOUTH CONSUME SPORT DRINKS?

It is sometimes suggested that youth athletes may benefit from the use of sport drinks containing simple sugars before, during, or after exercise (Rodriguez et al., 2009). These drinks may help young athletes fuel exercise, avoid glycogen depletion during exercise, and replenish glycogen stores after exercise. However, given the reduced insulin sensitivity that is characteristic of early and mid puberty, high-GI sport drinks should be used by adolescent athletes only with caution (Zakrzewski & Tolfrey, 2016). For most children involved in regular physical activity, the use of sport drinks, either during exercise or at other times, is unnecessary (American Academy of Pediatrics, 2011). For youth athletes who participate in events that are prolonged (i.e., last more than an hour) and involve vigorous exercise or take place in a hot and humid environment, it may be useful to use a sport drink containing carbohydrate and sodium chloride in order to maintain energy provision and electrolyte balance.

disease. However, the type of fat consumed is the most important factor in determining how fat affects an individual's health. In a recent Presidential Advisory statement, the American Heart Association (Sacks et al., 2017) concluded strongly that lowering one's intake of saturated fat and replacing saturated fat with unsaturated fat, particularly polyunsaturated fat, can lower the risk of cardiovascular disease. Thus youth fitness specialists must be acutely aware of the different types of fat contained in different foods and remain mindful that youth need adequate intake of "good" fat to support growth, maturation, and a physically active lifestyle.

Fats form a subcategory within the larger category of fat-soluble substances called **lipids**; other forms of lipids include oils and **cholesterol**. About 95 percent of the lipids in the human body and in food are triglycerides which are molecules in which a glycerol molecule is attached to three fatty acids (McLain & Conn, 2016). Consequently, as a more common and familiar term, *fat* is often used synonymously with *triglyceride* or *lipid*. Fats are categorized based on their chemical structure as either saturated or unsaturated. Saturated fats are sometimes referred to as "bad fats" because they play no known role in preventing chronic diseases; however, it is neither achievable nor desirable to completely remove these fats from the diet (Institute of Medicine, 2005). Saturated fats are solid at room temperature and are found in high amounts in animal foods (e.g., fatty red meats, high-fat dairy products, lard) and in some plant foods (e.g., coconuts, coconut oil, and palm oil).

Unsaturated fats can be further categorized as either monounsaturated or polyunsaturated. These kinds of fat tend to be liquid at room temperature and are predominantly found in foods sourced from plants. Monounsaturated fats are found in olive oil, avocados, and many nuts and seeds, whereas polyunsaturated fats are found in sunflower, soybean, and flaxseed oils, as well as fish and walnuts. Replacing saturated fats with polyunsaturated fats has been suggested as a way to improve health (Astrup et al., 2011), and increased consumption of polyunsaturated fats has been shown to improve blood lipid profiles (Mensink et al., 2003) and reduce the risk of heart disease (Mozaffarian et al., 2010), albeit in adults. Polyunsaturated fats are not stable when heated to high temperatures; therefore, oils that are higher in monounsaturated fats are recommended for cooking. Olive oil is a good choice for cooking because it consists of 85 percent unsaturated fat (75 percent monounsaturated, 10 percent polyunsaturated) and only 15 percent saturated fat.

Trans fat is created from polyunsaturated fat during an industrial process in which hydrogen is added in order to make fats harder. On food labels, trans fats are often referred to as "partially hydrogenated." Used to add taste and texture, they are inexpensive, long lasting, and able to withstand repeated heating without breaking down. As a result, they are added to many foods, especially foods that are processed, deep fried, or packaged. When polyunsaturated fats are converted to trans fats, they no longer provide their original benefits (McLain & Conn, 2016). In fact, trans fats provide no known health benefits and are associated with increased risk of disease; therefore, their consumption should be as low as possible (Institute of Medicine, 2005). A meta-analysis by Mozaffarian and colleagues (2006) showed that for each 2 percent of calories regularly consumed in the form of trans fat, the risk of coronary heart disease increases by 23 percent, and adverse effects are still apparent when the intake of trans fat falls below 3 percent of overall energy. This level equates to two to seven grams of trans fat per day for a person who consumes 2,000 kilocalories per day.

Teaching Tip

ESSENTIAL FATTY ACIDS

Although the body can produce most of the fatty acids it needs from carbohydrate and protein, the essential fatty acids omega-3 and omega-6 must be consumed in the diet. These polyunsaturated fats play a major role in the central nervous system and brain, aid visual development in infants, help maintain healthy skin and a healthy reproductive system, help regulate blood pressure, aid blood clotting, and help ensure a robust immune system (McLain & Conn, 2016). It has been recommended that omega-6 and omega-3 contribute at least 2.5 percent and 0.5 percent, respectively, of average energy intake (Nordic Council of Ministers, 2014). It has also been reported that the Western diet is very high in omega-6 and low in omega-3 and that changing the ratio between these essential fats can be favorable for disease prevention (Simopoulos, 2002). Consequently, youth fitness specialists should help ensure that youth consume adequate amounts of essential fatty acids, which can be found in oily fish (e.g., salmon, sardines, tuna), some oils (e.g., sunflower oil, flaxseed, soybean), nuts, and seeds.

Therefore, all youth should minimize consumption of foods that are high in trans fat.

Cholesterol is an essential building block of cell membranes; it is found in every cell in the body and provides the precursor for testosterone. Although cholesterol is vital for healthy development, excessive cholesterol is associated with increased cardiovascular disease. Cholesterol is found in foods, particularly eggs and liver, but the majority of cholesterol is produced by the body. Because cholesterol cannot travel in the blood on its own, it is combined with proteins to form lipoproteins, which allow cholesterol to move around the body. Low-density lipoproteins (LDLs) carry cholesterol from the liver around the body, but excessive LDL levels can lead to plaque deposits in the arteries (including the coronary artery), thus causing them to narrow. High-density lipoproteins (HDLs), on the other hand, take unused cholesterol from the bloodstream, and artery walls and return it to the liver for disposal, thereby acting as a protective mechanism.

Production of both LDL and HDL are influenced by consumption of saturated fat, unsaturated fat, and sugar. Higher consumption of saturated fat, trans fat, and sugar is associated with increased levels of circulating cholesterol and LDL (Institute of Medicine, 2005; Welsh et al., 2011). Replacing saturated fat with unsaturated fat has been shown to improve the ratio of HDL to total cholesterol (Mensink et al., 2003) and is a common nutritional recommendation for youth (Te Morenga & Montez, 2017). Therefore, it has been suggested that swapping saturated fat with unsaturated fat exerts a better effect on LDL and HDL than simply reducing intake of saturated fat (Mozaffarian et al., 2010; Nordic Council of Ministers, 2014).

Given the global obesity epidemic in youth, dietary fat has developed a bad reputation. However, fat is essential for healthy growth and development and plays a role in many important functions. In fact, it has been recently suggested that global dietary guidelines should be reconsidered given the emergence of evidence suggesting that fat intake shows little association with disease and mortality, whereas high carbohydrate intake has been associated with higher mortality (Dehghan et al., 2017). Clearly, not all fats are equal, and quality of fat needs to be considered as much as quantity. With the accumulation of evidence, public guidelines have evolved over recent decades to highlight a more positive role played by some fats. Fogelholm (2013) pointed out that between 1996 and 2012 the Nordic Nutrition Recommendations shifted from recommending that no more than 30 percent of calories come from fat to recommending a range from 25 percent to 40 percent with a target of 32 percent or 33 percent. The Dietary Guidelines for Americans recommend that fat contribute 25 percent to 35 percent of energy requirements (U.S. Department of Agriculture, 2015), and Public Health England (2016) provides reference guidelines based on fat contribution of 35 percent of total energy intake. These contemporary guidelines may reflect a slight shift away from previous policies promoting a low-fat, higher-carbohydrate diet.

Guidelines are consistent in their recommendations for youth to minimize consumption of trans fat, limit saturated fat to less than 10 percent of energy intake, and swap saturated fat for unsaturated fat, which can help promote good health. The diet must also contain adequate amounts of essential fatty acids, which cannot be produced by the body. Youth fitness specialists should help educate children, adolescents, and parents about making food choices that support the consumption of "good fats" while limiting the intake of the "bad fats" that raise cholesterol and LDL levels (i.e., saturated fats, sugars).

Protein

Protein is most often associated with its role in building skeletal muscle tissue. Skeletal muscle mass increases markedly during growth and maturation

---

Teaching Tip

FATS AND EXERCISE

Maturity influences the way in which macronutrients support the energy needed for physical activity. Prepubescent children are more reliant on fat oxidation during exercise than are adolescents or adults. This reliance may derive from a number of factors, including hormonal differences, lower levels of glycolytic enzymes, and lower levels of lactate production, which inhibits the mobilization of free fatty acids for energy. With a healthy diet, children hold adequate stores of fat to support exercise without accumulating the excessive fat storage associated with overweight and obesity. For highly active youth, there is no evidence that high-fat diets are effective in enhancing performance (McLain & Conn, 2016). Young athletes should follow guidelines for the general population, consuming enough (predominantly "good") fat to meet their energy requirements.

and can also increase in response to exercise and training, thus reflecting the adaptability of muscle when supported by adequate protein intake. In fact, protein is a major structural component of all cells in the body (Institute of Medicine, 2015) and is important for an array of other biological functions, including gene activity; transport of biological molecules; energy production; and synthesis of hormones, enzymes, and neurotransmitters (Escobar et al., 2016). If protein intake is inadequate, youth may experience reductions in linear growth (Semba et al., 2016) and muscle mass accumulation, as well as delayed sexual maturation (Story & Stang, 2005). In girls, protein intake may be particularly important in controlling fat mass gains during puberty (van Vught et al., 2009). In addition, youth athletes have greater protein needs than their less active peers (Petrie et al., 2004) due to the need to support exercise and recovery.

DO YOU KNOW?

Youth athletes have greater protein needs than their less active peers due to the need to support both exercise and recovery.

Children and adolescents need to achieve a positive protein balance in order to support growth, sexual maturation, and the deposition of new tissue. Positive protein balance also supports training by allowing for recovery and repair of skeletal tissue. Consequently, the relative protein needs of children are usually considered greater than those of adults, and the needs of active youth are greater than those of inactive youth.

Table 16.7 shows the RDA for protein needs of the general population based on recommendations from the Institute of Medicine (2005) and the Nordic Council of Ministers (2014). It has also been suggested that protein consumption should increase to 1.5 grams $\cdot$ kg^{-1}

$\cdot$ day^{-1} during the pubertal growth spurt (Petrie et al., 2004). Protein needs are higher for youth who are more physically active; specifically, Escobar and colleagues (2016) recommend an intake in the range of 1.0 to 1.5 grams $\cdot$ kg^{-1} $\cdot$ day^{-1} for youth involved in a resistance training program, 1.2 to 1.4 grams $\cdot$ kg^{-1} $\cdot$ day^{-1} for those involved in exhaustive endurance exercise, and 1.5 grams $\cdot$ kg^{-1} $\cdot$ day^{-1} or higher in youth athletes involved in heavy training and competition periods. In an international position statement, Jager and colleagues (2017) recommend intakes ranging from 1.4 to 2.0 grams $\cdot$ kg^{-1} $\cdot$ day^{-1} for exercising individuals and on up to 3.0 grams $\cdot$ kg^{-1} $\cdot$ day^{-1} in resistance-trained individuals. Although the recommendations of Jager and colleagues (2017) were not specific to youth, it seems reasonable to apply the findings to youth given the similar relative protein requirements of youth and adults.

Despite suggestions to the contrary from the popular media, evidence demonstrates that consuming protein above recommended limits does not lead to adverse renal or bone effects in healthy individuals (Escobar et al., 2016); hence, no tolerable upper limit is provided for protein in dietary guidelines (Institute of Medicine, 2005). However, youth fitness specialists should consider what upper limit of protein might be useful to promote adaptation and whether protein intake above that limit adds unwanted calories to the diet. Fox and colleagues (2011) and Escobar and colleagues (2016) pointed to a collection of evidence to support their recommendation of 2.0 grams $\cdot$ kg^{-1} $\cdot$ day^{-1} as the upper beneficial limit of protein consumption. The levels of protein consumption provided in table 16.7 should be easily achievable with a balanced diet and therefore should not require protein supplementation.

As with other macronutrients, it is not only the quantity of dietary protein that needs to be considered but also the quality. The building blocks of protein

TABLE 16.7   RECOMMENDED DAILY INTAKE OF PROTEIN FOR DIFFERENT POPULATIONS

Population	Recommended intake (g $\cdot$ kg^{-1} $\cdot$ day^{-1})
1-3 yr old	1.05-1.1[a,b]
4-13 yr old	0.95-1.1 [a,b]
14-18 yr old	0.85-1.1 [a,b]
≥19 yr old	0.80-1.1 [a,b]
Youth involved in sport	1.0-2.0[c,d]
Maximal beneficial limit in athletic populations	2.0-3.0[c,e,d]

Notes: RDA values for the general population are taken from [a]IOM (2005) and [b]Nordic Council of Ministers (2014). Data for "youth involved in sport" are based on recommendations from [c]Esbobar et al. (2016) and [d]Jager et al. (2017). Data for "maximal beneficial limit" are based on recommendations from [c]Escobar et al. (2016), [e]Fox et al. (2011), and [d]Jager et al. (2017).

Adapted from Institute of Medicine (2005); Nordic Council of Ministers (2014); Escobar, McLain, and Kerksick (2016); Jager, Kerksick, Campbell, et al. (2017); Fox, McDaniel, Breitbach, and Weiss (2011).

are amino acids, and the human body requires 20 of them in order to produce the protein it needs. Due to the number and sequencing of amino acids, the body creates proteins that vary in shape, size, and function, thus allowing for many types of protein to be synthesized. The eight **essential amino acids** are particularly important because they cannot be produced by the body and therefore must be consumed in the diet. They include isoleucine, leucine, lysine, methionine, phenylalanine, threonine, tryptophan, and valine. The nonessential amino acids, though important for function, do not have to be consumed in the diet, because the body can endogenously manufacture them. Nonessential amino acids play no role in the growth and building of muscle protein, a fact that highlights the importance of the essential amino acids in supporting growth, development, and physical activity in youth (Escobar et al., 2016).

DO YOU KNOW?

The essential amino acids are the building blocks of muscle protein and must be consumed in the diet.

Three of the essential amino acids—leucine, isoleucine, and valine—are classified as branched-chain amino acids (BCAAs), whose name describes their chemical structure. Whereas other amino acids are metabolized in the liver, BCAA are metabolized primarily in skeletal muscle and play a unique role in muscle protein metabolism. Leucine has the greatest metabolic activity, affecting muscle protein turnover, insulin resistance, and tissue sensitivity (Institute of Medicine, 2005). Of all of the amino acids, leucine is the most potent stimulator of muscle protein synthesis (Norton et, al., 2012). Therefore, consuming foods high in leucine is particularly important for youth but must be balanced with the ingestion of other amino acids to maximally stimulate muscle protein synthesis (Norton et al., 2012).

Youth fitness specialists should also consider the completeness of protein food sources—that is, the amount of essential amino acids present. If youth have a diet that consists of incomplete protein sources, it will challenge cellular and metabolic function, which over time can lead to protein malnutrition (Escobar et al., 2016). In this scenario, essential amino acids that are missing from the diet will be leached from body tissue (e.g., skeletal muscle) in an attempt to maintain function. Good sources of complete proteins, and therefore of BCAA, include animal-based foods such as meat, fish, poultry, and eggs. Plant-based foods contain protein but typically lack at least one of the essential amino acids and are therefore viewed as incomplete protein sources. Soybeans are one of the few plant foods that serve as a source of complete protein because they contain all essential amino acids, but they have only a low amount of the essential amino acid methionine.

Youth fitness specialists should prioritize the consumption of essential amino acids in the diet while also considering the overall nutrition needs of youth. For example, although processed meats may provide a source of complete animal protein, they are also likely to contain saturated fat and trans fat, high levels of sodium, and limited micronutrients. Ideally, therefore, they should be avoided.

Selected Micronutrients

Adequate intake of vitamins and minerals is needed in order to support many important aspects of growth and development and to maintain good health. Yet in both Europe and the United States, youth have been reported to consume inadequate amounts of some vitamins and minerals, including vitamins A, D, and E; calcium; iron; magnesium; and zinc (Story & Stang, 2005; Kaganov et al., 2015). In addition, research indicates that this trend is more pronounced in females than in males (Story & Stang 2005). It has been suggested that youth involved in sport tend to have better dietary practices and consume higher levels of micronutrients than their less active peers (Cupisti et al., 2002). However, the diet of many youth athletes may still be suboptimal. Gibson and colleagues (2011) reported that elite female youth soccer players had depleted vitamin D and iron status and consumed less than the recommended levels of vitamins B_5, B_9, and E, as well as calcium. It has also been shown that adolescent weightlifters consume lower than recommended amounts of calcium, magnesium, and potassium (Serairi Beji et al., 2016). Youth fitness specialists should be aware that the sheer fact of ready access to food does not ensure that youth are making healthy choices that meet their nutritional needs.

Vitamin D

Vitamin D is a steroid hormone that helps regulate the metabolism of several minerals (most notably calcium) and thereby helps to maintain skeletal health and growth. Consequently, a lack of vitamin D is associated with bone pathologies such as rickets and osteoporosis. Emerging evidence suggests that it may also help prevent cardiovascular disease, diabetes, immune disease, and cancer while also helping to improve strength and recovery from exercise (Schoenfeld & Aragon, 2016). Vitamin D is unique among other vitamins because it can be synthesized from exposure of the skin to

Teaching Tip

MEETING PROTEIN NEEDS WITH A VEGETARIAN OR VEGAN DIET

Muscle protein synthesis requires a plentiful supply of essential amino acids, and they are all contained in animal-based foods. However, some youth choose to follow a vegetarian or vegan diet, and it is important that they still achieve adequate intake of protein. Plant-based foods can provide protein but either lack or are very low in at least one essential amino acid. Even so, a diet that contains a variety of plant foods can ensure that all essential amino acids are included in the diet while also providing the additional benefit of supplying a wide range of micronutrients. For example, grains lack the amino acid lysine but are high in methionine, whereas legumes are low in methionine but high in lysine. It has also been suggested that vegetarians require greater overall levels of protein in the diet in order to compensate for the high intake of incomplete protein (Fink et al., 2012).

sunlight or consumed from food sources. In terms of intake, an RDA of 600 IU per day is given for youth of all ages (see table 16.4). However, the average intake in the general North American population is less than 400 IU per day (Ross et al., 2011), and vitamin D intake is also reported to be low in children across 16 European countries (Kaganov et al., 2015). Low levels of vitamin D intake reflect the fact that vitamin D occurs naturally in high amounts in only a few foods, such as oily fish (e.g., salmon, tuna, sardines), and these foods are consumed in low amounts in some Western diets. Consequently, vitamin D is often added to certain foods, such as cereals and milk.

One major source of vitamin D is sunlight. A recent report by the Institute of Medicine suggested that vitamin D inadequacy in the general population may have previously been overstated and that nearly all individuals have adequate serum vitamin D levels even with minimal sun exposure (Ross et al., 2011). That report also challenged the concept that "more is better," suggesting instead a lack of evidence to support the notion that higher vitamin D levels confer greater health benefits. The lack of consensus results partly from debate about the serum vitamin D level that represents sufficiency. The Institute of Medicine (Ross et al., 2011) has applied a value of more than 20 nanograms per milliliter (~50 nmol/L), whereas others have suggested a value of more than 30 nanograms per milliliter (Holick et al., 2011). Applying the higher threshold, Gibson and colleagues (2011) reported that more than half of 14- to 17-year-old elite female soccer players were vitamin D deficient, and Constantini and colleagues (2010) found that 73 percent of 10- to 30-year-old athletes and dancers fell below the threshold of 30 nanograms per milliliter. Even when applying the lower threshold of 20 nanograms per milliliter, Pekkinen and colleagues (2012) reported that 71 percent of girls and boys aged 7 to 19 years old were vitamin D deficient.

Schoenfeld and Aragon (2016) suggest that vitamin D may be a case where significantly exceeding the RDA is necessary in order to optimize several health benefits in youth, whereas Pekkinen and colleagues (2012) asserted an urgent need to increase vitamin D intake in order to optimize the bone health of children. However, it is accepted that too much vitamin D can be toxic, possibly leading to a number of negative health outcomes, although the level that constitutes toxicity is also debated (Holick et al., 2011; Ross et al., 2011). Youth fitness specialists should seek intervention from a qualified health care professional in order to diagnose vitamin D deficiency in youth athletes and to provide any subsequent prescription of a supplement to correct the deficiency. They should also be aware of youth who may be more at risk of vitamin D deficiency—for instance, those with poor nutrition, youth athletes on a calorie-restricted diet, those with minimal exposure to sunlight, and youth with dark skin pigmentation will all be at greater risk of vitamin D deficiency.

Calcium

Calcium is an important nutrient for skeletal health, particularly during childhood and adolescence, when bone growth is rapid. About 99 percent of calcium is found in the skeleton (Baker et al., 1999), and total skeletal calcium content increases from 25 grams at birth to 900 and 1200 grams for adult females and males, respectively (Bachrach, 2001). Because growth is particularly rapid during adolescence, calcium requirements are greater during this period than during childhood or adulthood. At peak height velocity, youth have achieved over 90 percent of their adult stature but less than 60 percent of their bone mineral content (Bailey et al., 1996), as maximal rates of bone mineral accrual lag behind peak height velocity by 6 to 12 months. About 45 percent of bone mass is attained during adolescence, and 90 percent is achieved by age 17 (Story & Stang, 2005).

This pattern means that around the time of the growth spurt, youth may have relatively undermineralized bones, which are therefore more susceptible to fracture. It also highlights the importance of adequate calcium intake to support bone mineralization; the hormonal changes that occur during puberty promote greater bone mineralization, which needs to be supported by sufficient calcium intake (Mesias et al., 2011). Childhood and adolescence represent windows of opportunity to optimize bone health through a combination of good nutrition and bone-loading physical activity; in contrast, failure to do so increases the risk of poor bone health into adulthood (Hoch et al., 2008). For example, Kalkwarf and colleagues (2003) found that women who consumed low levels of milk (which is naturally high in calcium) in childhood and adolescence had lower bone mineral density and increased risk of fracture in adulthood.

Worldwide, the majority of youth fail to consume the recommended amount of calcium (Mesias et al., 2011). In the United States, youth calcium intake falls below the recommended amount (Hess & Slavin, 2014) and is lower for girls than for boys at all ages (Story & Stang, 2005); specifically, only 14 percent of teenage girls and 36 percent of teenage boys meet the calcium RDA (Hoch et al., 2008). Lower calcium intake in girls may reflect the fact that dairy foods constitute the major source of dietary calcium for U.S. youth (Story & Stang, 2005) but may also be perceived as being "fattening" and therefore be avoided by girls who are body conscious. In any case, calcium intake in girls involved in gymnastics (Bernadot et al., 1989), figure skating (Ziegler et al., 1998), soccer (Gibson et al., 2011), and volleyball (Papadopoulou et al., 2002) have all been reported to be well below advocated levels for adolescents and youth athletes.

Supplementation of calcium may be an option to consider for youth who do not take in adequate calcium from food and drink, but a supplementation program should be prescribed by a registered health care professional. Any supplementation should be spread out over the day and limited to 500 milligrams per dose in order to maximize absorption (Hoch et al., 2008). Total intake should not exceed the upper limit of 2,500 milligrams per day for youth aged 4 to 8 years or 3,000 milligrams per day for 9- to 18-year-olds; above these levels, the risk for harm increases (Institute of Medicine, 2010). Ideally, youth fitness specialists encourage youth to meet their calcium requirements by consuming foods that are naturally high in calcium, including lower-fat and low-sugar dairy foods, as well as foods and beverages fortified with calcium.

Iron

Iron is vital for numerous cellular processes and is particularly important for enabling oxygen delivery in the blood and throughout the body; the majority of the body's iron is found in hemoglobin and myoglobin. Because exercise capacity depends on oxygen delivery, iron may be particularly important for supporting physical activity and sport performance in youth. With rapid increases in muscle mass and expansion of blood volume, iron needs increase markedly during adolescence, and the onset of menarche and the ensuing blood loss further increases the iron needs of girls beyond those of boys. Inadequate iron intake can be diagnosed as iron deficiency, and when this condition contributes to anemia it is termed *iron deficiency anemia*. Anemia is characterized by insufficient levels of hemoglobin or red blood cells, and in most populations the primary cause of anemia is iron deficiency resulting from sustained deterioration in iron stores (World Health Organization, 2011). Iron deficiency may negatively influence attentiveness, memory, academic performance, physical growth, the onset of menarche, immune status, and physical capacity in youth (World Health Organization, 2011). When youth fitness specialists help to identify and intervene with youth who are iron deficient, they can help improve overall health and well-being and prevent progression to an anemic state.

DO YOU KNOW?

Iron deficiency is the most common and widespread nutritional disorder in the world and is prevalent in youth in industrialized countries (World Health Organization, 2011).

Adolescent girls are subject to heightened risk for iron deficiency. Data from the United States show that only 56 percent of girls aged 14 to 18 years met the RDA for iron as compared with 98 percent of boys in the same age (Story & Stang, 2005). The risk is also higher in youth from low-income families and in youth who are overweight or obese (Nead et al., 2004). Infants and young children are also at risk of iron deficiency and anemia due to their rapid growth and the limited sources of dietary iron (Lozoff et al., 2006); this is a particular concern because iron is needed in order to support the rapid development of the central nervous system during this period. Worryingly, accumulating evidence suggests that iron deficiency and anemia in infancy and early childhood are associated with long-lasting impairments in cognitive and motor development, reduced academic performance, and behavioral issues, although it is difficult to unravel the confounding influence of low socioeconomic status (Grantham-McGregor & Ani, 2001).

Although the exact mechanisms are not understood, iron needs may also be further increased in youth athletes who regularly participate in intense or high-volume exercise. When reviewing available evidence, Schoenfeld and Aragon (2016) noted that a high prevalence of iron deficiency has been reported in young athletes across a wide variety of sports, including hockey, cross-country skiing, basketball, and softball. Research has also shown that short periods of intensive training or competition result in reductions in iron stores in prepubertal male swimmers (Spodaryk, 2002) and that elite youth athletes who expend greater energy are more likely to be iron depleted (Koehler et al., 2012).

Good dietary sources of iron include liver, lean beef and steak, baked beans, fortified cereals, prune juice, and spinach (Schoenfeld & Aragon, 2016). In youth who fail to consume adequate levels of iron, supplementation may provide a solution. However, iron supplementation programs adopted in several countries have been ineffective (World Health Organization, 2011), and excess supplementation poses a risk of iron toxicity and liver failure. The favored approach is for a youth fitness specialist to adopt a food-first framework and encourage youth athletes to meet dietary needs through a diverse diet.

Zinc

Zinc is associated with protein formation, gene expression, and many enzymes. Consequently, it plays an important role in a vast array of physiological functions, including immunity and skeletal development, hormone metabolism, and insulin secretion. Zinc requirements increase with growth in girls and boys (see table 16.4), and its interaction with many metabolic processes means that zinc deficiency can lead to impaired growth and delayed sexual maturation (Brandao-Neto et al., 1995; Institute of Medicine, 2001). Other symptoms of zinc deficiency in youth include defective immune function, dermatitis, diarrhea, impaired taste, and behavioral changes (International Zinc Nutrition Consultative Group, 2004). In the United States, only about two-thirds of boys and one-third of girls aged 11 to 18 years take in an adequate amount of zinc (Briefel et al., 2000), and comparable data from the UK show an increasing trend wherein 90 percent of boys and 85 percent of girls of the same age fail to achieve the RDI for zinc (Whitton et al., 2011). It has also been suggested that the zinc intake of youth athletes tends to be suboptimal, particularly in light of the fact that exercise and training can cause a chronic effect of suppressing zinc levels in youth athletes (Shoenfeld & Aragon, 2016).

Zinc is found in abundance in red meat, shellfish, wheat germ, and fortified cereals. As for plant-based sources of zinc, the indigestible fiber found in many plant-based sources of zinc can inhibit its absorption. Iron and zinc compete for absorption, and high levels of one can reduce the absorption of the other; as a result, youth who take an iron supplement may be at risk of developing mild zinc deficiency if iron intake is more than twice that of zinc (Story & Stang, 2005). Evidence is also equivocal with regard to whether zinc supplementation provides any performance gains for youth athletes (Shoenfeld & Aragon, 2016). Youth should be able to achieve adequate zinc levels through a healthy diet, but youth fitness specialists should be aware of symptoms of potential zinc deficiency and liaise with clinicians as necessary.

Sodium

Sodium is a mineral and electrolyte that contributes to many functions in the body, including regulation of fluid and acid–base balance, control of blood pressure, and propagation of nerve impulses to enable muscle contractions. It is needed in the diet in order to maintain function; during exercise, the process of sweating can lead to losses of sodium that need to be replenished. Sodium can be found naturally in many food sources but is most commonly associated with salt, which contains high levels of sodium. Salt is added to many **processed foods** as a preservative and to add taste by decreasing bitterness and increasing sweetness and other congruent flavors (Keast & Breslin, 2003). The increased consumption of processed foods with added salt has led to increased salt intake in youth populations (Centers for Disease Control and Prevention, 2016). Overconsumption of sodium increases with age and is greater in males than in females; boys aged 14 to 18 years consume more than 4,000 milligrams per day, well above the RDA of 2,300.

High sodium intake is undesirable due to its relationship with negative health outcomes. In reviewing available literature, Yang and colleagues (2012) summarized that high sodium intake is associated with high blood pressure in children, which in turn predisposes youth to develop hypertension in adulthood and increases the risk of cardiovascular disease and death. The influence of salt on blood pressure is further increased in overweight and obese youth (Yang et al., 2012). A review of controlled trials concluded that modest reductions in salt cause immediate reductions in blood pressure in children and adolescents (He & MacGregor, 2006). It was further suggested that reducing salt intake in youth would reduce the rise in blood pressure into adulthood.

DO YOU KNOW?

For most children, sodium intake exceeds dietary recommendations; major sources of dietary sodium include bread, cereal, and processed meats (Grimes et al., 2017).

Hydration

Water is essential for many physiological processes, including circulation, metabolism, temperature regulation, waste removal, and optimal brain function. Thus keeping youth hydrated is important for their physical health, cognitive function, and overall well-being. Recommended total water intake is 1.7 quarts (liters) per day for children aged 4 to 8 years, and it rises steadily to 2.3 liters per day and 3.3 liters per day for 14- to 18-year-old girls and boys, respectively, with 80 percent coming from drinks and 20 percent from foods (Institute of Medicine, 2004). Larger, more physically active youth need to drink more water because exercise and sweating increase water loss. Youth fitness specialists should also consider environmental factors, because higher temperature and humidity increase water loss and the need for fluid replacement.

DO YOU KNOW?

Inadequate hydration and even mild dehydration are associated with headache, irritability, poor physical performance, and reduced cognitive function (Kenney et al., 2015).

A recent study revealed that more than half of U.S. children and adolescents are not adequately hydrated; moreover, boys, adolescents, and black children were all found to be at higher risk (Kenney et al., 2015). Water should be the drink of choice for youth in order to remain hydrated because it provides a no-calorie, low-cost beverage that meets the body's needs in most circumstances. However, in a large sample of 6- to 19-year-old U.S. youth, nearly one-quarter reported consuming no plain water at all (Kenney et al., 2015). Youth may need reminders to drink water, because their thirst mechanism may be insufficient to maintain a hydrated state, particularly in the heat and during and after exercise (Kenney & Chiu, 2001). Water consumption in children increases when it is encouraged rather than consumed *ad libitum*, and *ad libitum* consumption is greater when flavored

water is available than when plain water is available (Kenney & Chiu, 2001). Youth fitness specialists should be proactive in making water readily accessible to youth, keeping water bottles and dispensers close by, establishing routines whereby water is regularly consumed during exercise sessions and throughout the day, and potentially offering flavored water as a more appealing option to youth. Practitioners should also set a good example by regularly consuming water in front of youth—and not sugar-sweetened beverages or diet sodas.

Youth typically consume a variety of beverages to meet their hydration needs. About 75 percent of youth drink plain water, 70 percent drink **sugar-sweetened beverages** (including soda and juice drinks), 67 percent to 75 percent drink milk, and about 25 percent drink 100 percent fruit juices (Kenney et al., 2015; Kit et al., 2011). Nutritional content for some of the most popular types of drinks are provided in table 16.8. Drinks other than water provide calories, which must be considered in planning overall energy consumption. However, it is not only the number of calories that should be considered but also the origin of the calories.

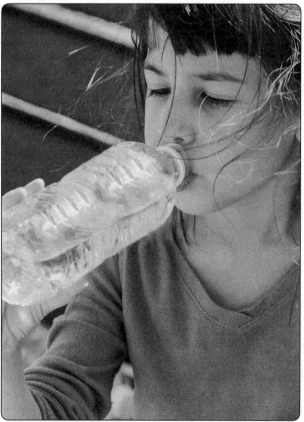

Water should be the drink of choice for youth in order to remain hydrated.

© Human Kinetics

Teaching Tip

HYDRATION OF YOUTH ATHLETES

Research shows that three-quarters of youth athletes arrive at training dehydrated (Arnaoutis et al., 2015). Instead, they should arrive well hydrated, having consumed 14 to 21 ounces (400 to 600 mL) of fluid in the two to three hours beforehand. During training and competition, youth should aim to match fluid loss and fluid intake by consuming 5 to 10 ounces (150 to 300 mL) of fluid every 15 to 20 minutes. If the event lasts less than one hour, then water is sufficient. However, for prolonged events lasting more than one hour and involving vigorous exercise or taking place in hot and humid environments, then a sport drink containing carbohydrate and sodium chloride may be useful for maintaining energy provision and electrolyte balance. After exercise, fluid should be replaced in proportion to any loss in body mass at the rate of 24 ounces per pound (1.5 L per kg) of weight lost during exercise (Leites & Meyer, 2016; Purcell & Canadian Paediatric Society Paediatric Sports and Exercise Medicine Section, 2013).

Milk and 100 percent fruit juices contain naturally occurring sugars, whereas the other drinks listed in table 16.8 are all high in added sugar (e.g., glucose, high fructose corn syrup). As discussed earlier in the chapter, intake of added sugar needs to be controlled and should contribute no more than 10 percent of daily energy intake. Nutritional information presented in table 16.8 is standardized to a serving size of 8 fluid ounces (235 mL), but youth fitness specialists should remember that commercial drinks are often packed in larger containers, and the average American child consumes two 8-ounce servings of sugar-sweetened beverage per day (Kenney et al., 2015). Thus a child can easily consume the daily limit of added sugar in a single serving of a carbonated drink or energy drink, which may also contain unwanted stimulants.

Low-fat milk and milk products are recommended in the Dietary Guidelines for Americans 2015 (U.S. Department of Agriculture, 2015) because they provide calcium, vitamin D, and other nutrients without excessive calorie or fat intake. Milk consumption is particularly important in childhood and adolescence to promote lifelong bone health (Greer et al., 2006; Kalkwarf et al., 2003). As shown in table 16.8, flavored milks contain added sugar, which increases calorie content. However, children and adolescents who consume flavored milk drinks have been shown to consume more overall milk than youth who drink only plain milk, thus achieving a similar level of nutrient intake without increasing the total amount of added sugar across the diet (Murphy et al., 2008). As with water, adding flavoring to low-fat milk may encourage youth to consume milk, thus giving them the additional benefit of increasing intake of other micronutrients. However, youth fitness specialists should be cognizant of the contribution that flavored milk drinks can make to total added sugar in the diet.

In the general population, children and adolescents are the highest consumers of fruit juice and juice drinks (Heyman et al., 2017). A fruit juice is a drink that contains 100 percent fruit, whereas a juice drink contains less fruit and also contains added sweeteners and flavorings; therefore, it is considered a sugar-sweetened beverage. Fruit juice can provide the same benefits as whole fruit in terms of many vitamins and minerals. Consequently, the American Dietary Guidelines (U.S. Department of Agriculture, 2015) allow for youth to consume up to half of their servings of fruit as fruit juice (but not as juice drink). Disadvantages of fruit juice include the fact that it lacks the dietary fiber content of whole fruit, can be consumed more quickly than whole fruit, does not promote eating behaviors associated with consumption of whole fruit, and may contribute excessive calorie intake if consumed in high volume (Heyman et al., 2017).

Sport drinks are intended to replace the carbohydrates, minerals, and electrolytes that are lost through exercise and sweating. In most instances, however, youth can likely achieve adequate hydration during sport participation simply by consuming water, along with a generally healthy diet that helps to maintain macro- and micronutrient stores. Energy drinks also contain nonnutritive stimulants such as caffeine, guarana, and taurine (Galemore, 2011). Both sport and energy drinks are popular with youth, and current data suggest that about 33 percent of adolescents consume sport drinks and 10 percent to 15 percent consume energy drinks (Larson et al., 2014). Concerns have been raised about the deleterious effects of caffeine and other stimulants on the developing neurological and cardiovascular systems (Galemore, 2011; Nawrot et al., 2003; Seifert et al., 2011). Youth fitness specialists should play a proactive role in preventing youth from consuming energy drinks and encouraging them to use sport drinks only to support prolonged, vigorous exercise. In all other circumstances, hydration should be achieved by consuming water or other nutritious, unsweetened beverages, such as low-fat milk and 100 percent fruit juice.

DO YOU KNOW?

Youth should not consume energy drinks, due to possible adverse effects on their developing neurological and cardiovascular systems (Nawrot et al., 2003).

Achieving a Healthy Diet

This chapter has discussed the role of the six essential nutrients in the diet of youth: carbohydrate (including dietary fiber), protein, fat, vitamins, minerals, and water. Suggestions have been made for preferable food and beverage choices to allow youth to achieve adequate intake of all nutrients. However, the essential nutrients occur in combination and in different amounts in different foods and drinks. Therefore, it can be challenging for youth, their parents, and youth fitness specialists to

TABLE 16.8   NUTRITIONAL CONTENT OF BEVERAGES POPULAR WITH CHILDREN AND ADOLESCENTS PER 8 FLUID OUNCES (240 ML)

Type	Calories (kcal)	Carbohydrate (g)	Total sugar (g)	Added sugar* (g)	Protein (g)	Vitamins	Minerals, electrolytes	Stimulants
Water	0	—	—	—	—	—	✓	—
Skim milk	84	12	12	—	8	✓	✓	—
Chocolate milk	130	24	22	10	8	✓	✓	—
100% fruit juice	110	26	22	—	2	✓	✓	—
Juice drink	60	12	12	12	—	✓	—	—
Carbonated drink	101	25	25	25	—		—	—
Sport drink	61	15	14	14	—		✓	—
Energy drink	113	29	26	26	—	✓	✓	✓

*Added sugar is estimated from the nutritional information and ingredients list.

Teaching Tip

MILK AS A RECOVERY DRINK

Milk has been suggested as a good choice of recovery drink for youth athletes who are involved in repeated training and competition events in close proximity (Desbrow et al., 2014). It can help replenish depleted macro- and micronutrient stores and provide the proteins needed to support muscle repair and recovery. In fact, low-fat chocolate milk has been found superior to formulated sport recovery drinks in aiding recovery in adult athletes (Pritchett et al., 2009) and has also been recommended for use by youth athletes (McDaniel & Fox, 2016; Sports Dietitians Australia, 2015). Low-fat flavored milk contains an ideal 3:1 ratio of carbohydrate to protein, as well as slow- and fast-digesting proteins and important vitamins and minerals such as calcium, vitamin D, and potassium (McDaniel & Fox, 2016).

achieve a diet that meets the individual's needs through food and drink choices that provide optimal intake of all essential nutrients. To overcome this challenge, public health organizations around the world have produced online resources that offer practical guidelines and interactive tools to help with planning a healthy diet. Perhaps the most comprehensive of these resources is MyPlate, which has been developed by the U.S. Department of Agriculture. The website www.choosemyplate. gov provides resources for a variety of audiences, including interactive pages designed specifically for youth (www.choosemyplate.gov/kids).

When making diet plans and recommendations, youth fitness specialists should consider the contribution of the five major food groups: grains, proteins, fruit, vegetables, and dairy—together with healthy oils and hydration. Achieving a good proportion of each food group, and good food choices within each group, ensures that youth meet their macro- and micronutrient needs. One common way to depict the contribution made by each food group is to present the groups in relative proportion on a plate, thus providing a visual similar to a pie chart. Examples include the following:

- MyPlate, published by the U.S. Department of Agriculture
- Healthy Eating Plate and Kid's Healthy Eating Plate, published by the Harvard School of Public Health
- Eatwell Plate/Guide, published by Public Health England
- Australian Healthy Eating Guide, published by the Australian Government and the National Health and Medical Research Council
- The Athlete's Plates, published by the United States Olympic Committee Sport Dietitians and the University of Colorado

The recommendations, guides, and plates provided by these and other organizations generally demonstrate good agreement with regard to the proportions and types of foods that contribute to a healthy diet. Figure 16.3 summarizes how the different food groups should contribute to the diet of youth aged two years and above. The depiction of a healthy eating plate has been used to encourage the general public to create healthy, balanced meals. Although guides are often depicted as plates, the intention is not that the proportions of food shown should necessarily be achieved at every meal; rather, the plate depicts an overall balanced diet. Thus youth fitness specialists should consider figure 16.3 and other available resources as general guides to help plan youth diets. They can be used to help prepare balanced meals and, more important, to

help promote a healthy diet throughout the day. Youth fitness specialists should consider how the different food groups contribute to the overall daily and weekly diet across all meals, snacks, and drinks.

Youth fitness specialists should consider both the relative contribution that each food group makes to the overall diet and the quality of the foods chosen in each group. Fruits and vegetables should contribute a substantial amount of the diet and include foods of different colors to maximize micronutrient intake. Juice can count toward fruit intake but must be 100 percent fruit juice and contain no added sugar while still allowing for at least half of fruit intake to come from whole fruits (U.S. Department of Agriculture, 2015).

DO YOU KNOW?

Most youth do not consume the recommended levels of fruit and vegetables. Replacing sugary snacks with fruit and vegetable alternatives is one way to help youth achieve a more balanced diet.

Contemporary data show that the general population often fails to achieve a diet with an optimal combination of the various food groups. Data from the United States routinely demonstrates that the general population has low intake of vegetables, particularly dark green and orange vegetables, as well as low intake of legumes (U.S. Department of Agriculture, 2015). Instead the predominant source of vegetable intake is potato, which is often eaten in the form of fries

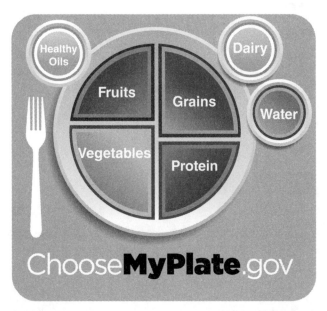

FIGURE 16.3 The proportion of the five food groups, which, together with healthy oils and water, make up a healthy diet.

USDA Center for Nutrition Policy and Promotion

or chips (Branum & Rossen, 2014). Consumption of whole grains is very low, and consumption of refined grains is very high; in addition, young children are particularly reliant on fruit juice to meet fruit intake requirements (U.S. Department of Agriculture, 2015). These examples demonstrate a common trend of poor dietary habits in the general population and more specifically in youth. Thus youth fitness specialists will routinely encounter youth who exhibit poor nutritional behaviors. An initial step for the practitioner is to understand those behaviors and why they occur. That information can then be used to help provide an integrated intervention that considers both nutrition and physical activity, as well as the influence of significant others (e.g., parents, coach) on changing dietary habits.

Supplements

As discussed earlier in this chapter, the use of supplements is generally discouraged in youth. Instead, practitioners should adopt a food-first approach that educates and encourages all youth to consume foods and drinks that allow them to achieve a balanced diet and meet their macro- and micronutrient needs (Desbrow et al., 2014). When youth consume a healthy diet, supplementation is unlikely to provide health benefits (Nordic Council of Ministers, 2012); moreover, in some instances, excess intake of micronutrients via supplementation may be harmful (Shenkin, 2006). Despite this risk, more than 30 percent of U.S. youth regularly consume supplements, the most popular of which include multivitamins and minerals (Picciano et al., 2007; Shaikh et al., 2009). Supplementation may be warranted when a vitamin or mineral deficiency has been identified by a medical professional and poses a risk to the health of the child. However, youth fitness specialists should take a food-first approach and encourage modifications in eating and drinking behaviors to allow youth to achieve a healthy, balanced diet.

Some sex differences appear in supplement usage in youth, as girls are more likely to take weight control products and boys more likely to opt for muscle-building and performance-enhancing supplements (Bell et al., 2004). This difference derives from the fact that adolescents are mostly motivated to take supplements in the search for what they believe to be the ideal body (Alves & Lima, 2009). The use of weight loss supplements is particularly concerning because they may contain stimulants and other active ingredients that can cause adverse health effects. Youth fitness specialists should recognize that adolescent females are more at risk of experimenting with weight loss supplements and that this risk increases for girls involved in weight-related sports such as gymnastics, dance, and running (Canadian Paediatric Society, 2004).

Youth athletes form a population that is particularly likely to engage in supplement use, and nearly 60 percent of U.S. youth regularly take supplements to enhance sport performance (Evans et al., 2012). The use of multivitamins, sport drinks, and energy drinks is popular among youth athletes regardless of age, gender, and sport (Parnell et al., 2016; Petroczi et al., 2008; Walsh et al., 2011). About 67 percent of school-age rugby players report using supplements; specifically, protein and creatine supplements are used by 44 percent and 29 percent of players, respectively (Walsh et al., 2011). Research demonstrates that youth athletes cite performance reasons, rather than benefits to health, as the primary reason for consuming supplements (Petroczi et al., 2008). This is the case despite the fact that only limited evidence supports the use of supplements to enhance athletic performance in youth athletes (Alves & Lima, 2009).

This discrepancy raises the question of where and how youth athletes acquire knowledge and make decisions about supplementation. In a study of elite youth athletes in the United Kingdom, Petroczi and colleagues (2008) reported that there was a worrying

Teaching Tip

ASSESSING YOUTH DIETARY HABITS AND NEEDS

Youth fitness specialists need to understand the current eating and drinking habits of the youth with whom they work in order to help identify where dietary improvements can be made. To help gather information, validated questionnaires are freely available—for example, the Youth Adolescent Food Frequency Questionnaire for 9- to 18-year-olds (Rockett et al., 2007). However, educating and empowering youth to make well-informed decisions about their lifestyle should be a primary goal, and it may be more effective to simply engage in discussion with youth about their dietary habits and knowledge. Practitioners can also provide youth with diaries (or use apps or solicit food and drink photos) to help them capture their drinking, eating, and snacking behaviors and to monitor weight, body composition, and energy levels. Gathering such information can help both the child and the practitioner reflect on how well the child's nutritional needs are being met and where changes need to be made.

trend for athletes to self-manage their supplementation without seeking professional advice. In the United States, only 15 percent of children taking supplements were doing so on the recommendation of a physician or other health care provider (Bailey et al., 2013). If adolescent boys seek advice from retailers, they are also likely to be misinformed; indeed, research has shown that sales assistants frequently recommended the use of creatine and testosterone boosters to youth (Herriman et al., 2017). This means that youth and young athletes are likely to be making ill-informed choices with regard to the need for supplementation, and practitioners can address this issue through education.

DO YOU KNOW?

For most adolescents, performance-enhancing supplements will not produce significant improvements above those attained with maturation and appropriate adherence to nutrition and training (LaBotz et al., 2016).

Nutritional supplements have also been suggested to act as a gateway to doping and illicit drug use in athletes and young adults (Backhouse et al., 2013; Hildebrandt et al., 2012). In one study of young adult athletes, Backhouse and colleagues (2013) reported that those who took nutritional supplements held more positive attitudes toward doping and were nearly four times more likely than nonusers to

be involved in doping. Similarly, the use of illicit appearance- and performance-enhancing drugs was found to be higher in undergraduate students who used supplements (Hildebrandt et al., 2012). These findings have led to the supposition that supplement use provides an initial pathway into doping. Thus supplement users can be considered an at-risk group for future doping, and doping prevention strategies should target youth who take legal supplements (Backhouse et al., 2013; Hildebrandt et al., 2012). Youth fitness specialists should be cognizant that supplement use provides a potential transition pathway to doping and take care to ensure that youth, parents, and coaches are fully aware of all of the risks and benefits of supplementation.

Recommended Changes to Achieve a Healthy Diet

It can be a daunting task to balance macro- and micronutrient needs across food groups in order to provide a healthy diet for youth in the real world. To help with this process, table 16.9 provides summary recommendations for making positive dietary changes to improve health and energy balance in youth. Children, parents, coaches, and youth fitness specialists can also use figure 16.4 as a prompt to help create meals and snacks that ensure a well-balanced diet. This guidance

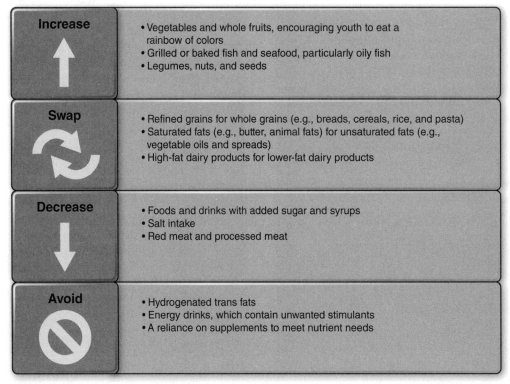

FIGURE 16.4   Recommended dietary changes to improve energy balance and health in youth.

Adapted from Nordic Council of Ministers (2014) and Gidding, Dennison, Birch, et al. (2005).

TABLE 16.9   EXAMPLES OF CUP AND WEIGHT NUTRITIONAL EQUIVALENTS FOR EACH FOOD GROUP

Fruits (1 cup equivalents)	Vegetables (1 cup equivalents)	Grains (1 oz, or 28 g, equivalents)	Protein (1 oz, or 28 g, equivalents)	Dairy (1 cup equivalents)
1 cup raw fruit 1 cup cooked fruit 1 cup fruit salad 1 cup fruit juice 1/2 cup dried fruit 1 large banana 32 grapes 1 small apple 8 large strawberries 1 orange	1 cup raw vegetable 1 cup cooked vegetable 1 cup vegetable juice 2 cups leafy salad greens 1 large sweet potato 12 baby carrots 1 cup cooked black beans 1 large pepper 2 cups raw spinach 1 large tomato	1/2 cup cooked rice or pasta 1 oz dry rice or pasta 1 regular slice of bread 1 cup cereal flakes 1/2 cup cooked bulgur wheat 1 mini bagel 5 whole-wheat crackers 1 small muffin 1 pancake 1 small tortilla	1 oz lean meat or poultry 1 oz seafood 1 slice sandwich turkey 1 egg 1/4 cup cooked beans 1/4 cup cooked tofu 1 tbsp peanut butter 1/2 oz nuts 1/2 oz seeds 2 tbsp hummus	1 cup milk 1 cup calcium fortified soy milk 8 oz (225 g) yogurt 1 1/2 oz (42 g) hard cheese 2 oz (57 g) processed cheese 1/2 cup shredded cheese 2 cups cottage cheese 1/2 cup ricotta cheese 1 cup milk pudding 1 1/2 cup ice cream

Compiled from U.S. Department of Agriculture (2015) and https://www.ChooseMyPlate.gov (2017).

should be coupled with the overriding principle that diet should reflect individual energy requirements, which vary depending on age, maturity, size, and physical activity levels.

Practical Recommendations and Examples for Achieving a Healthy Diet

There are many ways to achieve a healthy diet in youth. Although the general principles of healthy eating remain constant, the food and drink choices that can be used to achieve a healthy diet are limited only by the imagination. The American Dietary Guidelines (U.S. Department of Agriculture, 2015) provide target consumption levels for each food group at different calorie levels for individuals following a typical American, Mediterranean, vegetarian, or vegan diet, thus demonstrating that youth can achieve a healthy diet

in a variety of ways. Youth fitness specialists should recognize that the daily nutritional content of the diet is likely to vary somewhat from day to day. Thus, while the following sections provide useful tips and examples, they are by no means prescriptive or exhaustive.

Meal and Snack Planning

In order to achieve a heathy diet, good food choices from across and within the different food groups need to be consumed. Planning should look to combine foods from different groups in each meal and to incorporate a variety of foods from within each group across meals and snacks throughout the day and the week. Table 16.9 shows examples of foods in each group and can be used to help plan meals and snacks. The amounts are provided in cup or weight equivalents, which allow nutritionally similar portion sizes to be identified within a food group. For instance, one cup of cooked vegetables or two cups of raw spinach would be considered nutritionally similar.

Teaching Tip

ADD FLAVOR TO STIMULATE THE SENSES

Flavorings can encourage healthy eating behaviors in youth by making food and drinks more appealing. Use herbs and spices to add interest to meals and snacks and get kids involved in the food preparation process. Create dips that combine flavors and food groups—for instance, salsa, hummus, and avocado dip (add lemon and yogurt). Research shows that pairing dips with produce increases the amount of fruit and vegetables children eat (Savage et al., 2013). Also add unsweetened flavorings to water and low or nonfat milk to encourage youth to drink more and to avoid sugar-sweetened beverages.

The amount of food needed depends on the age, maturity, gender, size, and activity level of the child; two example scenarios are given in the next section. In table 16.9, the foods shown for fruits, vegetables, and dairy reflect common portion sizes, and it is easy to convert to smaller equivalents (e.g., by serving half of a portion). Grains and protein foods are shown in ounce equivalents but are typically served in larger portions. Grains are commonly served in 2- to 4-ounce equivalent servings, such as a sandwich with two slices of bread (2 oz), 1 cup of rice with a meal (2 oz), or a large bagel or tortilla (4 oz). Proteins are commonly served in 2- to 6-ounce portions—for instance, 1 cup of lentil or bean soup (2 oz), three-egg omelet (3 oz), one can of drained tuna (3-4 oz), one beef or salmon steak (4-6 oz).

Notwithstanding the need to consider individual energy needs, youth, parents, and practitioners can use table 16.9 to begin creating meal plans and menus. For example, a menu for one day might look like this:

- Breakfast: oatmeal made with milk and topped with almonds and raisins
- Lunch: turkey slice, Swiss cheese, and salad on whole-wheat bread made with mayonnaise; fruit
- Dinner: grilled fish, baked sweet potato, steamed vegetables, frozen yogurt
- Snacks: whole-wheat crackers with peanut butter and banana and carton of milk
- Other drinks: flavored water (not sweetened)

Youth fitness specialists can work with children and parents to expand table 16.9 and develop their own list of good choices in each food group. Practitioners, children, and parents should then be able to work creatively to develop meal and snack plans that are healthy but well-matched with the eating preferences and energy needs of the child. With this approach, children should begin to feel empowered and take ownership of their own meal planning.

Sample Scenarios and Plans

Youth fitness specialists are likely to work with youth who come from a diverse range of backgrounds and come with varying nutritional needs, ranging from overweight, obese, undernourished youth who need to lose weight to body-conscious girls on self-imposed calorie-restricted diets to youth athletes involved in high volumes of competition and training. Although it is beyond the scope of this chapter to provide sample plans for all of these scenarios, youth fitness specialists should be able to use the content from this chapter and the examples provided as a guide to suggesting a healthy diet for different individuals.

The sample scenario addressed here considers two 14-year-old adolescent boys of similar height and weight. One of the boys has a sedentary lifestyle, whereas the other boy is a highly active young athlete. The athlete typically trains twice per day—one session focused more on resistance training and physical conditioning and the other focused on team practice and technical performance. Although this is a simplified example it serves to highlight the effect of physical activity (or lack thereof) on nutritional requirements. The first step of the process is to identify the energy and the macro- and micronutrient needs of each boy. Table 16.10 shows the energy and micronutrient needs of each boy.

TABLE 16.10   DESCRIPTIVE CHARACTERISTICS WITH ENERGY AND MACRONUTRIENT REQUIREMENTS FOR TWO 14-YEAR-OLD BOYS OF SIMILAR SIZE BUT DIFFERENT PHYSICAL ACTIVITY LEVELS

	Boy A	Boy B
Lifestyle	Sedentary	Very Active
Age	14 yr	14 yr
Weight	108 lb (49.0 kg)	108 lb (49.1 kg)
Height	5 ft 3 in. (1.60 m)	5 ft 4 in. (1.63 m)
Energy requirements*	2,000 kcal/day	3,199 kcal/day
Carbohydrate requirements**	263 (225-300) g/day	420 (360-480) g/day
Fat requirements**	72 (56-89) g/day	116 (89-142) g/day
Protein requirements**	75 (50-100) g/day	120 (80-160) g/day

*Energy requirements are estimated from the IOM predictive equation shown earlier in table 16.3.

**Macronutrients are shown as the target amount (acceptable macronutrient distribution range). They are estimated from the target consumption and acceptable macronutrient density range shown earlier in figure 16.2 (Nordic Council of Ministers, 2014).

The next steps in the process are to identify the nutritional needs of both boys based on their individual energy and macronutrient requirements and then devise diet plans to match those requirements. The American Dietary Guidelines (U.S. Department of Agriculture, 2015) provide guidance regarding the amount of each food type required for children and adults based on energy requirements. Table 16.11 shows food requirements for youth at 12 calorie levels. Values for the boys in the example scenario are shown in the shaded columns, which indicate that the very active boy requires more fruit, vegetables, grains, protein, and oil. Youth fitness specialists should remember that fruit and vegetables of a variety of colors need to be consumed and at least half of dietary grains should be whole grains.

It can be seen from table 16.11 that each boy will still have some other available calories to complete his diet. This statement is based on the assumption that food choices have included nutrient-dense foods that are lean, low-fat, and prepared without added fats, sugars, refined starches, or salt. These discretionary calories can then be used to provide an allowance for the inclusion of small amounts of less desirable food sources, such as added sugar and hard fat (e.g., adding sugar to a cereal or mayonnaise to a sandwich). However, youth fitness specialists must ensure that the overall diet remains within a recommended range. This work includes ensuring that no more than 10 percent of calories come from added sugar and that less than 10 percent come from saturated fat. The additional calories can also be used to eat more than the recommended amount from a given food group. These discretionary calories may be particularly useful in allowing children some freedom to include foods for which they have the greatest preference. For the

very active boy it may be prudent to use some of the discretionary calories to increase the milk content of the diet, given that milk is a good postexercise recovery beverage.

The final step is to translate the food needs to a practical diet plan that considers the distribution and quantities of foods and nutrients consumed throughout the day and week. Meals and snacks should be planned to ensure that youth remain energized and hydrated throughout the day. Breakfast is an essential meal, and a review of available evidence showed that younger children who ate breakfast on a regular basis demonstrated better classroom behavior and achieved better school grades (Adolphus et al., 2013). However, the amount of food and energy allocated to each meal and snack can (and likely will) vary throughout the day and between days. This variation is normal, and Birch et al (1991) reported that in youth, the energy content of meals varied by about 40 percent from day to day, but overall daily energy intake was much more stable with only 10 percent variation.

Table 16.12 shows one example of how the diets for the sedentary and very active boy could be structured for one day, but youth fitness specialists should remember that food needs can be met in many different ways. For both boys, there is a focus on high-quality foods but with a use of discretionary calories to include small amounts of added fat and sugar. Youth fitness specialists should also be cognizant that it will be difficult and unrealistic to achieve exact macro- and micronutrient needs each day, but it is achievable over a longer time frame. Youth fitness specialists should aim to keep each macronutrient within the AMDR each day (see table 16.10 on page 340) but with a balance across macronutrients to keep overall energy intake

TABLE 16.11 RECOMMENDED AMOUNTS* FROM EACH FOOD GROUP AT DIFFERENT CALORIE LEVELS

Energy requirement (kcal)	1,000	1,200	1,400	1,600	1,800	2,000	2,200	2,400	2,600	2,800	3,000	3,200
Fruit (cups)	1	1	1.5	1.5	1.5	2	2	2	2	2.5	2.5	2.5
Vegetables (cups)	1	1.5	1.5	2	2.5	2.5	3	3	3.5	3.5	4	4
Grains (oz)	3	4	5	5	6	6	7	8	9	10	10	10
Healthy protein (oz)	2	3	4	5	5	5.5	6	6.5	6.5	7	7	7
Dairy (cups)	2	2.5	2.5	3	3	3	3	3	3	3	3	3
Oils (g)	15	17	17	22	24	27	29	31	34	36	44	51
Other available calories (kcal)**	150	100	110	130	170	270	280	350	380	400	470	610

*Amounts are shown as cup or weight equivalents (see table 16.9 for further information).

**If food choices are in nutrient-dense forms, are lean or low-fat, and are prepared without added fat, sugar, or refined starch, then some discretionary calories will remain within the overall calorie limit.

Adapted from U.S. Department of Agriculture (2015).

TABLE 16.12   SAMPLE DAILY MENU FOR A 14-YEAR-OLD SEDENTARY BOY AND A 14-YEAR-OLD VERY ACTIVE BOY OF SIMILAR SIZE

	Sedentary boy	Very active boy
Breakfast	Oatmeal cereal with fruit: 1 cup cereal flakes 1/2 cup low-fat milk 1 medium banana	Porridge with fruit, toast, and egg: 1 1/2 cup cereal flakes 1/2 cup low-fat milk 1 medium banana 1/2 cup raisins 1 slice whole-wheat toast 1 tsp margarine 1 boiled egg
Training	N/A	60 min of resistance training and physical conditioning
Snack		2 cups low-fat chocolate milk
Lunch	Tuna salad wrap: 1 tortilla wrap (whole wheat) 2 oz tuna 1 tbsp mayonnaise 1/2 cup shredded lettuce 1 sliced tomato 8 oz no-fat fruit yogurt	Tuna salad wrap: 2 tortilla wraps (whole wheat) 3 oz tuna 2 tbsp light mayonnaise 1 cup shredded lettuce 2 sliced tomatoes 8 oz no-fat fruit yogurt
Snack	1/2 cup carrot sticks 2 tbsp hummus	1 cup carrot sticks 4 tbsp hummus
Dinner	Beef stir fry: 3 oz roast lean beef 1/2 cup cabbage 1/4 cup bamboo shoots 1/2 cup sweet red peppers 1/2 cup green pepper 1 tbsp canola oil 1 cup cooked brown rice 1 scoop low-sugar ice-cream	Beef stir fry: 4 oz roast lean beef 3/4 cup cabbage 1/4 cup bamboo shoots 3/4 cup sweet red peppers 3/4 cup green pepper 1 tbsp canola oil 1 1/2 cups cooked brown rice 1 scoop low-sugar ice-cream
Training	N/A	1.5 hours team and technical training
Snack	1 cup low-fat milk	Turkey pita: 1 pita bread 1 12 oz roasted turkey slice 1/2 cup shredded mozzarella 1/2 cup 1 cup low-fat milk

Note: Plain or flavored water should be consumed at each meal and throughout the day unless an alternative drink is purposefully given.

close to target. By averaging the counts over the course of a week, youth fitness specialists should then be able to plan a diet where the average daily macronutrient consumption is close to target.

Nutrient timing may be particularly important for youth athletes, for whom food and drink are needed to support preparation for, engagement in, and recovery from training and competition. Athletes need to be adequately fueled and hydrated before training (and competition) and should also adopt a nutritional strategy that helps promote recovery afterward. In table 16.12 the additional energy and food needs of the very active boy have been used to increase portion sizes and the number of snacks. Ideally, youth athletes should allow two or three hours to digest meals before exercise; if eating closer to training, then the portion should be a smaller, predominantly carbohydrate-based snack (McDaniel & Fox, 2016). During training, hydration is the main focus, and the youth athlete should be encouraged to drink water every 15 to 20 minutes. Carbohydrate is not added to the fluids of the youth athlete in the example, because morning training lasts less than 60 minutes and evening training, though longer, is not intense.

Postexercise nutrition needs to include carbohydrate, protein, and fluid, the latter of which should be consumed at a rate of 1.5 times any losses in weight. Carbohydrate is needed to replenish depleted glycogen stores and protein to help with tissue repair and recovery. Athletes may experience suppressed appetite after an intense workout, and liquid nutrients may therefore be the best option. For this reason, the morning workout in the example is followed by a large, low-fat chocolate milk drink. This choice contains fluid, carbohydrate, and protein to aid recovery and should be supplemented by additional water consumption as needed. Following the lighter evening workout, a food snack is used to aid recovery and potentially help sleep. Protein is particularly important, because this snack is both postworkout and pre-bedtime and protein consumption at this time may increase overnight protein synthesis and recovery (Trommelen & van Loom, 2016).

Summary

To achieve a heathy lifestyle, children and adolescents should be habitually active and consume a varied, nutritious diet. When children are not active, it may be difficult to avoid a positive energy balance and unwanted weight gain. This is particularly the case with contemporary dietary habits, in which youth routinely consume calorie-dense foods that contain high amounts of added sugar, fat, and salt. Parents, caregivers, schools, clubs, and youth fitness specialists need to help each child achieve a diet that meets their energy and macro- and micronutrient needs through a diet that contains high-quality, nutrient-dense foods. These healthy eating habits should be established at a young age and reinforced by all individuals and organizations who are responsible for youths.

Energy and nutrient needs vary with age, maturity, size, and physical activity, and youth fitness specialists should consider all of these factors when determining the nutritional needs of a child. Macronutrient needs can be estimated using target contributions, the AMDR, micronutrient needs established from RDIs, and practical resources used to help convert these requirements to the amounts of food needed in the diet. The diet for each child should contain an appropriate quantity of nutrients from a variety of foods across and within the food groups. Simple changes—such as reducing salt intake, avoiding sugar-sweetened beverages, increasing fruit and vegetable consumption, and swapping out refined grains and animal fats for whole grains and plant fats—can all make a difference in youth health. Although the principles for maintaining a healthy diet are clear, youth fitness specialists should remember that the variety of food and drink choices available means that there are many practical solutions to achieving a healthy diet.

acanthosis nigricans—A dermatosis characterized by rough skin, irregular wrinkles, and hyperpigmentation that typically develops near the neck, armpits, and groin.

accelerated adaptation—Periods of rapid change in morphology of function.

acceleration—The phase of running that ends when the individual reaches maximum velocity.

acceptable macronutrient distribution range (AMDR)—A range of intakes for a particular energy source that is associated with reduced risk of chronic disease as well as adequate intake of essential nutrients.

accommodation—Failure to program variation into training, which leads to a blunted response of the biological system to a continued stimulus.

acetone—A colorless liquid ketone used as a solvent and found in diabetic urine.

active warm-up—Exercises and movement patterns that increase body temperature, blood flow, heart rate, and respiration rate.

acute fatigue—The disruption of an individual's homeostasis that leads to short-term performance decrements.

acute injury—An injury that occurs during a single traumatic event and typically consists of a fracture, sprain, strain, or concussion.

adaptation—Change in structure or function as a result of training, maturation, or an interaction of both; adaptation occurs in response to exercise with increased fitness when the stress is above a minimum intensity threshold.

added sugars—Sugars and syrups added to foods and beverages during the processing or preparation phase.

adenosine triphosphate (ATP)—A high-energy phosphate that is broken down to allow the contractile elements of skeletal muscle to produce mechanical work.

adequate intake (AI)—An estimation or approximation of the average daily intake that is adequate for apparently healthy individuals, used when the recommended daily allowance cannot be determined.

adolescence—The period from the end of late childhood until the attainment of adulthood.

adolescent awkwardness—A period of temporarily disrupted motor coordination, or clumsiness, caused by rapid growth of the long bones.

aerobic—Energy metabolism that requires the availability of oxygen.

agility—Rapid whole-body movements requiring changes in direction, velocity, or both in response to a stimulus.

allometric scaling—Adjusting physiological outcomes relative to a measure of body size raised to a power (the power law).

anabolic—A state in which chemical reactions synthesize complex molecules, such as muscle tissue.

anaerobic—Energy metabolism that does not require the availability of oxygen.

anaerobic capacity—An indirect measure of the total capacity of the anaerobic system (ATP-PC and glycolytic) to provide energy.

anaerobic glycolysis—The metabolism of glycogen or glucose to provide energy without the need for oxygen.

anaerobic power—An indirect measure of the maximal rate at which the anaerobic (ATP-PC) system can provide energy.

annual plan—The level of planning that reflects 12 months of programming and is dictated by the overarching goals of the multiyear plan.

anterior cruciate ligament injury—An injury to the ligamentous structures of the knee that results from collisions with another player or from noncontact situations such as cutting and pivoting movements.

assessment—Measurement of a range of physical, physiological, and psychosocial indices. In comparison to monitoring, assessment involves less frequent measurement (one to three times per year).

asthma—A respiratory condition characterized by bronchospasm that causes difficulty in breathing.

athleticism—The ability to move competently, confidently, and consistently in a variety of settings with speed, style, and precision.

athletic motor skill competencies—Targeted movements that act as component parts of more specialized motor skills and serve as the foundations for advanced training methods at a later stage of development.

ATP-PC system—A high-power, low-capacity system that provides energy in very intense exercise lasting approximately 10 seconds or less.

autogenic inhibition—A sudden relaxation in an agonist muscle following a muscle contraction.

autonomic nervous system—The system that regulates the internal organs, blood vessels, and glands.

average maturing—An individual who is biologically on time with their chronological age.

ballistic stretching—A type of stretch that involves rapid bouncing movements.

bio-banding—The grouping of youth athletes based on a descriptor of size or maturity rather than chronological age.

Blount's disease—A growth disorder of the tibia characterized by deformity resembling a bowleg.

body management—A training format designed to enhance a child's ability to orient and manage body weight, including a key focus on developing whole-body range of motion, stability, and basic strength.

body mass index—An estimate of body fatness calculated from height and weight.

bronchoconstriction—A narrowing of the bronchial air passages due to tightening of surrounding smooth muscle.

calcaneal apophysitis—An overuse-related injury in the heel that is typically experienced by youth, especially in boys. Also referred to as *Sever's disease*.

cardiopulmonary system—The system that consists of the heart and lungs.

cardiovascular system—The system that consists of the heart and the blood vessels that are distributed throughout the body.

catabolic—A state in which chemical reactions break down complex molecules, such as muscle tissue.

change-of-direction speed—The ability to change direction rapidly.

change-of-direction speed training—Training designed primarily to enhance the individual's ability to apply forces during acceleration, deceleration, and reacceleration.

childhood—The period from the first birthday to the onset of adolescence.

children—Boys and girls who have not yet developed secondary sex characteristics.

cholesterol—A type of lipid molecule and an essential building block of cell membranes; it is found in every cell in the body and provides the precursor for testosterone.

chronological age—Age measured as the time point away from birth.

cognitive age—A measure of one's ability to manage intellectual processes that require attention, alertness, memory, comprehension, application, judgment, and problem solving.

comorbidity—A disease or condition that occurs in the presence of another disease or disorder.

construct validity—The extent to which a test measures what it is supposed to measure.

content validity—The extent to which a test measures all elements of a construct. Sometimes referred to as *logical validity*.

creatine kinase—The enzyme that catalyzes the ATP-PC reaction.

criterion validity—Requires that results of a test agree with results from a gold standard measure (e.g., progressive 20-meter shuttle run test or $\dot{V}O_2$peak).

deceleration—A percentage decrease in velocity until the conclusion of the sprint.

degrees of freedom—The number of independent elements or components of a given task.

deliberate play—Reflects early exploratory activities that are intrinsically motivated and focused on maximizing enjoyment.

deliberate practice—Specific practice that entails both physical and cognitive contributions designed to improve performance and aid skill development.

deliberate preparation—The use of developmentally appropriate training modalities to help prepare youth for the demands of both deliberate play and deliberate practice.

detraining—A temporary or permanent reduction of the training stimulus.

development—The progress toward the adult state, which includes both biological and behavioral perspectives.

developmental milestone—Predictable behaviors or physical skills seen in infants and children as they grow and develop.

development models—Theoretical frameworks that can help youth fitness specialists structure the development pathways for children and adolescents in a given educational system or sport program.

diabetes mellitus—A group of metabolic disorders characterized by abnormally high blood glucose levels.

diabetic ketoacidosis—A serious complication of diabetes that occurs when the body produces high levels of ketones, which make blood more acidic.

differentiation—Proactive teaching or coaching that gives participants with different needs the opportunity to learn, engage, and participate effectively, regardless of ability or disability.

discriminative validity—The ability of a test to differentiate between different populations and subgroups of a population.

dynamic lower-extremity valgus—The combination of hip adduction and internal rotation, knee abduction, tibial external rotation and anterior translation, and ankle eversion.

dynamic stretching—A type of stretch that involves actively moving through a full range of motion in a controlled manner.

dynamic warm-up—Preparatory activities and whole-body movements that are specifically designed to prepare the body for exercise and sport.

dynapenia—A condition characterized by low levels of muscle strength and power and consequent functional limitations.

early maturing—An individual who is biologically ahead of their chronological age.

early specialization—Intensive year-round training in a single sport from a young age, which likely limits the child's exposure to a range of sporting activities.

ecological validity—The extent to which a test simulates the demands of the specific sport or task.

economy—The oxygen cost required to work at a given steady-state intensity.

efficiency—The percentage of physiological work that is converted to mechanical work.

ego orientation—Being motivated by social comparisons to others.

endochondral ossification—The process by which cartilage of the body is remodeled into bone.

endocrine system—A collection of glands that produce hormones to regulate the body's growth, metabolism, sexual development, and function.

energy balance—The difference between the amount of energy consumed and the amount of energy expended.

energy density—The amount of energy contained in a macronutrient, or food, per gram of weight.

environmental constraints—Constraints that exist outside of the body and can be easily manipulated to make a motor skill task more challenging.

epiphysis—The end part of a long bone.

essential amino acids—A group of eight amino acids that cannot be produced by the body and so must be consumed in the diet.

estimated average requirement (EAR)—The average daily nutrient intake that is estimated to meet the requirement of half of healthy individuals.

exercise—Planned, structured, repetitive movements intended to improve health-related fitness, skill-related physical fitness, or both.

exercise deficit disorder—A condition characterized by low levels of moderate to vigorous physical activity that are inconsistent with long-term health and well-being.

exercise-induced bronchospasm—A narrowing of the airways that occurs a few minutes after physical exertion with consequent shortness of breath, coughing, and wheezing.

external focus—An attentional cue that focuses on the effect or outcome of the movement.

external load—The objective measures of work performed by the athlete.

extrinsic motivation—Behavior that is driven by external rewards such as trophies or scholarships.

fine motor skills—Small movements that require accuracy and dexterity.

first-step quickness—The time required to cover the first five meters of a sprint.

fitness-fatigue model—Following exposure to training, an individual's level of preparedness is influenced by the dynamic and fluid interaction of the positive effects of fitness and the negative effects of fatigue.

flexibility training—Stretching exercises that increase joint range of motion.

functional overreaching—Intentional performance decrements resulting from training, which are greater than those experienced from acute fatigue alone and can take several days to several weeks to fully restore.

fundamental motor skill training—Training targeting the development of movement patterns inherent in successful execution of agility-related tasks, such as acceleration and deceleration mechanics, step patterns, cutting technique, backpedaling, and side-shuffling.

fundamental motor skills—The building blocks of future skill development, comprised of locomotion, manipulation, and stabilization skills.

fundamental movement skills—Basic movement patterns that involve locomotion, object control, or stability.

gallstone—A hard mass formed inside the gallbladder that can cause pain.

general adaptation syndrome—The physiological responses when the body is exposed to stress; this process has three stages: alarm phase, resistance phase, and exhaustion phase.

general warm-up—Preparatory activities that include nonspecific body movements such as low-intensity jogging.

glycated hemoglobin—A form of hemoglobin that can be measured to assess the average blood glucose concentration over the past two to three months.

goal orientation—Being motivated by personal improvement and task mastery.

gross motor skills—Whole-body movements or movements of large body parts.

growth—An increase in the size of the body or the size attained by specific parts of the body.

growth plate—The region of a long bone between the epiphysis and diaphysis where growth in bone length occurs.

health-related fitness— Measures of fitness associated with health or health risks, such as cardiorespiratory, muscular, and metabolic health.

holistic development—The philosophy of simultaneously promoting physical, social, and psychological development in youth in order to inspire and motivate lifelong participation in physical activity.

horizontal integration—The sequencing of training priorities so that, ideally, training progresses in a logical sequence in which one block lays the foundation for the next.

hyperglycemia—Abnormally high blood glucose levels.

hyperinsulinemia—The presence of excess insulin, relative to the level of glucose, circulating in the blood.

hypoglycemia—Abnormally low blood glucose levels.

hypogonadism—A reduction or absence of hormone secretions from the testes or ovaries.

indirect calorimetry—A noninvasive process that measures respiratory gases to accurately estimate energy expenditure and substrate use.

individual constraints—Constraints that exist within the body and are either *structural* (e.g., height, weight) or *functional* (e.g., motivation, fear) components that can affect performance.

individualization of training—The principle that because individuals differ in a number of ways, individuals differ in their ability to tolerate and respond to an exercise stimulus.

insulin resistance—A condition characterized by an impaired ability to achieve normal levels of blood glucose in response to insulin.

insulin sensitivity—A person's sensitivity to the effects of insulin; how much insulin they require to lower blood glucose.

integrative neuromuscular training—An approach to training that incorporates a variety of motor skill exercises, resistance training, coordination training, and exercises geared toward developing speed and agility.

intellectual disability—A neurodevelopmental disorder that becomes apparent before 18 years of age and is characterized by deficits in both intellectual functioning and adaptive behaviors, including physical functioning, social interactions, and communication skills.

internal focus—An attentional cue that focuses on a specific action or body part.

internal load—The relative physiological and psychological stressors experienced by an athlete.

intrinsic motivation—Behavior that is driven by internal rewards such as enjoyment and satisfaction.

ketoacidosis—A form of acidosis characterized by an increased accumulation of ketone bodies in the blood.

lactate dehydrogenase—The enzyme that catalyzes pyruvate to lactate.

lactate threshold—The exercise intensity where lactate starts to exponentially increase.

late maturing—An individual who is biologically behind their chronological age.

lipids—A collective term for fats, oils, and waxes.

Little League elbow—Injury to the elbow that is caused by excessive traction, compression, and shear forces around the elbow during repetitive throwing.

Little League shoulder—Injury to the shoulder that involves epiphysiolysis resulting from the high rotational stresses placed across the proximal humeral physis during overhead throwing.

local muscular endurance—The ability of specific muscle groups to sustain repeated actions for a given time period.

locomotion—Fundamental motor skills that involve using large, whole-body human movements to travel within their environment.

long-term plan—Programming that is focused on a longitudinal perspective and is built around training objectives specific to stage of development and technical ability.

lower-back pain—As with other regions of the body, the etiology of back pain may involve acute trauma or chronic overuse; however, overuse injuries appear to be more common and typically include spondylolysis, spondylolisthesis, apophyseal injury to the vertebral ring, disc degeneration or herniation, sacroiliac joint pain, and Scheuermann's disease.

macrocycle—Programming that spans a season and is traditionally divided into three distinct periods: preparation period, competition period, and transition period.

macronutrients—Energy-providing nutrients that are needed in large amounts in the diet.

manipulation—Fundamental motor skills that require an individual to use manipulative skills (typically hands or feet) to interact with an object.

mastery orientation—The belief that success is the result of effort and use of the appropriate strategies.

maturation—The process of becoming mature.

maximal velocity—The point where external forces are no longer changing velocity, which means that the individual is no longer accelerating.

menarche—The first menstrual cycle.

mesocycle—Programming that typically consists of a four- to six-week period, often referred to as a *block* of training.

metabolic conditioning—Training that will stimulate adaptation in either aerobic or anaerobic metabolism.

metabolic syndrome—A clustering of disease risk factors that has been linked with cardiovascular disease and type 2 diabetes.

metaphysis—The widened part of the bone shaft.

microcycle—Programming that typically covers a seven-day period, often referred to as the *training week*.

micronutrients—The collective term for vitamins and minerals; the elements and substances that are required in trace amounts for normal growth and development.

minute ventilation—The amount of air expired per minute.

mobility—The ability to move freely and effectively through an uninhibited range of motion with adequate flexibility, stability, and motor control.

modeling—Exhibiting the desired behavior with visual cues so that participants can see what they should do, how they should do it, and where it should be done.

monitoring—The routine evaluation of various physiological or perceptual metrics in order to determine the effectiveness of a training intervention, maximize performance, and minimize the risks of overtraining, injury, and illness.

motor skill competence—Proficiency displayed by an individual during goal-directed human movement.

multiyear plan—Planning that incorporates a series of annual plans (typically four to five sequential years).

muscle hyperplasia—An increase in the number of muscle fibers.

muscle hypertrophy—An increase in cellular size of muscle fibers due to increasing protein content.

muscular fitness—A collective term that includes the related but distinct aspects of muscular strength, muscular power, and local muscular endurance.

muscular power—The rate of performing work; a product of force and velocity.

muscular strength—The maximal amount of force that can be generated at a specified velocity.

needs analysis—Systematic gathering of information about the demands of the sport or physical activity and the characteristics and goals of the individual.

negative spiral of disengagement—Children with low motor competence are less likely to participate in physical activity and thus are not exposed to opportunities to improve their motor skills.

neural plasticity—The ability of the brain to modify and refine synaptic pathways continuously throughout an individual's life.

nonalcoholic fatty liver disease—A condition characterized by hepatic fat accumulation in the absence of excessive alcohol intake.

nonfunctional overreaching—Unintentional decrements in performance as a result of an imbalance between the training dosage and opportunities for recovery.

obesity—A body mass index at or above the 95th percentile in children and adolescents.

obstructive sleep apnea—A condition caused by complete or partial obstruction of the upper airways during sleep, which leads to fragmented sleep and intermittent hypoxia.

ontogenetic—The growth and development of an organism throughout the life course.

osteogenesis—The formation of bone.

osteoporosis—A substantially reduced bone mineral density (2.5 standard deviations below mean peak healthy adult bone mass).

outcome goal—The identified result that an individual wishes to achieve; outcome goals are largely out of an individual's control.

overtraining—Excessive training that leads to long-lasting decrements in performance and continual feelings of tiredness.

overuse injury—An injury caused by repetitive submaximal microtrauma to the musculoskeletal system in the absence of sufficient time for recovery and subsequent adaptation.

overweight—A body mass index at or above the 85th percentile but below the 95th percentile in children and adolescents.

passive warm-up—External techniques such as hot showers or saunas that that may increase body temperature without increasing metabolic demands.

peak aerobic power—The power output at the point of $\dot{V}O_2$peak in an incremental exercise test.

peak anaerobic power—The anaerobic power measured in watts.

peak height velocity—The maximal rate of growth in stature during the adolescent period.

peak oxygen uptake—The maximal rate at which energy can be supplied by aerobic metabolism.

peak weight velocity—The maximal rate of growth in body mass during the adolescent period.

pedagogy—The theory and practice of education; the term literally means "to lead the child."

pediatric exercise science—The application of scientific inquiry and principles as they relate to the exercising child and adolescent.

perceived competence—Self-perception of an individual in terms of capabilities and the ability to control the environment and situation.

perceptual and decision-making processes—Cognitive attributes that enable the individual to respond to an external stimulus in open and reactive tasks.

performance orientation—The belief that success is the judged by the result or outcome of an action or performance.

periodization—Manipulation of training variables in a logical, sequential, and integrative manner in order to optimize training outcomes and prevent overtraining.

peripheral nervous system (PNS)—The system that connects the central nervous system to the limbs and organs.

phenotype—Observable characteristics influenced by one's genotype and environmental factors.

phosphofructokinase—A key regulatory enzyme of glycolytic activity.

phylogenetic—Observable heritable traits related to genetic endowment.

physical activity—Movement produced by skeletal muscles that results in energy expenditure.

physical disability—A physical condition that limits mobility and daily functioning.

physical fitness—A state of well-being that relates to the ability to perform physical activities with energy, vigor, and enjoyment.

physical inactivity—Achieving less than the recommended amount of moderate to vigorous physical activity.

physical literacy—An inclusive concept that involves the motivation, confidence, competence, knowledge, and understanding to participate in physical activities for life.

physis—A segment of the bone where new bone growth takes place.

plyometric training—A specialized type of training that consists of quick, powerful actions that involve muscle lengthening immediately followed by rapid shortening of the same muscle.

polycystic ovary syndrome—A hormonal disorder in women characterized by hyperandrogenism and persistent menstrual disorders.

polydipsia—Excessive thirst that can be characteristic of diabetes mellitus.

polyuria—Excessive excretion of urine that can be characteristic of diabetes mellitus.

positive spiral of engagement—The tendency of children with high motor competence to engage in more physical activity and thus have greater opportunities for further motor skill development.

postactivation potentiation—An acute enhancement of muscle function as a direct result of its contractile history.

power ratio—The ratio of anaerobic power to aerobic power.

precocious puberty—The onset of puberty at an atypical age.

prediabetes—The precursor to diabetes mellitus characterized by slightly elevated blood glucose levels.

primordial prevention—Avoiding the development of clinical risk factors through healthy lifestyle behaviors.

process goal—The processes that must be repeated to increase the chances of achieving an outcome goal; process goals are controlled by the individual.

processed food—Food that has been altered in any way during preparation before the point of sale; this is often done to preserve the food and extend its shelf life.

process of motor skill performance—Subjective measures of the movement competency shown during a motor skill task.

product of motor skill performance—Objective measure of a motor skill task (e.g., time, distance).

proficiency barrier—The theory that early deficiency in fundamental motor skill competence likely impedes the learning of more complex movement patterns later in life.

programming—The process of constructing the training programs called for in the overall periodized plan.

progressive overload of training—A logical and progressive manipulation of training to disrupt the individual's current state of readiness (homeostasis) and elicit adaptation.

proprioceptive neuromuscular facilitation—A stretching technique that uses both stretching and muscle contraction to enhance range of motion.

puberty—The period of sexual development between childhood and adulthood.

rating of perceived exertion—A subjective measure of how hard a person feels they are working.

ratio scaling—A physiological outcome is divided by a measure of body size, most typically body mass.

reactive agility training—Training that requires children to perform agility-based tasks in response to an external stimulus.

reciprocal inhibition—Relaxation in an antagonist muscle group when contracting the agonist muscle group.

recommended daily allowance (RDA)—The average daily dietary nutrient intake level sufficient to meet the requirements of nearly all healthy individuals.

recommended daily intake—The nutrient reference values covered by the recommended daily allowance, adequate intake, upper limit, and estimated average requirement.

reflexive movements—Innate reflexes and spontaneous movements that are involuntary and controlled subcortically.

relative age effect—The birth date bias in youth sport by which participation is higher among those born early in the relevant selection period and correspondingly lower amongst those born late in the selection period.

reliability—The consistency (or stability) of results obtained from a test.

resistance training—A collective term that refers to methods of conditioning that involve the progression of a range of resistive loads, movement velocities, and training modalities.

resistance training skill competence—The process of developing and accessing movement patterns that are essential to mastery of a specific exercise.

reverse-dependency phenomenon—The process in which parents define their own self-worth in terms of their child's sport achievements.

reversibility of training—The loss of adaptations acquired from systematic training once training ceases.

rudimentary motor skills—As primitive and postural reflexes become inhibited, an infant begins to gain more voluntary control over movement, enabling more coordinated and concerted neuromuscular function.

sampling—An approach that encourages children to experience a number of different sports and activities or a number of different positions within a sport.

scaffolding—An instructional technique that connects past experiences to present actions.

sedentary behaviors—Any waking behavior characterized by an energy expenditure of 1.5 METs (metabolic equivalent units) or less.

self-efficacy—Confidence in one's ability to perform a specific task or succeed in reaching a goal.

sexual age—A rating of biological age based on the development of secondary sexual characteristics, such as breast, genital, and pubic hair development. Full sexual maturity is identified with fully functional reproductive capability.

skeletal age—A rating of biological age based on the progress of the skeleton from cartilage to bone. Full skeletal maturity is identified as a fully ossified skeleton.

skill-related fitness—Refers to measures of fitness associated with athleticism and qualities such as speed, power, agility, coordination, and balance.

slipped capital femoral epiphysis—A disorder of the proximal femur characterized by a fracture through the growth plate, which results in a slippage of the overlying end of the femur.

somatic age—A rating of biological age based on the progress toward full adult size and proportion. Full somatic maturity is identified as the achievement of final adult stature.

somatic nervous system—The system that controls voluntary skeletal muscle activation and mediates involuntary reflexes.

specialized motor skills—The combination of a number of fundamental motor skills to perform more complex, refined movement patterns in a variety of contexts, including competitive sport, recreational physical activity, and free play.

specific warm-up—Preparatory activities that consist of movement patterns similar to the upcoming sport or activity.

sport-related concussion—The clinical syndrome of traumatic brain injury induced by an event such as a direct blow to the head or neck, which transmits an impulsive force to the head.

spring-mass model—A model of the musculoskeletal system in which a spring represents the lower limb and the mass is the center of mass.

sprint performance—The combination of the acceleration and maximal velocity phases of sprinting.

stabilization—Fundamental motor skills that require an individual to demonstrate static or dynamic balance.

static stretching—A type of flexibility training that involves slowly lengthening a muscle to an elongated position and then holding this position for a predetermined period of time.

stature—A linear measurement of the distance from the floor to the vertex of the skull.

strength reserve—A resource of muscular strength that can be used to overcome physical challenges during daily life, exercise, and sport activities.

stretch–shortening cycle—A specific sequence of eccentric, isometric, and concentric muscle actions that enhance concentric force output.

stride frequency—The rate of lower limb movements as defined by the number of strides taken per second.

stride length—The distance travelled between alternate foot contacts.

sugar-sweetened beverages—Prepared drinks with added sugars.

supercompensation—Attaining a heightened level of baseline fitness after a bout of relatively intense training followed by sufficient recovery.

synergistic adaptation—The compatible relationship between specific adaptations to an imposed training demand and adaptations related to age and maturity.

talent development—The process of providing the best learning environment and support systems to develop identified talent.

talent identification—The process of identifying current participants who have the potential to excel in a given sport or activity.

tapering—Manipulation of training in the lead-up to an important event (i.e., competition), which typically involves reductions in training volume and a maintenance of training intensity.

task constraints—Manipulation of the rules, degree of challenge, or type of equipment involved in a given movement or activity.

task orientation—Refers to being motivated by task mastery.

technical competence—The proficiency displayed by an individual during goal-directed human movement; essentially the ability to perform movements with control and accuracy.

tidal volume—The amount of air inspired in each breath.

trainability—The responsiveness to exercise at different stages of growth and maturation.

training age—The number of years an individual has been engaged in a formalized training program.

training day—Programming that consists of daily activity dictated by the goals and objectives of the microcycle in which it resides.

training load—The sporting and nonsporting stress applied to the human body over varying time periods and magnitudes.

training relevance—The extent to which the exercise prescription (e.g., training mode, exercise selection) is relevant to the goal of the program.

training session—Programming that typically consists of a series of training components (e.g., warm-up, motor skills, speed and agility, strength and power).

training stress—The physical or psychological stress placed on the individual as a result of physical training or exercise that acts as a stimulus for adaptation; too much stress in the absence of recovery time can lead to maladaptive responses.

training variation—Ongoing manipulation of training to enable the development and mastery of skills.

trans fats—Fats created from polyunsaturated fats during an industrial process whereby hydrogen is added to make the fats harder.

ventilatory threshold—The point at which ventilation starts to increase at a faster rate than oxygen consumption during an incremental exercise test.

vertical integration—The notion that a number of fitness qualities need to be trained in order to maintain or improve existing levels; however, the fitness quality that most needs improvement should be prioritized.

vulnerable population—A group who may not fully understand information that is presented to them (e.g., children).

weightlifting—A sport that involves performing the snatch and clean-and-jerk lifts in competition.

weight training—A variety of multijoint movements, including modifications of weightlifting exercises.

Wingate anaerobic test—An all-out sprint test (normally lasting 30 seconds) on a cycle ergometer, where power is measured to provide an indirect measure of anaerobic power and capacity.

young athlete—Children and adolescents who are selected for, and routinely participate in, organized competitive sports.

youth—An umbrella term that encompasses both children and adolescents.

REFERENCES

Chapter 1 Physical Activity and Children's Health

Aadland, E., Andersen, L., Anderssen, S., Resaland, G., & Kvalheim, O. (2018). Associations of volumes and patterns of physical activity with metabolic health in children: A multivariate pattern analysis approach. *Preventive Medicine, 115*, 12-18.

American College of Sports Medicine. (2018). *ACSM's guidelines for exercise testing and prescription* (10th ed.). Baltimore, MD: Lippincott, Williams and Wilkins.

Arem, H., Moore, S., Patel, A., Hartge, P., Berrington de Gonzalez, A., Visvanathan, K., . . . Matthews, C. (2015). Leisure time physical activity and mortality: A detailed pooled analysis of the dose-response relationship. *JAMA Internal Medicine, 175*(6), 959-967.

Aubert, S., Barnes, J.D., Abdeta, C., Abi Nader, P., Adeniyi, A.F., Aguilar-Farias, N., . . . Tremblay, M.S. (2018). Global Matrix 3.0 physical activity report card grades for children and youth: Results and analysis from 49 countries. *Journal of Physical Activity and Health, 15*(S2), S251-S273.

Australian Government Department of Health. (n.d.). *Australia's physical activity and sedentary behaviour guidelines.* Retrieved from www.health.gov.au/internet/main/publishing.nsf/content/health-pubhlth-strateg-phys-act-guidelines#npa05

Bai, Y., Allums-Featherston, K., Saint-Maurice, P., Welk, G., & Candelaria, N. (2018). Evaluation of youth enjoyment toward physical activity and sedentary behavior. *Pediatric Exercise Science, 30*(2), 273-280.

Bangsbo, J., Krustrup, P., Duda, J., Hillman, C., Bo Andersen, L., Weiss, M., . . . Elbe, A. (2016). The Copenhagen Consensus Conference 2016: Children, youth, and physical activity in schools and during leisure time. *British Journal of Sports Medicine, 50*(19), 1177-1178.

Barnett, L., Van Beurden, E., Morgan, P., Brooks, L., & Beard, J. (2008). Does childhood motor skill proficiency predict adolescent fitness? *Medicine and Science in Sports and Exercise, 40*(12), 2137-2144.

Belcher, B., Berrigan, D., Dodd, K., Emken, A., Chou, C., & Spruijt-Metz, D. (2010). Physical activity in US youth: Effect of race/ethnicity, age, gender, and weight status. *Medicine and Science in Sports and Exercise, 42*(12), 2211-2221.

Berenson, G. (Ed.) (2011). *Evolution of cardio-metabolic risk from birth to middle age.* New York, NY: Springer.

Biddle, S., & Asare, M. (2011). Physical activity and mental health in children and adolescents: A review of reviews. *British Journal of Sports Medicine, 45*(11), 886-895.

Bjerregaard, L., Jensen, B., Ängquist, L., Osler, M., Sørensen, T., & Baker, J. (2018). Change in overweight from childhood to early adulthood and risk of type 2 diabetes. *New England Journal of Medicine, 378*(14), 1302-1312.

Black, R., Victora C.G., Walker, S., Bhutta, Z., Christian, P., de Onis, M., . . . Uauy, R. (2013). Maternal and child undernutrition and overweight in low-income and middle-income countries. *Lancet, 382*(9890), 427-451.

Blair, S. (2009). Physical inactivity: The biggest public health burden of the 21st century. *British Journal of Sports Medicine, 43*(1), 1-2.

Bloemen, M., Backx, F., Takken, T., Wittink, H., Benner, J., Mollema, J., & de Groot, J. (2015). Factors associated with physical activity in children and adolescents with a physical disability: A systematic review. *Developmental Medicine & Child Neurology, 57*(2), 137-148.

Bloemers, F., Collard, D., Paw, M., Van Mechelen, W., Twisk, J., & Verhagen, E. (2012). Physical inactivity is a risk factor for physical activity-related injuries in children. *British Journal of Sports Medicine, 46*(9), 669-674.

Boddy, L., Murphy, M., Cunningham, C., Breslin, G., Foweather, L., Gobbi, R., . . . Stratton, G. (2014). Physical activity, cardiorespiratory fitness, and clustered cardiometabolic risk in 10- to 12-year-old school children: The REACH Y6 study. *American Journal of Human Biology, 26*(4), 446-451.

Booth, F., & Lees, S. (2007). Fundamental questions about genes, inactivity, and chronic diseases. *Physiolical Genomics, 28*(2), 146-157.

Brenner, J., & Council on Sports Medicine and Fitness. (2016). Sports specialization and intensive training in young athletes. *Pediatrics, 138*(3), e20162148.

Brown, H., Pearson, N., Braithwaite, R., Brown, W., & Biddle, S. (2013). Physical activity interventions and depression in children and adolescents: A systematic review and meta-analysis. *Sports Medicine, 43*(3), 195-206.

Bukowsky, M., Faigenbaum, A., & Myer, G. (2014). FUNdamental Integrative Training (FIT) for physical education. *Journal of Physical Education Recreation and Dance, 85*(6), 23-30.

Cain, K., Gavand, K., Conway, T., Peck, E., Bracy, N., Bonilla, E., . . . Sallis, J. (2015). Physical activity in youth dance classes. *Pediatrics, 135*(6), 1066-1073.

Canadian Society for Exercise Physiology. (2012). *Canadian physical activity guidelines.* Retrieved from www.csep/ca/guidelines

Carson, V., Hunter, S., Kuzik, N., Gray, C., Poitras, V., Chaput, J., . . . Tremblay, M. (2016). Systematic review of sedentary behaviour and health indicators in school-aged children and youth: An update. *Applied Physiology Nutrition and Metabolism, 41*, S240-S265.

Cattuzzo, M., Dos Santos, H.R., Ré, A., de Oliveira, I., Melo, B., de Sousa Moura, M., . . . Stodden, D. (2016). Motor competence and health related physical fitness in youth: A systematic review. *Journal of Science and Medicine in Sport, 19*(2), 123-129.

Centers for Disease Control and Prevention. (2010). *The association between school based physical activity, including physical education, and academic performance.* Atlanta, GA: Author.

Centers for Disease Control and Prevention. (2011). *Diabetes success and opportunities for population-based prevention and control.* Retrieved from www.cdc.gov/diabetes

Cohen, D., Voss, C., Taylor, M., Delextrat, A., Ogunleye, A., & Sandercock, G. (2011). Ten-year secular changes in muscular fitness in English children. *Acta Paediatrica, 100*(10), e175-e177.

Colley, R., Garriguet, D., Janssen, I., Craig, C., Clarke, J., & Tremblay, M. (2011). Physical activity of Canadian children and youth: Accelerometer results from the 2007 to 2009 Canadian Health Measures Survey. *Health Reports, 22*(1), 15-23.

Collings, P., Wijndaele, K., Corder, K., Westgate, K., Ridgway C., Dunn, V., . . . Brage, S. (2014). Levels and patterns of objectively-measured physical activity volume and intensity distribution in UK adolescents: The ROOTS study. *International Journal of Behavior, Nutrition and Physical Activity, 11,* 23. doi:10.1186/1479-5868-11-23

Corder, K., Crespo, N., van Sluijs, E., Lopez, N., & Elder, J. (2012). Parent awareness of young children's physical activity. *Preventive Medicine, 55*(3), 201-205.

Corder, K., Sharp, S., Atkin, A., Andersen, L., Cardon, G., Page, A., . . . International Children's Accelerometry Database (ICAD) Collaborators. (2016). Age-related patterns of vigorous-intensity physical activity in youth: The International Children's Accelerometry Database. *Preventive Medicine Reports, 4,* 17-22.

Corder, K., van Sluijs, E., McMinn, A., Ekelund, U., Cassidy, A., & Griffin, S. (2010). Perception versus reality awareness of physical activity levels of British children. *American Journal of Preventative Medicine, 38*(1), 1-8.

Cote, A., Phillips, A., Harris, K., Sandor, G., Panagiotopoulos, C., & Devlin, A. (2015). Obesity and arterial stiffness in children: Systematic review and meta-analysis. *Arteriosclerosis, Thrombosis, and Vascular Biology, 35*(4), 1038-1044.

Council on Communications and Media. (2016). Media use by school-age children and adolescents. *Pediatrics, 138*(5), e20162592.

Craig, C., Shields, M., Leblanc, A., & Tremblay, M. (2012). Trends in aerobic fitness among Canadians, 1981 to 2007-2009. *Applied Physiology Nutrition and Metabolism, 37*(3), 511-519.

Daniels, S., Hassink, S., & Committee on Nutrition. (2015). The role of the pediatrician in primary prevention of obesity. *Pediatrics, 136*(1), e275-e292.

De Bock, F., Genser, B., Raat, H., Fischer, J., & Renz-Polster, H. (2013). A participatory physical activity intervention in preschools: A cluster randomized controlled trial. *American Journal of Preventative Medicine, 45*(1), 64-74.

De Meester, A., Stodden, D., Goodway, J., True, L., Brian, A., Ferkel, R., & Haerens, L. (2018). Identifying a motor proficiency barrier for meeting physical activity guidelines in children. *Journal of Science and Medicine in Sport, 21*(1), 58-62.

de Souza, M., de Chaves, R., Lopes, V., Malina, R., Garganta, R., Seabra, A., & Maia, J. (2014). Motor coordination, activity, and fitness at 6 years of age relative to activity and fitness at 10 years of age. *Journal of Physical Activity and Health, 11*(6), 1239-1247.

Department of Health Social Services and Public Safety. (2011). *Start active, stay active: A report on physical activity from the four home countries' Chief Medical Officers.* London, UK: Author.

Ding, D., Lawson, K., Kolbe-Alexander, T., Finkelstein, E., Katzmarzyk, P., van Mechelen, W., & Pratt, M. (2016). The economic burden of physical inactivity: A global analysis of major non-communicable diseases. *Lancet, 388*(10051), 1311-1324.

Dishman, R., McIver, K., Dowda, M., & Pate, R. (2018). Declining physical activity and motivation from middle school to high school. *Medicine and Science in Sports and Exercise, 50*(6), 1206-1215.

Donnelly, J., Hillman, C., Castelli, D., Etnier, J., Lee, S., Tomporowski, P., Szabo-Reed, A. (2016). Physical activity, fitness, cognitive function, and academic achievement in children: A systematic review. *Medicine and Science in Sports and Exercise, 48*(6), 1197-1222.

Eime, R., Young, J., Harvey, J., Charity, M., & Payne, W. (2013). A systematic review of the psychological and social benefits of participation in sport for children and adolescents: Informing development of a conceptual model of health through sport. *Int J Behav Nutr Phys Act, 10*(98). doi:10.1186/1479-5868-10-98

Ekstedt, M., Nyberg, G., Ingre, M., Ekblom, Ö., & Marcu, S.C. (2013). Sleep, physical activity and BMI in six to ten-year-old children measured by accelerometry: A cross-sectional study. *International Journal of Behavior, Nutrition and Physical Activity, 10*(82). doi:10.1186/1479-5868-10-82

Ericsson, I., & Karlsson, M. (2012). Motor skills and school performance in children with daily physical education in school: A 9-year intervention study. *Scandinavian Journal of Medicine and Science in Sport, 24*(2), 273-278.

Esteban-Cornejo, I., Rodriguez-Ayllon, M., Verdejo-Roman, J., Cadenas-Sanchez, C., Mora-Gonzalez, J., Chaddock-Heyman, L., . . . Hillman, C. (2019). Physical fitness, white matter volume and academic performance in children: Findings from the ActiveBrains and FITKids2 Projects. *Frontiers in Psychology, 10,* 208.

Faigenbaum, A., Farrell, A., Fabiano, M., Radler, T., Naclerio, F., Ratamess, N., . . . Myer, G. (2011). Effects of integrated neuromuscular training on fitness performance in children. *Pediatric Exercise Science, 23,* 573-584.

Faigenbaum, A., Lloyd, R., MacDonald, J., & Myer, G. (2016). Citius, Altius, Fortius: Beneficial effects of resistance training for young athletes: Narrative review. *British Journal of Sports Medicine, 50*(1), 3-7.

Faigenbaum, A., & Myer, G. (2012). Exercise deficit disorder in youth: Play now or play later. *Current Sports Medicine Reports, 11*(4), 196-200.

Faigenbaum, A., & Rial, T. (2018). Understanding physical literacy in youth. *Strength and Conditioning Journal, 40*(6), 90-94.

Faigenbaum, A., Rial Rebullido, T., & MacDonald, J. (2018). Pediatric inactivity triad: A risky PIT. *Current Sports Medicine Reports, 17*(2), 1-3.

Farooq, M., Parkinson, K., Adamson, A., Pearce, M., Reilly, J., Hughes, A., . . . Reilly, J. (2018). Timing of the decline in physical activity in childhood and adolescence: Gateshead Millennium Cohort Study. *British Journal of Sports Medicine, 52*(15), 1002-1006.

Finkelstein, E., Graham, W., & Malhotra, R. (2014). Lifetime direct medical costs of childhood obesity. *Pediatrics, 133*(5), 854-862.

Fletcher, G.F., Landolfo, C., Niebauer, J., Ozemek, C., Arena, R., & Lavie, C.J. (2018). Promoting physical activity and exercise; JACC health promotion series. *Journal of American College of Cardiology, 72*(14), 1622-1639.

Francis, S., Morrissey, J., Letuchy, E., Levy, S., & Janz, K. (2013). Ten-year objective physical activity tracking: Iowa bone development study. *Medicine and Science in Sports and Exercise, 45*(8), 1508-1514.

Fransen, J., Deprez, D., Pion, J., Tallir, I., D'Hondt, E., Vaeyens, R., . . . Philippaerts, R. (2014). Changes in physical fitness and sports participation among children with different levels of motor competence: A 2-year longitudinal study. *Pediatric Exercise Science, 26*(1), 1-21.

Fyfe-Johnson, A., Ryder, J., Alonso, A., MacLehose, R., Rudser, K., Fox , C., . . . Kelly, A. (2018). Ideal cardiovascular health and adiposity: Implications in youth. *Journal of the American Heart Association, 7*(8), e007467.

Galland, B., & Mitchell, E. (2010). Helping children sleep. *Archives of Disease in Childhood, 95*(10), 850-853.

García-Hermoso, A., Ramírez-Campillo, R., & Izquierdo M. (2019). Is muscular fitness associated with future health benefits in children and adolescents? A systematic review and meta-analysis of longitudinal studies. *Sports Medicine*, doi: 10.1007/s40279-019-01098-6.

Granacher, U., Lesinski, M., Busch, D., Muehlbauer. T., Prieske, O., Puta, C., . . . Behm, D. (2016). Effects of resistance training in youth athletes on muscular fitness and athletic performance: A conceptual model for long-term athlete development. *Frontiers in Physiology, 7*(164).

Guagliano, J., Rosenkranz, R., & Kolt, G. (2013). Girls' physical activity levels during organized sports in Australia. *Medicine and Science in Sports and Exercise, 45*(1), 116-122.

Guthold, R., Cowan, M., Autenrieth, C., Kann, L., & Riley, L. (2010). Physical activity and sedentary behavior among schoolchildren: A 34-country comparison. *Journal of Pediatrics, 157*(1), 43-49.

Gutin, B., & Owens, S. (2011). The influence of physical activity on cardiometabolic biomarkers in youths: A review. *Pediatric Exercise Science, 23*(2), 169-185.

Hallal, P., Andersen, L., Bull, F., Guthold, R., Haskell, W., Ekelund, U., & Lancet Physical Activity Series Working Group. (2012). Global physical activity levels: Surveillance progress, pitfalls, and prospects. *Lancet, 380*(9838), 247-257.

Hallal, P., Victora, C., Azevedo, M., & Wells, J. (2006). Adolescent physical activity and health: A systematic review. *Sports Medicine, 36*(12), 1019-1030.

Hamer, M., & Stamatakis, E. (2018). Relative proportion of vigorous physical activity, total volume of moderate to vigorous activity, and body mass index in youth: The Millennium Cohort Study. *International Journal of Obesity (Lond), 42*(6), 1239-1242.

Hardy, L., Barnett, L., Espinel, P., & Okely, A. (2013). Thirteen-year trends in child and adolescent fundamental movement skills: 1997-2010. *Medicine and Science in Sports and Exercise, 45*(10), 1965-1970.

Henrique, R., Bustamante, A., Freitas, D., Tani, G., Katzmarzyk, P., & Maia, J. (2018). Tracking of gross motor coordination in Portuguese children. *Journal of Sports Science, 36*(2), 220-228.

Hillman, C., & Biggan, J. (2017). A review of childhood physical activity, brain, and cognition: perspectives on the future. *Pediatric Exercise Science, 29*(2), 170-176.

Hillman, C., Pontifex, M., Castelli, D., Khan, N., Raine, L., Scudder, M., . . . Kamijo, K. (2014). Effects of the FITKids randomized controlled trial on executive control and brain function. *Pediatrics, 134*(4), e1083-e1071.

Hivert, M., Arena, R., Forman, D., Kris-Etherton, P., McBride, P., Pate, R., . . . Council on Cardiovascular and Stroke Nursing. (2016). Medical training to achieve competency in lifestyle counseling: An essential foundation for prevention and reatment of cardiovascular diseases and other chronic medical conditions: A scientific statement from the American Heart Association. *Circulation, 134*(15), e308-e327.

Hollingworth, W., Hawkins, J., Lawlor, D., Brown, M., Marsh, T., & Kipping, R. (2012). Economic evaluation of lifestyle interventions to treat overweight or obesity in children. *International Journal of Obesity (Lond), 36*(4), 559-566.

Howie, E., & Pate, R. (2012). Physical activity and academic achievement in children: A historical perspective *Journal of Sport and Health Science, 1*(3), 160-169.

Institute of Medicine. (2011). *Early childhood obesity prevention policies: Goals, recommendations, and potential actions.* Washington, DC: National Academies Press.

Institute of Medicine. (2015). *Physical activity: Moving toward obesity solutions.* Washington, DC: National Academies Press.

Janz, K., Kwon, S., Letuchy, E., Eichenberger Gilmore, J., Burns, T., Torner, J., . . . Levy, S. (2009). Sustained effect of early physical activity on body fat mass in older children. *American Journal of Preventative Medicine, 37*(1), 35-40.

Juonala, M., Magnussen, C., Venn, A., Dwyer, T., Burns, T., Davis, P., . . . Raitakari, O. (2010). Influence of age on associations between childhood risk factors and carotid intima-media thickness in adulthood: The Cardiovascular Risk in Young Finns Study, the Childhood Determinants of Adult Health Study, the Bogalusa Heart Study, and the Muscatine Study for the International Childhood Cardiovascular Cohort (i3C) Consortium. *Circulation, 122*(24), 2514-2520.

Kallio, P., Pahkala, K., Heinonen, O., Tammelin, T., Hirvensalo, M., Telama, R., . . . Raitakari, O. (2018). Physical inactivity from youth to adulthood and risk of impaired glucose metabolism. *Medicine and Science in Sports and Exercise, 50*(6), 1192-1198.

Kalman, M., Inchley, J., Sigmundova, D., Iannotti, R., Tynjälä, J., Hamrik, Z., . . . Bucksch, J. (2015). Secular trends in moderate-to-vigorous physical activity in 32 countries from 2002 to 2010: A cross-national perspective. *European Journal of Public Health,* Suppl 2, 37-40.

Kambas, A., Michalopoulou, M., Fatouros, I., Christoforidis, C., Manthou, E., Giannakidou, D., . . . Zimmer, R. (2012). The relationship between motor proficiency and pedometer-determined physical activity in young children. *Pediatric Exercise Science, 24*(1), 34-44.

Kanazawa, H., Kawai, M., Niwa, F., Hasegawa, T., Iwanaga, K., Ohata, K., . . . Heike, T. (2014). Subcutaneous fat accumulation in early infancy is more strongly associated with motor development and delay than muscle growth. *Acta Paediatrica, 103*(6), e262-e267.

Katzmarzyk, P., Barreira, T., Broyles, S., Champagne, C., Chaput, J., Fogelholm, M., . . . Church T. (2015). Physical activity, sedentary time, and obesity in an international sample of children. *Medicine and Science in Sports, 47*(10), 2062-2069.

Kehler, D., Stammers, A., Susser, S., Hamm, N., Kimber, D., Hlynsky, M., & Duhamel, T. (2014). Cardiovascular complications of type 2 diabetes in youth. *Biochemistry Cell Biology, 93*(5), 496-510.

Kohl, H., Craig, C., Lambert, E., Inoue, S., Alkandari, J., Leetongin, G., . . . Lancet Physical Activity Series Working Group. (2012). The pandemic of physical inactivity: Global action for public health. *Lancet, 380,* 294-305.

Konstabel, K., Veidebaum, T., Verbestel, V., Moreno, L., Bammann, K., Tornaritis, M., . . . Pitsiladis, Y. (2014). Objectively measured physical activity in European children: The IDEFICS study. *International Journal of Obesity (Lond), 38*(Suppl 2), S135-S143.

Kraus, H., & Raab, W. (1961). *Hypokinetic disease.* Springfield, IL: Charles C. Thomas.

Kraus, W., Bittner, V., Appel, L., Blair, S., Church, T., Després, J., . . . Whitsel, L. (2015). The National Physical Activity Plan: A call to action from the American Heart Association: A science advisory from the American Heart Association. *Circulation, 131*(21), 1932-1940.

Laguna, M., Ruiz, J., Lara, M., & Aznar, S. (2013). Recommended levels of physical activity to avoid adiposity in Spanish children. *Pediatric Obesity, 8*(1), 62-69.

Laitinen, T., Pahkala, K., Magnussen, C., Viikari, J., Oikonen, M., Taittonen, L., . . . Juonala, M. (2012). Ideal cardiovascular health in childhood and cardiometabolic outcomes in adulthood: The Cardiovascular Risk in Young Finns Study. *Circulation, 125*(16), 1971-1978.

Lang, J., Tremblay, M., Léger, L., Olds, T., & Tomkinson, G. (2018). International variability in 20 m shuttle run performance in children and youth: Who are the fittest from a 50-country comparison? A systematic literature review with pooling of aggregate results. *British Journal of Sports Medicine, 52*(4), 276.

LaPrade, R., Agel, J., Baker, J., Brenner, J., Cordasco, F., Côté, J., . . . Provencher, M. (2016). AOSSM early sport specialization consensus statement. *Orthopedic Journal of Sports Medicine, 4*(4), 2325967116644241.

Lauersen, J., Bertelsen, D., & Andersen, L. (2014). The effectiveness of exercise interventions to prevent sports injuries: a systematic review and meta-analysis of randomised controlled trials. *British Journal of Sports Medicine, 48*(11), 871-877.

Lee, B., Adam, A., Zenkov, E., Hertenstein, D., Ferguson, M., Wang, P., . . . Brown, S. (2017). Modeling the economic and health impact of increasing children's physical activity in the United States. *Health Affairs (Millford), 36*(5), 902-908.

Lee, I., Shiroma, E., Lobelo, F., Puska, P., Blair, S., Katzmarzyk, P., & Lancet Physical Activity Series Working Group. (2012). Effect of physical inactivity on major non-communicable diseases worldwide: An analysis of burden of disease and life expectancy. *Lancet, 380*(9838), 219-229.

Leek, D., Carlson, J., Cain, K., Henrichon, S., Rosenberg, D., Patrick, K., & Sallis, J.F. (2010). Physical activity during youth sports practices. *Archives of Pediatric and Adolescent Medicine, 165*(4), 294-299.

Li, K., Haynie, D., Lipsky, L., Iannotti, R., Pratt, C., & Simons-Morton, B. (2016). Changes in moderate-to-vigorous physical activity among older adolescents. *Pediatrics, 138*(6), e20161372.

Ligthart, S., van Herpt, T., Leening, M., Kavousi, M., Hofman, A., Stricker, B., . . . Dehghan, A. (2016). Lifetime risk of developing impaired glucose metabolism and eventual progression from prediabetes to type 2 diabetes: A prospective cohort study. *Lancet Diabetes Endocrinology, 4*(1), 44-51.

Lloyd, R., & Oliver, J. (2012). The youth physical development model: A new approach to long-term athletic development. *Strength and Conditioning, 34*(3), 61-72.

Lopes, V., Rodriques, L., Maia, A., & Malina, R. (2011). Motor coordination as a predictor of physical activity in childhood. *Scandinavian Journal of Medicine and Science in Sport, 21*, 663-669.

Lubans, D., Morgan, P., Cliff, D., & Barnett, L. (2010). Fundamental movement skills in children and adolescents. *Sports Medicine, 40*(12), 1019-1035.

Lubans, D., Richards, J., Hillman, C., Faulkner, G., Beauchamp, M., Nilsson, M., . . . Biddle, S. (2016). Physical activity for cognitive and mental health in youth: A systematic review of mechanisms. *Pediatrics, 138*(3), e20161642.

Malina, R., Bouchard, C., & Bar-Or, O. (2004). *Growth, maturation, and physical activity* (2nd ed.). Champaign, IL: Human Kinetics.

Martikainen, S., Pesonen, A., Lahti, J., Heinonen, K., Feldt, K., Pyhälä, R., . . . Räikkönen, K. (2013). Higher levels of physical activity are associated with lower hypothalamic-pituitary-adrenocortical axis reactivity to psychosocial stress in children. *Journal of Clinical Endocrinology and Metabolism, 98*(4), e619-e627.

Matthews, C., Chen, K., Freedson, P., Buchowski, M., Beech, B., Pate, R., & Troiano, R. (2008). Amount of time spent in sedentary behaviors in the United States, 2003-2004. *American Journal of Epidemiology, 167*(7), 875-881.

May, A., Kuklina, E., & Yoon, P. (2012). Prevalence of cardiovascular disease risk factors among US adolescents, 1999-2008. *Pediatrics, 129*(6), 1035-1041.

McCrindle, B. (2015). Cardiovascular consequences of childhood obesity. *Canadian Journal of Cardiology, 31*(2), 124-130.

McMahon, E., Corcoran, P., O'Regan, G., Keeley, H., Cannon, M., Carli, V., . . . Wasserman, D. (2017). Physical activity in European adolescents and associations with anxiety, depression and well-being. *European Child & Adolescent Psychiatry, 26*(1), 111-121.

Metcalf, B., Hosking, J., Jeffery, A., Henley, W., & Wilkin, T. (2015). Exploring the adolescent fall in physical activity: A 10-yr cohort study (EarlyBird 41). *Medicine and Science in Sports and Exercise, 47*(10), 2084-2092.

Morgan, P., Barnett, L., Cliff, D., Okely, A., Scott, H., Cohen, K., & Lubans, D. (2013). Fundamental movement skill interventions in youth: A systematic review and meta-analysis. *Pediatrics, 132*(5), e1361-e1683.

Myer, G., Faigenbaum, A., Chu, D., Falkel, J., Ford, K., Best, T., & Hewett, T. (2011). Integrative training for children and adolescents: Techniques and practices for reducing sports-related injuries and enhancing athletic performance. *Physician and Sports Medicine, 39*(1), 74-84.

Myer, G., Faigenbaum, A., Edwards, E., Clark. J., Best, T., & Sallis, R. (2015). 60 minutes of what? A developing brain perspective for activating children with an integrative approach. *British Journal of Sports Medicine, 49*(12), 1510-1516.

Myer, G., Faigenbaum, A., Ford, K., Best, T., Bergeron, M., & Hewett, T. (2011). When to initiate integrative neuromuscular training to reduce sports-related injuries and enhance health in youth? *Current Sports Medicine Reports, 10*(3), 155-166.

Myer, G., Faigenbaum, A., Stracciolini, A., Hewett, T., Micheli, L., & Best, T. (2013). Exercise deficit disorder in youth: A paradigm shift towards disease prevention and comprehensive care. *Current Sports Medicine Reports, 12*(4), 248-255.

National Association for Sport and Physical Education. (2009). *Active Start: A statement of physical activity guidelines for children birth to five years.* Reston, VA: American Alliance for Health, Physical Education, Recreation and Dance. Retrieved from www.aahperd.org/naspe

National Association for Sport and Physical Education & American Heart Association. (2016). *2016 shape of the nation report: Status of physical education in the USA.* Reston, VA: American Alliance for Health, Physical Education, Recreation and Dance.

Nauta, J., Martin-Diener, E., Martin, B., van Mechelen, W., & Verhagen, E. (2014). Injury risk during different physical activity behaviours in children: A systematic review with bias assessment. *Sports Medicine, 45*(3), 327-336.

Nyberg, G., Nordenfelt, A., Ekelund, U., & Marcus, C. (2009). Physical activity patterns measured by accelerometry in 6- to 10-yr-old children. *Medicine and Science in Sports and Exercise, 41*(10), 1842-1848.

O'Donovan, G., Blazevich, A., Boreham, C.A., Cooper, A., Crank, H., Ekelund, U., . . . Stamatakis, E. (2010). The ABC of physical activity for health: A consensus statement from the British Association of Sport and Exercise Sciences. *Journal of Sports Sciences, 28*(6), 573-591.

O'Neill, J., Williams, H., Pfeiffer, K., Dowda, M., McIver, K., Brown, W., & Pate, R. (2014). Young children's motor skill performance: Relationships with activity types and parent perception of athletic competence. *Journal of Science and Medicine in Sport, 17*, 607-610.

Oliver, J., & Lloyd, R. (2014). Physical training as a potential form of abuse. In M. Lang & M. Hartill (Eds.), *Safeguarding, child protection and abuse in sport: International perspectives in research, policy and practice* (pp. 163-171). Oxon, UK: Routledge.

Olshansky, S., Passaro, D., Hershow, R., Layden, J., Carnes, B., Brody, J., . . . Ludwig, D. (2005). A potential decline in life expectancy in the United States in the 21st century. *New England Journal of Medicine, 352*(11), 1138-1145.

Ortega, F., Ruiz, J., Castillo, M., & Sjostrom, M. (2008). Physical fitness in children and adolescence: A powerful marker of health. *International Journal of Obesity, 32*, 1-11.

Pahkala, K., Hietalampi, H., Laitinen, T., Viikari, J., Ronnemaa, T., Niinikoski, H., . . . Raitakari, O. (2013). Ideal cardiovascular health in adolescence: Effect of lifestyle intervention and association with vascular intima-media thickness and elasticity (the Special Turku Coronary Risk Factor Intervention Project for Children [STRIP] study). *Circulation, 127*, 2088-2096.

ParticipACTION. (2018). *Canadian kids need to move more to boost their brain health: The 2018 ParticipACTION report card on physical activity for children and youth.* Toronto, Canada: ParticipACTION.

Pate, R., Brown, W., Pfeiffer, K., Howie, E., Saunders, R., Addy, C., & Dowda, M. (2016). An intervention to increase physical activity in children: A randomized controlled trial with 4-year-olds in preschools. *American Journal of Preventative Medicine, 51*(1), 12-22.

Pate, R., O'Neill, J., Brown, W., Pfeiffer, K., Dowda, M., & Addy, C. (2015). Prevalence of compliance with a new physical activity guideline for preschool-age children. *Childhood Obesity, 11*(4), 415-420.

Pesce, C., Faigenbaum, A., Goudas, M., & Tomporowski, P. (2018). Coupling our plough of thoughtful moving to the star of children's right to play. In R. Meeusen, S. Schaefer, P. Tomporowski, & R. Bailey (Eds.), *Physical activity and education achievement* (pp. 247-274). Oxon, UK: Routledge.

Poitras, V., Gray, C., Borghese, M., Carson, V., Chaput, J., Janssen, I., . . . Tremblay, M. (2016). Systematic review of the relationships between objectively measured physical activity and health indicators in school-aged children and youth. *Applied Physiology Nutrition and Metabolism, 41*, S197-S239.

Ridley, K., Zabeen, S., & Lunnay, B. (2018). Children's physical activity levels during organised sports practices. *Journal of Science and Medicine in Sport, 21*(9), 930-934.

Rowland, T. (1990). *Exercise and children's health.* Champaign, IL: Human Kinetics.

Rowland, T. (2005). *Children's exercise physiology.* Champaign, IL: Human Kinetics.

Rowland, T. (2007). Promoting physical activity for children's health. *Sports Medicine, 37*, 929-936.

Runhaar, J., Collard, D., Singh, A., Kemper, H., van Mechelen, W., & Chinapaw, M. (2010). Motor fitness in Dutch youth: differences over a 26-year period (1980-2006). *Journal of Science and Medicine in Sport, 13*(3), 323-328.

Sallis, R., Baggish, A., Franklin, B., & Whitehead, J. (2016). The call for a physical activity vital sign in clinical practice. *American Journal of Medicine, 129*(9), 903-905.

Sallis, R., Matuszak, J., Baggish, A., Franklin, B., Chodzko-Zajko, W., Fletcher, B., . . . Williams, J. (2016). Call to action on making physical activity assessment and prescription a medical standard of care. *Current Sports Medicine Reports, 15*(3), 207-214.

Schwarzfischer, P., Gruszfeld, D., Stolarczyk, A., Ferre, N., Escribano, J., Rousseaux, D., . . . Grote, V. (2019). Physical activity and sedentary behaviour from ages 6 to 11 years. *Pediatrics, 143*(1), e20180994.

Seefeldt, V. (1980). Developmental motor patterns: Implications for elementary school physical education. In K. Nadeau, K. Newell, & G. Roberts (Eds.), *Psychology of motor behavior and sport* (pp. 314-323). Champaign, IL: Human Kinetics.

Shay, C., Ning, H., Daniels, S., Rooks, C., Gidding, S., & Lloyd-Jones, D. (2013). Status of cardiovascular health in US adolescents: Prevalence estimates from the National Health and Nutrition Examination Surveys (NHANES) 2005-2010. *Circulation, 127*(13), 1369-1376.

Shields, N., King, M., Corbett, M., & Imms, C. (2014). Is participation among children with intellectual disabilities in outside school activities similar to their typically developing peers? A systematic review. *Developmental Neurorehabilitation, 17*(1), 64-71.

Sit, C., McKenzie, T., Cerin, E., Chow, B., Huang, W., & Yu, J. (2017). Physical activity and sedentary time among children with disabilities at school. *Medicine and Science in Sports and Exercise, 49*(2), 292-297.

Slining, M., Adair, L., Goldman, B., Borja, J., & Bentley, M. (2010). Infant overweight is associated with delayed motor development. *Journal of Pediatrics, 157*(1), 20-25.

Spittaels, H., Van Cauwenberghe, E., Verbestel, V., De Meester, F., Van Dyck, D., Verloigne, M., . . . De Bourdeaudhuij, I. (2012). Objectively measured sedentary time and physical activity time across the lifespan: A cross-sectional study in four age groups. *International Journal of Behavior, Nutrition and Physical Activity, 18*(9), 149.

Society of Health and Physical Educators. (2014). *National Standards & Grade Level Outcomes for K-12 Physical Education.* Champaign, IL: Human Kinetics.

Steinberger, J., Daniels, S., Hagberg, N., Isasi, C., Kelly, A., Lloyd-Jones, D., . . . Stroke Council. (2016). Cardiovascular health promotion in children: Challenges and opportunities for 2020 and beyond. *Circulation, 134*(12), e236-e255.

Stodden, D., True, L., Langendorfer, S., & Gao, Z. (2013). Associations among selected motor skills and health-related fitness: Indirect evidence for Seefeldt's proficiency barrier theory in young adults? *Research Quarterly in Exercise and Sport, 84*, 397-403.

Stracciolini, A., Myer, G., & Faigenbaum, A. (2013). Exercise deficit disorder in youth: Are we ready to make the diagnosis? *Physician and Sports Medicine, 41*(1), 94-101.

Strong, J., Malcom, G., McMahan, C., Tracy, R., Newman, W., Herderick, E., & Cornhill, J. (1999). Prevalence and extent of atherosclerosis in adolescents and young adults: Implications for prevention from the Pathobiological Determinants of Atherosclerosis in Youth Study. *Journal of the American Medical Association, 24*(8), 727-735.

Sugimoto, D., Myer, G., Barber Foss, K., & Hewett, T. (2015). Specific exercise effects of preventive neuromuscular training intervention on anterior cruciate ligament injury risk reduction in young females: Meta-analysis and subgroup analysis. *British Journal of Sports Medicine, 49*(5), 282-289.

Tanrikulu, M., Agirbasli, M., & Berenson, G. (2017). Primordial prevention of cardiometabolic risk in childhood. *Advances in Experimental Medicine and Biology, 956*, 489-496.

Telama, R., Yang, X., Leskinen, E., Kankaanpää, A., Hirvensalo, M., Tammelin, T., . . . Raitakari, O. (2014). Tracking of physical activity from early childhood through youth into adulthood. *Medicine and Science in Sports and Exercise, 46*(5), 955-962.

Thornton, J., Frémont, P., Khan, K., Poirier, P., Fowles, J., Wells, G., & Frankovich, R. (2016). Physical activity prescription: A critical opportunity to address a modifiable risk factor for the prevention and management of chronic disease: A position statement by the Canadian Academy of Sport and Exercise Medicine. *Clinical Journal of Sports Medicine, 26*(4), 259-265.

Tremblay, M., Barnes, J., González, S., Katzmarzyk, P., Onywera, V., Reilly, J., . . . Global Matrix 2.0 Research Team. (2016). Global Matrix 2.0: Report card grades on the physical activity of children and youth comparing 38 countries. *Journal of Physical Activity and Health, 13*(Suppl 2), S343-S366.

Tremblay, M., Chaput, J., Adamo, K., Aubert, S., Barnes, J., Choquette, L., . . . Carson, V. (2017). Canadian 24-hour movement guidelines for the early years (0-4 years): An integration of physical activity, sedentary behaviour, and sleep. *BMC Public Health, 17*(Suppl 5), 874.

Tremblay, M., Gray, C., Akinroye, K., Harrington, D., Katzmarzyk, P., Lambert, E., . . . Tomkinson, G. (2014). Physical activity of children: A global matrix of grades comparing 15 countries. *Journal of Physical Activity and Health, 11*(supp 1), S113-S125.

Tremblay, M., Leblanc, A., Janssen, I., Kho, M., Hicks, A., Murumets, K., . . . Duggan, M. (2011). Canadian sedentary behaviour guidelines for children and youth. *Applied Physiology Nutrition and Metabolism, 36*(1), 59-64.

Tremblay, M., Warburton, D.E., Janssen, I., Paterson, D.H., Latimer, A.E., Rhodes, E.R., . . . Duggan, M. (2011). New Canadian physical activity guidelines. *Applied Physiology Nutrition and Metabolism, 36*, 36-46.

Tudor-Locke, C., Johnson, W., & Katzmarzyk, P. (2010). Accelerometer-determined steps per day in US children and youth. *Medicine and Science in Sports and Exercise, 42*(12), 2244-2250.

United States Department of Health and Human Services. (2018). *Physical activity guidelines for Americans, 2nd edition.* Washington, DC: Author.

United States Department of Health and Human Services. (2012). *Physical activity guidelines for Americans Midcourse report: Strategies to increase physical activity.* Washington, DC: Author.

United States Department of Health and Human Services. (2016). *Healthy people 2020: Physical activity objectives.* Retrieved from www.healthypeople.gov/2020/topics-objectives.

Utesch, T., Bardid, F., Büsch, D., & Strauss, B. (2019). The relationship between motor competence and physical fitness from early childhood to early adulthood: A meta-analysis. *Sports Medicine, 49*(4), 541-551.

Walker, G., Stracciolini, A., Faigenbaum, A., & Myer, G. (2018). Physical inactivity in youth. Can exercise deficit disorder alter the way we view preventive care? *ACSM's Health and Fitness Journal, 22*(2), 42-46.

Weiler, R., Allardyce, S., Whyte, G., & Stamatakis, E. (2014). Is the lack of physical activity strategy for children complicit mass child neglect? *British Journal of Sports Medicine, 48*(13), 1010-1013.

Weintraub, W., Daniels, S., Burke, L., Franklin, B., Goff, D., Hayman, L., . . . Council on Clinical Cardiology. (2011). Value of primordial and primary prevention for cardiovascular disease: A policy statement from the American Heart Association. *Circulation, 124*(8), 967-990.

Wilson, P., Haegele, J., & Zhu, X. (2016). Mobility status as a predictor of obesity, physical activity, and screen time use among children aged 5-11 years in the United States. *Journal of Pediatrics, 176*, 23-29.

World Health Organization. (2010). *Global recommendations on physical activity for health.* Geneva, Switzerland: WHO Press.

World Health Organization. (2018). *Global action plan on physical activity 2018-2030: More active people for a healthier world.* Geneva, Switzerland: WHO Press.

Yu, S., Yarnell, J., Sweetnam, P., & Murray, L. (2003). What level of physical activity protects against premature cardiovascular death? The Caerphilly study. *Heart, 89*(5), 502-506.

Zecevic, C., Trembla, Y.L., Lovsin, T., & Michel, L. (2010). Parental influence on young children's physical activity. *International Journal of Pediatrics, 468526*.

Zhao, G., Li, C., Ford, E., Fulton, J., Carlson, S., Okoro, C., . . . Balluz, L. (2014). Leisure-time aerobic physical activity, muscle-strengthening activity and mortality risks among US adults: The NHANES linked mortality study. *British Journal of Sports Medicine, 48*(3), 244-249.

Chapter 2 Principles of Pediatric Exercise Science

Aaltonen, S., Latvala, A., Rose, R.J., Pulkkinen, L., Kujala, U.M., Kaprio, J., & Silventoinen, K. (2015). Motor development and physical activity: A longitudinal discordant twin-pair study. *Medicine and Science in Sports and Exercise, 47*(10), 2111-2118.

Alvarez-San Emeterio, C., Antunano, N.P., Lopez-Sobaler, A.M., & Gonzalez-Badillo, J.J. (2011). Effect of strength training and the practice of Alpine skiing on bone mass density, growth, body composition, and the strength and power of the legs of adolescent skiers. *Journal of Strength and Conditioning Research, 25*(10), 2879-2890.

American Academy of Pediatrics. (2000). Intensive training and sports specialization in young athletes. *Pediatrics, 106*(1), 154-157.

Andrew, G.M., Becklake, M.R., Guleria, J.S., & Bates, D.V. (1972). Heart and lung functions in swimmers and nonathletes during growth. *Journal of Applied Physiology, 32*(2), 245-251.

Armstrong, N., & Barker, A.R. (2011). Endurance training and elite young athletes. In N. Armstrong & A.M. McManus (Eds.), *The elite young athlete* (pp. 59-83). Basel: Karger.

Armstrong, N., & Fawkner, S.G. (2008). Exercise metabolism. In N. Armstrong & W. van Mechelen (Eds.), *Paediatric exercise science and medicine* (pp. 213-226). Oxford, UK: Oxford University Press.

Armstrong, N., & Welsman, J.R. (2000). Development of aerobic fitness during childhood and adolescence. *Pediatric Exercise Science, 12*, 128-149.

Bailey, D.A. (1997). The Saskatchewan pediatric bone mineral accrual study: Bone mineral acquisition during the growing years. *International Journal of Sports Medicine, 18*(Suppl 3), S191-S194.

Bailey, D.A., McKay, H.A., Mirwald, R.L., Crocker, P.R., & Faulkner, R.A. (1999). A six-year longitudinal study of the relationship of physical activity to bone mineral accrual in growing children: The university of Saskatchewan bone mineral accrual study. *Journal of Bone and Mineral Research, 14*(10), 1672-1679.

Bailey, R. (2012). So what is developmentally appropriate sport? Retrieved from www.sportscoachuk.org/blog/so-what-developmentally-appropriate-sport-richard-bailey

Barker, A.R., Welsman, J.R., Fulford, J., Welford, D., & Armstrong, N. (2008). Muscle phosphocreatine kinetics in children and adults at the onset and offset of moderate-intensity exercise. *Journal of Applied Physiology, 105*(2), 446-456.

Barnett, L.M., Van Beurden, E., Morgan, P.J., Brooks, L.O., & Beard, J.R. (2008). Does childhood motor skill proficiency predict adolescent fitness? *Medicine and Science in Sports and Exercise, 40*(12), 2137-2144.

Bar-Or, O., & Rowland, T. (2004). *Pediatric Exercise Medicine: From Physiological Principles to Health Care Applications.* Champaign, IL: Human Kinetics.

Bass, S.L. (2000). The prepubertal years: A uniquely opportune stage of growth when the skeleton is most responsive to exercise? *Sports Medicine, 30*(2), 73-78.

Bass, S., Pearce, G., Bradney, M., Hendrich, E., Delmas, P.D., Harding, A., & Seeman, E. (1998). Exercise before puberty may confer residual benefits in bone density in adulthood: Studies in active prepubertal and retired female gymnasts. *Journal of Bone and Mineral Research, 13*(3), 500-507.

Beggs, S. (2013). Swimming training for asthma in children and adolescents aged 18 years and under. *Journal of Evidence-Based Medicine, 6*(3), 199.

Behm, D.G., Young, J.D., Whitten, J.H.D., Reid, J.C., Quigley, P.J., Low, J., . . . Granacher, U. (2017). Effectiveness of traditional strength vs. power training on muscle strength, power and speed with youth: A systematic review and meta-analysis. *Frontiers in Physiology, 8*, 423.

Behringer, M., Vom Heede, A., Matthews, M., & Mester, J. (2011). Effects of strength training on motor performance skills in children and adolescents: A meta-analysis. *Pediatric Exercise Science, 23*(2), 186-206.

Behringer, M., Vom Heede, A., Yue, Z., & Mester, J. (2010). Effects of resistance training in children and adolescents: A meta-analysis. *Pediatrics, 126*(5), e1199-1210.

Berg, A., Kim, S.S., & Keul, J. (1986). Skeletal muscle enzyme activities in healthy young subjects. *International Journal of Sports Medicine, 7*(4), 236-239.

Bergeron, M.F., Mountjoy, M., Armstrong, N., Chia, M., Cote, J., Emery, C.A., . . . Engebretsen, L. (2015). International Olympic Committee consensus statement on youth athletic development. *British Journal of Sports Medicine, 49*(13), 843-851.

Binzoni, T., Bianchi, S., Hanquinet, S., Kaelin, A., Sayegh, Y., Dumont, M., & Jequier, S. (2001). Human gastrocnemius medialis pennation angle as a function of age: From newborn to the elderly. *Journal of Physiological Anthropology and Applied Human Science, 20*(5), 293-298.

Blazevich, A.J., Waugh, C., & Korff, T. (2013). Development of musculoskeletal stiffness. In M.B.A. De Ste Croix & T. Korff (Eds.), *Paediatric biomechanics and motor control: Theory and application.* Abingdon, UK: Routledge.

Blimkie, C.J. (1989). Age- and sex-associated variation in strength during childhood: Anthropometric, morphologic, neurologic, iomechanical, endocrinologic, genetic, and physical activity correlates. In C.V. Gisolfi (Ed.), *Perspectives in exercise science and sports medicine* (pp. 99-163). Indianapolis, IN: Benchmark Press.

Blimkie, C.J., Rice, S., Webber, C.E., Martin, J., Levy, D., & Gordon, C.L. (1996). Effects of resistance training on bone mineral content and density in adolescent females. *Canadian Journal of Physiology and Pharmacology, 74*(9), 1025-1033.

Boisseau, N., & Delamarche, P. (2000). Metabolic and hormonal responses to exercise in children and adolescents. *Sports Medicine, 30*(6), 405-422.

Bradney, M., Pearce, G., Naughton, G., Sullivan, C., Bass, S., Beck, T., . . . Seeman, E. (1998). Moderate exercise during growth in prepubertal boys: Changes in bone mass, size, volumetric density, and bone strength: A controlled prospective study. *Journal of Bone and Mineral Research, 13*(12), 1814-1821.

Brenner, J.S. (2016). Sports specialization and intensive training in young athletes. *Pediatrics, 138*(3).

Burger, E.H., & Klein-Nulend, J. (1999). Mechanotransduction in bone—Role of the lacuno-canalicular network. *FASEB Journal, 13*(Suppl), S101-S112.

Cadefau, J., Casademont, J., Grau, J.M., Fernandez, J., Balaguer, A., Vernet, M., . . . Urbano-Marquez, A. (1990). Biochemical and histochemical adaptation to sprint training in young athletes. *Acta Physiologica Scandinavica, 140*(3), 341-351.

Clark, P.A., & Rogol, A.D. (1996). Growth hormones and sex steroid interactions at puberty. *Endocrinology and Metabolism Clinics of North America, 25*(3), 665-681.

Conroy, B.P., Kraemer, W.J., Maresh, C.M., Fleck, S.J., Stone, M.H., Fry, A.C., . . . Dalsky, G.P. (1993). Bone mineral density in elite junior Olympic weightlifters. *Medicine and Science in Sports and Exercise, 25*(10), 1103-1109.

Cooper, D.M., Kaplan, M.R., Baumgarten, L., Weiler-Ravell, D., Whipp, B.J., & Wasserman, K. (1987). Coupling of ventilation and CO2 production during exercise in children. *Pediatric Research, 21*(6), 568-572.

Cutler, G.B., Jr. (1997). The role of estrogen in bone growth and maturation during childhood and adolescence. *Journal of Steroid Biochemestry and Molecular Biology, 61*(3-6), 141-144.

Davies, J.H., Evans, B.A., & Gregory, J.W. (2005). Bone mass acquisition in healthy children. *Archives of Disease in Childhood, 90*(4), 373-378.

Deighan, M., De Ste Croix, M., Grant, C., & Armstrong, N. (2006). Measurement of maximal muscle cross-sectional area of the elbow extensors and flexors in children, teenagers and adults. *Journal of Sports Sciences, 24*(5), 543-546.

De Ste Croix, M.B.A. (2008). Muscle Strength. In N. Armstrong & W. van Mechelen (Eds.), *Paediatric exercise science and medicine* (pp. 199-211). Oxford, UK: Oxford University Press.

De Ste Croix, M.B., Priestley, A.M., Lloyd, R.S., & Oliver, J.L. (2014). ACL injury risk in elite female youth soccer: Changes in neuromuscular control of the knee following soccer-specific fatigue. *Scandinavian Journal of Medicine & Science in Sports, 25*(5), e531-e538.

DiFiori, J.P., Benjamin, H.J., Brenner, J.S., Gregory, A., Jayanthi, N., Landry, G.L., & Luke, A. (2014). Overuse injuries and burnout in youth sports: A position statement from the American Medical Society for Sports Medicine. *British Journal of Sports Medicine, 48*(4), 287-288.

Di Luigi, L., Baldari, C., Gallotta, M.C., Perroni, F., Romanelli, F., Lenzi, A., & Guidetti, L. (2006). Salivary steroids at rest and after a training load in young male athletes: Relationship with chronological age and pubertal development. *International Journal of Sports Medicine, 27*(9), 709-717.

Dotan, R., Mitchell, C., Cohen, R., Klentrou, P., Gabriel, D., & Falk, B. (2012). Child-adult differences in muscle activation—A review. *Pediatric Exercise Science, 24*(1), 2-21.

Eliakim, A., Brasel, J.A., Mohan, S., Barstow, T.J., Berman, N., & Cooper, D.M. (1996). Physical fitness, endurance training, and the growth hormone-insulin-like growth factor I system in adolescent females. *Journal of Clinical Endocrinology and Metabolism, 81*(11), 3986-3992.

Eliakim, A., Brasel, J.A., Mohan, S., Wong, W.L., & Cooper, D.M. (1998). Increased physical activity and the growth hormone-IGF-I axis in adolescent males. *American Journal of Physiology, 275*(1 Pt 2), R308-R314.

Eliakim, A., Cooper, D.M., & Nemet, D. (2014). The GH-IGF-I response to typical field sports practices in adolescent athletes: A summary. *Pediatric Exercise Science, 26*(4), 428-433.

Eliakim, A., Portal, S., Zadik, Z., Rabinowitz, J., Adler-Portal, D., Cooper, D.M., . . . Nemet, D. (2009). The effect of a volleyball practice on anabolic hormones and inflammatory markers in elite male and female adolescent players. *Journal of Strength and Conditioning Research, 23*(5), 1553-1559.

Eriksson, B.O. (1980). Muscle metabolism in children: A review. *Acta Paediatricaica Scandinavica Supplement, 283*, 20-28.

Eriksson, B.O., Gollnick, P.D., & Saltin, B. (1973). Muscle metabolism and enzyme activities after training in boys 11-13 years old. *Acta Physiologica Scandinavica, 87*(4), 485-497.

Eriksson, B.O., & Koch, G. (1973). Effect of physical training on hemodynamic response during submaximal and maximal exercise in 11-13-year old boys. *Acta Physiologica Scandinavica, 87*(1), 27-39.

Eriksson, O., & Saltin, B. (1974). Muscle metabolism during exercise in boys aged 11 to 16 years compared to adults. *Acta Paediatricaica Belgica, 28 suppl*, 257-265.

Falk, B., & Eliakim, A. (2014). Endocrine response to resistance training in children. *Pediatric Exercise Science, 26*(4), 404-422.

Fawkner, S.G. (2008). Pulmonary Function. In N. Armstrong & W. van Mechelen (Eds.), *Paediatric exercise science and medicine* (pp. 243-253). Oxford, UK: Oxford University Press.

Foure, A., Nordez, A., & Cornu, C. (2010). Plyometric training effects on Achilles tendon stiffness and dissipative properties. *Journal of Applied Physiology, 109*(3), 849-854.

Fournier, M., Ricci, J., Taylor, A.W., Ferguson, R.J., Montpetit, R.R., & Chaitman, B.R. (1982). Skeletal muscle adaptation in adolescent boys: Sprint and endurance training and detraining. *Medicine and Science in Sports and Exercise, 14*(6), 453-456.

Frisancho, A.R. (1981). New norms of upper limb fat and muscle areas for assessment of nutritional status. *American Journal of Clinical Nutrition, 34*(11), 2540-2545.

Frost, G., Bar-Or, O., Dowling, J., & Dyson, K. (2002). Explaining differences in the metabolic cost and efficiency of treadmill locomotion in children. *Journal of Sports Sciences, 20*(6), 451-461.

Fuchs, R.K., Bauer, J.J., & Snow, C.M. (2001). Jumping improves hip and lumbar spine bone mass in prepubescent children: A randomized controlled trial. *Journal of Bone and Mineral Research, 16*(1), 148-156.

Fukunaga, T., Funato, K., & Ikegawa, S. (1992). The effects of resistance training on muscle area and strength in prepubescent age. *The Annals of Physiological Anthropology, 11*(3), 357-364.

Gilsanz, V., & Ratib, O. (2005). *Hand bone age, a digital atlas of skeletal maturity*. Berlin, Germany: Springer.

Gogtay, N., Giedd, J.N., Lusk, L., Hayashi, K.M., Greenstein, D., Vaituzis, A.C., . . . Thompson, P.M. (2004). Dynamic mapping of human cortical development during childhood through early adulthood. *Proceedings of the National Academy of Sciences of the United States of America, 101*(21), 8174-8179.

Gomez-Bruton, A., Montero-Marin, J., Gonzalez-Aguero, A., Garcia-Campayo, J., Moreno, L.A., Casajus, J.A., & Vicente-Rodriguez, G. (2016). The effect of swimming during childhood and adolescence on bone mineral density: A systematic review and meta-analysis. *Sports Medicine, 46*(3), 365-379.

Granacher, U., Goesele, A., Roggo, K., Wischer, T., Fischer, S., Zuerny, C., . . . Kriemler, S. (2011). Effects and mechanisms of strength training in children. *International Journal of Sports Medicine, 32*(5), 357-364.

Grosset, J.F., Mora, I., Lambertz, D., & Perot, C. (2005). Age-related changes in twitch properties of plantar flexor muscles in prepubertal children. *Pediatric Research, 58*(5), 966-970.

Grosset, J.F., Mora, I., Lambertz, D., & Perot, C. (2007). Changes in stretch reflexes and muscle stiffness with age in prepubescent children. *Journal of Applied Physiology, 102*(6), 2352-2360.

Gutin, B., Barbeau, P., Litaker, M.S., Ferguson, M., & Owens, S. (2000). Heart rate variability in obese children: Relations to total body and visceral adiposity, and changes with physical training and detraining. *Obesity Research, 8*(1), 12-19.

Haapasalo, H., Kannus, P., Sievanen, H., Pasanen, M., Uusi-Rasi, K., Heinonen, A., . . . Vuori, I. (1998). Effect of long-term unilateral activity on bone mineral density of female junior tennis players. *Journal of Bone and Mineral Research, 13*(2), 310-319.

Hamilton, P., & Andrew, G.M. (1976). Influence of growth and athletic training on heart and lung functions. *European Journal of Applied Physiology and Occupational Physiology, 36*(1), 27-38.

Haralambie, G. (1982). Enzyme activities in skeletal muscle of 13-15 years old adolescents. *Bulletin Europeen de Physiopathologie Respiratoire, 18*(1), 65-74.

Heinonen, A., Sievanen, H., Kannus, P., Oja, P., Pasanen, M., & Vuori, I. (2000). High-impact exercise and bones of growing girls: A 9-month controlled trial. *Osteoporosis International, 11*(12), 1010-1017.

Hemper, H.C.G. (2008). Physical activity, physical exercise, and bone health. In N. Armstrong & W. van Mechelen (Eds.), *Paediatric exercise science and medicine* (pp. 365-374). Oxford, UK: Oxford University Press.

Hernandez, D.J. (2012). *Double jeopardy how third grade reading skills and poverty influence high school graduation*. Baltimore, MD: Annie E. Casey Foundation.

Hollmann, W., Bouchard, C., & Herkenrath, G. (1967). Die leistungsentwicklung des kindes und jugendlichen unter besonderer berücksichtigung des biologischen alter. *Ärztliche Jugendkunde, 58*, 198-203.

Hume, P., & Russell, K. (2014). Overuse injuries and injury prevention strategies for youths. In R.S. Lloyd & J.L. Oliver (Eds.), *Strength and conditioning for young athletes: Science and application* (pp. 200-212). Abingdon, UK: Routledge.

Institute of Medicine (2010). *Report brief: Dietary reference intakes or calcium and vitamin D.* Washington D.C.: National Academy of Sciences.

Johnson, S.B., Blum, R.W., & Giedd, J.N. (2009). Adolescent maturity and the brain: The promise and pitfalls of neuroscience research in adolescent health policy. *Journal of Adolescent Health, 45*(3), 216-221.

Jurimae, T., & Jurimae, J. (2008). Hormonal responses and adaptations. In N. Armstrong & W. van Mechelen (Eds.), *Paediatric exercise science and medicine* (pp. 503-512). Oxford, UK: Oxford University Press.

Kannus, P., Haapasalo, H., Sankelo, M., Sievanen, H., Pasanen, M., Heinonen, A., . . . Vuori, I. (1995). Effect of starting age of physical activity on bone mass in the dominant arm of tennis and squash players. *Annals of Internal Medicine, 123*(1), 27-31.

Kaplowitz, P.B., Slora, E.J., Wasserman, R.C., Pedlow, S.E., & Herman-Giddens, M.E. (2001). Earlier onset of puberty in girls: Relation to increased body mass index and race. *Pediatrics, 108*(2), 347-353.

Kraemer, R.R., Acevedo, E.O., Synovitz, L.B., Hebert, E.P., Gimpel, T., & Castracane, V.D. (2001). Leptin and steroid hormone responses to exercise in adolescent female runners over a 7-week season. *European Journal of Applied Physiology, 86*(1), 85-91.

Kuno, S., Takahashi, H., Fujimoto, K., Akima, H., Miyamaru, M., Nemoto, I., . . . Katsuta, S. (1995). Muscle metabolism during exercise using phosphorus-31 nuclear magnetic resonance spectroscopy in adolescents. *European Journal of Applied Physiology and Occupational Physiology, 70*(4), 301-304.

Leclair, E., Berthoin, S., Borel, B., Thevenet, D., Carter, H., Baquet, G., & Mucci, P. (2013). Faster pulmonary oxygen uptake kinetics in children vs adults due to enhancements in oxygen delivery and extraction. *Scandinavian Journal of Medicine & Science in Sports, 23*(6), 705-712.

Lehmann, M., Keul, J., & Korsten-Reck, U. (1981). The influence of graduated treadmill exercise on plasma catecholamines, aerobic and anaerobic capacity in boys and adults. *European Journal of Applied Physiology and Occupational Physiology, 47*(3), 301-311.

Lenroot, R.K., & Giedd, J.N. (2006). Brain development in children and adolescents: Insights from anatomical magnetic resonance imaging. *Neuroscience and Biobehavioral Reviews, 30*(6), 718-729.

Levitt, P. (2009). Key concepts: Brain architecture. Retrieved from http://developingchild.harvard.edu/key_concepts/brain_architecture

Lexell, J., Sjostrom, M., Nordlund, A.S., & Taylor, C.C. (1992). Growth and development of human muscle: A quantitative morphological study of whole vastus lateralis from childhood to adult age. *Muscle Nerve, 15*(3), 404-409.

Lloyd, R.S., Faigenbaum, A.D., Stone, M.H., Oliver, J.L., Jeffreys, I., Moody, J.A., . . . Myer, G.D. (2014). Position statement on youth resistance training: The 2014 international consensus. *British Journal of Sports Medicine, 48*(7), 498-505.

Lloyd, R.S., Oliver, J.L., Hughes, M.G., & Williams, C.A. (2012). Age-related differences in the neural regulation of stretch-shortening cycle activities in male youths during maximal and sub-maximal hopping. *Journal of Electromyography and Kinesiology, 22*(1), 37-43.

Lopes, V.P., Rodrigues, L.P., Maia, J.A., & Malina, R.M. (2011). Motor coordination as predictor of physical activity in childhood. *Scandinavian Journal of Medicine & Science in Sports, 21*(5), 663-669.

MacKelvie, K.J., Khan, K.M., & McKay, H.A. (2002). Is there a critical period for bone response to weight-bearing exercise in children and adolescents? A systematic review. *British Journal of Sports Medicine, 36*(4), 250-257.

MacKelvie, K.J., McKay, H.A., Khan, K.M., & Crocker, P.R. (2001). A school-based exercise intervention augments bone mineral accrual in early pubertal girls. *Journal of Pediatrics, 139*(4), 501-508.

MacKelvie, K.J., McKay, H.A., Petit, M.A., Moran, O., & Khan, K.M. (2002). Bone mineral response to a 7-month randomized controlled, school-based jumping intervention in 121 prepubertal boys: Associations with ethnicity and body mass index. *Journal of Bone and Mineral Research, 17*(5), 834-844.

Mahon, A.D., Marjerrison, A.D., Lee, J.D., Woodruff, M.E., & Hanna, L.E. (2010). Evaluating the prediction of maximal heart rate in children and adolescents. *Research Quarterly for Exercise and Sport, 81*(4), 466-471.

Malina, R.M. (2006). Weight training in youth-growth, maturation, and safety: An evidence-based review. *Clinical Journal of Sport Medicine, 16*(6), 478-487.

Malina, R.M., Bouchard, C., & Bar-Or, O. (2004). *Growth, maturation and physical activity* Champaign, IL: Human Kinetics.

Mandigout, S., Melin, A., Fauchier, L., N'Guyen, L.D., Courteix, D., & Obert, P. (2002). Physical training increases heart rate variability in healthy prepubertal children. *European Journal of Clinical Investigation, 32*(7), 479-487.

Marin, G., Domene, H.M., Barnes, K.M., Blackwell, B.J., Cassorla, F.G., & Cutler, G.B., Jr. (1994). The effects of estrogen priming and puberty on the growth hormone response to standardized treadmill exercise and arginine-insulin in normal girls and boys. *Journal of Clinical Endocrinology and Metabolism, 79*(2), 537-541.

Martha, P.M., Jr., Rogol, A.D., Veldhuis, J.D., Kerrigan, J.R., Goodman, D.W., & Blizzard, R.M. (1989). Alterations in the pulsatile properties of circulating growth hormone concentrations during puberty in boys. *Journal of Clinical Endocrinology and Metabolism, 69*(3), 563-570.

Matos, N.F., Winsley, R.J., & Williams, C.A. (2011). Prevalence of nonfunctional overreaching/overtraining in young English athletes. *Medicine and Science in Sports and Exercise, 43*(7), 1287-1294.

McKay, H.A., MacLean, L., Petit, M., MacKelvie-O'Brien, K., Janssen, P., Beck, T., & Khan, K.M. (2005). "Bounce at the Bell": A novel program of short bouts of exercise improves proximal femur bone mass in early pubertal children. *British Journal of Sports Medicine, 39*(8), 521-526.

McKay, H.A., Petit, M.A., Schutz, R.W., Prior, J.C., Barr, S.I., & Khan, K.M. (2000). Augmented trochanteric bone mineral density after modified physical education classes: A randomized school-based exercise intervention study in prepubescent and early pubescent children. *Journal of Pediatrics, 136*(2), 156-162.

Meyers, R.W., Oliver, J.L., Hughes, M.G., Cronin, J.B., & Lloyd, R.S. (2015). Maximal sprint speed in boys of increasing maturity. *Pediatric Exercise Science, 27*(1), 85-94.

Miller, A.E., MacDougall, J.D., Tarnopolsky, M.A., & Sale, D.G. (1993). Gender differences in strength and muscle fiber characteristics. *European Journal of Applied Physiology and Occupational Physiology, 66*(3), 254-262.

Mitchell, C., Cohen, R., Dotan, R., Gabriel, D., Klentrou, P., & Falk, B. (2011). Rate of muscle activation in power- and endurance-trained boys. *International Journal of Sports Physiology and Performance, 6*(1), 94-105.

Moran, J.J., Sandercock, G.R., Ramirez-Campillo, R., Meylan, C.M., Collison, J.A., & Parry, D.A. (2017). Age-related variation in male youth athletes' countermovement jump after plyometric training: A meta-analysis of controlled trials. *Journal of Strength and Conditioning Research, 31*(2), 552-565.

Morris, F.L., Naughton, G.A., Gibbs, J.L., Carlson, J.S., & Wark, J.D. (1997). Prospective ten-month exercise intervention in premenarcheal girls: Positive effects on bone and lean mass. *Journal of Bone and Mineral Research, 12*(9), 1453-1462.

Nagai, N., Hamada, T., Kimura, T., & Moritani, T. (2004). Moderate physical exercise increases cardiac autonomic nervous system activity in children with low heart rate variability. *Child's Nervous System, 20*(4), 209-214.

Nagai, N., Matsumoto, T., Kita, H., & Moritani, T. (2003). Autonomic nervous system activity and the state and development of obesity in Japanese school children. *Obesity Research, 11*(1), 25-32.

Nagai, N., & Moritani, T. (2004). Effect of physical activity on autonomic nervous system function in lean and obese children. *International Journal of Obesity and Related Metabolic Disorders, 28*(1), 27-33.

Naughton, G., Farpour-Lambert, N.J., Carlson, J., Bradney, M., & Van Praagh, E. (2000). Physiological issues surrounding the performance of adolescent athletes. *Sports Medicine, 30*(5), 309-325.

Nemet, D., & Eliakim, A. (2010). Growth hormone-insulin-like growth factor-1 and inflammatory response to a single exercise bout in children and adolescents. *Medicine and Sport Science, 55*, 141-155.

Nemet, D., Eliakim, A., Mills, P.J., Meckal, Y., & Cooper, D.M. (2009). Immunological and growth mediator response to cross-country training in adolescent females. *Journal of Pediatric Endocrinology & Metabolism, 22*(11), 995-1007.

Nottin, S., Nguyen, L.D., Terbah, M., & Obert, P. (2004). Left ventricular function in endurance-trained children by tissue Doppler imaging. *Medicine and Science in Sports and Exercise, 36*(9), 1507-1513.

Nottin, S., Vinet, A., Stecken, F., N'Guyen, L.D., Ounissi, F., Lecoq, A.M., & Obert, P. (2002). Central and peripheral cardiovascular adaptations to exercise in endurance-trained children. *Acta Physiologica Scandinavica, 175*(2), 85-92.

Nourry, C., Deruelle, F., Guinhouya, C., Baquet, G., Fabre, C., Bart, F., . . . Mucci, P. (2005). High-intensity intermittent running training improves pulmonary function and alters exercise breathing pattern in children. *European Journal of Applied Physiology, 94*(4), 415-423.

NSW Department of Education and Training. (2000). *Get skilled: Get active. A K-6 resource to support the teaching of fundamental movement skills.* Moorebank, NSW: Author.

Obert, P., Mandigout, S., Vinet, A., N'Guyen, L.D., Stecken, F., & Courteix, D. (2001). Effect of aerobic training and detraining on left ventricular dimensions and diastolic function in prepubertal boys and girls. *International Journal of Sports Medicine, 22*(2), 90-96.

Obert, P., Mandigouts, S., Nottin, S., Vinet, A., N'Guyen, L.D., & Lecoq, A.M. (2003). Cardiovascular responses to endurance training in children: Effect of gender. *European Journal of Clinical Investigation, 33*(3), 199-208.

O'Brien, T.D., Reeves, N.D., Baltzopoulos, V., Jones, D.A., & Maganaris, C.N. (2010a). In vivo measurements of muscle specific tension in adults and children. *Experimental Physiology, 95*(1), 202-210.

O'Brien, T.D., Reeves, N.D., Baltzopoulos, V., Jones, D.A., & Maganaris, C.N. (2010b). Muscle-tendon structure and dimensions in adults and children. *Journal of Anatomy, 216*(5), 631-642.

Ohuchi, H., Suzuki, H., Yasuda, K., Arakaki, Y., Echigo, S., & Kamiya, T. (2000). Heart rate recovery after exercise and cardiac autonomic nervous activity in children. *Pediatric Research, 47*(3), 329-335.

Oliver, J.L., & Smith, P.M. (2010). Neural control of leg stiffness during hopping in boys and men. *Journal of Electromyography and Kinesiology, 20*(5), 973-979.

Ozmun, J.C., Mikesky, A.E., & Surburg, P.R. (1994). Neuromuscular adaptations following prepubescent strength training. *Medicine and Science in Sports and Exercise, 26*(4), 510-514.

Pomerants, T., Tillmann, V., Karelson, K., Jurimae, J., & Jurimae, T. (2006). Ghrelin response to acute aerobic exercise in boys at different stages of puberty. *Hormone and Metabolic Research, 38*(11), 752-757.

Ramsay, J.A., Blimkie, C.J., Smith, K., Garner, S., MacDougall, J.D., & Sale, D.G. (1990). Strength training effects in prepubescent boys. *Medicine and Science in Sports and Exercise, 22*(5), 605-614.

Ratel, S., Duche, P., Hennegrave, A., Van Praagh, E., & Bedu, M. (2002). Acid-base balance during repeated cycling sprints in boys and men. *Journal of Applied Physiology, 92*(2), 479-485.

Ratel, S., & Williams, C.A. (2008). Children's musculoskeletal system: new research perspectives. In N.P. Beaulieu (Ed.), *Physical activity and children: New research.* Hauppauge, NY: Nova Science.

Ratel, S., Williams, C.A., Oliver, J., & Armstrong, N. (2004). Effects of age and mode of exercise on power output profiles during repeated sprints. *European Journal of Applied Physiology, 92*(1-2), 204-210.

Roemmich, J.N., & Sinning, W.E. (1997a). Weight loss and wrestling training: Effects on growth-related hormones. *Journal of Applied Physiology, 82*(6), 1760-1764.

Roemmich, J.N., & Sinning, W.E. (1997b). Weight loss and wrestling training: Effects on nutrition, growth, maturation, body composition, and strength. *Journal of Applied Physiology, 82*(6), 1751-1759.

Round, J.M., Jones, D.A., Honour, J.W., & Nevill, A.M. (1999). Hormonal factors in the development of differences in strength between boys and girls during adolescence: A longitudinal study. *Annals of Human Biology, 26*(1), 49-62.

Rowland, T. W. (1989). Welcome to Pediatric Exercise Science! *Pediatric Exercise Science, 1*(1), 1.

Rowland, T. (1996). *Developmental exercise physiology*. Champaign, IL: Human Kinetics.

Rowland, T.W. (2005). *Children's exercise physiology*. Champaign; IL: Human Kinetics.

Rowland, T. (2008). Cardiovascular function. In N. Armstrong & W. van Mechelen (Eds.), *Paediatric exercise science and medicine* (pp. 255-267). Oxford, UK: Oxford University Press.

Rowland, T.W., & Boyajian, A. (1995). Aerobic response to endurance exercise training in children. *Pediatrics, 96*(4 Pt 1), 654-658.

Rowland, T.W., Maresh, C.M., Charkoudian, N., Vanderburgh, P.M., Castellani, J.W., & Armstrong, L.E. (1996). Plasma norepinephrine responses to cycle exercise in boys and men. *International Journal of Sports Medicine, 17*(1), 22-26.

Rowland, T., & Saltin, B. (2008). Learning from children: The emergence of pediatric exercise science. *Journal of Applied Physiology, 105*(1), 322-324.

Rowland, T., Unnithan, V., Fernhall, B., Baynard, T., & Lange, C. (2002). Left ventricular response to dynamic exercise in young cyclists. *Medicine and Science in Sports and Exercise, 34*(4), 637-642.

Rumpf, M.C., Cronin, J.B., Pinder, S.D., Oliver, J., & Hughes, M. (2012). Effect of different training methods on running sprint times in male youth. *Pediatric Exercise Science, 24*(2), 170-186.

Scammon, R.E., "The Measurement of the Body in Childhood," in *The Measurement of Man*, edited by J.A. Harris et al. (Minneapolis: University of Minnesota Press, 1930), 193.

Society of Health and Physical Educators–SHAPE America. (2011). *Physical Education for Lifelong Fitness*. Champaign, IL: Human Kinetics.

Stephens, B.R., Cole, A.S., & Mahon, A.D. (2006). The influence of biological maturation on fat and carbohydrate metabolism during exercise in males. *International Journal of Sport Nutrition and Exercise Metabolism, 16*(2), 166-179.

Stratton, G., & Oliver, J.L. (2014). The impact of growth and maturation on physical performance. In R.L. Lloyd & J.L. Oliver (Eds.), *Strength and cnditioning for young athletes: science and application* (pp. 3-18). Abingdon, UK: Routledge.

Taylor, D.J., Kemp, G.J., Thompson, C.H., & Radda, G.K. (1997). Ageing: Effects on oxidative function of skeletal muscle in vivo. *Molecular and Cellular Biochemistry, 174*(1-2), 321-324.

Timmons, B.W., Bar-Or, O., & Riddell, M.C. (2003). Oxidation rate of exogenous carbohydrate during exercise is higher in boys than in men. *Journal of Applied Physiology, 94*(1), 278-284.

Tsolakis, C., Messinis, D., Stergioulas, A., & Dessypris, A. (2000). Hormonal responses after strength training and detraining in prepubertal and pubertal boys. *Journal of Strength and Conditioning Research, 14*(4), 399-404.

Tsolakis, C., Xekouki, P., Kaloupsis, S., Karas, D., Messinis, D., Vagenas, G., & Dessypris, A. (2003). The influence of exercise on growth hormone and testosterone in prepubertal and early-pubertal boys. *Hormones (Athens), 2*(2), 103-112.

Turner, C.H. (1998). Three rules for bone adaptation to mechanical stimuli. *Bone, 23*(5), 399-407.

Valdimarsson, O., Linden, C., Johnell, O., Gardsell, P., & Karlsson, M.K. (2006). Daily physical education in the school curriculum in prepubertal girls during 1 year is followed by an increase in bone mineral accrual and bone width—Data from the prospective controlled Malmo pediatric osteoporosis prevention study. *Calcified Tissue International, 78*(2), 65-71.

Vingren, J.L., Kraemer, W.J., Ratamess, N.A., Anderson, J.M., Volek, J.S., & Maresh, C.M. (2010). Testosterone physiology in resistance exercise and training: The up-stream regulatory elements. *Sports Medicine, 40*(12), 1037-1053.

Viru, A., Laaneots, L., Karelson, K., Smirnova, T., & Viru, M. (1998). Exercise-induced hormone responses in girls at different stages of sexual maturation. *European Journal of Applied Physiology and Occupational Physiology, 77*(5), 401-408.

Waugh, C.M., Blazevich, A.J., Fath, F., & Korff, T. (2012). Age-related changes in mechanical properties of the Achilles tendon. *Journal of Anatomy, 220*(2), 144-155.

Waugh, C.M., Korff, T., Fath, F., & Blazevich, A.J. (2013). Rapid force production in children and adults: Mechanical and neural contributions. *Medicine and Science in Sports and Exercise, 45*(4), 762-771.

Waugh, C.M., Korff, T., Fath, F., & Blazevich, A.J. (2014). Effects of resistance training on tendon mechanical properties and rapid force production in prepubertal children. *Journal of Applied Physiology, 117*(3), 257-266.

Weaver, C.M., Gordon, C.M., Janz, K.F., Kalkwarf, H.J., Lappe, J.M., Lewis, R., . . . Zemel, B.S. (2016). The National Osteoporosis Foundation's position statement on peak bone mass development and lifestyle factors: A systematic review and implementation recommendations. *Osteoporosis International, 27*(4), 1281-1386.

Weeks, B.K., Young, C.M., & Beck, B.R. (2008). Eight months of regular in-school jumping improves indices of bone strength in adolescent boys and girls: The POWER PE study. *Journal of Bone and Mineral Research, 23*(7), 1002-1011.

Weise, M., Eisenhofer, G., & Merke, D.P. (2002). Pubertal and gender-related changes in the sympathoadrenal system in healthy children. *Journal of Clinical Endocrinology and Metabolism, 87*(11), 5038-5043.

Welsman, J.R., Fawkner, S.G., & Armstrong, N. (2001). Ventilatory response and arterial blood gases during exercise in children. *Pediatric Exercise Science, 13*, 263-264.

Williams, C.A., Cobb, M., Rowland, T., & Winter, E. (2011). The BASES expert statement on the ethics and participation in research of young people. *The Sport and Exercise Scientist, 29*, 12-13.

Witzke, K.A., & Snow, C.M. (2000). Effects of plyometric jump training on bone mass in adolescent girls. *Medicine and Science in Sports and Exercise, 32*(6), 1051-1057.

Yan, X., Zhu, M.J., Dodson, M.V., & Du, M. (2013). Developmental programming of fetal skeletal muscle and adipose tissue development. *Journal of Genomics, 1*, 29-38.

Yu, C.C., Sung, R.Y., So, R.C., Lui, K.C., Lau, W., Lam, P.K., & Lau, E.M. (2005). Effects of strength training on body composition and bone mineral content in children who are obese. *Journal of Strength and Conditioning Research, 19*(3), 667-672.

Zanconato, S., Buchthal, S., Barstow, T.J., & Cooper, D.M. (1993). 31P-magnetic resonance spectroscopy of leg muscle metabolism during exercise in children and adults. *Journal of Applied Physiology, 74*(5), 2214-2218.

Zinman, R., & Gaultier, C. (1986). Maximal static pressures and lung volumes in young female swimmers. *Respiration Physiology, 64*(2), 229-239.

Chapter 3 Growth, Maturation, and Physical Fitness

Armstrong, N., & Welsman, J.R. (1994). Assessment and interpretation of aerobic fitness in children and adolescents. *Exercise and Sport Sciences Reviews, 22,* 435-476.

Baker, J., Janning, C., Wong, H., Cobley, S., & Schorer, J. (2014). Variations in relative age effects in individual sports: Skiing, figure skating and gymnastics. *European Journal of Sport Science, 14*(Suppl 1), S183-S190.

Barker, A.R., Welsman, J.R., Fulford, J., Welford, D., & Armstrong, N. (2008). Muscle phosphocreatine kinetics in children and adults at the onset and offset of moderate-intensity exercise. *Journal of Applied Physiology, 105*(2), 446-456.

Beunen, G., Ostyn, M., Simons, J., Renson, R., Claessens, A.L., Vanden Eynde, B., . . . van't Hof, M.A. (1997). Development and tracking in fitness components: Leuven longitudinal study on lifestyle, fitness and health. *International Journal of Sports Medicine, 18*(Suppl 3), S171-S178.

Bielicki, T., Koniarek, J., & Malina, R.M. (1984). Interrelationships among certain measures of growth and maturation rate in boys during adolescence. *Annals of Human Biology, 11*(3), 201-210.

Blimkie, J.R., & Sale, D.G. (1998). Strength development and trainability during childhood. In E. Van Praagh (Ed.), *Pediatric anaerobic performance* (pp. 193-224). Champaign, IL: Human Kinetics.

Bond, L., Clements, J., Bertalli, N., Evans-Whipp, T., McMorris, B.J., Patton, G.C., . . . Catalano, R.F. (2006). A comparison of self-reported puberty using the Pubertal Development Scale and the Sexual Maturation Scale in a school-based epidemiologic survey. *Journal of Adolescence, 29*(5), 709-720.

Boucher, J.L., & Mutimer, B.T. (1994). The relative age phenomenon in sport: a replication and extension with ice-hockey players. *Research Quarterly for Exercise and Sport, 65*(4), 377-381.

Caine, D., Purcell, L., & Maffulli, N. (2014). The child and adolescent athlete: A review of three potentially serious injuries. *BMC Sports Science, Medicine & Rehabilitation, 6,* 22.

Cameron, N., Griffiths, P.L., Wright, M.M., Blencowe, C., Davis, N.C., Pettifor, J.M., & Norris, S.A. (2004). Regression equations to estimate percentage body fat in African prepubertal children aged 9 y. *American Journal of Clinical Nutrition, 80*(1), 70-75.

Carskadon, M.A., & Acebo, C. (1993). A self-administered rating scale for pubertal development. *Journal of Adolescent Health, 14*(3), 190-195.

Catley, M.J., & Tomkinson, G.R. (2013). Normative health-related fitness values for children: Analysis of 85347 test results on 9-17-year-old Australians since 1985. *British Journal of Sports Medicine, 47*(2), 98-108.

Christiansen, K. (2001). Behavioural effects of androgen in men and women. *Journal of Endocrinology, 170*(1), 39-48.

Cole, T.J., Rousham, E.K., Hawley, N.L., Cameron, N., Norris, S.A., & Pettifor, J.M. (2015). Ethnic and sex differences in skeletal maturation among the Birth to Twenty cohort in South Africa. *Archives of Disease in Childhood, 100*(2), 138-143.

Cole, T.J., & Wright, C.M. (2011). A chart to predict adult height from a child's current height. *Annals of Human Biology, 38*(6), 662-668.

Cornier, M.A., Despres, J.P., Davis, N., Grossniklaus, D.A., Klein, S., Lamarche, B., . . . Stroke, C. (2011). Assessing adiposity: A scientific statement from the American Heart Association. *Circulation, 124*(18), 1996-2019.

Cumming, S.P., Lloyd, R.S., Oliver, J.L., Eisenmann, J.C., & Malina, R.M. (2017). Bio-banding in sport: Applications to competition, talent identification, and strength and conditioning of youth athletes. *Strength and Conditioning Journal, 39*(2), 34-47.

Del Campo, D.G.D., J.C.P., V., Villora, S.G., & Jordan, O.R.C. (2010). The relative age effect in youth soccer players from Spain. *Journal of Sports Science and Medicine, 9,* 190-198.

Deprez, D., Coutts, A.J., Fransen, J., Deconinck, F., Lenoir, M., Vaeyens, R., & Philippaerts, R. (2013). Relative age, biological maturation and anaerobic characteristics in elite youth soccer players. *International Journal of Sports Medicine, 34*(10), 897-903.

Duke, P.M., Litt, I.F., & Gross, R.T. (1980). Adolescents' self-assessment of sexual maturation. *Pediatrics, 66*(6), 918-920.

Duke, S.A., Balzer, B.W., & Steinbeck, K.S. (2014). Testosterone and its effects on human male adolescent mood and behavior: A systematic review. *Journal of Adolescent Health, 55*(3), 315-322.

Epstein, L.H., Valoski, A.M., Kalarchian, M.A., & McCurley, J. (1995). Do children lose and maintain weight easier than adults: A comparison of child and parent weight changes from six months to ten years. *Obesity Research, 3*(5), 411-417.

Faria, E.R., Franceschini Sdo, C., Peluzio Mdo, C., Sant'Ana, L.F., & Priore, S.E. (2013). Methodological and ethical aspects of the sexual maturation assessment in adolescents. *Revista Paulista de Pediatria, 31*(3), 398-405.

Fisher, A., Reilly, J.J., Kelly, L.A., Montgomery, C., Williamson, A., Paton, J.Y., & Grant, S. (2005). Fundamental movement skills and habitual physical activity in young children. *Medicine and Science in Sports and Exercise, 37*(4), 684-688.

Fransen, J., Bush, S., Woodcock, S., Novak, A., Deprez, D., Baxter-Jones, A.D.G., . . . Lenoir, M. (2018). Improving the prediction of maturity from anthropometric variables using a maturity ratio. *Pediatric Exercise Science, 30*(2), 296-307.

Fransen, J., Deprez, D., Pion, J., Tallir, I.B., D'Hondt, E., Vaeyens, R., . . . Philippaerts, R.M. (2014). Changes in physical fitness and sports participation among children with different levels of motor competence: A 2-year longitudinal study. *Pediatric Exercise Science, 26*(1), 11-21.

Gil, S.M., Badiola, A., Bidaurrazaga-Letona, I., Zabala-Lili, J., Gravina, L., Santos-Concejero, J., . . . Granados, C. (2014). Relationship between the relative age effect and anthropometry, maturity and performance in young soccer players. *Journal of Sports Sciences, 32*(5), 479-486.

Gilsanz, V., & Ratib, O. (2005). *Hand bone age: A digital atlas of skeletal maturity.* Berlin, Germany: Springer-Verlang.

Greulich, W. W., & Pyle, S. I. (1959). *Radiographic atlas of skeletal development of the hand and wrist. 2nd edition.* Stanford, California: Stanford University Press.

Griffiths, L.J., Cortina-Borja, M., Sera, F., Pouliou, T., Geraci, M., Rich, C., . . . Dezateux, C. (2013). How active are our children? Findings from the Millennium Cohort Study. *BMJ Open, 3*(8), e002893.

Hardy, L.L., King, L., Farrell, L., Macniven, R., & Howlett, S. (2010). Fundamental movement skills among Australian preschool children. *Journal of Science and Medicine in Sport, 13*(5), 503-508.

Hergenroeder, A.C., Hill, R.B., Wong, W.W., Sangi-Haghpeykar, H., & Taylor, W. (1999). Validity of self-assessment of pubertal maturation in African American and European American adolescents. *Journal of Adolescent Health, 24*(3), 201-205.

Khamis, H.J., & Roche, A.F. (1994). Predicting adult stature without using skeletal age: The Khamis-Roche method. *Pediatrics, 94*(4 Pt 1), 504-507.

Koo, M.M., & Rohan, T.E. (1997). Accuracy of short-term recall of age at menarche. *Annals of Human Biology, 24*(1), 61-64.

Koziel, S.M., & Malina, R.M. (2018). Modified maturity offset prediction equations: Validation in independent longitudinal samples of boys and girls. *Sports Medicine, 48*(1), 221-236.

Lloyd, R.S., Oliver, J.L., Faigenbaum, A.D., Myer, G.D., & De Ste Croix, M.B. (2014). Chronological age vs. biological maturation: Implications for exercise programming in youth. *Journal of Strength and Conditioning Research, 28*(5), 1454-1464.

Lopes, V.P., Rodrigues, L.P., Maia, J.A., & Malina, R.M. (2011). Motor coordination as predictor of physical activity in childhood. *Scandinavian Journal of Medicine & Science in Sports, 21*(5), 663-669.

Lubans, D.R., Morgan, P.J., Cliff, D.P., Barnett, L.M., & Okely, A.D. (2010). Fundamental movement skills in children and adolescents: Review of associated health benefits. *Sports Medicine, 40*(12), 1019-1035.

Luo, Z.C., Albertsson-Wikland, K., & Karlberg, J. (1998). Target height as predicted by parental heights in a population-based study. *Pediatric Research, 44*(4), 563-571.

Malina, R.M. (2011). Skeletal age and age verification in youth sport. *Sports Medicine, 41*(11), 925-947.

Malina, R.M., Bouchard, C., & Bar-Or, O. (2004). *Growth, maturation and physical activity* Champaign, IL: Human Kinetics.

Malina, R.M., Chamorro, M., Serratosa, L., & Morate, F. (2007). TW3 and Fels skeletal ages in elite youth soccer players. *Annals of Human Biology, 34*(2), 265-272.

Malina, R.M., Coelho, E.S.M.J., Figueiredo, A.J., Carling, C., & Beunen, G.P. (2012). Interrelationships among invasive and non-invasive indicators of biological maturation in adolescent male soccer players. *Journal of Sports Sciences, 30*(15), 1705-1717.

Malina, R.M., Cumming, S.P., Morano, P.J., Barron, M., & Miller, S.J. (2005). Maturity status of youth football players: A noninvasive estimate. *Medicine and Science in Sports and Exercise, 37*(6), 1044-1052.

Malina, R.M., Dompier, T.P., Powell, J.W., Barron, M.J., & Moore, M.T. (2007). Validation of a noninvasive maturity estimate relative to skeletal age in youth football players. *Clinical Journal of Sport Medicine, 17*(5), 362-368.

Malina, R.M., & Koziel, S.M. (2014a). Validation of maturity offset in a longitudinal sample of Polish boys. *Journal of Sports Sciences, 32*(5), 424-437.

Malina, R.M., & Koziel, S.M. (2014b). Validation of maturity offset in a longitudinal sample of Polish girls. *Journal of Sports Sciences, 32*(14), 1374-1382.

Meyers, R.W., Oliver, J.L., Hughes, M.G., Lloyd, R.S., & Cronin, J.B. (2017). Influence of age, maturity, and body size on the spatiotemporal determinants of maximal sprint speed in boys. *Journal of Strength and Conditioning Research, 31*(4), 1009-1016.

Mirwald, R.L., Baxter-Jones, A.D., Bailey, D.A., & Beunen, G.P. (2002). An assessment of maturity from anthropometric measurements. *Medicine and Science in Sports and Exercise, 34*(4), 689-694.

Moore, S.A., McKay, H.A., Macdonald, H., Nettlefold, L., Baxter-Jones, A.D., Cameron, N., & Brasher, P.M. (2015). Enhancing a somatic maturity prediction model. *Medicine and Science in Sports and Exercise, 47*(8), 1755-1764.

Nagahara, R., Takai, Y., Haramura, M., Mizutani, M., Matsuo, A., Kanehisa, H., & Fukunaga, T. (2018). Age-related differences in spatiotemporal variables and ground reaction forces during sprinting in boys. *Pediatric Exercise Science*, 1-10.

Navarro, J.J., Garcia-Rubio, J., & Olivares, P.R. (2015). The relative age effect and its influence on academic performance. *PLoS One, 10*(10), e0141895.

Nevill, A., & Burton, R.F. (2018). Commentary on the article "Improving the prediction of maturity from anthropometric variables using a Maturity ratio." *Pediatric Exercise Science, 30*(2), 308-310.

Okely, A.D., & Booth, M.L. (2004). Mastery of fundamental movement skills among children in New South Wales: Prevalence and sociodemographic distribution. *Journal of Science and Medicine in Sport, 7*(3), 358-372.

Petersen, A.C., Crockett, L., Richards, M., & Boxer, A. (1988). A self-report measure of pubertal status: Reliability, validity and initial norms. *Journal of Youth and Adolescence, 17*, 117-133.

Philippaerts, R.M., Vaeyens, R., Janssens, M., Van Renterghem, B., Matthys, D., Craen, R., . . . Malina, R.M. (2006). The relationship between peak height velocity and physical performance in youth soccer players. *Journal of Sports Sciences, 24*(3), 221-230.

Quatman-Yates, C.C., Quatman, C.E., Meszaros, A.J., Paterno, M.V., & Hewett, T.E. (2012). A systematic review of sensorimotor function during adolescence: A developmental stage of increased motor awkwardness? *British Journal of Sports Medicine, 46*(9), 649-655.

Rasmussen, A.R., Wohlfahrt-Veje, C., Tefre de Renzy-Martin, K., Hagen, C.P., Tinggaard, J., Mouritsen, A., . . . Main, K.M. (2015). Validity of self-assessment of pubertal maturation. *Pediatrics, 135*(1), 86-93.

Roberts, S.J., Boddy, L.M., Fairclough, S.J., & Stratton, G. (2012). The influence of relative age effects on the cardiorespiratory fitness levels of children age 9 to 10 and 11 to 12 years of age. *Pediatric Exercise Science, 24*(1), 72-83.

Robertson, E.B., Skinner, M.L., Love, M.M., Elder, G.H., Conger, R.D., Dubas, J.S., & Petersen, A.C. (1992). The pubertal development scale: A rural and suburban comparison. *Journal of Early Adolescence, 12*(2), 174-186.

Robinson, L.E., Stodden, D.F., Barnett, L.M., Lopes, V.P., Logan, S.W., Rodrigues, L.P., & D'Hondt, E. (2015). Motor competence and its effect on positive developmental trajectories of health. *Sports Medicine, 45*(9), 1273-1284.

Roche, A.F., Chumlea, W.C., & Thissen, D. (1988). *Assessing the skeletal maturity of the hand-wrist: Fels method.* Springfield, IL: Charles C Thomas.

Roche, A.F., Wellens, R., Attie, K.M., & Siervogel, R.M. (1995). The timing of sexual maturation in a group of US white youths. *Journal of Pediatric Endocrinology & Metabolism, 8*(1), 11-18.

Rodriguez, G., Moreno, L.A., Blay, M.G., Blay, V.A., Fleta, J., Sarria, A., . . . Group, A.V.-Z.S. (2005). Body fat measurement in adolescents: Comparison of skinfold thickness equations with dual-energy X-ray absorptiometry. *European Journal of Clinical Nutrition, 59*(10), 1158-1166.

Romann, M., & Cobley, S. (2015). Relative age effects in athletic sprinting and corrective adjustments as a solution for their removal. *PLoS One, 10*(4), e0122988.

Rowland, T.W. (2005). *Children's exercise physiology*. Champaign; IL: Human Kinetics.

Roy, M.A., Bernard, D., Roy, B., & Marcotte, G. (1989). Body checking in Pee Wee hockey. *The Physician and Sportsmedicine, 17*, 119-126.

Schlossberger, N.M., Turner, R.A., & Irwin, C.E., Jr. (1992). Validity of self-report of pubertal maturation in early adolescents. *Journal of Adolescent Health, 13*(2), 109-113.

Sherar, L.B., Baxter-Jones, A.D., Faulkner, R.A., & Russell, K.W. (2007). Do physical maturity and birth date predict talent in male youth ice hockey players? *Journal of Sports Sciences, 25*(8), 879-886.

Sherar, L.B., Mirwald, R.L., Baxter-Jones, A.D., & Thomis, M. (2005). Prediction of adult height using maturity-based cumulative height velocity curves. *Journal of Pediatrics, 147*(4), 508-514.

Slaughter, M.H., Lohman, T.G., Boileau, R.A., Horswill, C.A., Stillman, R.J., Van Loan, M.D., & Bemben, D.A. (1988). Skinfold equations for estimation of body fatness in children and youth. *Human Biology, 60*(5), 709-723.

Society of Health and Physical Educators–SHAPE America. (2014). *National standards & grade-level outcomes for K-12 physical education*. Champaign, IL: Human Kinetics.

Stratton, G., McWhannell, N., Foweather, L., Henagen, J., Graves, L., Ridgers, N.D., & Hepples, J. (2009). *The A-CLASS project research findings: Executive summary*. Liverpool, UK: Sportslinx.

Stratton, G., & Oliver, J.L. (2014). The impact of growth and maturation on physical performance. In R.S. Lloyd & J.L. Oliver (Eds.), *Strength and conditioning for young athletes: Science and application* (pp. 3-18). Abingdon, UK: Routledge.

Sun, S.S., Schubert, C.M., Chumlea, W.C., Roche, A.F., Kulin, H.E., Lee, P.A., . . . Ryan, A.S. (2002). National estimates of the timing of sexual maturation and racial differences among US children. *Pediatrics, 110*(5), 911-919.

Tanner, J.M. (1962). *Growth at adolescence*. Oxford: Blackwell.

Tanner, J.M. (1990). *Foetus into man: Physical growth from conception to maturity*. Cambridge, MA: Harvard University Press.

Tanner, J.M., Goldstein, H., & Whitehouse, R.H. (1970). Standards for children's height at age 2 to 9 years allowing for height of parents. *Archives of Disease in Childhood, 45*(244), 819.

Tanner, J.M., Healy, M.J.R., Goldstein, H., & Cameron, N. (2001). *Assessment of skeletal maturity and prediction of adult height (TW3 Method)*. London, UK: Saunders.

Tanner, J.M., Whitehouse, R.H., Cameron, N., Marshall, W.A., Healy, M.J.R., & Goldstein, H. (1975). *Assessment of skeletal maturity and prediction of adult height (TW2 method)*. New York, NY: Academic Press.

Tanner, J.M., Whitehouse, R.H., & Healy, M.J.R. (1962). *A new system for estimating maturity from the hand and wrist, with standards derived from a study of 2,600 healthy British children*. Paris, France: International Children's Centre.

Tonson, A., Ratel, S., Le Fur, Y., Cozzone, P., & Bendahan, D. (2008). Effect of maturation on the relationship between muscle size and force production. *Medicine and Science in Sports and Exercise, 40*(5), 918-925.

Viru, A., Loko, J., Harrow, M., Volver, A., Laaneots, L., & M, V. (1999). Critical periods in the development of performance capacity during childhood and adolescence. *Europeam Journal of Physical Education, 4*, 75-119.

Whithall, J. (2003). Development of locomotor co-ordination and control in children. In G.J.P. Savelsberg, K. Davids, & J. Van Der Kamp (Eds.), *Development of movement co-ordination in children* (pp. 251-270). London, UK: Routledge.

World Heath Organization. (2015). Adolescent health. Retrieved May 2015 from www.who.int/topics/adolescent_health/en

Zhang, A., Sayre, J.W., Vachon, L., Liu, B.J., & Huang, H.K. (2009). Racial differences in growth patterns of children assessed on the basis of bone age. *Radiology, 250*(1), 228-235.

Chapter 4 Long-Term Athletic Development

American Academy of Pediatrics (1983). Weight training and weight lifting: Information for the pediatrician. *The Physician and Sportsmedicine, 11*(3), 157-161.

Bailey, R. (2006). Physical education and sport in schools: A review of benefits and outcomes. *Journal of School Health, 76*(8), 397-401. doi:10.1111/j.1746-1561.2006.00132.x

Bailey, R., & Morley, D. (2006). Towards a model of talent development in physical education. *Sport, Education and Society, 11*(3), 211-230.

Balyi, I., & Hamilton, A. (2004). *Long-term athlete development: Trainability in childhood and adolescence. Windows of Opportunity. Optimal trainability*. Victoria, British Columbia, Canada: National Coaching Institute & Advanced Training and Performance.

Barnes, J.D., Colley, R.C., Borghese, M., Janson, K., Fink, A., & Tremblay, M.S. (2013). Results from the active healthy kids Canada 2012 report card on physical activity for children and youth. *Paediatrics & Child Health, 18*(6), 301-304.

Barynina, I.I. & Vaitsekhovskii, S.M. (1992). The aftermath of early sports specialization for highly qualified swimmers. *Fitness and Sports Review International, 27*(4), 132–133.

Behringer, M., Vom Heede, A., Matthews, M., & Mester, J. (2011). Effects of strength training on motor performance skills in children and adolescents: A meta-analysis. *Pediatric Exercise Science, 23*(2), 186-206.

Bergeron, M.F., Mountjoy, M., Armstrong, N., Chia, M., Cote, J., Emery, C.A., . . . Engebretsen, L. (2015). International Olympic Committee consensus statement on youth athletic development. *British Journal of Sports Medicine, 49*(13), 843-851. doi:10.1136/bjsports-2015-094962

Berry, J., Abernethy, B., & Cote, J. (2008). The contribution of structured activity and deliberate play to the development of expert perceptual and decision-making skill. *Journal of Sport & Exercise Psychology, 30*(6), 685-708.

Bloemers, F., Collard, D., Paw, M.C., Van Mechelen, W., Twisk, J., & Verhagen, E. (2012). Physical inactivity is a risk factor for physical activity-related injuries in children. *British Journal of Sports Medicine, 46*(9), 669-674. doi:10.1136/bjsports-2011-090546

Bompa, T.O. (2000). *Total training for young champions*. Champaign, IL: Human Kinetics.

Brenner, J.S., & Council on Sports Medicine & Fitness. (2016). Sports specialization and intensive training in young athletes. *Pediatrics, 138*(3). doi:10.1542/peds.2016-2148.

Capranica, L., & Millard-Stafford, M.L. (2011). Youth sport specialization: How to manage competition and training? *International Journal of Sports Physiology and Performance, 6*(4), 572-579.

Cattuzzo, M.T., Dos Santos Henrique, R., Re, A.H., de Oliveira, I.S., Melo, B.M., de Sousa Moura, M., . . . Stodden, D. (2016). Motor competence and health related physical fitness in youth: A systematic review. *Journal of Science and Medicine in Sport, 19*(2), 123-129. doi:10.1016/j.jsams.2014.12.004

Chaouachi, A., Hammami, R., Kaabi, S., Chamari, K., Drinkwater, E.J., & Behm, D.G. (2014). Olympic weightlifting and plyometric training with children provides similar or greater performance improvements than traditional resistance training. *Journal of Strength and Conditioning Research, 28*(6), 1483-1496. doi:10.1519/JSC.0000000000000305

Cohen, D.D., Voss, C., Taylor, M.J., Delextrat, A., Ogunleye, A.A., & Sandercock, G.R. (2011). Ten-year secular changes in muscular fitness in English children. *Acta Paediatrica, 100*(10), e175-177. doi:10.1111/j.1651-2227.2011.02318.x

Côté, J., Baker, J., & Abernethy, B. (2007). Practice to play in the development of sport expertise. In R. Eklund & G. Tenenbaum (Eds.), *Handbook of sport psychology* (pp. 184-202). Hoboken, NJ: Wiley.

Côté, J., Lidor, R., & Hackfort, D. (2009). ISSP position stand: to sample or to specialize? Seven postulates about youth sport activities that lead to continued participation and elite performance. *International Journal of Sport and Exercise Psychology, 9*, 7-17.

D'Hondt, E., Deforche, B., Gentier, I., De Bourdeaudhuij, I., Vaeyens, R., Philippaerts, R., & Lenoir, M. (2013). A longitudinal analysis of gross motor coordination in overweight and obese children versus normal-weight peers. *International Journal of Obesity, 37*(1), 61-67. doi:10.1038/ijo.2012.55

D'Hondt, E., Deforche, B., Gentier, I., Verstuyf, J., Vaeyens, R., De Bourdeaudhuij, I., . . . Lenoir, M. (2014). A longitudinal study of gross motor coordination and weight status in children. *Obesity (Silver Spring), 22*(6), 1505-1511. doi:10.1002/oby.20723

De Ste Croix, M.B., Priestley, A.M., Lloyd, R.S., & Oliver, J.L. (2014). ACL injury risk in elite female youth soccer: Changes in neuromuscular control of the knee following soccer-specific fatigue. *Scandinavian Journal of Medicine & Science in Sports, 25*, e531-538. doi:10.1111/sms.12355

Deli, E., Bakle, I., & Zachopoulou, E. (2006). Implementing intervention movement programs for kindergarten children. *Journal of Early Childhood Research, 4*, 5-18.

DiFiori, J.P., Benjamin, H.J., Brenner, J., Gregory, A., Jayanthi, N., Landry, G.L., & Luke, A. (2014). Overuse injuries and burnout in youth sports: A position statement from the American Medical Society for Sports Medicine. *Clin J Sport Med, 24*(1), 3-20. doi:10.1097/JSM.0000000000000060

Edwards, L.C., Bryant, A.S., Keegan, R.J., Morgan, K., Cooper, S.M., & Jones, A.M. (2018). "Measuring" physical literacy and related constructs: A systematic review of empirical findings. *Sports Medicine, 48*(3), 659-682. doi:10.1007/s40279-017-0817-9

Edwards, L.C., Bryant, A.S., Keegan, R.J., Morgan, K., & Jones, A.M. (2017). Definitions, foundations and associations of physical literacy: A systematic review. *Sports Medicine, 47*(1), 113-126. doi:10.1007/s40279-016-0560-7

Ericsson, K.A. (2013). Training history, deliberate practice and elite sports performance: An analysis in response to Tucker and Collins review—What makes champions? *British Journal of Sports Medicine, 47*(9), 533-535. doi:10.1136/bjsports-2012-091767

Ericsson, K.A., Krampe, R.T., & Tesch-Römer, C. (1993). The role of deliberate practice in the acquisition of expert performance. *Psychological Review, 100*(3), 363-406.

Faigenbaum, A.D., Lloyd, R.S., MacDonald, J., & Myer, G.D. (2016). Citius, Altius, Fortius: Beneficial effects of resistance training for young athletes: Narrative review. *British Journal of Sports Medicine, 50*, 3-7. doi:10.1136/bjsports-2015-094621

Fathi, A., Hammami, R., Moran, J., Borji, R., Sahli, S., & Rebai, H. (2018). Effect of a 16 week combined strength and plyometric training program followed by a detraining period on athletic performance in pubertal Volleyball players. *Journal of Strength and Conditioning Research.* doi:10.1519/JSC.0000000000002461

Feeley, B.T., Agel, J., & LaPrade, R.F. (2016). When is it too early for single sport specialization? *American Journal of Sports Medicine, 44*(1), 234-241. doi:10.1177/0363546515576899

Fleisig, G.S., Andrews, J.R., Cutter, G.R., Weber, A., Loftice, J., McMichael, C., . . . Lyman, S. (2011). Risk of serious injury for young baseball pitchers: A 10-year prospective study. *American Journal of Sports Medicine, 39*(2), 253-257. doi:10.1177/0363546510384224

Ford, P., De Ste Croix, M., Lloyd, R., Meyers, R., Moosavi, M., Oliver, J., . . . Williams, C. (2011). The long-term athlete development model: physiological evidence and application. *Journal of Sports Sciences, 29*(4), 389-402. doi:10.1080/02640414.2010.536849

Fransen, J., Deprez, D., Pion, J., Tallir, I.B., D'Hondt, E., Vaeyens, R., . . . Philippaerts, R.M. (2014). Changes in physical fitness and sports participation among children with different levels of motor competence: A 2-year longitudinal study. *Pediatric Exercise Science, 26*(1), 11-21. doi:10.1123/pes.2013-0005

Fransen, J., Pion, J., Vandendriessche, J., Vandorpe, B., Vaeyens, R., Lenoir, M., & Philippaerts, R.M. (2012). Differences in physical fitness and gross motor coordination in boys aged 6-12 years specializing in one versus sampling more than one sport. *Journal of Sports Sciences, 30*(4), 379-386. doi:10.1080/026 40414.2011.642808

Gabbett, T.J. (2016). The training-injury prevention paradox: should athletes be training smarter and harder? *British Journal of Sports Medicine, 50*(5), 273-280. doi:10.1136/bjsports-2015-095788

Gagné, F. (1993). Constructs and models pertaining to exceptional human abilities. In K.A. Heller, Monks, F.J., Passow, A.H. (Ed.), *International Handbook of Research and Development of Giftedness and Talent.* Oxford, United Kingdom: Pergamon Press.

Gould, D., Udry, E., Tuffey, S., & Loehr, J. (1996). Burnout in competitive junior tennis players: pt. 1. A quantitative psychological assessment. *Sport Psychologist, 10*(4), 322-340.

Hall, R., Barber Foss, K., Hewett, T.E., & Myer, G.D. (2015). Sport specialization's association with an increased risk of developing anterior knee pain in adolescent female athletes. *Journal of Sport Rehabilitation, 24*(1), 31-35. doi:10.1123/jsr.2013-0101

Hardy, L.L., Reinten-Reynolds, T., Espinel, P., Zask, A., & Okely, A.D. (2012). Prevalence and correlates of low fundamental movement skill competency in children. *Pediatrics, 130*(2), e390-398. doi:10.1542/peds.2012-0345

Holt, N. (2011). Sport and positive youth development. In I. Stafford (Ed.), *Coaching children in sport* (pp. 256-266). Oxon, UK: Routledge.

Hulteen, R.M., Morgan, P.J., Barnett, L.M., Stodden, D.F., & Lubans, D.R. (2018). Development of foundational movement skills: A conceptual model for physical activity across the lifespan. *Sports Medicine, 48*(7), 1533-1540. doi:10.1007/s40279-018-0892-6

Iyer, R.S., Thapa, M.M., Khanna, P.C., & Chew, F.S. (2012). Pediatric bone imaging: Imaging elbow trauma in children—A review of acute and chronic injuries. *American Journal of Roentgenology, 198*(5), 1053-1068. doi:10.2214/AJR.10.7314

Kalman, M., Inchley, J., Sigmundova, D., Iannotti, R.J., Tynjala, J.A., Hamrik, Z., . . . Bucksch, J. (2015). Secular trends in moderate-to-vigorous physical activity in 32 countries from 2002 to 2010: A cross-national perspective. *European Journal of Public Health, 25*(Suppl 2), 37-40. doi:10.1093/eurpub/ckv024

Katch, V.L. (1983). Physical conditioning of children. *Journal of Adolescent Health Care, 3*(4), 241-246.

LaPrade, R.F., Agel, J., Baker, J., Brenner, J.S., Cordasco, F.A., Cote, J., . . . Provencher, M.T. (2016). AOSSM early sport specialization consensus statement. *Orthopaedic Journal of Sports Medicine, 4*(4), 2325967116644241. doi:10.1177/2325967116644241

Law, M., Côté, J., & Ericsson, K.A. (2007). Characteristics of expert development in rhythmic gymnastics: a retrospective study. *International Journal of Sport and Exercise Psychology 5*(1), 82-103.

Lloyd, R.S., Cronin, J.B., Faigenbaum, A.D., Haff, G.G., Howard, R., Kraemer, W.J., . . . Oliver, J.L. (2016). National Strength and Conditioning Association position statement on long-term athletic development. *Journal of Strength and Conditioning Research, 30*(6), 1491-1509. doi:10.1519/JSC.0000000000001387

Lloyd, R.S., Faigenbaum, A.D., Stone, M.H., Oliver, J.L., Jeffreys, I., Moody, J.A., . . . Myer, G.D. (2014). Position statement on youth resistance training: The 2014 International Consensus. *British Journal of Sports Medicine, 48*(7), 498-505. doi:10.1136/bjsports-2013-092952

Lloyd, R.S., & Oliver, J.L. (2012). The youth physical development model: A new approach to long-term athletic development. *Strength and Conditioning Journal, 34*(3), 61-72.

Lloyd, R.S., Oliver, J.L., Faigenbaum, A.D., Howard, R., De Ste Croix, M.B., Williams, C.A., . . . Myer, G.D. (2015a). Long-term athletic development, part 1: A pathway for all youth. *Journal of Strength and Conditioning Research, 29*(5), 1439-1450. doi:10.1519/JSC.0000000000000756

Lloyd, R.S., Oliver, J.L., Faigenbaum, A.D., Howard, R., De Ste Croix, M.B., Williams, C.A., . . . Myer, G.D. (2015b). Long-term athletic development, part 2: Barriers to success and potential solutions. *Journal of Strength and Conditioning Research, 29*(5), 1451-1464. doi:10.1519/01.JSC.0000465424.75389.56

Lloyd, R.S., Oliver, J.L., Faigenbaum, A.D., Myer, G.D., & De Ste Croix, M.B. (2014). Chronological age vs. biological maturation: Implications for exercise programming in youth. *Journal of Strength and Conditioning Research, 28*(5), 1454-1464. doi:10.1519/JSC.0000000000000391

Lloyd, R.S., Radnor, J.M., De Ste Croix, M.B., Cronin, J.B., & Oliver, J.L. (2016). Changes in sprint and jump performances after traditional, plyometric, and combined resistance training in male youth pre- and post-peak height velocity. *Journal of Strength and Conditioning Research, 30*(5), 1239-1247. doi:10.1519/JSC.0000000000001216

Lopes, V.P., Stodden, D.F., Bianchi, M.M., Maia, J.A., & Rodrigues, L.P. (2012). Correlation between BMI and motor coordination in children. *Journal of Science and Medicine in Sport, 15*(1), 38-43. doi:10.1016/j.jsams.2011.07.005

Lubans, D.R., Morgan, P.J., Cliff, D.P., Barnett, L.M., & Okely, A.D. (2010). Fundamental movement skills in children and adolescents: Review of associated health benefits. *Sports Medicine, 40*(12), 1019-1035. doi:10.2165/11536850-000000000-00000

McNarry, M., Barker, A.R., Lloyd, R.S., Buchheit, M., Williams, C.A., & Oliver, J.L. (2014). The BASES expert statement on trainability during childhood and adolescence. *The Sport Exercise Scientist, 41*, 22-23.

Meylan, C.M., Cronin, J.B., Oliver, J.L., Hopkins, W.G., & Contreras, B. (2014). The effect of maturation on adaptations to strength training and detraining in 11-15-year-olds. *Scandinavian Journal of Medicine & Science in Sports, 24*(3), e156-164. doi:10.1111/sms.12128

Moesch, K., Elbe, A.M., Hauge, M.L., & Wikman, J.M. (2011). Late specialization: The key to success in centimeters, grams, or seconds (CGS) sports. *Scandinavian Journal of Medicine & Science in Sports, 21*(6), e282-290. doi:10.1111/j.1600-0838.2010.01280.x

Moliner-Urdiales, D., Ruiz, J.R., Ortega, F.B., Jimenez-Pavon, D., Vicente-Rodriguez, G., Rey-Lopez, J.P., . . . Groups, H.S. (2010). Secular trends in health-related physical fitness in Spanish adolescents: The AVENA and HELENA studies. *Journal of Science and Medicine in Sport, 13*(6), 584-588. doi:10.1016/j.jsams.2010.03.004

Myer, G.D., Jayanthi, N., Difiori, J.P., Faigenbaum, A.D., Kiefer, A.W., Logerstedt, D., & Micheli, L.J. (2015). Sport specialization, part I: Does early sports specialization Increase negative outcomes and reduce the opportunity for success in young athletes? *Sports Health, 7*(5), 437-442. doi:10.1177/1941738115598747

Myer, G.D., Kushner, A.M., Faigenbaum, A.D., Kiefer, A., Kashikar-Zuck, S., & Clark, J.F. (2013). Training the developing brain, part I: Cognitive developmental considerations for training youth. *Current Sports Medicine Reports, 12*(5), 304-310. doi:10.1097/01.CSMR.0000434106.12813.69

Olsen, S.J., 2nd, Fleisig, G.S., Dun, S., Loftice, J., & Andrews, J.R. (2006). Risk factors for shoulder and elbow injuries in adolescent baseball pitchers. *American Journal of Sports Medicine, 34*(6), 905-912. doi:10.1177/0363546505284188

Radnor, J.M., Lloyd, R.S., & Oliver, J.L. (2017). Individual response to different forms of resistance training in school-aged boys. *Journal of Strength and Conditioning Research, 31*(3), 787-797. doi:10.1519/JSC.0000000000001527

Ratel, S., Duche, P., & Williams, C.A. (2006). Muscle fatigue during high-intensity exercise in children. *Sports Medicine, 36*(12), 1031-1065.

Riordan, J. (1977). *Sport in Soviet society.* Cambridge: Cambridge University Press.

Roberts, W.O. (2007). Can children and adolescents run marathons? *Sports Medicine, 37*(4-5), 299-301.

Robinson, L.E., Stodden, D.F., Barnett, L.M., Lopes, V.P., Logan, S.W., Rodrigues, L.P., & D'Hondt, E. (2015). Motor competence and its effect on positive developmental trajectories of health. *Sports Medicine, 45*(9), 1273-1284. doi:10.1007/s40279-015-0351-6

Rodrigues, L.P., Stodden, D.F., & Lopes, V.P. (2016). Developmental pathways of change in fitness and motor competence are related to overweight and obesity status at the end of primary school. *Journal of Science and Medicine in Sport, 19*(1), 87-92. doi:10.1016/j.jsams.2015.01.002

Rumpf, M.C., Cronin, J.B., Pinder, S.D., Oliver, J., & Hughes, M. (2012). Effect of different training methods on running sprint times in male youth. *Pediatric Exercise Science, 24*(2), 170-186.

Runhaar, J., Collard, D.C., Singh, A.S., Kemper, H.C., van Mechelen, W., & Chinapaw, M. (2010). Motor fitness in Dutch youth: Differences over a 26-year period (1980-2006). *Journal of Science and Medicine in Sport, 13*(3), 323-328. doi:10.1016/j.jsams.2009.04.006

Sands, W.A., & McNeal, J. (2013). Mobility and flexibility development in youths. In R.S. Lloyd & J.L. Oliver (Eds.), *Strength and conditioning for young athletes: Science and application* (pp. 132-146). Oxon, England: Routledge.

Seifert, L., Button, C., & Davids, K. (2013). Key properties of expert movement systems in sport: An ecological dynamics perspective. *Sports Medicine, 43*(3), 167-178. doi:10.1007/s40279-012-0011-z

Society of Health and Physical Educators–SHAPE America. (2016). *Shape of the nation 2016: Status of physical education in the USA.* Reston, VA: Author.

Stamatakis, E., & Chaudhury, M. (2008). Temporal trends in adults' sports participation patterns in England between 1997 and 2006: The Health Survey for England. *British Journal of Sports Medicine, 42*(11), 901-908. doi:10.1136/bjsm.2008.048082

Stein, C.J., & Micheli, L.J. (2010). Overuse injuries in youth sports. *The Physician and Sportsmedicine, 38*(2), 102-108. doi:10.3810/psm.2010.06.1787

Stodden, D., Langendorfer, S., & Roberton, M.A. (2009). The association between motor skill competence and physical fitness in young adults. *Research Quarterly for Exercise and Sport, 80*(2), 223-229. doi:10.1080/02701367.2009.10599556

Stodden, D.F., True, L.K., Langendorfer, S.J., & Gao, Z. (2013). Associations among selected motor skills and health-related fitness: Indirect evidence for Seefeldt's proficiency barrier in young adults? *Research Quarterly for Exercise and Sport, 84*(3), 397-403. doi:10.1080/02701367.2013.814910

Stovitz, S.D., & Johnson, R.J. (2006). "Underuse" as a cause for musculoskeletal injuries: Is it time that we started reframing our message? *British Journal of Sports Medicine, 40*(9), 738-739. doi:10.1136/bjsm.2006.029975

Thompson, W.R. (2016). Worldwide survey of fitness trends for 2016. *ACSM's Health & Fitness Journal, 19*(6), 9-18.

Tinning, R., Kirk, D., Evans, J. (1993). *Learning to teach physical education.* Sydney, Australia: Prentice Hall.

Tomkinson, G.R., Leger, L.A., Olds, T.S., & Cazorla, G. (2003). Secular trends in the performance of children and adolescents (1980-2000): An analysis of 55 studies of the 20m shuttle run test in 11 countries. *Sports Medicine, 33*(4), 285-300.

Vaeyens, R., Lenoir, M., Williams, A.M., & Philippaerts, R.M. (2008). Talent identification and development programmes in sport: Current models and future directions. *Sports Medicine, 38*(9), 703-714.

Wall, M. & Côté, J. (2007). Developmental activities that lead to dropout and investment in sport. *Physical Education and Sport Pedagogy, 12*(1), 77-87.

Whitehead, M. (2001). The concept of physical literacy. *European Journal of Physical Education, 6*(2), 127-138.

World Health Organization. (2010). *Global recommendations on physical activity for health.* Retrieved from www.who.int/diet-physicalactivity/publications/9789241599979/en

Chapter 5 Pedagogy for Youth Fitness Specialists

Ames, C. (1995). Achievement goals, motivational climate, and motivational processes. In G. Roberts (Ed.), *Motivation in sport and exercise* (pp. 161-176). Champaign, IL: Human Kinetics.

Armour, K., & Chambers, F. (2014). "Sport and exercise pedagogy": The case for a new integrative sub-discipline in the field of sport & exercise sciences/kinesiology/human movement sciences. *Sport, Education and Society, 19*(7), 855-868.

Barr-Anderson, D, Neumark-Sztainer, D, Schmitz, K, Ward, D, Conway, T, Pratt, C, Baggett, C, Lytle, L, Pate, R. (2008). But I like PE: factors associated with enjoyment of physical education class in middle school girls. *Research Quarterly for Exercise and Sport, 79*(1): 18-27.

Benjaminse, A., Gokeler, A., Dowling, A., Faigenbaum, A., Ford, K., Hewett, T., . . . Myer, G. (2015). Optimization of the anterior cruciate ligament injury prevention paradigm: Novel feedback techniques to enhance motor learning and reduce injury risk. *Journal of Orthopaedic and Sports Physical Therapy, 45*(3), 170-182.

Boixados, M., Cruz, J., Torregrosa, M., & Valiente, L. (2004). Relationships among motivational climate, satisfaction, perceived ability, and fair play attitudes in young soccer players. *Journal of Applied Sport Psychology, 16*, 301-317.

Bond, B., Weston, K., Williams, C., & Barker, A. (2017). Perspectives on high-intensity interval exercise for health promotion in children and adolescents. *Open Access Journal of Sports Medicine, 8*, 243-265.

Brink, M., Visscher, C., Coutts, A., & Lemmink, K. (2012). Changes in perceived stress and recovery in overreached young elite soccer players. *Scandinavian Journal of Medicine and Science in Sport, 22*(2), 285-292.

Bulger, S., Mohr, D., & Walls, R. (2002). Stack the deck in favor of your students by using the four aces of effective teaching *Journal of Effective Teaching, 5*(2).

Centers for Disease Control and Prevention. (n.d.). Developmental milestones. Retrieved from www.cdc.gov/actearly

Chan, D., Lonsdale, C., & Fung, H. (2012). Influences of coaches, parents, and peers on the motivational patterns of child and adolescent athletes. *Scandinavian Journal of Medicine and Science in Sport, 22*(4), 558-568.

Child Protection in Sport Unit. (2012). *Physical contact and young people in sport.* London, United Kingdom.

Chiviacowsky, S., Wulf, G., & Lewthwaite, R. (2012). Self-controlled learning: the importance of protecting perceptions of competence. *Frontiers in Psychology, 3*(458). doi:10.3389/fpsyg.2012.00458

Collins, D., Macnamara, A., & McCarthy, N. (2016). Putting the bumps in the rocky road: Optimizing the pathway to excellence. *Frontiers in Psychology, 7*(1482), 1-6.

Curran, T., Hill, A., Hall, H., & Jowett, G. (2015). Relationships between the coach-created motivational climate and athlete engagement in youth sport. *Journal of Sport and Exercise Psychology, 37*(2), 193-198.

De Bock, F., Genser, B, Raat, H, Fischer, J, & Renz-Polster, H. (2013). A participatory physical activity intervention in preschools: A cluster randomized controlled trial. *American Journal of Preventative Medicine, 45*(1), 64-74.

Deci, E., Koestner, R., & Ryan, R. (1999). A meta-analytic review of experiments examining the effects of extrinsic rewards on intrinsic motivation. *Psychological Bulletin, 125*(6), 627-668.

Dishman, R., Motl, R., Saunders, R., Felton, G., Ward, D., Dowda, M., & Pate, R. (2005). Enjoyment mediates effects of a school-based physical activity intervention. *Medicine and Science in Sports and Exercise, 37*, 478-487.

Epstein, J. (1989). Family structures and student motivation: A developmental perspective. In C. Ames & R. Ames (Eds.), *Research on motivation in education* (Vol. 3, pp. 259-295). New York, NY: Academic Press.

Faigenbaum, A., Bush, J., McLoone, R., Kreckel, M., Farrell, A., Ratamess, N., & Kang, J. (2015). Benefits of strength and skill based training during primary school physical education. *Journal of Strength and Conditioning Research, 29*(5), 1255-1262.

Faigenbaum, A., & Meadors, L. (2016). A coaches dozen: An update on building healthy, strong and resiliant young athletes. *Strength and Conditioning, 39*(2), 27-33.

Faigenbaum, A., & Rial Rebullido, T. (2018). Understanding physical literacy in youth. *Strength and Conditioning Journal* 40(6): 90-94..

Faude, O., Rössler, R., Petushek, E., Roth, R., Zahner, L., & Donath, L. (2017). Neuromuscular adaptations to multimodal injury prevention programs in youth sports: A systematic review with meta-analysis of randomized controlled trials. *Frontiers in Physiology, 8*, 791.

Fuller, C., Thiele, E., Flores, M., Junge, A., Netto, D., & Dvorak, J. (2015). A successful nationwide implementation of the "FIFA 11 for Health" programme in Brazilian elementary schools. *British Journal of Sports Medicine, 49*(9), 623-629.

Gogtay, N., Giedd, J., Lusk, L., Hayashi, K., Greenstein, D., Vaituzis, A., . . . Thompson, P. (2004). Dynamic mapping of human cortical development during childhood through early adulthood. *Proceedings of the National Academy of Sciences of the United States of America, 101*(21), 8174-8179.

Graham, G. (2008). *Teaching children physical education.* Champaign, IL: Human Kinetics.

Graham, G., Holt/Hale, S., & Parker, M. (2013). *Children moving. A reflective approach to teaching physical education* (9th ed.). New York, NY: McGraw Hill.

Granero-Gallegos, A., Gómez-López, M., Rodríguez-Suárez, N., Abraldes, J., Alesi, M., & Bianco, A. (2017). Importance of the motivational climate in goal, enjoyment, and the causes of success in handball players. *Frontiers in Psychology, 8*, 2081.

Gutiérrez, M., & Ruiz, L. (2009). Perceived motivational climate, sportsmanship, and students' attitudes toward physical education classes and teachers. *Perceptual and Motor Skills, 108*(1), 308-326.

Haff, G. (2014). Periodization strategies for youth development. In R. Lloyd & J. Oliver (Eds.), *Strength and conditioning for young athletes: Science and application* (pp. 149-168). Oxford, UK: Routledge Publishing.

Hagan, J., Shaw, J., & Duncan, P. (Eds.). (2008). *Bright futures: Guidelines for health supervision of infants, children and adolescents* (3rd ed.). Elk Grove Village, IL: American Academy of Pediatrics.

Handford, C., Davids, K., Bennett, S., & Button, C. (1997). Skill acquisition in sport: Some applications of an evolving practice ecology. *Journal of Sports Science, 15*(6), 621-640.

Haywood, K., & Getchell, N. (2014). *Lifespan motor development.* Champaign, IL: Human Kinetics.

Heather, P., Garratt, D., & Taylor, B. (2013). Hands off! The practice and politics of touch in physical education and sports coaching. *Sport, Education and Society, 18*(5), 575-582.

Hodges, N., & Franks, I. (2002). Modelling coaching practice: the role of instruction and demonstration. *Journal of Sport Sciences, 20*(10), 793-811.

Institute of Medicine. (2013). *Educating the student body: Taking physical activity and physical education to school.* Washington, DC: The National Academies Press.

Ismail, F., Fatemi, A., Johnston, M. Cerebral plasticity: Windows of opportunity in the developing brain. *European Journal of Paediatric Neurology, 21*(1): 23-48.

Janelle, C., Champenoy, J., Coombes, S., & Mousseau, M. (2003). Mechanisms of attentional cueing during observational learning to facilitate motor skill acquisition. *Journal of Sports Science, 21*(10), 825-838.

Johnson, S., Blum, R., & Giedd, J. (2009). Adolescent maturity and the brain: The promise and pitfalls of neuroscience research in adolescent health policy. *Journal of Adolescent Health, 45*(3), 216-221.

Jones, M., Dunn, J., Holt, N., Sullivan, P., & Bloom, G. (2011). Exploring the "5Cs" of positive youth development in sport. *Journal of Sport Behavior.* Retrieved from www.highbeam.com/doc/1G1-263992245.html

Jonsson, L., Berg, C., Larsson, C., Korp, P., & Lindgren, E. (2017). Facilitators of physical activity: Voices of adolescents in a disadvantaged community. *International Journal of Environmental Research and Public Health, 14*(8), e839.

Kal, E., van der Kamp, J., & Houdijk, H. (2013). External attentional focus enhances movement automatization: a comprehensive test of the constrained action hypothesis. *Human Movement Science, 32*(4), 527-539.

Karageorghis, C., & Terry, P. (2011). *Inside sport psychology.* Champaign, IL: Human Kinetics.

Kibbe, D., Hackett, J., Hurley, M., McFarland, A., Schubert, K., Schultz, A., & Harris, S. (2011). Ten years of TAKE 10!(®): Integrating physical activity with academic concepts in elementary school classrooms. *Preventive Medicine, 52*(Suppl 1), S43-S50.

Kim, K. (2011). The creativity crisis: the decrease in creative thinking scores on the Torrance Tests of Creative Thinking. *Creativity Research Journal, 23*(4), 285-295.

Kushner, A., Kiefer, A., Lesnick, S., Faigenbaum, A., Kashikar-Zuck, S., & Myer, G. (2015). Training the developing brain, part II: Cognitive considerations for youth instruction and feedback. *Current Sports Medicine Reports, 14*(3), 235-243.

Laguna, P. (2008). Task complexity and sources of task-related information during the observational learning process. *Journal of Sport Sciences, 26*(10), 1097-1113.

Latorre Román, P., Pinillos, F., Pantoja Vallejo, A., & Berrios Aguayo, B. (2017). Creativity and physical fitness in primary school-aged children. *Pediatrics International, 59*(11), 1194-1199.

Lerner, R., Lerner, J., Almerigi, J., Theokas, C., Phelps, E., Gestsdottir, S., . . . von Eye, A. (2005). Positive youth development, participation in community youth development programs, and community contributions of fifth-grade adolescents: Findings from the first wave of the 4-H study of positive youth development *The Journal of Early Adolescence, 25*(1), 17-71.

Lloyd, R., Cronin, J., Faigenbaum, A., Haff, G., Howard, R., Kraemer, W., . . . Oliver, J. (2016). The National Strength and Conditioning Association position statement on long-term athletic development. *Journal of Strength and Conditioning Research, 30*(6), 1491-1509.

Lloyd, R., Faigenbaum, A., Stone, M., Oliver, J., Jeffreys, I., Moody, J., . . . Myer, G. (2014). Position statement on youth resistance training: the 2014 International Consensus. *British Journal of Sports Medicine, 48*(7), 498-505.

Martens, R. (2004). *Successful coaching* (3rd ed.). Champaign, IL: Human Kinetics.

McKenzie, T., & Lounsbery, M. (2013). Physical education teacher effectiveness in a public health context. *Research Quarterly in Exercise and Sport, 84*(4), 419-430.

Mesquita, I., Coutinho, P., De Martin-Silva, L., Parente, B., Faria, M., & Afonso, J. (2015). The value of indirect teaching strategies in enhancing student-coaches' learning engagement. *Journal of Sports Science and Medicine, 14*(3), 657-668.

Metzler, M. (2005). *Instructional models for physical education.* Scottsdale, AZ: Holcomb Hathaway.

Mooses, K., Pihu, M., Riso, E., Hannus, A., Kaasik, P., & Kull, M. (2017). Physical education increases daily moderate to vigorous physical activity and reduces sedentary time. *Journal of School Health, 87*(8), 602-607.

Myer, G., Faigenbaum, A., Edwards, E., Clark. J., Best, T., & Sallis, R. (2015). 60 minutes of what? A developing brain perspective for activation children with an integrative approach. *British Journal of Sports Medicine, 49*(12), 1510-1516.

Myer, G., Kushner, A., Faigenbaum, A., Kiefer, A., Kashikar-Zuck, S., & Clark, J. (2013). Training the developing brain, part I: Cognitive developmental considerations for training youth. *Current Sports Medicine Reports, 12*(5), 304-310.

National Association for Sport and Physical Education. (2011). *Physical education for lifelong fitness.* Champaign, IL: Human Kinetics.

Nicaise, V., Bois, J., Fairclough, S., Amorose, A., & Cogérino, G. (2007). Girls' and boys' perceptions of physical education teachers' feedback: Effects on performance and psychological responses. *Journal of Sports Science, 25*(8), 915-926.

Oliver, J., Lloyd, J., & Meyers, R. (2011). Training elite child athletes: Promoting welfare and well-being. *Strength and Conditioning, 33*(4), 73-79.

Ommundsen, Y., Roberts, G., Lemyre, P., & Miller, B. (2006). Parental and coach support or pressure on psychosocial outcomes of pediatric athletes in soccer. *Clinical Journal of Sports Medicine, 16*(6), 522-526.

Parish, L., Rudisill, M., & St Onge, P. (2007). Mastery motivational climate: influence on physical play and heart rate in African American toddlers. *Research Quarterly in Exercise and Sport, 78*(3), 171-178.

Parish, L., & Treasure, D. (2003). Physical activity and situational motivation in physical education: influence of the motivational climate and perceived ability. *Research Quarterly in Exercise and Sport, 74*(2), 173-182.

ParticipACTION. (2018). *Canadian kids need to move more to boost their brain health. The 2018 ParticipACTION report card on physical activity for children and youth.* Toronto, Canada: ParticipACTION.

Pate, R., Brown, W., Pfeiffer, K., Howie, E., Saunders, R., Addy, C., & Dowda, M. (2016). An intervention to increase physical activity in children: A randomized controlled trial with 4-year-olds in preschools. *American Journal of Preventative Medicine, 51*(1), 12-22.

Pesce, C., Faigenbaum, A., Goudas, M., & Tomporowski, P. (2018). Coupling our plough of thoughtful moving to the star of children's right to play. In R. Meeusen, S. Schaefer, P. Tomporowski, & R. Bailey (Eds.), *Physical acitivty and education achievement* (pp. 247-274). Oxon, UK: Routledge.

Robbins L, Wen F, Ling J. (2019). Mediators of physical activity behavior change in the "Girls on the Move" intervention. *Nursing Research* doi: 10.1097/NNR.0000000000000359

Roberts, G., Treasure, D., & Conroy, D. (2007). Understanding the dynamics of motivation in sport and physical activity: An achievement goal interpretation. In G. Tenenbaum & R. Eclund (Eds.), *Handbook of research in sport psychology* (pp. 3-30). New York, NY: Wiley.

Robinson, L., Palmer, K., Webster, E., Logan, S., & Chinn, K. (2018). The effect of CHAMP on physical activity and lesson context in preschoolers: A feasibility study. *Research Quarterly in Exercise and Sport, 89*(2), 265-271.

Saw, A., Main, L., & Gastin, P. (2016). Monitoring the athlete training response: Subjective self-reported measures trump commonly used objective measures: A systematic review. *British Journal of Sports Medicine, 50*(5), 281-291.

Saxena, S., & Caroni, P. (2007). Mechanisms of axon degeneration: from development to disease. *Progress in Neurobiology, 83*, 174-191.

Schickedanz, J., Schickedanz, D., Forsyth, P., & Forsyth, G. (2000). *Understanding children and adolescents* (4th ed.). Boston, MA: Allyn and Bacon.

Silva, D., Chaput, J., Katzmarzyk, P., Fogelholm, M., Hu, G., Maher, C., . . . Tremblay, M. (2018). Physical education classes, physical activity, and sedentary behavior in children. *Medicine and Science in Sports and Exercise, 50*, 995-1004.

Smith, R., Smoll, F., & Cumming, S. (2007). Effects of a motivational climate intervention for coaches on young athletes' sport performance anxiety. *Journal of Sports and Exercise Psychology, 29*(1), 39-59.

Thelen, E. (1995). Motor development: A new synthesis. *American Psychologist, 50*, 79-95.

Tomporowski, P., McCullick, B., & Horvat, M. (2011). The role of contextual interference and mental engagement on learning. In F. Edvardsen & H. Kulle (Eds.), *Education games: Design, learning and application* (pp. 127-155). Hauppauge, NY: Nova Science.

Treasure, D. (2001). Enhancing young people's motivation in youth sport: An achievement goal approach. In G. Roberts (Ed.), *Advances in Motivation in Sport and Exercise* (pp. 79-100). Champaign, IL: Human Kinetics.

Ungerleider, L., Doyon, J., & Karni, A. (2002). Imaging brain plasticity during motor skill learning. *Neurobiology of Learning and Memory, 78*(3), 553-564.

United States Department of Health and Human Services. (2012). *Physical activity guidelines for Americans midcourse report: Strategies to increase physical activity.* Washington, DC: Author.

Valentini, N. (2004). Visual cues, verbal cues and child development. *Strategies, 17*(3), 21-23.

Vallerand, R., & Losier, G. (1999). An integrative analysis of intrinsic and extrinsic motivation in sport. *Journal of Applied Sport Psychology, 11*, 142-169.

Visek, A., Achrati, S., Manning, H., McDonnell, K., Harris, B., & Dipietro, L. (2015). The Fun Integration Theory: Towards sustaining children and adolescents sport participation. *Journal of Physical Activity and Health, 12*(3), 424-433.

Watson, L., Baker, M., & Chadwick, P. (2016). Kids just wanna have fun: Children's experiences of a weight management programme. *British Journal of Health Psychology, 21*(2), 407-420.

Weiss, J., & American Academy of Pediatrics Committee on Injury, Violence, and Poison Prevention. (2010). Prevention of drowning. *Pediatrics, 126*(1), e253-e262.

Weiss, M. (2011). Teach the children well: A holistic approach to developing psychosocial and behavioral competencies through physical education. *Quest, 63*(1), 55-65.

Whitehead, M. (2010). The concept of physical literacy. In M. Whitehead (Ed.), *Physical literacy through the lifecourse* (pp. 10-20). London, UK: Routledge.

Wilks, T., Gerber, R., & Erdie-Lalena, C. (2010). Developmental milestones: Cognitive development. *Pediatrics in Review, 31*(9), 267-277.

Wulf, G., Dufek, J., Lozano, L., & Pettigrew, C. (2010). Increased jump height and reduced EMG activity with an external focus. *Human Movement Science, 29*(3), 440-448.

Wulf, G., Shea, C., & Lewthwaite, R. (2010). Motor skill learning and performance: A review of influential factors. *Medical Education, 44*(1), 75-84.

Zhou, Y., Lin, F., Du, Y., Qin, L., Zhao, Z., Xu, J., & Lei, H. (2011). Gray matter abnormalities in internet addiction: A voxel-based morphometry study. *European Journal of Radiology, 79*(1), 92-95.

Chapter 6 Assessing Youth Fitness

ALPHA. (2009). *The ALPHA Health-Related Fitness Test Battery for Children and Adolescents test manual.* Retrieved from www.thealphaproject.net

Armstrong, N. (1995). Health-related physical activity in the national curriculum. In M. Darmody & G. O'Donovan (Eds.), *Physical education at the crossroads* (pp. 44-48). Limerick, Ireland: PEAI.

Armstrong, N., & Welsman, J.R. (2000). Development of aerobic fitness during childhood and adolescence. *Pediatric Exercise Science, 12*, 128-149.

Armstrong, N., & Barker, A. R. (2011). Endurance Training and Elite Young Athletes. In N. Armstrong & A. M. McManus (Eds.), *The Elite Young Athlete* (pp. 59-83). Basel: Karger.

Atlantis, E., Barnes, E.H., & Singh, M.A. (2006). Efficacy of exercise for treating overweight in children and adolescents: A systematic review. *International Journal of Obesity, 30*(7), 1027-1040.

Australian Sports Commission. (2018). *The draft Australian physical literacy standard.* Canberra, Australia: Author.

Baquet, G., van Praagh, E., & Berthoin, S. (2003). Endurance training and aerobic fitness in young people. *Sports Medicine, 33*(15), 1127-1143.

Barnett, L.M., Minto, C., Lander, N., & Hardy, L.L. (2014). Inter-rater reliability assessment using the Test of Gross Motor Development–2. *Journal of Science and Medicine in Sport, 17*(6), 667-670.

Barnett, L., Reynolds, J., Faigenbaum, A.D., Smith, J.J., Harries, S., & Lubans, D.R. (2015). Rater agreement of a test battery designed to assess adolescents' resistance training skill competency. *Journal of Science and Medicine in Sport, 18*(1), 72-76.

Behringer, M., Vom Heede, A., Yue, Z., & Mester, J. (2010). Effects of resistance training in children and adolescents: A meta-analysis. *Pediatrics, 126*(5), e1199-1210.

Biddle, S.J., Gorely, T., Pearson, N., & Bull, F.C. (2011). An assessment of self-reported physical activity instruments in young people for population surveillance: Project ALPHA. *International Journal of Behavioral Nutrition and Physical Activity, 8*, 1.

Boreham, C., & Riddoch, C. (2001). The physical activity, fitness and health of children. *Journal of Sports Sciences, 19*(12), 915-929.

Boyer, C., Tremblay, M., Saunders, T.J., McFarlane, A., Borghese, M., Lloyd, M., & Longmuir, P. (2013). Feasibility, validity and reliability of the plank isometric hold as a field-based assessment of torso muscular endurance for children 8-12 years of age. *Pediatric Exercise Science, 25*(3), 407-422.

Cale, L., & Harris, J. (2005). *Exercise and young people: Issues, implications and initiatives.* Basingstoke, UK: Palgrave Macmillan.

Cale, L., Harris, J., & Chen, M.H. (2007). More than 10 years after "the horse is dead . . .": surely it must be time to "dismount"?! *Pediatric Exercise Science, 19*(2), 115-123.

CAPL. (2015). Are children physically literate? Quick and easy screening tasks. Retrieved from www.capl-ecsfp.ca/physical-literacy-screening-tasks

CAPL. (2017). Manual for Test Administration, Second Edition. Retrieved from www.capl-eclp.ca/capl-manual/

Caspersen, C.J., Powell, K.E., & Christenson, G.M. (1985). Physical activity, exercise, and physical fitness: Definitions and distinctions for health-related research. *Public Health Reports, 100*(2), 126-131.

Castagna, C., Manzi, V., Impellizzeri, F., Weston, M., & Barbero Alvarez, J.C. (2010). Relationship between endurance field tests and match performance in young soccer players. *Journal of Strength and Conditioning Research, 24*(12), 3227-3233.

Castro-Piñero, J., Artero, E.G., España-Romero, V., Ortega, F.B., Sjostrom, M., Suni, J., & Ruiz, J.R. (2010). Criterion-related validity of field-based fitness tests in youth: A systematic review. *British Journal of Sports Medicine, 44*(13), 934-943.

Catley, M.J., & Tomkinson, G.R. (2013). Normative health-related fitness values for children: Analysis of 85347 test results on 9-17-year-old Australians since 1985. *British Journal of Sports Medicine, 47*(2), 98-108.

Chillón, P., Castro-Piñero, J., Ruiz, J.R., Soto, V.M., Carbonell-Baeza, A., Dafos, J., . . . Ortega, F.B. (2010). Hip flexibility is the main determinant of the back-saver sit-and-reach test in adolescents. *Journal of Sports Sciences, 28*(6), 641-648.

Chinapaw, M.J., Mokkink, L.B., van Poppel, M.N., van Mechelen, W., & Terwee, C.B. (2010). Physical activity questionnaires for youth: A systematic review of measurement properties. *Sports Medicine, 40*(7), 539-563.

Clarke, H. (1971). Basic understanding of physical fitness. *The President's Council on Physical Fitness and Sports Research Digest, 1*(1).

Cook, G., Burton, L., & Hogenboom, B. (2006). The use of fundamental movements as an assessment of function: Part 1. *North American Journal of Sports Physical Therapy, 1*, 62-72.

Cooper, A.R., Page, A.S., Wheeler, B.W., Hillsdon, M., Griew, P., & Jago, R. (2010). Patterns of GPS measured time outdoors after school and objective physical activity in English children: The PEACH project. *International Journal of Behavioral Nutrition and Physical Activity, 7*, 31.

Corbin, C.B., Pangrazi, R.P., & Franks, D. (2000). Definitions: Health, fitness, and physical fitness. *The President's Council on Physical Fitness and Sports Research Digest, 3*(9).

Crocker, P.R., Bailey, D.A., Faulkner, R.A., Kowalski, K.C., & McGrath, R. (1997). Measuring general levels of physical activity: Preliminary evidence for the Physical Activity Questionnaire for Older Children. *Medicine and Science in Sports and Exercise, 29*(10), 1344-1349.

Cumming, S., Eisenmann, J.C., Lloyd, R.S., Malina, R.M., & Oliver, J.L. (in press). New directions in the study and practice of bio-banding: applications in competition, talent identification and training. *Strength and Conditioning Journal*.

Cumming, S.P., Lloyd, R.S., Oliver, J.L., Eisenmann, J.C., & Malina, R.M. (2017). Bio-banding in sport: Applications to competition, talent identification, and strength and conditioning of youth athletes. *Strength and Conditioning Journal, 39*(2), 34-47.

Deprez, D., Coutts, A.J., Lenoir, M., Fransen, J., Pion, J., Philippaerts, R., & Vaeyens, R. (2014). Reliability and validity of the Yo-Yo intermittent recovery test level 1 in young soccer players. *Journal of Sports Sciences, 32*(10), 903-910.

Donaldson, L. (2010). *2009 annual report of the chief medical officer*. UK: Department of Health.

Duncan, J.S., Badland, H.M., & Schofield, G. (2009). Combining GPS with heart rate monitoring to measure physical activity in children: A feasibility study. *Journal of Science and Medicine in Sport, 12*(5), 583-585.

Ekelund, U., Anderssen, S.A., Froberg, K., Sardinha, L.B., Andersen, L.B., Brage, S., & European Youth Heart Study Group. (2007). Independent associations of physical activity and cardiorespiratory fitness with metabolic risk factors in children: The European youth heart study. *Diabetologia, 50*(9), 1832-1840.

Ekelund, U., Brage, S., Froberg, K., Harro, M., Anderssen, S.A., Sardinha, L.B., . . . Andersen, L.B. (2006). TV viewing and physical activity are independently associated with metabolic risk in children: The European Youth Heart Study. *PLoS Medicine, 3*(12), e488.

España-Romero, V., Artero, E.G., Jimenez-Pavon, D., Cuenca-Garcia, M., Ortega, F.B., Castro-Piñero, J., . . . Ruiz, J.R. (2010). Assessing health-related fitness tests in the school setting: Reliability, feasibility and safety; the ALPHA Study. *International Journal of Sports Medicine, 31*(7), 490-497.

España-Romero, V., Artero, E.G., Santaliestra-Pasias, A.M., Gutierrez, A., Castillo, M.J., & Ruiz, J.R. (2008). Hand span influences optimal grip span in boys and girls aged 6 to 12 years. *Journal of Hand Surgery, 33*(3), 378-384.

Faigenbaum, A.D., Milliken, L.A., & Westcott, W.L. (2003). Maximal strength testing in healthy children. *Journal of Strength and Conditioning Research, 17*(1), 162-166.

Faigenbaum, A.D., & Myer, G.D. (2012). Exercise deficit disorder in youth: Play now or pay later. *Current Sports Medicine Reports, 11*(4), 196-200.

Farrokhi, A., Zareh Zadeh, M., Karimi Alvar, L., Kazemnejad, A., & Ilbeigi, S. (2014). Reliability and validity of the test of gross motor development-2 among 3-10 aged children of Tehran City. *Journal of Physical Education and Sports Management, 5*, 18-28.

Fjortoft, I. (2000). Motor fitness in pre-primary school children: The EUROFIT motor fitness test explored on 5-7 year old children. *Pediatric Exercise Science, 12*, 424-436.

Foweather, L. (2010). *Fundamental movement skill competence among 10-11 year old children: Year 2 PEPASS Physical Activity Project*. Liverpool, UK: Liverpool John Moores University.

Francis, C. E., Longmuir, P. E., Boyer, C., Andersen, L. B., Barnes, J. D., Boiarskaia, E., . . . Tremblay, M. S. (2016). The Canadian Assessment of Physical Literacy: Development of a Model of Children's Capacity for a Healthy, Active Lifestyle Through a Delphi Process. *Journal of Physical Activity & Health, 13*(2), 214-222.

Gomes, T.N., Dos Santos, F.K., Katzmarzyk, P.T., & Maia, J. (2016). Active and strong: Physical activity, muscular strength, and metabolic risk in children. *American Journal of Human Biology*. doi:10.1002/ajhb.22904

Hagströmer, M., Bergman, P., De Bourdeaudhuij, I., Ortega, F.B., Ruiz, J.R., Manios, Y., . . . Group, H.S. (2008). Concurrent validity of a modified version of the International Physical Activity Questionnaire (IPAQ-A) in European adolescents: The HELENA Study. *International Journal of Obesity, 32*(Suppl 5), S42-S48.

Harris, J., & Cale, L. (2006). A review of children's fitness testing. *European Physical Education Review, 12*, 201-225.

Hillman, C.H., Castelli, D.M., & Buck, S.M. (2005). Aerobic fitness and neurocognitive function in healthy preadolescent children. *Medicine and Science in Sports and Exercise, 37*(11), 1967-1974.

Hillman, C.H., Pontifex, M.B., Castelli, D.M., Khan, N.A., Raine, L.B., Scudder, M.R., . . . Kamijo, K. (2014). Effects of the FITKids randomized controlled trial on executive control and brain function. *Pediatrics, 134*(4), e1063-1071.

Hume, C., Okely, A., Bagley, S., Telford, A., Booth, M., Crawford, D., & Salmon, J. (2008). Does weight status influence associations between children's fundamental movement skills and physical activity? *Research Quarterly for Exercise and Sport, 79*(2), 158-165.

Institute of Medicine. (2012). *Fitness measures and health outcomes in youth*. Washington, DC: National Academic Press.

Janssen, I., & Leblanc, A.G. (2010). Systematic review of the health benefits of physical activity and fitness in school-aged children and youth. *International Journal of Behavioral Nutrition and Physical Activity, 7*, 40.

Kennedy, J.F. (1960). The soft American. *Sports Illustrated, 13*, 15-17.

Kowalski, K.C., Crocker, P.R., & Faulkner, R.A. (1997). Validation of the physical activity questionnaire for older children. *Pediatric Exercise Science, 9*, 174-186.

Kowalski, K.C., Crocker, P.R., & Kowalski, N.P. (1997). Convergent validity of the physical activity questionnaire for adolescents. *Pediatric Exercise Science, 9*(342-352).

Kraus, H., & Hirschland, R.P. (1954). Minimum muscular fitness tests in school children. *The Research Quarterly, 25*, 178-188.

Larouche, R., Boyer, C., Tremblay, M.S., & Longmuir, P. (2014). Physical fitness, motor skill, and physical activity relationships in grade 4 to 6 children. *Applied Physiology, Nutrition, and Metabolism, 39*(5), 553-559.

Laurson, K.R., Saint-Maurice, P.F., Welk, G.J., & Eisenmann, J.C. (2016). Reference curves for field tests of musculoskeletal fitness in U.S. children and adolescents: The 2012 NHANES National Youth Fitness Survey. *Journal of Strength and Conditioning Research*. doi:10.1519/JSC.0000000000001678

Leger, L.A., Mercier, D., Gadoury, C., & Lambert, J. (1988). The multistage 20 metre shuttle run test for aerobic fitness. *Journal of Sports Sciences, 6*(2), 93-101.

Lemos, A.G., Avigo, E.L., & Barela, J.A. (2012). Physical education in kindergarten promotes fundamental motor skill development. *Advances in Physical Education, 2*, 17-21.

Lesinski, M., Prieske, O., & Granacher, U. (2016). Effects and dose-response relationships of resistance training on physical performance in youth athletes: A systematic review and meta-analysis. *British Journal of Sports Medicine, 50*(13), 781-795.

Lloyd, M., Colley, R.C., & Tremblay, M.S. (2010). Advancing the debate on "fitness testing" for children: Perhaps we're riding the wrong animal. *Pediatric Exercise Science, 22*(2), 176-182.

Lloyd, M., & Tremblay, M.S. (2010). Physical literacy measurement: The missing piece. *Physical and Health Education, Spring*, 26-30.

Lloyd, R.S., Faigenbaum, A.D., Stone, M.H., Oliver, J.L., Jeffreys, I., Moody, J.A., . . . Myer, G.D. (2014). Position statement on youth resistance training: The 2014 international consensus. *British Journal of Sports Medicine, 48*(7), 498-505.

Lloyd, R.S., Oliver, J.L., Radnor, J.M., Rhodes, B.C., Faigenbaum, A.D., & Myer, G.D. (2015). Relationships between functional movement screen scores, maturation and physical performance in young soccer players. *Journal of Sports Sciences, 33*(1), 11-19.

Lochbaum, M., Kallinen, V., & Konttinen, N. (2017). Task and ego goal orientations across the youth sport experience. *Studia Sportiva, 11*(2), 99-105.

Longmuir, P.E., Boyer, C., Lloyd, M., Borghese, E.K., Saunders, T.J., Boiarskaia, E., . . . Tremblay, M.S. (2015). Canadian Agility and Movement Skill Assessment (CAMSA): Validity, objectivity, and reliability for children 8-12 years of age. *Journal of Sport and Health Science*, 1-10.

Longmuir, P.E., Boyer, C., Lloyd, M., Yang, Y., Boiarskaia, E., Zhu, W., & Tremblay, M.S. (2015). The Canadian Assessment of Physical Literacy: Methods for children in grades 4 to 6 (8 to 12 years). *BMC Public Health, 15*(1), 767.

Lubans, D.R., Morgan, P.J., Cliff, D.P., Barnett, L.M., & Okely, A.D. (2010). Fundamental movement skills in children and adolescents: Review of associated health benefits. *Sports Medicine, 40*(12), 1019-1035.

Lubans, D.R., Smith, J.J., Harries, S.K., Barnett, L.M., & Faigenbaum, A.D. (2014). Development, test-retest reliability, and construct validity of the resistance training skills battery. *Journal of Strength and Conditioning Research, 28*(5), 1373-1380.

Mac Donncha, C., Watson, A.W.S., McSweeney, T., & O'Donovan, D.J. (1999). Reliability of Eurofit physical fitness items for adolescent males with and without mental retardation. *Adapted Physical Activity Quarterly, 16*, 86-95.

Malina, R.M., Bouchard, C., & Bar-Or, O. (2004). *Growth, maturation and physical activity* Champaign, IL: Human Kinetics.

McKenzie, T.L. (2002). Use of direct observation to assess physical activity. In G.J. Welk (Ed.), *Physical activity assessments for health-related research* (pp. 179-195). Champaign, IL: Human Kinetics.

McKenzie, T.L., Cohen, D.A., Sehgal, A., Williamson, S., & Golinelli, D. (2006). System for Observing Play and Recreation in Communities (SOPARC): Reliability and feasibility measures. *Journal of Physical Activity & Health, 3*(Suppl 1), S208-S222.

Meredith, M.D., & Welk, G.J. (2013). *FitnessGram/ActivityGram test administration manual* (4th ed.). Champaign, IL: Human Kinetics.

Moeskops, S., Oliver, J.L., Read, P.J., Cronin, J.B., Myer, G.D., Haff, G.G., & Lloyd, R.S. (2018). Within and between-session reliability of the isometric midthigh pull in young female athletes. *Journal of Strength and Conditioning Research, 32*(7), 1892-1901.

Morrow, J.R., Zhu, W., & Mahar, M.T. (2013). Physical fitness standards for children. In S.A. Plowman & M.D. Meredith (Eds.), *FitnessGram/ActivityGram reference guide* (4th ed., pp. 4-1-12). Dallas, TX: The Cooper Institute.

Myer, G.D., Lloyd, R.S., Brent, J.L., & Faigenbaum, A.D. (2013). How young is "too young" to start training? *ACSM's Health & Fitness Journal, 17*(5), 14-23.

Naughton, G.A., Carlson, J.S., & Greene, D.A. (2006). A challenge to fitness testing in primary schools. *Journal of Science and Medicine in Sport, 9*(1-2), 40-45.

Ng, M., Fleming, T., Robinson, M., Thomson, B., Graetz, N., Margono, C., . . . Gakidou, E. (2014). Global, regional, and national prevalence of overweight and obesity in children and adults during 1980-2013: A systematic analysis for the Global Burden of Disease Study 2013. *Lancet, 384*(9945), 766-781.

NSW Department of Education and Training. (2000). *Get skilled: Get active. A K-6 resource to support the teaching of fundamental movement skills*. Moorebank, NSW: Author.

Okely, A.D., & Booth, M.L. (2004). Mastery of fundamental movement skills among children in New South Wales: Prevalence and sociodemographic distribution. *Journal of Science and Medicine in Sport, 7*(3), 358-372.

Oliver, J.L., Brady, A., & Lloyd, R.S. (2014). Well-being of youth athletes. In R.S. Lloyd & J.L. Oliver (Eds.), *Strength and conditioning for young athletes: Science and application* (pp. 213-225). Abingdon, UK: Routledge.

Ortega, F.B., Cadenas-Sanchez, C., Sanchez-Delgado, G., Mora-Gonzalez, J., Martinez-Tellez, B., Artero, E.G., . . . Ruiz, J.R. (2015). Systematic review and proposal of a field-based physical fitness-test battery in preschool children: The PREFIT battery. *Sports Medicine, 45*(4), 533-555.

Ortega, F.B., Ruiz, J.R., Castillo, M.J., & Sjostrom, M. (2008). Physical fitness in childhood and adolescence: A powerful marker of health. *International Journal of Obesity, 32*(1), 1-11.

Parsonage, J.R., Williams, R.S., Rainer, P., McKeown, I., & Williams, M.D. (2014). Assessment of conditioning-specific movement tasks and physical fitness measures in talent identified under 16-year-old rugby union players. *Journal of Strength and Conditioning Research, 28*(6), 1497-1506.

Pate, R.R., Welk, G.J., & McIver, K.L. (2013). Large-scale youth physical fitness testing in the United States: A 25-year retrospective review. *Pediatric Exercise Science, 25*(4), 515-523.

Plowman, S.A., & Meredith, M.D. (Eds.). (2013). *FitnessGram/ActivityGram reference guide* (4th ed.). Dallas, TX: The Cooper Institute.

Plowman, S.A., Meredith, M.D., Sterling, C.L., Corbin, C.B., Welk, G.J., & Morrow, J.R. (2013). The history of FitnessGram. In S.A. Plowman & M.D. Meredith (Eds.), *FitnessGram/ActivityGram reference guide* (4th ed., pp. 1-22). Dallas, TX: The Cooper Institute.

Presidential Youth Fitness Program. (2015). *Monitoring student fitness levels*. Retrieved from http://pyfp.org/doc/monitoring-fitness.pdf

Rogers, S. A., Hassmen, P., Roberts, A. H., Alcock, A., Gilleard, W. L., & Warmenhoven, J. S. (2019). Development and Reliability of an Athlete Introductory Movement Screen for Use in Emerging Junior Athletes. *Pediatric Exercise Science*, 1-10.

Rowland, T. (1995). "The horse is dead; let's dismount." *Pediatric Exercise Science, 7*, 117-120.

Rowlands, A.V., Ingledew, D.K., & Eston, R.G. (2000). The effect of type of physical activity measure on the relationship between body fatness and habitual physical activity in children: A meta-analysis. *Annals of Human Biology, 27*(5), 479-497.

Ruiz, J.R., Castro-Piñero, J., España-Romero, V., Artero, E.G., Ortega, F.B., Cuenca, M.M., . . . Castillo, M.J. (2011). Field-based fitness assessment in young people: The ALPHA health-related fitness test battery for children and adolescents. *British Journal of Sports Medicine, 45*(6), 518-524.

Ruiz, J.R., Cavero-Redondo, I., Ortega, F.B., Welk, G.J., Andersen, L.B., & Martinez-Vizcaino, V. (2016). Cardiorespiratory fitness cut points to avoid cardiovascular disease risk in children and adolescents; what level of fitness should raise a red flag? A systematic review and meta-analysis. *British Journal of Sports Medicine.*

Ruiz, J.R., España-Romero, V., Ortega, F.B., Sjostrom, M., Castillo, M.J., & Gutierrez, A. (2006). Hand span influences optimal grip span in male and female teenagers. *Journal of Hand Surgery, 31*(8), 1367-1372.

Safrit, M. (1990). Reliabiltiy of fitness tests for children: A review. *Pediatric Exercise Science, 2,* 9-28.

Sallis, J.F., Patterson, T.L., Buono, M.J., & Nader, P.R. (1988). Relation of cardiovascular fitness and physical activity to cardiovascular disease risk factors in children and adults. *American Journal of Epidemiology, 127*(5), 933-941.

Secomb, J.L., Nimphius, S., Farley, O.R., Lundgren, L.E., Tran, T.T., & Sheppard, J.M. (2015). Relationships between lower-body muscle structure and, lower-body strength, explosiveness and eccentric leg stiffness in adolescent athletes. *Journal of Sports Science & Medicine, 14*(4), 691-697.

Seefeldt, V. (1980). Developmental motor patterns: Implications for elementary school physical eduction. In C. Naeau, W. Holliwell, K. Newell, & G. Roberts (Eds.), *Psychology of motor behavior and sport* (pp. 314-323). Champaign, IL: Human Kinetics.

Silverman, S., Keating, X.D., & Phillips, S.R. (2008). A lasting impression: A pedagogical perspective on youth fitness testing. *Measurement in Physical Education and Exercise Science, 12,* 146-166.

Sirard, J.R., & Pate, R.R. (2001). Physical activity assessment in children and adolescents. *Sports Medicine, 31*(6), 439-454.

Society of Health and Physical Educators–SHAPE America. (2010). *Appropriate uses of fitness measurement position statement.* Reston, VA: Author.

Society of Health and Physical Educators–SHAPE America. (2016). *Shape of the nation, status of physical education in the USA.* Reston, VA: Author.

Stratton, G., McWhannell, N., Foweather, L., Henagen, J., Graves, L., Ridgers, N.D., & Hepples, J. (2009). *The A-CLASS project resaerch findings: Executive summary.* Liverpool, UK: Sportslinx.

Tomkinson, G.R., Carver, K.D., Atkinson, F., Daniell, N.D., Lewis, L.K., Fitzgerald, J.S., . . . Ortega, F.B. (2017). European normative values for physical fitness in children and adolescents aged 9-17 years: Results from 2 779 165 Eurofit performances representing 30 countries. *British Journal of Sports Medicine.* doi:10.1136/bjsports-2017-098253

Tomkinson, G.R., Lang, J.J., Tremblay, M.S., Dale, M., LeBlanc, A.G., Belanger, K., . . . Leger, L. (2016). International normative 20 m shuttle run values from 1 142 026 children and youth representing 50 countries. *British Journal of Sports Medicine.* doi:10.1136/bjsports-2016-095987

Tomkinson, G.R., & Olds, T.S. (2008). Field tests of fitness. In N. Armstrong & W. van Mechelen (Eds.), *Paediatric exercise science and medicine* (pp. 109-128). Oxford, UK: Oxford University Press.

Ulrich, D.A. (2000). *Test of gross motor development* (2nd ed.). Austin, TX: Pro-Ed.

Ulrich, D.A., Webster, E.K., & Pitchford, E.A. (2015). *The psychometric properties of the TGMD-3 in a sample of children from the USA.* Paper presented at the European Congress of Sport Psychology, Bern, Switzerland.

Welk, G.J. (2008). The role of physical activity assessments for school-based physical activity promotion. *Measurement in Physical Education and Exercise Science, 12,* 184-206.

Welk, G.J., Dzewaltowski, D.A., & Hill, J.L. (2004). Comparison of the computerized AcitivityGram instrument and the previous day physical activity recall for assessing physical activity in children. *Research Quarterly for Exercise and Sport, 75*(4), 370-380.

Welk, G.J., Mahar, M.T., & Morrow, J.R. (2013). Physical activity assessment. In S.A. Plowman & M.D. Meredith (Eds.), *FitnessGram/ActivityGram reference guide* (4th ed., pp. 5-1-19). Dallas, TX: The Cooper Institute.

Welk, G.J., & Wood, K. (2000). Physical activity assessments in physical education: A practical review of instruments and their use in the curriculum. *Journal of Physical Education, Recreation and Dance, 71,* 30-40.

Whitehead, M. (2016). International Physical Literacy Association homepage. Retrieved from www.physical-literacy.org.uk

Wiart, L., & Darrah, J. (2001). Review of four tests of gross motor development. *Developmental Medicine and Child Neurology, 43*(4), 279-285.

Wiersma, L.D., & Sherman, C.P. (2008). The responsible use of youth fitness testing to enhance student motivation, enjoyment, and performance. *Measurement in Physical Education, 12,* 167-183.

Williams, C.A., Oliver, J.L., & Faulkner, J. (2011). Seasonal monitoring of sprint and jump performance in a soccer youth academy. *International Journal of Sports Physiology and Performance, 6*(2), 264-275.

Williams, H.G., Pfeiffer, K.A., Dowda, M., Jeter, C., Jones, S., & Pate, R.R. (2009). A field-based testing Protocol for assessing gross motor skills in preschool children: The CHAMPS Motor Skills Protocol (CMSP). *Measurement in Physical Education and Exercise Science, 13*(3), 151-165.

Woods, C.T., Keller, B.S., McKeown, I., & Robertson, S. (2016). A comparison of athletic movement between talent identified juniors from different football codes in Australia: Implications for talent development. *Journal of Strength and Conditioning Research, 30*(9), 2440-2445.

Woods, J.A., Pate, R.R., & Burgess, M.L. (1992). Correlates to performance on field tests of muscular strength. *Pediatric Exercise Science, 4*(4), 302-311.

World Health Organization. (2011). *Global recommendations on physical activity for health.* Geneva, Switzerland: Author.

Zuvela, F., Bozanic, A., & Miletic, D. (2011). POLYGON: A new fundamental movement skills test for 8 year old children: Construction and validation. *Journal of Sports Science & Medicine, 10*(1), 157-163.

Chapter 7 Dynamic Warm-Up and Flexibility

Abade, E., Sampaio, J., Gonçalves, B., Baptista, J., Alves, A., & Viana, J. (2017). Effects of different re-warm up activities in football players' performance. *PLoS ONE, 12*(6), e0180152.

Akbulut, T., & Agopyan, A. (2015). Effects of an eight-week proprioceptive neuromuscular facilitation stretching program on kicking speed and range of motion in young male soccer players. *Journal of Strength and Conditioning Research, 29*(12), 3412-3423.

Allen, B., Hannon, J., Burns, R., & Williams, S. (2014). Effect of a core conditioning intervention on tests of trunk muscular endurance in school-aged children. *Journal of Strength and Conditioning Research, 28*(7), 2063-2070.

American College of Sports Medicine. (2018). *ACSM's guidelines for exercise testing and prescription* (10th ed.). Baltimore, MD: Lippincott, Williams and Wilkins.

Apostolopoulos, N., Metsios, G., Flouris, A., Koutedakis, Y., & Wyon, M. (2015). The relevance of stretch intensity and position-a systematic review. *Frontiers in Psychology, 6*, 1128.

Ayala, F., Moreno-Pérez, V., Vera-Garcia, F., Moya, M., Sanz-Rivas, D., & Fernandez-Fernandez, J. (2016). Acute and time-course effects of traditional and dynamic warm-up routines in young elite junior tennis players. *PLoS ONE, 11*(4), e0152790.

Bazett-Jones, D., Winchester, J., & McBride, J. (2005). Effect of potentiation and stretching on maximal force, rate of force development, and range of motion. *Journal of Strength and Conditioning Research, 19*(2), 421-426.

Behm, D., Blazevich, A., Kay, A., & McHugh, M. (2016). Acute effects of muscle stretching on physical performance, range of motion, and injury incidence in healthy active individuals: a systematic review. *Applied Physiology Nutrition and Metabolism, 41*(1), 1-11.

Behm, D., & Chaouachi, A. (2011). A review of the acute effects of static and dynamic stretching on performance. *European Journal of Applied Physiology, 111*(11), 2633-2651.

Bergeron, M., Mountjoy, M., Armstrong, N., Chia, M., Côté, J., Emery, C., . . . Engebretsen, L. (2015). International Olympic Committee consensus statement on youth athletic development. *British Journal of Sports Medicine, 49*(13), 843-851.

Brunner-Ziegler, S., Strasser, B., & Haber, P. (2011). Comparison of metabolic and biomechanic responses to active vs. passive warm-up procedures before physical exercise. *Journal of Strength and Conditioning Research, 25*(4), 909-914.

Chaouachi, A., Castagna, C., Chtara, M., Brughelli, M., Turki, O., Galy, O., . . . Behm, D. (2010). Effect of warm-ups involving static or dynamic stretching on agility, sprinting, and jumping performance in trained individuals. *Journal of Strength and Conditioning Research, 24*(8), 2001-2011.

Chatzopoulos, D., Galazoulas, C., Patikas, D., & Kotzamanidis, C. (2014). Acute effects of static and dynamic stretching on balance, agility, reaction time and movement time. *Journal of Sports Science and Medicine, 13*(2), 403-409.

Dallas, G., Smirniotou, A., Tsiganos, G., Tsopani, D., Di Cagno, A., & Tsolakis, C. (2014). Acute effect of different stretching methods on flexibility and jumping performance in competitive artistic gymnasts. *Journal of Sports Medicine and Physical Fitness, 54*(6), 683-690.

Edholm, P., Krustrup, P., & Randers, M. (2014). Half-time re-warm up increases performance capacity in male elite soccer players. *Scandinavian Journal of Medicine and Science in Sport, 25*(2), e40-49.

Emery, C., Roy, T., Whittaker, J., Nettel-Aguirre, A., & van Mechelen, W. (2015). Neuromuscular training injury prevention strategies in youth sport: A systematic review and meta-analysis. *British Journal of Sports Medicine, 49*(13), 865-870.

Faigenbaum, A. (2012). Dynamic warm-up. In J. Hoffman (Ed.), *NSCA's guide to program design* (pp. 51-70). Champaign, IL: Human Kinetics.

Faigenbaum, A., Bellucci, M., Bernieri, A., Bakker, B., & Hoorens, K. (2005). Acute effects of different warm-up protocols on fitness performance in children. *Journal of Strength and Conditioning Research, 19*(2), 376-381. doi:10.1519/R-15344.1

Faigenbaum, A., & Bruno, L. (2017). A fundamental approach for treating pediatric dynapenia in kids. *ACSM's Health and Fitness Journal, 21*(4), 18-24.

Faigenbaum, A., Kang, J., & McFarland, J. (2006). Acute effects of different warm-up protocols on anaerobic performance in teenage athletes. *Pediatric Exercise Science, 17*, 64-75.

Faigenbaum, A., & McFarland, J. (2007). Guidelines for implementing a dynamic warm-up for physical education. *Journal of Physical Education Recreation and Dance, 78*, 25-28.

Faigenbaum, A., McFarland, J., Kelly, N., Ratamess, N., Kang, J., & Hoffman, J. (2010). Influence of recovery time on warm-up effects in adolescent athletes. *Pediatric Exercise Science, 22*(2), 266-277.

Faigenbaum, A., McFarland, J., Schwerdtman, J., Ratamess, N., Kang, J., & Hoffman, J. (2006). Dynamic warm-up protocols, with and without a weighted vest, and fitness performance in high school female athletes. *Journal of Athletic Training, 41*(4), 357-363.

Foss, K., Thomas, S., Khoury, J., Myer, G., & Hewett, T. (2018). A school-based neuromuscular training program and sport-related injury incidence: A prospective randomized controlled clinical trial. *Journal of Athletic Training, 53*(1), 20-28.

Frikha, M., Chaâri, N., Derbel, M., Elghoul, Y., Zinkovsky A., & Chamari, K. (2016). Acute effect of stretching modalities and time-pressure on accuracy and consistency of throwing darts among 12-13 year-old schoolboys. *Journal of Sports Medicine and Physical Fitness.* 57(9): 1089-1097. doi: 10.23736/S0022-4707.16.06521-X

Garber, C., Blissmer, B., Deschenes, M., Franklin, B., Lamonte, M., Lee, I., . . . American College of Sports Medicine. (2011). American College of Sports Medicine position stand. Quantity and quality of exercise for developing and maintaining cardiorespiratory, musculoskeletal, and neuromotor fitness in apparently healthy adults: Guidance for prescribing exercise. *Medicine and Science in Sports, 43*(7), 1334-1359.

Geladas, N., Nassis, G., & Pavlicevic, S. (2005). Somatic and physical traits affecting sprint swimming performance in young swimmers. *International Journal of Sports Medicine, 26*(2), 139-144.

Hägglund, M., Atroshi, I., Wagner, P., & Waldén, M. (2013). Superior compliance with a neuromuscular training programme is associated with fewer ACL injuries and fewer acute knee injuries in female adolescent football players: Secondary analysis of an RCT. *British Journal of Sports Medicine, 47*(15), 974-979.

Hammami, A., Zois, J., Slimani, M., Russel, M., & Bouhlel, E. (2018). The efficacy and characteristics of warm-up and re-warm-up practices in soccer players: A systematic review. *Journal of Sports Medicine and Physical Fitness, 58*(1-2), 135-149.

Hindle, K., Whitcomb, T., Briggs, W., & Hong, J. (2012). Proprioceptive neuromuscular facilitation (PNF): Its mechanisms and effects on range of motion and muscular function. *Journal of Human Kinetics, 31*, 105-113.

Jeffreys, I. (2007). Warm-up revisited: The ramp method of optimizing warm-ups. *Professional Strength and Conditioning, 6*, 12-18.

Jeffreys, I. (2019). The Warm-Up. Champaign, IL; Human Kinetics, 2019

Kallerud, H., & Gleeson, N. (2013). Effects of stretching on performances involving stretch-shortening cycles. *Sports Medicine, 43*(8), 733-750.

Kamandulis, S., Emeljanovas, A., & Skurvydas, A. (2013). Stretching exercise volume for flexibility enhancement in secondary school children. *Journal of Sports Medicine and Physical Fitness, 53*(6), 687-692.

Kay, A., & Blazevich, A. (2012). Effect of acute static stretch on maximal muscle performance: a systematic review. *Medicine and Science in Sports, 44*(1), 154-164.

Keats, M., Emery, C., & Finch, C. (2012). Are we having fun yet? Fostering adherence to injury preventive exercise recommendations in young athletes. *Sports Medicine, 42*(3), 175-184.

Kilding, A., Tunstall, H., & Kuzmic, D. (2008). Suitability of FIFA's "The 11" training programme for young football players: Impact on physical performance. *Journal of Sports Science and Medicine, 7*(3), 320-326.

Kilduff, L., Bevan, H., Kingsley, M., Owen, N., Bennett, M., Bunce, P., . . . Cunningham, D. (2007). Postactivation potentiation in professional rugby players: Optimal recovery. *Journal of Strength and Conditioning Research, 21*(4), 1134-1138.

Kokkonen, J., Nelson, A., Eldredge, C., & Winchester, J.B. (2007). Chronic static stretching improves exercise performance. *Medicine and Science in Sports and Exercise, 39*(10), 1825-1831.

LaBella, C., Huxford, M., Grissom, J., Kim, K., Peng J, & Christoffel, K. (2011). Effect of neuromuscular warm-up on injuries in female soccer and basketball athletes in urban public high schools: Cluster randomized controlled trial. *Archives of Pediatric and Adolescent Medicine, 165*(11), 1033-1040.

Lauersen, J., Bertelsen, D., & Andersen, L. (2014). The effectiveness of exercise interventions to prevent sports injuries: A systematic review and meta-analysis of randomised controlled trials. *British Journal of Sports Medicine, 48*(11), 871-877.

Lorenz, D. (2011). Postactivation potentiation: An introduction. *The International Journal of Sports Physical Therapy, 6*(3), 234-240.

Maddigan, M, Peach, A, Behm, D. (2012). A comparison of assisted and unassisted proprioceptive neuromuscular facilitation techniques and static stretching. *Journal of Strength and Conditioning Research, 26*(5): 1238-1244.

Malina, R., Bouchard, C., & Bar-Or, O. (2004). *Growth, maturation and physical activity* (2nd ed.). Champaign, IL: Human Kinetics.

Maloney, S., Turner, A., & Fletcher, I. (2014). Ballistic exercise as a pre-activation stimulus: A review of the literature and practical applications. *Sports Medicine, 44*(10), 1347-1359.

McCrary, J., Ackermann, B., & Halaki, M. (2015). A systematic review of the effects of upper body warm-up on performance and injury. *British Journal of Sports Medicine, 49*(14), 935-942.

McGowan, C., Pyne, D., Thompson, K., & Rattray, B. (2015). Warm-up strategies for sport and exercise: Mechanisms and applications. *Sports Medicine, 45* 1523-1546.

McKay, C., Steffen, K., Romiti, M., Finch, C., & Emery, C. (2014). The effect of coach and player injury knowledge, attitudes and beliefs on adherence to the FIFA 11+ programme in female youth soccer. *British Journal of Sports Medicine, 48*(7), 1281-1286.

McNeal, J., & Sands, W. (2003). Acute static stretching reduces lower extremity power in trained children. *Pediatric Exercise Science, 15*, 139-145.

Medeiros, D., Cini, A., Sbruzzi, G., & Lima, C. (2016). Influence of static stretching on hamstring flexibility in healthy young adults: Systematic review and meta-analysis. *Physiotherapy Theory and Practice, 32*(6), 438-445.

Mediate, P., & Faigenbaum, A. (2007). *Medicine ball for all kids.* Monterey, CA: Healthy Learning.

Myer, G., Sugimoto, D., Thomas, S., & Hewett, T. (2013). The influence of age on the effectiveness of neuromuscular training to reduce anterior cruciate ligament injuries in female athletes: A meta analysis. *The American Journal of Sports Medicine, 41*(1), 203-215.

National Association for Sport and Physical Education. (2011). *Physical education for lifelong fitness.* Champaign, IL: Human Kinetics.

Needham, R., Morse, C., & Degens, H. (2009). The acute effect of different warm-up protocols on anaerobic performance in elite youth soccer players. *Journal of Strength and Conditioning Research, 23*(9), 2614-2620.

O'Brien, J., Young, W., & Finch, C. (2017). The use and modification of injury prevention exercises by professional youth soccer teams. *Scandinavian Journal of Medicine and Science in Sport.* 27(11): 1337-1346 doi: 10.1111/sms.1275

Olsen, O., Myklebust, G., & Engebretsen, L. (2005). Exercises to prevent lower limb injuries in youth sports: Cluster randomised controlled trial. *British Medical Journal, 330,* 449.

Opplert, J., & Babault, N. (2018). Acute Effects of Dynamic Stretching on Muscle Flexibility and Performance: An Analysis of the Current Literature. Sports Medicine, 48(2): 299-325.

Owoeye, O., Akinbo, S., Tella, B., & Olawale, O. (2014). Efficacy of the FIFA 11+ warm-up programme in male youth football: A cluster randomised controlled trial. *Journal of Sports Science and Medicine, 13*(2), 321-328.

Paradisis, G., Pappas, P., Theodorou, A., Zacharogiannis, E., Skordilis, E., & Smirniotou, A. (2014). Effects of static and dynamic stretching on sprint and jump performance in boys and girls. *Journal of Strength and Conditioning Research, 28*(1), 154-160.

Peck E, Chomko G, Gaz DV, Farrell AM. (2014). The effects of stretching on performance. *Current Sports Medicine Reports*, 13(3): 179-185.

Popp, J., Bellar, D., Hoover, D., Craig, B., Leitzelar, B., Wanless, E., & Judge, L. (2017). Pre- and post-activity stretching practices of collegiate athletic trainers in the United States. *Journal of Strength and Conditioning Research.* 31(9), 2347-2354.

Rassier, D., & MacIntosh, B. (2000). Coexistence of potentiation and fatigue in skeletal muscle. *Brazilian Journal of Medical and Biological Research, 33,* 499-508.

Ratamess, N. (2012). *ACSM's Foundations of strength training and conditioning.* Philadelphia, PA: Lippincott, Williams and Wilkins.

Richmond, S., Kang, J., Doyle-Baker, P., Nettel-Aguirre, A., & Emery, C. (2016). A school-based injury prevention program to reduce sport injury risk and improve healthy outcomes in youth: A pilot cluster-randomized controlled trial. *Clinical Journal of Sports Medicine, 26*(4), 291-298.

Robbins, D. (2006). Postactivation potentiation and its practical application: A brief review. *Journal of Strength and Conditioning Research, 19,* 453-458.

Rössler, R., Donath, L., Bizzini, M., & Faude, O. (2016). A new injury prevention programme for children's football—FIFA 11+ Kids—can improve motor performance: A cluster-randomised controlled trial. *Journal of Sports Science, 34*(6), 549-556.

Rössler, R, Junge, A, Bizzini, M, Verhagen, E, Chomiak, J, Aus der Fünten, K, Meyer, T, Dvorak, J, Lichtenstein, E, Beaudouin, F, Faude. O. (2018). A multinational cluster randomised controlled trial to assess the efficacy of '11+ Kids': A warm-up programme to prevent injuries in children's football. *Sports Medicine,* 48 (6): 1493-1505.

Rössler R, Verhagen E, Rommers N, Dvorak J, Junge A, Lichtenstein E, Donath L, Faude O. (2019). Comparison of the '11+ Kids' injury prevention programme and a regular warmup in children's football (soccer): a cost effectiveness analysis. British Journal of Sports Medicine. 53(5):309-314.

Russell, M., West, D., Briggs, M., Bracken, R., Cook, C., Giroud, T., . . . Kilduff, L. (2015). A passive heat maintenance strategy implemented during a simulated half-time improves lower body power output and repeated sprint ability in professional Rugby Union players. *PLoS ONE, 10*(3), e0119374.

Sakata, J., Nakamura, E., Suzuki, T., Suzukawa, M., Akaike, A., Shimizu, K., & Hirose, N. (2018). Efficacy of a prevention program for medial elbow injuries in youth baseball players. *American Journal of Sports Medicine, 46*(2), 460-469.

Sands, W., & McNeal, J. (2014). Mobility development and flexibility in youths. In R. Lloyd & J. Oliver (Eds.), *Strength and conditioning for young athletes* (pp. 132-146). London, UK: Routledge.

Santonja Medina, F., Sainz De Baranda Andújar, P., Rodríguez García, P., López Miñarro, P., & Canteras Jordana, M. (2007). Effects of frequency of static stretching on straight-leg raise in elementary school children. *Journal of Sports Medicine and Physical Fitness, 47*(3), 304-308.

Seitz, L., & Haff, G. (2016). Factors modulating post-activation potentiation of jump, sprint, throw, and upper-body ballistic performances: A systematic review with meta-analysis. *Sports Medicine, 46*(2), 231-240.

Siatras, T., Papadopoulos, G., Mameletzi, D., Gerodimos, V., & Kellis, S. (2003). Static and dynamic acute stretching effect on gymnasts' speed in vaulting. *Pediatric Exercise Science, 15,* 383-391.

Silva, L., Neiva, H., Marques, M., Izquierdo, M., & Marinho, D. (2018). Effects of warm-up, post-warm-up, and re-warm-up strategies on explosive efforts in team sports: A systematic review. *Sports Medicine.* 48(10: 2285-2299 doi: 10.1007/s40279-018-0958-5

Silvers-Granelli, H., Bizzini, M., Arundale, A., Mandelbaum, B., & Snyder-Mackler, L. (2017). Does the FIFA 11+ injury prevention program reduce the incidence of ACL injury in male soccer players? *Clinical Orthopaedics and Related Research, 475*(10), 2447-2455.

Simic, L., Sarabon, N., & Markovic, G. (2013). Does pre-exercise static stretching inhibit maximal muscular performance? A meta-analytical review. *Scandinavian Journal of Medicine and Science in Sport, 23*(2), 131-148.

Slauterbeck, J., Reilly, A., Vacek, P., Choquette, R., Tourville, T., Mandelbaum, B., . . . Beynnon, B. (2017). Characterization of prepractice injury prevention exercises of high school athletic teams. *Sports Health, 9*(6), 511-517.

Soligard, T., Myklebust, G., Steffen, K., Holme, I., Silvers, H., Bizzini, M., . . . Andersen, T.E. (2008). Comprehensive warm-up programme to prevent injuries in young female footballers: Cluster randomised controlled trial. *BMJ, 337,* a2469.

Steffen, K., Emery, C., Romiti, M., Kang, J., Bizzini, M., Dvorak, J., . . . Meeuwisse, W. (2013). High adherence to a neuromuscular injury prevention programme (FIFA 11+) improves functional balance and reduces injury risk in Canadian youth female football players: A cluster randomised trial. *British Journal of Sports Medicine, 47*(12), 794-802.

Stodden, D., Fleisig, G., McLean, S., Lyman, S., & Andrews, J. (2001). Relationship of pelvis and upper torso kinematics to pitched baseball velocity. *Journal Applied Biomechanics, 17,* 164-172.

Sugimoto, D., Myer, G., Barber Foss, K., & Hewett, T. (2015). Specific exercise effects of preventive neuromuscular training intervention on anterior cruciate ligament injury risk reduction in young females: meta-analysis and subgroup analysis. *British Journal of Sports Medicine, 49*(5), 282-289.

Taylor, K., Sheppard, J., Lee, H., & Plummer, N. (2009). Negative effect of static stretching restored when combined with a sport specific warm-up component. *Journal of Science and Medicine in Sport, 12*(6), 657-661.

Tillin, N., & Bishop, D. (2009). Factors modulating post-activation potentiation and its effect on performance of subsequent explosive activities. *Sports Medicine, 39*(2), 147-166.

Waldén, M., Atroshi, I., Magnusson, H., Wagner, P., & Hägglund, M. (2012). Prevention of acute knee injuries in adolescent female football players: Cluster randomised controlled trial. *British Medical Journal, 344,* e3042.

Wilson, J., Duncan, N., Marin, P., Brown, L., Loenneke, J., Wilson, S., . . . Ugrinowitsch, C. (2013). Meta-analysis of postactivation potentiation and power: effects of conditioning activity, volume, gender, rest periods, and training status. *Journal of Strength and Conditioning Research, 27*(3), 854-859.

Zakaria, A., Kiningham, R., & Sen, A. (2015). Effects of static and dynamic stretching on injury prevention in high school soccer athletes: A randomized trial. *Journal of Sports Rehabilitation, 24*(3), 229-235.

Zarei, M., Abbasi, H., Daneshjoo, A., Barghi, T., Rommers, N., Faude, O., & Rössler, R. (2018). Long-term effects of the 11+ warm-up injury prevention programme on physical performance in adolescent male football players: A cluster-randomised controlled trial. *Journal of Sport Sciences,* 36(12): 2447-2454.

Zebis, M., Andersen, L., Brandt, M., Myklebust, G., Bencke, J., Lauridsen, H., . . . Aagaard, P. (2016). Effects of evidence-based prevention training on neuromuscular and biomechanical risk factors for ACL injury in adolescent female athletes: A randomised controlled trial. *British Journal of Sports Medicine, 50*(9), 552-557.

Chapter 8 Motor Skill Training

ACSM. (2014). *ACSM's guidelines for exercise testing and prescription* (9th ed.). Philadelphi, PA: Lippincott Williams & Wilkins.

Alhassan, S., Nwaokelemeh, O., Ghazarian, M., Roberts, J., Mendoza, A., & Shitole, S. (2012). Effects of locomotor skill program on minority preschoolers' physical activity levels. *Pediatric Exercise Science, 24*(3), 435-449.

Ames, C. (1992). Classrooms: Goals, structures, and student motivation. *Journal of Educational Psychology, 84*(3), 261-271.

Bailey, R.C., Olson, J., Pepper, S.L., Porszasz, J., Barstow, T.J., & Cooper, D.M. (1995). The level and tempo of children's physical activities: An observational study. *Medicine and Science in Sports and Exercise, 27*(7), 1033-1041.

Barnett, L.M., Van Beurden, E., Morgan, P.J., Brooks, L.O., & Beard, J.R. (2008). Does childhood motor skill proficiency predict adolescent fitness? *Medicine and Science in Sports and Exercise, 40*(12), 2137-2144. doi:10.1249/MSS.0b013e31818160d3

Behringer, M., Vom Heede, A., Matthews, M., & Mester, J. (2011). Effects of strength training on motor performance skills in children and adolescents: A meta-analysis. *Pediatric Exercise Science, 23*(2), 186-206.

Bergeron, M.F., Mountjoy, M., Armstrong, N., Chia, M., Cote, J., Emery, C.A., . . . Engebretsen, L. (2015). International Olympic Committee consensus statement on youth athletic development. *British Journal of Sports Medicine, 49*(13), 843-851. doi:10.1136/bjsports-2015-094962

Booth, M.L., Okely, T., McLellan, L., Phongsavan, P., Macaskill, P., Patterson, J., . . . Holland, B. (1999). Mastery of fundamental motor skills among New South Wales school students: Prevalence and sociodemographic distribution. *Journal of Science and Medicine in Sport, 2*(2), 93-105.

Bryant, E.S., Duncan, M.J., & Birch, S.L. (2014). Fundamental movement skills and weight status in British primary school children. *European Journal of Sport Science, 14*(7), 730-736. doi: 10.1080/17461391.2013.870232

Butler, R. (1987). Task-involving and ego-involving properties of evaluation: Effects of different feedback conditions on motivational perceptions, interest, and performance. *Journal of Educational Psychology, 79*(4), 474-482.

Casey, B.J., Giedd, J.N., & Thomas, K.M. (2000). Structural and functional brain development and its relation to cognitive development. *Biological Psychology, 54*(1-3), 241-257.

Casey, B.J., Tottenham, N., Liston, C., & Durston, S. (2005). Imaging the developing brain: What have we learned about cognitive development? *Trends in Cognitive Sciences, 9*(3), 104-110. doi:10.1016/j.tics.2005.01.011

Cattuzzo, M.T., Dos Santos Henrique, R., Re, A.H., de Oliveira, I.S., Melo, B.M., de Sousa Moura, M., . . . Stodden, D. (2016). Motor competence and health related physical fitness in youth: A systematic review. *Journal of Science and Medicine in Sport, 19*(2), 123-129. doi:10.1016/j.jsams.2014.12.004

Christou, M., Smilios, I., Sotiropoulos, K., Volaklis, K., Pilianidis, T., & Tokmakidis, S.P. (2006). Effects of resistance training on the physical capacities of adolescent soccer players. *Journal of Strength and Conditioning Research, 20*(4), 783-791. doi:10.1519/R-17254.1

Cohen, K.E., Morgan, P.J., Plotnikoff, R.C., Callister, R., & Lubans, D.R. (2015). Physical activity and skills intervention: SCORES cluster randomized controlled trial. *Medicine and Science in Sports and Exercise, 47*(4), 765-774. doi:10.1249/MSS.0000000000000452

Comfort, P., Stewart, A., Bloom, L., & Clarkson, B. (2014). Relationships between strength, sprint, and jump performance in well-trained youth soccer players. *Journal of Strength and Conditioning Research, 28*(1), 173-177. doi:10.1519/JSC.0b013e318291b8c7

Cools, W., Martelaer, K.D., Samaey, C., & Andries, C. (2009). Movement skill assessment of typically developing preschool children: A review of seven movement skill assessment tools. *Journal of Sports Science & Medicine, 8*(2), 154-168.

Crane, J.R., Naylor, P.J., Cook, R., & Temple, V.A. (2015). Do perceptions of competence mediate the relationship between fundamental motor skill proficiency and physical activity levels of children in kindergarten? *Journal of Physical Activity & Health, 12*(7), 954-961. doi:10.1123/jpah.2013-0398

de Souza, M.C., de Chaves, R.N., Lopes, V.P., Malina, R.M., Garganta, R., Seabra, A., & Maia, J. (2014). Motor coordination, activity, and fitness at 6 years of age relative to activity and fitness at 10 years of age. *Journal of Physical Activity & Health, 11*(6), 1239-1247. doi:10.1123/jpah.2012-0137

Elliott, E.S., & Dweck, C.S. (1988). Goals: An approach to motivation and achievement. *Journal of Personality and Social Psychology, 54*(1), 5-12.

Ericsson, I., & Karlsson, M.K. (2014). Motor skills and school performance in children with daily physical education in school—A 9-year intervention study. *Scandinavian Journal of Medicine & Science in Sports, 24*(2), 273-278. doi:10.1111/j.1600-0838.2012.01458.x

Eston, R., Byrne, C., & Twist, C. (2003). Muscle function after exercise-induced muscle damage: Considerations for athletic performance in children and adults. *Journal of Exercise Science and Fitness, 1*(2), 85-96.

Faigenbaum, A.D., Bush, J.A., McLoone, R.P., Kreckel, M.C., Farrell, A., Ratamess, N.A., & Kang, J. (2015). Benefits of strength and skill-based training during primary school physical education. *Journal of Strength and Conditioning Research, 29*(5), 1255-1262. doi:10.1519/JSC.0000000000000812

Faigenbaum, A.D., Farrell, A., Fabiano, M., Radler, T., Naclerio, F., Ratamess, N.A., . . . Myer, G.D. (2011). Effects of integrative neuromuscular training on fitness performance in children. *Pediatric Exercise Science, 23*(4), 573-584.

Faigenbaum, A.D., Farrell, A.C., Fabiano, M., Radler, T.A., Naclerio, F., Ratamess, N.A., . . . Myer, G.D. (2013). Effects of detraining on fitness performance in 7-year-old children. *Journal of Strength and Conditioning Research, 27*(2), 323-330. doi:10.1519/JSC.0b013e31827e135b

Faigenbaum, A.D., Lloyd, R.S., MacDonald, J., & Myer, G.D. (2016). Citius, Altius, Fortius: Beneficial effects of resistance training for young athletes: Narrative review. *British Journal of Sports Medicine, 50*, 3-7. doi:10.1136/bjsports-2015-094621

Faigenbaum, A.D., Lloyd, R.S., & Myer, G.D. (2013). Youth resistance training: Past practices, new perspectives, and future directions. *Pediatric Exercise Science, 25*(4), 591-604.

Faigenbaum, A.D., McFarland, J.E., Keiper, F.B., Tevlin, W., Ratamess, N.A., Kang, J., & Hoffman, J.R. (2007). Effects of a short-term plyometric and resistance training program on fitness performance in boys age 12 to 15 years. *Journal of Sports Science & Medicine, 6*(4), 519-525.

Faigenbaum, A.D., & Myer, G.D. (2012). Exercise deficit disorder in youth: Play now or pay later. *Current Sports Medicine Reports, 11*(4), 196-200. doi:10.1249/JSR.0b013e31825da961

Foulkes, J.D., Knowles, Z., Fairclough, S.J., Stratton, G., O'Dwyer, M., Ridgers, N.D., & Foweather, L. (2015). Fundamental movement skills of preschool children in northwest England. *Perceptual and Motor Skills, 121*(1), 260-283. doi:10.2466/10.25.PMS.121c14x0

Fransen, J., Deprez, D., Pion, J., Tallir, I.B., D'Hondt, E., Vaeyens, R., . . . Philippaerts, R.M. (2014). Changes in physical fitness and sports participation among children with different levels of motor competence: A 2-year longitudinal study. *Pediatric Exercise Science, 26*(1), 11-21. doi:10.1123/pes.2013-0005

Fry, A.C. (2004). The role of resistance exercise intensity on muscle fibre adaptations. *Sports Medicine, 34*(10), 663-679.

Gallahue, D.L., Ozmun, J.C., & Goodway, J.D. (2012). *Understanding motor development*. New York, NY: McGraw-Hill.

Gonzalez-Badillo, J.J., & Sanchez-Medina, L. (2010). Movement velocity as a measure of loading intensity in resistance training. *International Journal of Sports Medicine, 31*(5), 347-352. doi:10.1055/s-0030-1248333

Granacher, U., Muehlbauer, T., Doerflinger, B., Strohmeier, R., & Gollhofer, A. (2011). Promoting strength and balance in adolescents during physical education: Effects of a short-term resistance training. *Journal of Strength and Conditioning Research, 25*(4), 940-949. doi:10.1519/JSC.0b013e3181c7bb1e

Hardy, L.L., Barnett, L., Espinel, P., & Okely, A.D. (2013). Thirteen-year trends in child and adolescent fundamental movement skills: 1997-2010. *Medicine and Science in Sports and Exercise, 45*(10), 1965-1970. doi:10.1249/MSS.0b013e318295a9fc

Hardy, L.L., Reinten-Reynolds, T., Espinel, P., Zask, A., & Okely, A.D. (2012). Prevalence and correlates of low fundamental movement skill competency in children. *Pediatrics, 130*(2), e390-e398. doi:10.1542/peds.2012-0345

Hulteen, R.M., Morgan, P.J., Barnett, L.M., Stodden, D.F., & Lubans, D.R. (2018). Development of foundational movement skills: A conceptual model for physical activity across the lifespan. *Sports Medicine, 48*(7), 1533-1540. doi:10.1007/s40279-018-0892-6

Hutchison, B.L., Stewart, A.W., & Mitchell, E.A. (2009). Characteristics, head shape measurements and developmental delay in 287 consecutive infants attending a plagiocephaly clinic. *Acta Paediatrica, 98*(9), 1494-1499. doi:10.1111/j.1651-2227.2009.01356.x

Hutchison, B.L., Stewart, A.W., & Mitchell, E.A. (2011). Deformational plagiocephaly: A follow-up of head shape, parental concern and neurodevelopment at ages 3 and 4 years. *Archives of Disease in Childhood, 96*(1), 85-90. doi:10.1136/adc.2010.190934

Hutchison, B.L., Thompson, J.M., & Mitchell, E.A. (2003). Determinants of nonsynostotic plagiocephaly: A case-control study. *Pediatrics, 112*(4), e316.

Iivonen, K.S., Saakslahti, A.K., Mehtala, A., Villberg, J.J., Tammelin, T.H., Kulmala, J.S., & Poskiparta, M. (2013). Relationship between fundamental motor skills and physical activity in 4-year-old preschool children. *Perceptual and Motor Skills, 117*(2), 627-646. doi:10.2466/10.06.PMS.117x22z7

Largo, R.H., Molinari, L., Weber, M., Comenale Pinto, L., & Duc, G. (1985). Early development of locomotion: Significance of prematurity, cerebral palsy and sex. *Developmental Medicine and Child Neurology, 27*(2), 183-191.

Laukkanen, A., Pesola, A., Havu, M., Saakslahti, A., & Finni, T. (2014). Relationship between habitual physical activity and gross motor skills is multifaceted in 5- to 8-year-old children. *Scandinavian Journal of Medicine & Science in Sports, 24*(2), e102-e110. doi:10.1111/sms.12116

Lemos, A.G., Avigo, E.L., & Barela, J.A. (2012). Physical education in kindergarten promotes fundamental motor skill development. *Advances in Physical Education, 2*(1), 17-21.

Lloyd, M., Saunders, T.J., Bremer, E., & Tremblay, M.S. (2014). Long-term importance of fundamental motor skills: A 20-year follow-up study. *Adapted Physical Activity Quarterly, 31*(1), 67-78. doi:10.1123/apaq:2013-0048

Lloyd, R.S., Cronin, J.B., Faigenbaum, A.D., Haff, G.G., Howard, R., Kraemer, W.J., . . . Oliver, J.L. (2016). National Strength and Conditioning Association position statement on long-term athletic development. *Journal of Strength and Conditioning Research, 30*(6), 1491-1509. doi:10.1519/JSC.0000000000001387

Lloyd, R.S., Faigenbaum, A.D., Stone, M.H., Oliver, J.L., Jeffreys, I., Moody, J.A., . . . Myer, G.D. (2014). Position statement on youth resistance training: The 2014 international consensus. *British Journal of Sports Medicine, 48*(7), 498-505. doi:10.1136/bjsports-2013-092952

Lloyd, R.S., & Oliver, J.L. (2012). The youth physical development model: A new approach to long-term athletic development. *Strength and Conditioning Journal, 34*(3), 61-72.

Lloyd, R.S., Oliver, J.L., Faigenbaum, A.D., Howard, R., De Ste Croix, M.B., Williams, C.A., . . . Myer, G.D. (2015a). Long-term athletic development, part 1: A pathway for all youth. *Journal of Strength and Conditioning Research, 29*(5), 1439-1450. doi:10.1519/JSC.0000000000000756

Lloyd, R.S., Oliver, J.L., Faigenbaum, A.D., Howard, R., De Ste Croix, M.B., Williams, C.A., . . . Myer, G.D. (2015b). Long-term athletic development, part 2: Barriers to success and potential solutions. *Journal of Strength and Conditioning Research, 29*(5), 1451-1464. doi:10.1519/01.JSC.0000465424.75389.56

Lloyd, R.S., Oliver, J.L., Meyers, R.W., Moody, J.A., & Stone, M.H. (2012). Long-term athletic development and its application to youth weightlifting. *Strength and Conditioning Journal, 34*(4), 55-66.

Lloyd, R.S., Oliver, J.L., Radnor, J.M., Rhodes, B.C., Faigenbaum, A.D., & Myer, G.D. (2015). Relationships between functional movement screen scores, maturation and physical performance in young soccer players. *Journal of Sports Sciences, 33*(1), 11-19. doi:10.1080/02640414.2014.918642

Logan, S.W., Robinson, L.E., Wilson, A.E., & Lucas, W.A. (2012). Getting the fundamentals of movement: A meta-analysis of the effectiveness of motor skill interventions in children. *Child: Care, Health and Development, 38*(3), 305-315. doi:10.1111/j.1365-2214.2011.01307.x

Logan, S.W., Ross, S.M., Chee, K., Stodden, D.F., & Robinson, L.E. (2017). Fundamental motor skills: A systematic review of terminology. *Journal of Sports Sciences,* 1-16. doi:10.1080/02640414.2017.1340660

Lopes, V.P., Rodrigues, L.P., Maia, J.A., & Malina, R.M. (2011). Motor coordination as predictor of physical activity in childhood. *Scandinavian Journal of Medicine & Science in Sports, 21*(5), 663-669. doi:10.1111/j.1600-0838.2009.01027.x

Lopes, V.P., Stodden, D.F., Bianchi, M.M., Maia, J.A., & Rodrigues, L.P. (2012). Correlation between BMI and motor coordination in children. *Journal of Science and Medicine in Sport, 15*(1), 38-43. doi:10.1016/j.jsams.2011.07.005

Loprinzi, P.D., Davis, R.E., & Fu, Y.C. (2015). Early motor skill competence as a mediator of child and adult physical activity. *Preventive Medicine Reports, 2,* 833-838. doi:10.1016/j.pmedr.2015.09.015

Lubans, D.R., Morgan, P.J., Cliff, D.P., Barnett, L.M., & Okely, A.D. (2010). Fundamental movement skills in children and adolescents: Review of associated health benefits. *Sports Medicine, 40*(12), 1019-1035. doi:10.2165/11536850-000000000-00000

Malina, R.M. (2004). Motor development during infancy and early childhood: Overview and suggested directions for research. *Journal of Sport and Health ScienceInternational Journal of Sport and Health Science, 2*, 50-66.

Malina, R.M., Bouchard, C., & Bar-Or, O. (2004). *Growth, maturation and physical activity.* Champaign, IL: Human Kinetics.

Malina, R.M., Cumming, S.P., & Coelho, E.S.M.J. (2016). Physical activity and movement Proficiency: The need for a biocultural approach. *Pediatric Exercise Science, 28*(2), 233-239. doi:10.1123/pes.2015-0271

Meece, J.L., Blumenfeld, P.C., & Hoyle, R.H. (1988). Students' goal orientations and cognitive engagement in classroom activities. *Journal of Educational Psychology, 80*(4), 514-523.

Moody, J.A., Naclerio, F., Green, P., & Lloyd, R.S. (2013). Motor skill development in youths. In R.S. Lloyd & J.L. Oliver (Eds.), *Strength and conditioning for young athletes: Science and application* (pp. 49-65). Oxon, UK: Routledge.

Morgan, P.J., Barnett, L.M., Cliff, D.P., Okely, A.D., Scott, H.A., Cohen, K.E., & Lubans, D.R. (2013). Fundamental movement skill interventions in youth: A systematic review and meta-analysis. *Pediatrics, 132*(5), e1361-1383. doi:10.1542/peds.2013-1167

Myer, G.D., Faigenbaum, A.D., Edwards, N.M., Clark, J.F., Best, T.M., & Sallis, R.E. (2015). Sixty minutes of what? A developing brain perspective for activating children with an integrative exercise approach. *British Journal of Sports Medicine.* doi:10.1136/bjsports-2014-093661

Myer, G.D., Faigenbaum, A.D., Ford, K.R., Best, T.M., Bergeron, M.F., & Hewett, T.E. (2011). When to initiate integrative neuromuscular training to reduce sports-related injuries and enhance health in youth? *Current Sports Medicine Reports, 10*(3), 155-166. doi:10.1249/JSR.0b013e31821b1442

Myer, G.D., Lloyd, R.S., Brent, J.L., & Faigenbaum, A.D. (2013). How young is "too young" to start training? *ACSM's Health & Fitness Journal, 17*(5), 14-23. doi:10.1249/FIT.0b013e3182a06c59

K.M. Newell, "Constraints on the Development of Coordination," in *Motor Development in Children: Aspects of Coordination and Control,* edited by M. G. Wade and H.T. A. Whiting (Dordrecht: Springer Netherlands, 1986), 341-360.

Nicholls, J.G., Patashnick, M., & Nolen, S.B. (1985). Adolescents' theories of education. *Journal of Educational Psychology, 77*(6), 683-692.

Okely, A.D., & Booth, M.L. (2004). Mastery of fundamental movement skills among children in New South Wales: Prevalence and sociodemographic distribution. *Journal of Science and Medicine in Sport, 7*(3), 358-372.

Palmer, K.K., Chinn, K.M., & Robinson, L.E. (2017). Using achievement goal theory in motor skill instruction: A systematic review. *Sports Medicine.* doi:10.1007/s40279-017-0767-2

Piek, J.P., Hands, B., & Licari, M.K. (2012). Assessment of motor functioning in the preschool period. *Neuropsychology Review, 22*(4), 402-413. doi:10.1007/s11065-012-9211-4

Ratel, S., Williams, C.A., Oliver, J., & Armstrong, N. (2006). Effects of age and recovery duration on performance during multiple treadmill sprints. *International Journal of Sports Medicine, 27*(1), 1-8. doi:10.1055/s-2005-837501

Robinson, L.E. (2011a). Effect of a mastery climate motor program on object control skills and perceived physical competence in preschoolers. *Research Quarterly for Exercise and Sport, 82*(2), 355-359. doi:10.1080/02701367.2011.10599764

Robinson, L.E. (2011b). The relationship between perceived physical competence and fundamental motor skills in preschool children. *Child: Care, Health and Development, 37*(4), 589-596. doi:10.1111/j.1365-2214.2010.01187.x

Robinson, L.E., Palmer, K.K., & Bub, K.L. (2016). Effect of the Children's Health Activity Motor Program on motor skills and self-regulation in Head Start preschoolers: An efficacy trial. *Front Public Health, 4*, 173. doi:10.3389/fpubh.2016.00173

Robinson, L.E., Stodden, D.F., Barnett, L.M., Lopes, V.P., Logan, S.W., Rodrigues, L.P., & D'Hondt, E. (2015). Motor competence and its effect on positive developmental trajectories of health. *Sports Medicine, 45*(9), 1273-1284. doi:10.1007/s40279-015-0351-6

Robinson, L.E., Veldman, S.L.C., Palmer, K.K., & Okely, A.D. (2017). A ball skills Intervention in preschoolers: The CHAMP randomized controlled trial. *Medicine and Science in Sports and Exercise, 49*(11), 2234-2239. doi:10.1249/MSS.0000000000001339

Robinson, L.E., Webster, E.K., Logan, S.W., Lucas, W.A., & Barber, L.T. (2012). Teaching practices that promote motor skills in early childhood settings. *Early Childhood Education Journal, 40*(2), 79-86.

Seefeldt, V. (1980). Developmental motor patterns: Implications for elementary school physical education. In C. Nadeau, W. Holliwell, K. Newell, & G. Robert (Eds.), *Psychology of motor behavior and sport* (pp. 314-323). Champaign: IL: Human Kinetics.

Seiler, K.S., & Kjerland, G.O. (2006). Quantifying training intensity distribution in elite endurance athletes: Is there evidence for an "optimal" distribution? *Scandinavian Journal of Medicine & Science in Sports, 16*(1), 49-56. doi:10.1111/j.1600-0838.2004.00418.x

Society of Health and Physical Educators–SHAPE America. (2016). *Shape of the nation 2016: Status of physical education in the USA.* Reston, VA: Author.

Stodden, D.F., Gao, Z., Goodway, J.D., & Langendorfer, S.J. (2014). Dynamic relationships between motor skill competence and health-related fitness in youth. *Pediatric Exercise Science, 26*(3), 231-241. doi:10.1123/pes.2013-0027

Stodden, D., Langendorfer, S., & Roberton, M.A. (2009). The association between motor skill competence and physical fitness in young adults. *Research Quarterly for Exercise and Sport, 80*(2), 223-229. doi:10.1080/02701367.2009.10599556

Stratton, G., McWhannell, N., Foweather, L., Henaghan, J., Graves, L., Ridgers, N.D., & Hepples, J. (2009). *The A-CLASS Project research findings: Executive summary.* Liverpool, UK:

Tveter, A.T., & Holm, I. (2010). Influence of thigh muscle strength and balance on hop length in one-legged hopping in children aged 7-12 years. *Gait & Posture, 32*(2), 259-262. doi:10.1016/j.gaitpost.2010.05.009

Weiler, R., Allardyce, S., Whyte, G.P., & Stamatakis, E. (2014). Is the lack of physical activity strategy for children complicit mass child neglect? *British Journal of Sports Medicine, 48*(13), 1010-1013. doi:10.1136/bjsports-2013-093018

World Health Organization. (2010). *Global recommendations on physical activity for health.* Geneva, Switzerland: Author.

Wrotniak, B.H., Epstein, L.H., Dorn, J.M., Jones, K.E., & Kondilis, V.A. (2006). The relationship between motor proficiency and physical activity in children. *Pediatrics, 118*(6), e1758-1765. doi:10.1542/peds.2006-0742

Zafeiriou, D.I. (2004). Primitive reflexes and postural reactions in the neurodevelopmental examination. *Pediatric Neurology, 31*(1), 1-8. doi:10.1016/j.pediatrneurol.2004.01.012

Chapter 9 Strength and Power Training

Allen, B., Hannon, J., Burns, R., & Williams, S. (2014). Effect of a core conditioning intervention on tests of trunk muscular endurance in school-aged children. *Journal of Strength and Conditioning Research, 28*(7), 2063-2070.

Alves, A., Marta, C., Neiva, H., Izquierdo, M., & Marques, M. (2016). Concurrent training in prepubescent children: the effects of eight weeks of strength and aerobic training on explosive strength and VO2max. *Journal of Strength and Conditioning Research, 30*(7), 2019-2032.

American Academy of Pediatrics. (2008). Strength training by children and adolescents. *Pediatrics, 121*, 835-840.

American College of Sports Medicine. (2018). *ACSM's guidelines for exercise testing and prescription* (10th ed.). Baltimore, MD: Lippincott, Williams and Wilkins.

American Council on Exercise, IHRSA, & Club Intel. (2015). *International fitness industry trend report. Whats all the rage? Executive summary.* Retrieved from https://acewebcontent.azureedge.net/assetportfoliodownloads/Industry-Trends-2015.pdf

Annesi, J.J., Westcott, W.L., Faigenbaum, A.D., & Unruh, J.L. (2005). Effects of a 12-week physical activity protocol delivered by YMCA after-school counselors (Youth Fit for Life) on fitness and self-efficacy changes in 5-12-year-old boys and girls. *Research Quarterly for Exercise and Sport, 76*(4), 468-476.

Assunção, A., Bottaro, M., Cardoso, E., Dantas da Silva., D., Ferraz, M., Vieira, C., & Gentil, P. (2018). Effects of a low-volume plyometric training in anaerobic performance of adolescent athletes. *Journal of Sports Medicine and Physical Fitness, 58*(5), 570-575.

Augustsson, S., & Ageberg, E. (2017). Weaker lower extremity muscle strength predicts traumatic knee injury in youth female but not male athletes. *BMJ Open Sport & Exercise Medicine, 3*(1), e000222.

Australian Strength and Conditioning Association. (2007). Resistance training for children and youth: A position stand from the Australian Strength and Conditioning Association. Retrieved June 17, 2009, from www.strengthandconditioning.org

Babic, M., Morgan, P., Plotnikoff, R., Lonsdale, C., White, R., & Lubans, D. (2014). Physical activity and physical self-concept in youth: Systematic review and meta-analysis. *Sports Medicine, 44*(11), 1589-1601.

Balsamo, S., Tibana, R., Nascimento, D.C., Franz, C., Lyons, S., Faigenbaum, A., & Prestes, J. (2013). Exercise order influences number of repetitions and lactate levels but not perceived exertion during resistance exercise in adolescents. *Journal of Strength and Conditioning Research, 21*(4), 293-304.

Bangsbo, J., Krustrup, P., Duda, J., Hillman, C., Bo Andersen, L., Weiss, M., . . . Elbe, A. (2016). The Copenhagen Consensus Conference 2016: Children, youth, and physical activity in schools and during leisure time. *British Journal of Sports Medicine, 50*(19), 1177-1178.

Barnett, L., Reynolds, J., Faigenbaum, A., Smith, J., Harries, S., & Lubans, D. (2015). Rater agreement of a test battery designed to assess adolescents' resistance training skill competency. *Journal of Science and Medicine in Sport, 18*(1), 72-76.

Bass, R., & Eneli, I. (2015). Severe childhood obesity: an under-recognised and growing health problem. *Postgraduate Medicine, 91*(1081), 639-645.

Bea, J., Blew, R., Howe, C., Hetherington-Rauth, M., & Going, S. (2017). Resistance training effects on metabolic function among youth: A systematic review. *Pediatric Exercise Science, 29*(3), 297-315.

Beck, N., Lawrence, J., Nordin, J., DeFor, T., & Tompkins, M. (2017). ACL tears in school-aged children and adolescents over 20 years. *Pediatrics, 139*(3), e20161877.

Bedoya, A., Miltenberger, M., & Lopez, R. (2015). Plyometric training effects on athletic performance in youth soccer athletes: A systematic review. *Journal of Strength and Conditioning Research, 29*(8), 2351-2360.

Behm, D.G., Faigenbaum, A.D., Falk, B., & Klentrou, P. (2008). Canadian Society for Exercise Physiology position paper: Resistance training in children and adolescents. *Applied Physiology Nutrition and Metabolism, 33*(3), 547-561.

Behm, D., Young, J., Whitten, J., Reid, J., Quigley, P., Low, J., . . . Granacher, U. (2017). Effectiveness of traditional strength versus power training on muscle strength, power and speed with youth: A systematic review and meta-analysis. *Frontiers in Physiology.* doi:10.3389/fphys.2017.00423

Behringer, M., Gruetzner, S., McCourt, M., & Mester, J. (2014). Effects of weight-bearing activities on bone mineral content and density in children and adolescents: A meta-analysis. *Journal of Bone and Mineral Research, 29*(2), 467-478.

Behringer, M., Neuerburg, S., Matthews, M., & Mester, J. (2013). Effects of two different resistance-training programs on mean tennis-serve velocity in adolescents. *Pediatric Exercise Science, 25*(3), 370-384.

Behringer, M., Vom Heede, A., Matthews, M., & Mester, J. (2011). Effects of strength training on motor performance skills in children and adolescents: A meta-analysis. *Pediatric Exercise Science, 23*(2), 186-206.

Behringer, M., Vom Heede, A., Yue, Z., & Mester, J. (2010). Effects of resistance training in children and adolescents: A meta-analysis. *Pediatrics, 126*(5), e1199-e1210.

Bergeron, M., Mountjoy, M., Armstrong, N., Chia, M., Côté, J., Emery, C., . . . Engebretsen, L. (2015). International Olympic Committee consensus statement on youth athletic development. *British Journal of Sports Medicine, 49*(13), 843-851.

Blagrove, R., Howe, L., Cushion, E., Spence, A., Howatson, G., Pedlar, C., & Hayes, P. (2018). Effects of strength training on postpubertal adolescent distance runners. *Medicine and Science in Sports and Exercise, 50*(6), 1224-1232.

Blanksby, B.A., & Gregor, J. (1981). Anthropometric, strength, and physiological changes in male and female swimmers with progressive resistance training. *Australian Journal of Sports Science, 1*, 3-6.

Bloemers, F., Collard, D., Paw, M., Van Mechelen, W., Twisk, J., & Verhagen, E. (2012). Physical inactivity is a risk factor for physical activity-related injuries in children. *British Journal of Sports Medicine, 46*(9), 669-674.

Bompa, T., & Haff, G. (2009). *Periodization: Theory and methodology of training.* Champaign, IL: Human Kinetics.

Bottaro, M., Brown, L., Celes, R., Martorelli, S., Carregaro, R., & de Brito Vidal, J. (2011). Effect of rest interval on neuromuscular and metabolic responses between children and adolescents. *Pediatric Exercise Science, 23*(3), 311-321.

Burt, L., Ducher, G., Naughton, G., Courteix, D., & Greene, D. (2013). Gymnastics participation is associated with skeletal benefits in the distal forearm: A 6-month study using peripheral quantitative computed tomography. *Journal of Musculoskeletal & Neuronal Interactions, 13*(4), 395-404.

Campbell, C., Carson, J., Diaconescu, E., Celebrini, R., Rizzardo, M., Godbout, V., . . . Canadian Academy of Sport and Exercise Medicine. (2014). Canadian Academy of Sport and Exercise Medicine position statement: Neuromuscular training programs can decrease anterior cruciate ligament injuries in youth soccer players. *Clinical Journal of Sports Medicine, 24*(3), 263-267.

Casey, B., Tottenham, N., Liston, C., & Durston, S. (2005). Imaging the developing brain: What have we learned about cognitive development? *Trends in Cognitive Science, 9*(3), 104-110.

Cattuzzo, M., Dos Santos, H.R., Ré, A., de Oliveira, I., Melo, B., de Sousa Moura, M., . . . Stodden, D. (2016). Motor competence and health related physical fitness in youth: A systematic review. *Journal of Science and Medicine in Sport.* 19(2): 123-129 . doi: 10.1016/j.jsams.2014.12.004

Channell, B.T., & Barfield, J.P. (2008). Effect of Olympic and traditional resistance training on vertical jump improvement in high school boys. *J Strength Cond Res, 22*(5), 1522-1527. doi:10.1519/JSC.0b013e318181a3d0

Chaouachi, A., Ben Othman, A., Makhlouf, I., Young, J., Granacher, U., & Behm, D. (2018). Global training effects of trained and untrained muscles with youth can be maintained during 4 weeks of detraining. *Journal of Strength and Conditioning Research.* doi: 10.1519/JSC.0000000000002606

Chaouachi, A., Hammami, R., Kaabi, S., Chamari, K., Drinkwater, E., & Behm, D. (2014). Olympic weightlifting and plyometric training with children provides similar or greater performance improvements than traditional resistance training. *Journal of Strength and Conditioning Research.* 28(6): 1483-1496. doi: 10.1519/JSC.0000000000000305

Chaouachi, A., Othman, A., Hammami, R., Drinkwater, E., & Behm, D. (2014). The combination of plyometric and balance training improves sprint and shuttle run performances more often than plyometric-only training with children. *Journal of Strength and Conditioning Research, 28*(2), 401-412.

Chu, D., & Myer, G. (2013). *Plyometrics.* Champaign, IL: Human Kinetics.

Clark, B., & Manini , T. (2008). Sarcopenia ≠ dynapenia. *The Journals of Gerontology. Series A, Biological Sciences and Medical Sciences, 63*(8), 829-834.

Cohen, D., Gómez-Arbeláez, D., Camacho, P., Pinzon, S., Hormiga, C., Trejos-Suarez, J., . . . Lopez-Jaramillo, P. (2014). Low muscle strength is associated with metabolic risk factors in Colombian children: The ACFIES study. *PLoS ONE, 9*(4), e93150.

Cohen, D., López-Jaramillo, P., Fernández-Santos, J., Castro-Piñero, J., & Sandercock, G. (2017). Muscle strength is associated with lower diastolic blood pressure in schoolchildren. *Preventive Medicine, 95*, 1-6.

Conroy, B.P., Kraemer, W.J., Maresh, C.M., Fleck, S.J., Stone, M.H., Fry, A.C., . . . Dalsky, G.P. (1993). Bone mineral density in elite junior Olympic weightlifters. *Medicine and Science in Sports and Exercise, 25*(10), 1103-1109.

Contreras, B., Vigotsky, A., Schoenfeld, B., Beardsley, C., McMaster, D., Reyneke, J., & Cronin, J. (2017). Effects of a six-week hip thrust vs. front squat resistance training program on performance in adolescent males: A randomized-controlled trial. *Journal of Strength and Conditioning Research.* 31(4): 999-1008 doi: 10.1519/JSC.0000000000001510.

Cormie, P., McGuigan, M., & Newton, R. (2011). Developing maximal neuromuscular power: Part 2—Training considerations for improving maximal power production. *Sports Medicine, 41*(2), 125-146.

De Meester, A., Stodden, D., Goodway, J., True, L., Brian, A., Ferkel, R., & Haerens, L. (2018). Identifying a motor proficiency barrier for meeting physical activity guidelines in children. *Journal of Science and Medicine in Sport, 21*(1), 58-62.

de Salles, B., Simão, R., Miranda, F., Novaes Jda, S., Lemos, A., & Willardson , J. (2009). Rest interval between sets in strength training. *Sports Medicine, 39*(9), 765-777.

DeRenne, C., Hetzler, R.K., Buxton, B., & Ho, K.K. (1996). Effects of training frequency on strength maintenance in pubescent baseball players. *Journal of Strength and Conditioning Research, 10*, 8-14.

Diallo, O., Dore, E., Duche, P., & Van Praagh, E. (2001). Effects of plyometric training followed by a reduced training program on physical performance in prepubescent soccer players. *Journal of Sports Medicine and Physical Fitness, 41*, 342-348.

Dias, I., Farinatti, P., de Souza, M., Manhanini, D., Balthazar, E., Dantas, D., . . . Kraemer-Aguiar, L. (2015). Effects of resistance training on obese adolescents. *Medicine and Science in Sports and Exercise, 47*(12), 2636-2644.

Difiori, J., Benjamin, H., Brenner, J., Gregory, A., Jayanthi, N., Landry, G., & Luke, A. (2014). Overuse injuries and burnout in youth sports: A position statement from the American Medical Society for Sports Medicine. *Clinical Journal of Sports Medicine, 24*(1), 3-20.

Docherty, D., Wenger, H.A., & Collis, M.L. (1987). The effects of resistance training on aerobic and anaerobic power of young boys. *Medicine and Science in Sports and Exercise, 19*(4), 389-392.

Dorgo, S., King, G., Candelaria, N., Bader, J., Brickey, G., & Adams, C. (2009). Effects of manual resistance training on fitness in adolescents. *Journal of Strength and Conditioning Research, 23*(8), 2287-2294.

Duncan, M., Eyre, E., & Oxford, S. (2017). The effects of 10 weeks integrated neuromuscular training on fundamental movement skills and physical self-efficacy in 6-7 year old children. *Journal of Strength and Conditioning Research, epub before print.*

Emery, C., Roy, T., Whittaker, J., Nettel-Aguirre, A., & van Mechelen, W. (2015). Neuromuscular training injury prevention strategies in youth sport: A systematic review and meta-analysis. *British Journal of Sports Medicine, 49*(13), 865-870.

Faigenbaum, A., & Bruno, L. (2017). A fundamental approach for treating pediatric dynapenia in kids. *ACSM's Health and Fitness Journal, 21*(4), 18-24.

Faigenbaum, A., Bush, J., McLoone, R., Kreckel, M., Farrell, A., Ratamess, N., & Kang, J. (2015). Benefits of strength and skill based training during primary school physical education. *Journal of Strength and Conditioning Research, 29*(5), 1255-1262.

Faigenbaum, A., Farrell, A., Fabiano, M., Radler, T., Naclerio, F., Ratamess, N., . . . Myer, G. (2011). Effects of integrated neuromuscular training on fitness performance in children. *Pediatric Exercise Science, 23*, 573-584.

Faigenbaum, A., Farrell, A., Fabiano, M., Radler, T., Naclerio, F., Ratamess, N., . . . Myer, G. (2013). Effects of detraining on fitness performance in 7-year-old children. *Journal of Strength and Conditioning Research, 27*(2), 323-330.

Faigenbaum, A., Farrell, A., Radler, T., Zbojovsky, D., Chu, D., Ratamess, N., Hoffman, J. (2009). Plyo Play: A novel program of short bouts of moderate and high intensity exercise improves physical fitness in elementary school children. *The Physical Educator, 69,* 37-44.

Faigenbaum, A., Kang, J., Ratamess, N., Farrell, A., Ellis, N., Vought, I., & Bush, J. (2018). Acute cardiometabolic responses to medicine ball interval training in children. *International Journal of Exercise Science, 11*(4), 886-899.

Faigenbaum, A., Kang, J., Ratamess, N., Farrell, A., Golda, S., Stranieri, A., Bush, J. (2018). Acute cardiometabolic responses to battling rope exercise in children. *Journal of Strength and Conditioning Research, 32*(5), 1197-1206.

Faigenbaum, A., Kraemer, W., Blimkie, C., Jeffreys, I., Micheli, L., Nitka, M., & Rowland, T. (2009). Youth resistance training: Updated position statement paper from the National Strength and Conditioning Association. *Journal of Strength and Conditioning Research, 23*(Suppl 5), S60-S79.

Faigenbaum, A., Lloyd, R., MacDonald, J., & Myer, G. (2016). Citius, Altius, Fortius: Beneficial effects of resistance training for young athletes: Narrative review. *British Journal of Sports Medicine, 50*(1), 3-7.

Faigenbaum, A., Lloyd, R., & Myer, G. (2013). Youth resistance training: Past practices, new perspectives and future directions. *Pediatric Exercise Science, 25,* 591-604.

Faigenbaum, A.D., Loud, R.L., O'Connell, J., Glover, S., & Westcott, W.L. (2001). Effects of different resistance training protocols on upper-body strength and endurance development in children. *Journal of Strength and Conditioning Research, 15*(4), 459-465.

Faigenbaum, A., & MacDonald, J. (2017). Dynapenia: It's not just for grown-ups anymore. *Acta Paediatrica, 106,* 696-697.

Faigenbaum A, MacDonald J, Haff G. (2019). Are young athletes strong enough for sport? DREAM On. *Current Sports Medicine Reports,* 18(1): 6-8.

Faigenbaum, A., & McFarland, J. (2016). Youth resistance training: Right from the start. *ACSM's Health and Fitness Journal, 20*(5), 16-22.

Faigenbaum, A., McFarland, J., Herman, R., Naclerio, F., Ratamess, N., Kang, J., & Myer, G. (2012). Reliability of the one-repetition-maximum power clean test in adolescent athletes. *Journal of Strength and Conditioning Research, 26*(2), 432-437.

Faigenbaum, A., McFarland, J., Johnson, L., Kang, J., Bloom, J., Ratamess, N., & Hoffman, J. (2007). Preliminary evaluation of an after-school resistance training program for improving physical fitness in middle school-age boys. *Perceptual and Motor Skills, 104*(2), 407-415.

Faigenbaum, A., McFarland, J., Keiper, F., Tevlin, W., Ratamess, N., Kang, J., & Hoffman, J. (2007). Effects of a short term plyometric and resistance training program on fitness performance in boys age 12 to 15 years. *Journal of Sports Science and Medicine, 6,* 519-525.

Faigenbaum, A., & Mediate, P. (2006). The effects of medicine ball training on physical fitness in high school physical education students. *The Physical Educator, 63,* 160-167.

Faigenbaum, A., Milliken, L., & Westcott, W. (2003). Maximal strength testing in healthy children. *Journal of Strength and Conditioning Research, 17*(1), 162-166.

Faigenbaum, A., & Myer, G. (2010a). Pediatric resistance training: Benefits, concerns and program design considerations. *Current Sports Medicine Reports, 9*(3), 161-168.

Faigenbaum, A., & Myer, G. (2010b). Resistance training among young athletes: Safety, efficacy and injury prevention effects. *British Journal of Sports Medicine, 44,* 56-63.

Faigenbaum, A., Myer, G., Naclerio, F., & Casas, A. (2011). Injury trends and prevention in youth resistance training. *Strength and Conditioning, 33*(3), 36-41.

Faigenbaum, A., Ratamess, N., McFarland, J., Kaczmarek, J., Coraggio, M., Kang, J., & Hoffman, J. (2008). Effect of rest interval length on bench press performance in boys, teens, and men. *Pediatric Exercise Science, 20*(4), 457-469.

Faigenbaum, A., Westcott, W., Micheli, L., Outerbridge, A., Long, C., LaRosa-Loud, R., & Zaichkowsky, L. (1996). The effects of strength training and detraining on children. *Journal of Strength and Conditioning Research, 10*(2), 109-114.

Faigenbaum, A., Zaichkowsky, L., Westcott, W., Micheli, L., & Fehlandt, A. (1993). The effects of a twice per week strength training program on children. *Pediatric Exercise Science, 5,* 339-346.

Falk, B., & Dotan, R. (2006). Child-adult differences in the recovery from high-intensity exercise. *Exercise and Sport Science Reviews, 34*(3), 107-112. doi:00003677-200607000-00004

Falk, B., & Eliakim, A. (2003). Resistance training, skeletal muscle and growth. *Pediatric Endocrinology Reviews, 1*(2), 120-127.

Fernandez-Fernandez, J., de Villarreal, E., Sanz-Rivas, D., & Moya, M. (2016). The effects of 8-week plyometric training on physical performance in young tennis players. *Pediatric Exercise Science, 28*(1), 77-86.

Ferry, B., Lespessailles, E., Rochcongar, P., Duclos, M., & Courteix, D. (2013). Bone health during late adolescence: Effects of an 8-month training program on bone geometry in female athletes. *Joint, Bone, Spine, 80*(1), 57-63.

Fleck, S., & Kraemer, W. (2014). *Designing resistance training programs* (4th ed.). Champaign, IL: Human Kinetics.

Foss, K., Thomas, S., Khoury, J., Myer, G., & Hewett, T. (2018). A school-based neuromuscular training program and sport-related injury incidence: A prospective randomized controlled clinical trial. *Journal of Athletic Training, 53*(1), 20-28.

Francis, S., Morrissey, J., Letuchy, E., Levy, S., & Janz, K. (2013). Ten-year objective physical activity tracking: Iowa bone development study. *Medicine and Science in Sports and Exercise, 45*(8), 1508-1514.

Fransen, J., Deprez, D., Pion, J., Tallir, I., D'Hondt, E., Vaeyens, R., . . . Philippaerts, R. (2014). Changes in physical fitness and sports participation among children with different levels of motor competence: A 2-year longitudinal study. *Pediatric Exercise Science, 26*(1), 1-21.

Fraser, B., Huynh, Q., Schmidt, M., Dwyer, T., Venn, A., & Magnussen, C. (2016). Childhood muscular fitness phenotypes and adult metabolic syndrome. *Medicine and Science in Sports and Exercise, 48*(9), 1715-1722.

Fripp, R., & Hodgson, J. (1987). Effect of resistive training on plasma lipid and lipoprotein levels in male adolescents. *Journal of Pediatrics, 111,* 926-931.

Fritz, J., Rosengren, B., Dencker, M., Karlsson, C., & Karlsson, M. (2016). A seven-year physical activity intervention for children increased gains in bone mass and muscle strength. *Acta Paediatrica, 105*(10), 1216-1224.

Fröberg, A., Alricsson, M., & Ahnesjö, J. (2014). Awareness of current recommendations and guidelines regarding strength training for youth. *International Journal of Adolescent Medicine and Health, 26*(4), 517-523.

García-Hermoso A, Ramírez-Campillo R, Izquierdo M. (2019). Is Muscular Fitness Associated with Future Health Benefits in Children and Adolescents? A Systematic Review and Meta-Analysis of Longitudinal Studies. *Sports Medicine*, doi: 10.1007/s40279-019-01098-6 epub before print

Gomes, T., Dos Santos, F., Katzmarzyk, P., & Maia, J. (2017). Active and strong: physical activity, muscular strength, and metabolic risk in children. *American Journal of Human Biology, 29*(1).

Gómez-Bruton, A., Matute-Llorente, Á., González-Agüero, A., Casajús, J., & Vicente-Rodríguez, G. (2017). Plyometric exercise and bone health in children and adolescents: A systematic review. *World Journal of Pediatrics, 13*(2), 112-121.

Gordon, J., Dolinsky, V., Mughal, W., Gordon, G., & McGavock, J. (2015). Targeting skeletal muscle mitochondria to prevent type 2 diabetes in youth. *Biochemistry and Cell Biology, 93*(5), 452-465.

Granacher, U., Goesele, A., Roggo, K., Wischer, T., Fischer, S., Zuerny, C., . . . Kriemer, S. (2011). Effects and mechanisms of strength training in children. *International Journal of Sports Medicine, 32*, 357-364.

Granacher, U., Lesinski, M., Busch, D., Muehlbauer. T., Prieske, O., Puta, C., . . . Behm, D. (2016). Effects of resistance training in youth athletes on muscular fitness and athletic performance: A conceptual model for long-term athlete development. *Frontiers in Physiology, 7*(164).

Granacher, U., Schellbach, J., Klein, K., Prieske, O., Baeyens, J., & Muehlbauer, T. (2014). Effects of core strength training using stable versus unstable surfaces on physical fitness in adolescents: A randomized controlled trial. *BMC Sports Science, Medicine & Rehabilitation, 6*(1), 40.

Grøntved, A., Ried-Larsen, M., Christian Møller, N., Lund Kristensen, P., Froberg, K., Brage, S., & Bo Andersen, L. (2015). Muscle strength in youth and cardiovascular risk in young adulthood (the European Youth Heart Study). *British Journal of Sports Medicine, 49*, 90-94.

Guagliano, J., Rosenkranz, R., & Kolt, G. (2013). Girls' physical activity levels during organized sports in Australia. *Medicine and Science in Sports and Exercise, 45*(1), 116-122.

Gumbs, V., Segal, D., Halligan, J., & Lower, G. (1982). Bilateral distal radius and ulnar fractures in adolescent weightlifters. *American Journal of Sports Medicine, 10*, 375-379.

Gunter, K., Almstedt, H., & Janz, K. (2012). Physical activity in childhood may be the key to optimizing lifespan skeletal health. *Exercise and Sport Science Reviews, 40*(1), 13-21.

Haff, G. (2014). Periodization strategies for youth development. In R. Lloyd & J. Oliver (Eds.), *Strength and conditioning for young athletes: Science and application.* (pp. 149-168). Oxford, UK: Routledge Publishing.

Haff, G., & Nimphius, S. (2012). Training principles for power. *Strength and Conditioning Journal, 34*(6), 2-12.

Hagberg, J., Ehsani, A., Goldring, D., Hernandez, A., Sinacore, D., & Holloszy, J. (1984). Effect of weight training on blood pressure and hemodynamics in hypertensive adolescents. *Journal of Pediatrics, 104*, 147-151.

Harries, S., Lubans, D., & Callister, R. (2012). Resistance training to improve power and sports performance in adolescent athletes: A systematic review and meta-analysis. *Journal of Science and Medicine in Sport, 15*(6), 532-540.

Henriksson, H., Henriksson, P., Tynelius, P., & Ortega, F. (2018). Muscular weakness in adolescence is associated with disability 30 years later: A population-based cohort study of 1.2 million men. *British Journal of Sports Medicine, epub before print.*

Hewett, T.E., Myer, G.D., & Ford, K.R. (2004). Decrease in neuromuscular control about the knee with maturation in female athletes. *J Bone Joint Surg Am, 86-A*(8), 1601-1608. doi:86/8/1601

Hooper, D., Szivak, T., Comstock, B., Dunn-Lewis, C., Apicella, J., Kelly, N., . . . Kraemer, W. (2014). Effects of fatigue from resistance training on barbell back squat biomechanics. *Journal of Strength and Conditioning Research, 28*(4), 1127-1134.

Hulteen, R., Morgan, P., Barnett, L., Stodden, D., & Lubans, D. (2018). Development of foundational movement skills: A conceptual model for physical activity across the lifespan. *Sports Medicine, 48*(7), 1533-1540.

Ignjatovic, A., Markovic, Z., & Radovanovic, D. (2012). Effects of 12-week medicine ball training on muscle strength and power in young female handball players. *Journal of Strength and Conditioning Research, 26*(8), 2166-2173.

Ingle, L., Sleap, M., & Tolfrey, K. (2006). The effect of a complex training and detraining programme on selected strength and power variables in early prepubertal boys. *Journal of Sport Sciences, 24*, 987-997.

Ishikawa, S., Kim, Y., Kang, M., & Morgan, D. (2013). Effects of weight-bearing exercise on bone health in girls: A meta-analysis. *Sports Medicine, 43*(9), 875-892.

Janz, K., Letuchy, E., Francis, S., Metcalf, K., Burns, T., & Levy, S. (2014). Objectively measured physical activity predicts hip and spine bone mineral content in children and adolescents ages 5-15 years: Iowa bone development study. *Frontiers in Endocrinology, 5*(112).

Jenkins, N., & Mintowt-Czyz, W. (1986). Bilateral fracture separations of the distal radial epiphyses during weight-lifting. *British Journal of Sports Medicine, 20*, 72-73.

Kindler, J., Lewis, R., & Hamrick, M. (2015). Skeletal muscle and pediatric bone development. *Current Opinion in Endocrinology, Diabetes, and Obesity, 22*(6), 467-474.

Klentrou, P. (2016). Influence of exercise and training on critical stages of bone growth and development. *Pediatric Exercise Science, 28*(2), 178-186.

Komi, P. (2003). Stretch-shortening cycle. In P. Komi (Ed.), *Strength and power in sport* (pp. 184-202). Oxford, UK: Blackwell Scientific.

Kraemer, W., Fry, A., Frykman, P., Conroy, B., & Hoffman, J. (1989). Resistance training and youth. *Pediatric Exercise Science, 1*, 336-350.

Larsen, M., Nielsen, C., Helge, E., Madsen, M., Manniche, V., Hansen, L., . . . Krustrup, P. (2018). Positive effects on bone mineralisation and muscular fitness after 10 months of intense school-based physical training for children aged 8-10 years: The FIT FIRST randomised controlled trial. *British Journal of Sports Medicine, 52*, 254-260.

Lauersen, J., Bertelsen, D., & Andersen, L. (2014). The effectiveness of exercise interventions to prevent sports injuries: A systematic review and meta-analysis of randomised controlled trials. *British Journal of Sports Medicine, 48*(11), 871-877.

Lazaridis, S., Bassa, E., Patikas, D., Hatzikotoulas, K., Lazaridis, F., & Kotzamanidis, C. (2013). Biomechanical comparison in different jumping tasks between untrained boys and men. *Pediatric Exercise Science, 25*(1), 101-113.

Leek, D., Carlson, J., Cain, K., Henrichon, S., Rosenberg, D., Patrick, K., & Sallis, J.F. (2010). Physical activity during youth sports practices. *Archives of Pediatric and Adolescent Medicine, 165*(4), 294-299.

Lesinski, M., Prieske, O., & Granacher, U. (2016). Effects and dose–response relationships of resistance training on physical performance in youth athletes: A systematic review and meta-analysis. *British Journal of Sports Medicine, 50*(13), 781-795.

Lillegard, W.A., Brown, E.W., Wilson, D.J., Henderson, R., & Lewis, E. (1997). Efficacy of strength training in prepubescent to early postpubescent males and females: Effects of gender and maturity. *Pediatric Rehabilitation, 1*(3), 147-157.

Lloyd, R., Cronin, J., Faigenbaum, A., Haff, G., Howard, R., Kraemer, W., . . . Oliver, J. (2016). The National Strength and Conditioning Association position statement on long-term athletic development. *Journal of Strength and Conditioning Research, 30*(6), 1491-1509.

Lloyd, R., Faigenbaum, A., Stone, M., Oliver, J., Jeffreys, I., Moody, J., . . . Myer, G. (2014). Position statement on youth resistance training: The 2014 International Consensus. *British Journal of Sports Medicine, 48*(7), 498-505.

Lloyd, R., Meyers, R., & Oliver, J. (2011). The natural developmentand trainability of plyometric ability during childhood. *Strength and Conditioning, 33*(2), 23-32.

Lloyd, R., Oliver, J., Faigenbaum, A., Howard, R., De Ste Croix, M., Williams, C., . . . Myer, G. (2015). Long-term physical development: Barriers to success and potential solutions—Part 2. *Journal of Strength and Conditioning Research, 29*(5), 1451-1464.

Lloyd, R., Oliver, J., Hughes, M., & Williams, C. (2012). Effects of 4-weeks plyometric training on reactive strength index and leg stiffness in male youths. *Journal of Strength and Conditioning Research, 26*(10), 2812-2819.

Lloyd, R., Radnor, J., De Ste Croix, M., Cronin, J., & Oliver, J. (2015). Changes in sprint and jump performance following traditional, plyometric and combined resistance training in male youth pre- and post-peak height velocity. *Journal of Strength and Conditioning Research, 30*(5), 1239-1247.

Lloyd, R., Radnor, J., De Ste Croix, M., Cronin, J., & Oliver, J. (2016). Changes in sprint and jump performances after traditional, plyometric, and combined resistance training in male youth pre- and post-peak height velocity. *Journal of Strength and Conditioning Research, 30*(5), 1239-1247.

Lobstein, T., Jackson-Leach, R., Moodie, M., Hall, K., Gortmaker, S., Swinburn, B., . . . McPherson, K. (2015). Child and adolescent obesity: Part of a bigger picture. *Lancet, 385*(9986), 2510-2520.

Löfgren, B., Daly, R., Nilsson, J., Dencker, M., & Karlsson, M. (2013). An increase in school-based physical education increases muscle strength in children. *Medicine and Science in Sports and Exercise, 45*(5), 997-1003.

Loturco, I., Nakamura, F., Kobal, R., Gil, S., Abad, C., Cuniyochi, R., . . . Roschel, H. (2015). Training for power and speed: effects of increasing or decreasing jump squat velocity in elite young soccer players. *Journal of Strength and Conditioning Research, 29*(10), 2771-2779.

Lubans, D., Smith, J., Harries, S., Barnett, L., & Faigenbaum, A. (2014). Development, test-retest reliability, and construct validity of the resistance training skills battery. *Journal of Strength and Conditioning Research, 28*(5), 1373-1380.

Malina, R. (2006). Weight training in youth—Growth, maturation, and safety: An evidence-based review. *Clinical Journal of Sports Medicine, 16*(6), 478-487.

Malina, R., Baxter-Jones, A., Armstrong, N., Beunen, G., Caine, D., Daly, R., . . . Russell, K. (2013). Role of intensive training in the growth and maturation of artistic gymnasts. *Sports Medicine, 43*(9), 783-802.

Malina, R., Bouchard, C., & Bar-Or, O. (2004). *Growth, maturation and physical activity* (2nd ed.). Champaign, IL: Human Kinetics.

Marshall, D., Lopatina, E., Lacny, S., & Emery, C. (2016). Economic impact study: Neuromuscular training reduces the burden of injuries and costs compared to standard warm-up in youth soccer. *British Journal of Sports Medicine, 50*(22), 1388-1393.

Mascarin, N., de Lira, C., Vancini, R., de Castro Pochini, A., da Silva, A., & Andrade Mdos, S. (2016). Strength training using elastic band improves muscle power and throwing performance in young female handball players. *Journal of Sport Rehabilitation, 26*(3), 245-252.

Matos, N., Winsley, R., & Williams, C. (2011). Prevalence of nonfunctional overreaching/overtraining in young English athletes. *Medicine and Science in Sports, 43*(7), 1287-1294.

Mayer-Davis E, Dabelea D, Lawrence J. et al (2017). Incidence trends of Type 1 and Type 2 diabetes among Youths, 2002-2012. *New England Journal of Medicine, 376*(15): 1419-1429.

McGladrey, B., Hannon, J., Faigenbaum, A., Shultz, B., & Shaw, J. (2014). High school physical educators' and sport coaches' knowledge of resistance training principles and methods. *Journal of Strength and Conditioning Research, 28*(5), 1433-1442.

McKay, H., Tsang, G., Heinonen, A., MacKelvie, K., Sanderson, D., & Khan, K.M. (2005). Ground reaction forces associated with an effective elementary school based jumping intervention. *British Journal of Sports Medicine, 39*, 10-14.

McNitt-Gray, J., Hester, D., Mathiyakom, W., & Munkasy, B. (2001). Mechanical demand on multijoint control during landing depend on orientation of the body segments relative to the reaction force. *Journal of Biomechanics, 34*, 1471-1482.

Meinhardt, U., Witassek, F., Petrò, R., Fritz, C., & Eiholzer, U. (2013). Strength training and physical activity in boys: A randomized trial. *Pediatrics, 132*(6), 1105-1111.

Meylan, C., Cronin, J., Oliver, J., Hopkins, W., & Contreras, B. (2014). The effect of maturation on adaptations to strength training and detraining in 11-15-year-olds. *Scandinavian Journal of Medicine and Science in Sport, 24*(3), e156-e164.

Micheli, L. (1988). Strength training in the young athlete. In E. Brown & C. Branta (Eds.), *Competitive sports for children and youth* (pp. 99-105). Champaign, IL: Human Kinetics.

Moraes, E., Fleck, S., Ricardo Dias, M., & Simão, R. (2013). Effects on strength, power, and flexibility in adolescents of nonperiodized vs. daily nonlinear periodized weight training. *Journal of Strength and Conditioning Research, 27*(12), 3310-3321.

Moran, J., Sandercock, G., Ramirez-Campillo, R., Clark, C., Fernandes, J., & Drury, B. (2018). A meta-analysis of resistance training in female youth: Its effect on muscular trength, and shortcomings in the literature. *Sports Medicine, 48*(7), 1661-1671.

Murphy, J., Button, D., Chaouachi, A., & Behm, D. (2014). Prepubescent males are less susceptible to neuromuscular fatigue following resistance exercise. *European Journal of Applied Physiology, 114*(4), 825-835.

Myer, G., Chu, D., Brent, J., & Hewett, T. (2008). Trunk and hip control neuromuscular training for the prevention of knee joint injury. *Clinical Journal of Sports Medicine, 27*(3), 425-448.

Myer, G., Faigenbaum, A., Edwards, E., Clark. J., Best, T., & Sallis, R. (2015). 60 minutes of what? A developing brain perspective for activation children with an integrative approach. *British Journal of Sports Medicine, 49*(12), 1510-1516.

Myer, G., Jayanthi, N., DiFiori, J., Faigenbaum, A., Kiefer, A., Logerstedt, D., & Micheli, L. (2015). Sports specialization, part II: Alternative solutions to early sport specialization in youth athletes. *Sports Health, 8*(1), 65-73.

Myer, G., Quatman, C., Khoury, J., Wall, E., & Hewett, T. (2009). Youth vs. adult "weightlifting" injuries presented to United States Emergengy Rooms: Accidental vs. non-accidental injury mechanisms. *Journal of Strength and Conditioning Research, 23*(7), 2054-2060.

Nasri, R., Hassen Zrour, S., Rebai, H., Fadhel Najjar, M., Neffeti, F., Bergaoui, N., . . . Tabka, Z. (2013). Grip strength is a predictor of bone mineral density among adolescent combat sport athletes. *Journal of Clinical Densitometry, 16*(1), 92-97.

National Strength and Conditioning Association. (1985). Position paper on prepubescent strength training. *National Strength and Conditioning Association Journal, 7*, 27-31.

Ortega, F., Silventoinen, K., Tynelius, P., & Rasmussen, F. (2012). Muscular strength in male adolescents and premature death: Cohort study of one million participants. *BMJ, 345*, e7279.

Owoeye, O., Palacios-Derflingher, L., & Emery, C. (2018). Prevention of ankle sprain injuries in youth soccer and basketball: Effectiveness of a neuromuscular training program and examining risk factors. *Clinical Journal of Sports Medicine, 28*(4), 325-331.

Ozmen, T., & Aydogmus, M. (2016). Effect of core strength training on dynamic balance and agility in adolescent badminton players. *Journal of Bodywork and Movement Therapies, 20*(3), 565-570.

Ozmun, J.C., Mikesky, A.E., & Surburg, P.R. (1994). Neuromuscular adaptations following prepubescent strength training. *Medicine and Science in Sports and Exercise, 26*(4), 510-514.

Peitz, M, Behringer, M, Granacher, U. A systematic review on the effects of resistance and plyometric training on physical fitness in youth- What do comparative studies tell us? (2018). *PLoS One*, 13(10): e0205525. doi: 10.1371/journal.pone.0205525.

Peterson, M., Zhang, P., Saltarelli, W., Visich, P., & Gordon, P. (2016). Low muscle strength thresholds for the detection of cardiometabolic risk in adolescents. *American Journal of Preventive Medicine, 50*(5), 593-599.

Pfeiffer, R., & Francis, R. (1986). Effects of strength trianing on muscle development in prepubescent, pubescent and postpubescent males. *Physician and Sports Medicine, 14*(9), 134-143.

Piazza, M., Battaglia, C., Fiorilli, G., Innocenti, G., Iuliano, E., Aquino, G., . . . Di Cagno A. (2014). Effects of resistance training on jumping performance in pre-adolescent rhythmic gymnasts: A randomized controlled study. *Italian Journal of Anatomy and Embryology, 119*(1), 10-19.

Prieske, O., Muehlbauer, T., Borde, R., Gube, M., Bruhn, S., Behm, D., & Granacher, U. (2016). Neuromuscular and athletic performance following core strength training in elite youth soccer: Role of instability. *Scandinavian Journal of Medicine and Science in Sport, 26*(1), 48-56.

Racil, G., Zouhal, H., Elmontassar, W., Ben Abderrahmane, A., De Sousa, M., Chamari, K., . . . Coquart, J. (2016). Plyometric exercise combined with high-intensity interval training improves metabolic abnormalities in young obese females more so than interval training alone. *Applied Physiology Nutrition and Metabolism, 41*(1), 103-109.

Ramírez-Campillo, R., Meylan, C., Alvarez, C., Henríquez-Olguín, C., Martínez, C., Cañas-Jamett, R., . . . Izquierdo, M. (2014). Effects of in-season low-volume high-intensity plyometric training on explosive actions and endurance of young soccer players. *Journal of Strength and Conditioning Research, 28*(5), 1335-1342.

Ramsay, J.A., Blimkie, C.J., Smith, K., Garner, S., MacDougall, J.D., & Sale, D.G. (1990). Strength training effects in prepubescent boys. *Medicine and Science in Sports and Exercise, 22*(5), 605-614.

Ratamess, N. (2012). *ACSM's foundations of strength training and conditioning*. Philadelphia, PA: Lippincott, Williams and Wilkins.

Renstrom, P., Ljungqvist, A., Arendt, E., Beynnon, B., Fukubayashi, T., Garrett, W., . . . Engebretsen, L. (2016). Non-contact ACL injuries in female athletes: An International Olympic Committee current concepts statement. *British Journal of Sports Medicine, 42*(6), 394-412.

Rians, C.B., Weltman, A., Cahill, B.R., Janney, C.A., Tippett, S.R., & Katch, F.I. (1987). Strength training for prepubescent males: Is it safe? *Am J Sports Med, 15*(5), 483-489.

Richmond, S., Kang, J., Doyle-Baker, P., Nettel-Aguirre, A., & Emery, C. (2016). A school-based injury prevention program to reduce sport injury risk and improve healthy outcomes in youth: A pilot cluster-randomized controlled trial. *Clinical Journal of Sports Medicine, 26*(4), 291-298.

Ridley, K., Zabeen, S., & Lunnay, B. (2018). Children's physical activity levels during organised sports practices. *Journal of Science and Medicine in Sport*. 21(9): 930-934 doi: 10.1016/j.jsams.2018.01.019

Rivière, M., Louit, L., Strokosch, A., & Seitz, L. (2016). Variable resistance training promotes greater strength and power adaptations than traditional resistance training in elite youth rugby league players. *Journal of Strength and Conditioning Research, 31*(4), 947-955.

Robinson, L., Stodden, D., Barnett, L., Lopes, V., Logan, S., Rodrigues, L., & D'Hondt, E. (2015). Motor competence and its effect on positive developmental trajectories of health. *Sports Medicine, 45*(9), 1273-1284.

Robinson, L., Veldman, S., Palmer, K., & Okely, A. (2017). A ball skills intervention in preschoolers: The CHAMP randomized controlled trial. *Medicine and Science in Sports and Exercise, 49*(11), 2234-2239.

Rowe, P.H. (1979). Colles fracture due to weightlifting. *British Journal of Sports Medicine, 13*(3), 130-131.

Ruas, C., Punt, C., Pinto, R., & Oliveira, M. (2014). Strength and power in children with low motor performance scores: A descriptive analysis. *Brazilian Journal of Motor Behavior, 8*(1), 1-8.

Rumpf, M., Cronin, J., Pinder, S., Oliver, J., & Hughes, M. (2012). Effect of different training methods on running sprint times in male youth. *Pediatric Exercise Science, 24*(2), 170-186.

Ryan, J., & Salciccioli, G. (1976). Fractures of the distal radial epiphysis in adolescent weight lifters. *American Journal of Sports Medicine, 4*, 26-27.

Sander, A., Keiner, M., Wirth, K., & Schmidtbleicher, D. (2013). Influence of a 2-year strength training programme on power performance in elite youth soccer players. *European Journal of Sport Science, 13*(5), 445-451.

Santos, E., & Janeira, M. (2008). Effects of complex training on explosive strength in adolescent male basketball players. *Journal of Strength and Conditioning Research, 22*, 903-909.

Santos, E., & Janeira, M. (2009). Effects of reduced training and detraining on upper and lower body explosive strength in adolescent male basketball players. *Journal of Strength and Conditioning Research, 23*(6), 1737-1744.

Schranz, N., Tomkinson, G., Parletta, N., Petkov, J., & Olds, T. (2014). Can resistance training change the strength, body composition and self-concept of overweight and obese adolescent males? A randomised controlled trial. *British Journal of Sports Medicine, 48*(20), 1482-1488.

Sigal, R., Alberga, A., Goldfield, G., Prud'homme, D., Hadjiyannakis, S., Gougeon, R., . . . Kenny, G. (2014). Effects of aerobic training, resistance training, or both on percentage body fat and cardiometabolic risk markers in obese adolescents: The healthy eating aerobic and resistance training in youth randomized clinical trial. *JAMA Pediatrics, 168*(11), 1006-1014.

Smith, J., Eather, N., Morgan, P., Plotnikoff, R., Faigenbaum, A., & Lubans, D. (2014). The health benefits of muscular fitness for children and adolescents: A systematic review and meta-analysis. *Sports Medicine, 44*(9), 1209-1223.

Smith, J, Eather, N, Weaver, R, Riley, N, Beets, M, Lubans, D. (2019). Behavioral correlates of muscular fitness in children and adolescents: A systematic review. *Sports Medicine,* doi: 10.1007/s40279-019-01089-7. Epub before print

Society of Health and Physical Educators–SHAPE America. (2014). *National standards & grade level outcomes for K-12 physical education.* Champaign, IL: Human Kinetics.

Sommi, C., Gill, F., Trojan, J., & Mulcahey, M. (2018). Strength and conditioning in adolescent female athletes. *Physician and Sports Medicine.* 46(4): 420-426 doi: 10.1080/00913847.2018.1486677

Specker, B., Thiex, N., & Sudhagoni, R. (2015). Does exercise influence pediatric bone? A systematic review. *Clinical Orthopedics and Related Research, 473*(11), 3658-3672.

Suchomel, T., Nimphius, S., & Stone, M. (2016). The importance of muscular strength in athletic performance. *Sports Medicine, 46*(10), 1419-1449.

Sugimoto, D., Myer, G., Barber Foss, K., & Hewett, T. (2015). Specific exercise effects of preventive neuromuscular training intervention on anterior cruciate ligament injury risk reduction in young females: meta-analysis and subgroup analysis. *British Journal of Sports Medicine, 49*(5), 282-289.

Sugimoto, D., Myer, G., Barber Foss, K., Pepin, M., Micheli, L., & Hewett, T. (2016). Critical components of neuromuscular training to reduce ACL injury risk in female athletes: Meta-regression analysis. *British Journal of Sports Medicine, 50*(20), 1259-1266.

Sugimoto, D., Myer, G., Foss, K., & Hewett, T. (2015). Specific exercise effects of preventive neuromuscular training intervention on anterior cruciate ligament injury risk reduction in young females: Meta-analysis and subgroup analysis. *British Journal of Sports Medicine, 49*(5), 282-289.

Sung, R.Y., Yu, C.W., Chang, S.K., Mo, S.W., Woo, K.S., & Lam, C.W. (2002). Effects of dietary intervention and strength training on blood lipid level in obese children. *Archives of Disease in Childhood, 86*(6), 407-410.

Tarp, J, Bugge, A, Møller, NC, Klakk, H, Rexen, CT, Grøntved, A, Wedderkopp, N . (2019). Muscle fitness changes during childhood associates with improvements in cardiometabolic risk factors: A prospective study. *Journal of Physical Activity and Health.* 16(2): 108-115.

ten Hoor, G., Sleddens, E., Kremers, S., Schols, A., Kok, G., & Plasqui, G. (2015). Aerobic and strength exercises for youngsters aged 12 to 15: What do parents think? *BMC Public Health, 15,* 994.

Thomas, K., French, D., & Hayes, P. (2009). The effect of two plyometric training techniques on muscular power and agility in youth soccer players. *Journal of Strength and Conditioning Research, 23*(1), 332-335.

Thompson-Kolesar, J., Gatewood, C., Tran, A., Silder, A., Shultz, R., Delp, S., & Dragoo, J. (2018). Age influences biomechanical changes after participation in an anterior cruciate ligament injury prevention program. *American Journal of Sports Medicine, 46*(3), 598-606.

Tibana, R., Prestes, J., ,, Nascimento, D., Martins, O., De Santana, F., & Balsamo, S. (2012). Higher muscle performance in adolescents compared with adults after a resistance training session with different rest intervals. *Journal of Strength and Conditioning Research, 26*(4), 1027-1032.

Tsolakis, C., Vagenas, G., & Dessypris, A. (2004). Strength adaptations and hormonal responses to resistance training and detraining in preadolescent males. *Journal of Strength and Conditioning Research, 18*(3), 625-629.

Tveit, M., Rosengren, B., Nilsson, J., & Karlsson, M. (2015). Exercise in youth: High bone mass, large bone size, and low fracture risk in old age. *Scandinavian Journal of Medicine and Science in Sport, 25*(4), 453-461.

Utesch, T, Bardid, F, Büsch, D, Strauss, B. (2019). The relationship between motor competence and physical fitness from early childhood to early adulthood: A meta-analysis. *Sports Medicine,* 49(4): 541-551.

Van der Heijden, G., Wang, Z., Chu, Z., Toffolo, G., Manesso, E., Sauer, P., & Sunehag, A. (2010). Strength exercise improves muscle mass and hepatic insulin sensitivity in obese youth. *Medicine and Science in Sports and Exercise, 42*(11), 1973-1980.

Virvidakis, K., Georgiu, E., Korkotsidis, A., Ntalles, A., & Proukakis, C. (1990). Bone mineral content of junior competitive weightlifters. *International Journal of Sports Medicine, 11,* 244-246.

Vrijens, F. (1978). Muscle strength development in the pre and post pubescent age. *Medicine and Sport Science, 11,* 152-158.

Waugh, C., Korff, T., Fath F., & Blazevich, A. (2014). Effects of resistance training on tendon mechanical properties and rapid force production in prepubertal children. *Journal of Applied Physiology, 117,* 257-266.

Weaver, C., Gordon, C., Janz, K., Kalkwarf, H., Lappe, J., Lewis, R., . . . Zemel, B. (2016). The National Osteoporosis Foundation's position statement on peak bone mass development and lifestyle factors: A systematic review and implementation recommendations. *Osteoporosis International, 27*(4), 1281-1386.

Webster, K., Hewett, T., Meta-analysis of meta-analyses of anterior cruciate ligament injury reduction training programs (2018). *Journal of Orthopaedic Research, 36*(10): 2696-2708.

Weltman, A., Janney, C., Rians, C., Strand, K., & Katch, F. (1987). Effects of hydraulic-resistance strength training on serum lipids in prepubertal boys. *American Journal of Diseases in Children, 141,* 777-780.

Westcott, W. (1979). Female response to weight training. *The Journal of Physical Education, 77*(2), 31-33.

World Health Organization. (2010). *Global recommendations on physical activity for health*. Geneva, Switzerland: Author.

Zouch, M., Vico, L., Frere, D., Tabka, Z., & Alexandre, C. (2014). Young male soccer players exhibit additional bone mineral acquisition during the peripubertal period: 1-year longitudinal study. *European Journal of Pediatrics, 173*(1), 53-61.

Chapter 10 Speed and Agility Training

Abernethy, B., Baker, J., & Cote, J. (2005). Transfer of pattern recall skills may contribute to the development of sport expertise. *Applied Cognitive Psychology , 19*, 705-718.

Alcaraz, P.E., Palao, J.M., & Elvira, J.L. (2009). Determining the optimal load for resisted sprint training with sled towing. *Journal of Strength and Conditioning Research, 23*(2), 480-485. doi:10.1519/JSC.0b013e318198f92c

Asadi, A., Arazi, H., Ramirez-Campillo, R., Moran, J., & Izquierdo, M. (2017). Influence of maturation stage on agility performance Gains after plyometric training: A systematic review and meta-analysis. *Journal of Strength and Conditioning Research, 31*(9), 2609-2617. doi:10.1519/JSC.0000000000001994

Bachero-Mena, B., & Gonzalez-Badillo, J.J. (2014). Effects of resisted sprint training on acceleration with three different loads accounting for 5, 12.5, and 20% of body mass. *Journal of Strength and Conditioning Research, 28*(10), 2954-2960. doi:10.1519/JSC.0000000000000492

Baker, J., Cote, J., & Abernethy, B. (2003). Sport-specific practice and the development of expert decision-making in team ball sports. *Journal of Applied Psychology, 15*, 12-25.

Baquet, G., van Praagh, E., & Berthoin, S. (2003). Endurance training and aerobic fitness in young people. *Sports Medicine, 33*(15), 1127-1143.

Bar-Or, O., & Rowland, T.W. (2004). *Pediatric exercise medicine: From physiological principles to health care application*. Champaign, IL: Human Kinetics.

Bedoya, A.A., Miltenberger, M.R., & Lopez, R.M. (2015). Plyometric training effects on athletic performance in youth soccer athletes: A systematic review. *Journal of Strength and Conditioning Research, 29*(8), 2351-2360. doi:10.1519/JSC.0000000000000877

Behringer, M., Vom Heede, A., Yue, Z., & Mester, J. (2010). Effects of resistance training in children and adolescents: A meta-analysis. *Pediatrics, 126*(5), e1199-e1210. doi:10.1542/peds.2010-0445

Besier, T.F., Lloyd, D.G., Cochrane, J.L., & Ackland, T.R. (2001). External loading of the knee joint during running and cutting maneuvers. *Medicine and Science in Sports and Exercise, 33*(7), 1168-1175.

Bloomfield, J., Ackland, T.R., & Elliot, B.C. (1994). *Applied anatomy and biomechanics in sport*. Melbourne, Victoria: Blackwell Scientific.

Bret, C., Rahmani, A., Dufour, A.B., Messonnier, L., & Lacour, J.R. (2002). Leg strength and stiffness as ability factors in 100 m sprint running. *Journal of Sports Medicine and Physical Fitness, 42*(3), 274-281.

Buchheit, M., Samozino, P., Glynn, J.A., Michael, B.S., Al Haddad, H., Mendez-Villanueva, A., & Morin, J.B. (2014). Mechanical determinants of acceleration and maximal sprinting speed in highly trained young soccer players. *Journal of Sports Sciences, 32*(20), 1906-1913. doi:10.1080/02640414.2014.965191

Casey, B.J., Giedd, J.N., & Thomas, K.M. (2000). Structural and functional brain development and its relation to cognitive development. *Biological Psychology, 54*(1-3), 241-257.

Casey, B.J., Tottenham, N., Liston, C., & Durston, S. (2005). Imaging the developing brain: What have we learned about cognitive development? *Trends in Cognitive Sciences, 9*(3), 104-110. doi:10.1016/j.tics.2005.01.011

Catley, M.J., & Tomkinson, G.R. (2013). Normative health-related fitness values for children: Analysis of 85347 test results on 9-17-year-old Australians since 1985. *British Journal of Sports Medicine, 47*(2), 98-108. doi:10.1136/bjsports-2011-090218

Chaouachi, A., Chtara, M., Hammami, R., Chtara, H., Turki, O., & Castagna, C. (2014). Multidirectional sprints and small-sided games training effect on agility and change of direction abilities in youth soccer. *Journal of Strength and Conditioning Research, 28*(11), 3121-3127. doi:10.1519/JSC.0000000000000505

Chaouachi, A., Hammami, R., Kaabi, S., Chamari, K., Drinkwater, E., & Behm, D. (2014). Olympic weightlifting and plyometric training with children provides similar or greater performance improvements than traditional resistance training. *Journal of Strength and Conditioning Research*.

Chelly, S.M., & Denis, C. (2001). Leg power and hopping stiffness: Relationship with sprint running performance. *Medicine and Science in Sports and Exercise, 33*(2), 326-333.

Chiodera, P., Volta, E., Gobbi, G., Milioli, M.A., Mirandola, P., Bonetti, A., . . . Vitale, M. (2008). Specifically designed physical exercise programs improve children's motor abilities. *Scandinavian Journal of Medicine & Science in Sports, 18*(2), 179-187. doi:10.1111/j.1600-0838.2007.00682.x

Cooper, D.M. (1995). New horizons in pediatric exercise research. In C.J.R. Blimkie & O. Bar-Or (Eds.), *New horizons in pediatric exercise science* (pp. 1-24). Champaign, IL: Human Kinetics.

Cormie, P., McGuigan, M.R., & Newton, R.U. (2011a). Developing maximal neuromuscular power: Part 1—Biological basis of maximal power production. *Sports Medicine, 41*(1), 17-38. doi:10.2165/11537690-000000000-00000

Cormie, P., McGuigan, M.R., & Newton, R.U. (2011b). Developing maximal neuromuscular power: Part 2—Training considerations for improving maximal power production. *Sports Medicine, 41*(2), 125-146. doi:10.2165/11538500-000000000-00000

Cronin, J.B., & Hansen, K.T. (2005). Strength and power predictors of sports speed. *Journal of Strength and Conditioning Research, 19*(2), 349-357. doi:10.1519/14323.1

Delaney, J.A., Scott, T.J., Ballard, D.A., Duthie, G.M., Hickmans, J.A., Lockie, R.G., & Dascombe, B.J. (2015). Contributing factors to change-of-direction ability in professional Rugby League players. *Journal of Strength and Conditioning Research, 29*(10), 2688-2696. doi:10.1519/JSC.0000000000000960

Dotan, R., Mitchell, C., Cohen, R., Klentrou, P., Gabriel, D., & Falk, B. (2012). Child-adult differences in muscle activation—A review. *Pediatric Exercise Science, 24*(1), 2-21.

Eisenmann, J.C., & Malina, R.M. (2003). Age- and sex-associated variation in neuromuscular capacities of adolescent distance runners. *Journal of Sports Sciences, 21*(7), 551-557. doi:10.1080/0264041031000101845

Faigenbaum, A.D., Farrell, A., Fabiano, M., Radler, T., Naclerio, F., Ratamess, N.A., . . . Myer, G.D. (2011). Effects of integrative neuromuscular training on fitness performance in children. *Pediatric Exercise Science, 23*(4), 573-584.

Faigenbaum, A.D., & McFarland, J.E. (2014). Criterion repetion maximum testing. *Strength and Conditioning Journal, 36*(1), 88-91.

Faigenbaum, A.D., McFarland, J.E., Keiper, F.B., Tevlin, W., Ratamess, N.A., Kang, J., & Hoffman, J.R. (2007). Effects of a short-term plyometric and resistance training program on fitness performance in boys age 12 to 15 years. *Journal of Sports Science & Medicine, 6*(4), 519-525.

Farley, C.T., & Gonzalez, O. (1996). Leg stiffness and stride frequency in human running. *Journal of Biomechanics, 29*(2), 181-186.

Figueiredo, A.J., Goncalves, C.E., Coelho, E.S.M.J., & Malina, R.M. (2009). Youth soccer players, 11-14 years: Maturity, size, function, skill and goal orientation. *Annals of Human Biology, 36*(1), 60-73. doi:10.1080/03014460802570584

Forbes, H., Bullers, A., Lovell, A., McNaughton, L.R., Polman, R.C., & Siegler, J.C. (2009). Relative torque profiles of elite male youth footballers: Effects of age and pubertal development. *International Journal of Sports Medicine, 30*(8), 592-597. doi:10.1055/s-0029-1202817

Gallahue, D.L., Ozmun, J.C., & Goodway, J.D. (2012). *Understanding motor development*. New York, NY: McGraw-Hill.

Garcia-Pinillos, F., Martinez-Amat, A., Hita-Contreras, F., Martinez-Lopez, E.J., & Latorre-Roman, P.A. (2014). Effects of a contrast training program without external load on vertical jump, kicking speed, sprint, and agility of young soccer players. *Journal of Strength and Conditioning Research, 28*(9), 2452-2460. doi:10.1519/JSC.0000000000000452

Gogtay, N., Giedd, J.N., Lusk, L., Hayashi, K.M., Greenstein, D., Vaituzis, A.C., . . . Thompson, P.M. (2004). Dynamic mapping of human cortical development during childhood through early adulthood. *Proceedings of the National Academy of Sciences of the United States of America, 101*(21), 8174-8179. doi:10.1073/pnas.0402680101

Hammami, M., Negra, Y., Billaut, F., Hermassi, S., Shephard, R.J., & Chelly, M.S. (2017). Effects of lower-limb strength training on agility, repeated sprinting with changes of direction, leg peak power, and neuromuscular adaptations of soccer players. *Journal of Strength and Conditioning Research.* doi:10.1519/JSC.0000000000001813

Hammami, M., Negra, Y., Shephard, R.J., & Chelly, M.S. (2017). The effect of standard strength vs. contrast strength training on the development of sprint, agility, repeated change of direction, and jump in junior male soccer players. *Journal of Strength and Conditioning Research, 31*(4), 901-912. doi:10.1519/JSC.0000000000001815

Harrison, A.J., & Bourke, G. (2009). The effect of resisted sprint training on speed and strength performance in male rugby players. *Journal of Strength and Conditioning Research, 23*(1), 275-283. doi:10.1519/JSC.0b013e318196b81f

Hatamoto, Y., Yamada, Y., Sagayama, H., Higaki, Y., Kiyonaga, A., & Tanaka, H. (2014). The relationship between running velocity and the energy cost of turning during running. *PLoS One, 9*(1), e81850. doi:10.1371/journal.pone.0081850

Hausdorff, J.M., Zemany, L., Peng, C., & Goldberger, A.L. (1999). Maturation of gait dynamics: Stride-to-stride variability and its temporal organization in children. *Journal of Applied Physiology, 86*(3), 1040-1047.

Hill-Haas, S.V., Dawson, B., Impellizzeri, F.M., & Coutts, A.J. (2011). Physiology of small-sided games training in football: A systematic review. *Sports Medicine, 41*(3), 199-220. doi:10.2165/11539740-000000000-00000

Hirose, N., & Seki, T. (2015). Two-year changes in anthropometric and motor ability values as talent identification indexes in youth soccer players. *Journal of Science and Medicine in Sport.* doi:10.1016/j.jsams.2015.01.004

Hunter, J.P., Marshall, R.N., & McNair, P.J. (2004). Interaction of step length and step rate during sprint running. *Medicine and Science in Sports and Exercise, 36*(2), 261-271. doi:10.1249/01.MSS.0000113664.15777.53

Ingle, L., Sleap, M., & Tolfrey, K. (2006). The effect of a complex training and detraining programme on selected strength and power variables in early pubertal boys. *Journal of Sports Sciences, 24*(9), 987-997. doi:10.1080/02640410500457117

Jakovljevic, S.T., Karalejic, M.S., Pajic, Z.B., Macura, M.M., & Erculj, F.F. (2012). Speed and agility of 12- and 14-year-old elite male basketball players. *Journal of Strength and Conditioning Research, 26*(9), 2453-2459. doi:10.1519/JSC.0b013e31823f2b22

Jones, P., Bampouras, T.M., & Marrin, K. (2009). An investigation into the physical determinants of change of direction speed. *Journal of Sports Medicine and Physical Fitness, 49*(1), 97-104.

Jullien, H., Bisch, C., Largouet, N., Manouvrier, C., Carling, C.J., & Amiard, V. (2008). Does a short period of lower limb strength training improve performance in field-based tests of running and agility in young professional soccer players? *Journal of Strength and Conditioning Research, 22*(2), 404-411. doi:10.1519/JSC.0b013e31816601e5

Junge, A., Rosch, D., Peterson, L., Graf-Baumann, T., & Dvorak, J. (2002). Prevention of soccer injuries: A prospective intervention study in youth amateur players. *The American Journal of Sports Medicine, 30*(5), 652-659.

Kawamori, N., Newton, R., & Nosaka, K. (2014). Effects of weighted sled towing on ground reaction force during the acceleration phase of sprint running. *Journal of Sports Sciences, 32*(12), 1139-1145. doi:10.1080/02640414.2014.886129

Keiner, M., Sander, A., Wirth, K., & Schmidtbleicher, D. (2014). Long-term strength training effects on change-of-direction sprint performance. *Journal of Strength and Conditioning Research, 28*(1), 223-231. doi:10.1519/JSC.0b013e318295644b

Kotzamanidis, C., D. Chatzopoulos, C. Michailidis, G. Papaiakovou, and D. Patikas. 2005. The effect of a combined high-intensity strength and speed training program on the running and jumping ability of soccer players. *Journal of Strength and Conditioning Research, 19* (2):369-75.

Kuitunen, S., Avela, J., Kyrolainen, H., Nicol, C., & Komi, P.V. (2002). Acute and prolonged reduction in joint stiffness in humans after exhausting stretch-shortening cycle exercise. *European Journal of Applied Physiology, 88*(1-2), 107-116. doi:10.1007/s00421-002-0669-2

Lenroot, R.K., & Giedd, J.N. (2006). Brain development in children and adolescents: Insights from anatomical magnetic resonance imaging. *Neuroscience & Biobehavioral Reviews, 30*(6), 718-729. doi:10.1016/j.neubiorev.2006.06.001

Lesinski, M., Prieske, O., & Granacher, U. (2016). Effects and dose-response relationships of resistance training on physical performance in youth athletes: A systematic review and meta-analysis. *British Journal of Sports Medicine, 50*(13), 781-795. doi:10.1136/bjsports-2015-095497

Lloyd, R.S., & Oliver, J.L. (2012). The youth physical development model: A new approach to long-term athletic development. *Strength and Conditioning Journal, 34*(3), 61-72.

Lloyd, R.S., Radnor, J.M., De Ste Croix, M.B., Cronin, J.B., & Oliver, J.L. (2016). Changes in sprint and jump performances after traditional, plyometric, and combined resistance training in male youth pre- and post-peak height velocity. *Journal of*

Strength and Conditioning Research, 30(5), 1239-1247. doi:10.1519/ JSC.0000000000001216

Lloyd, R.S., Read, P., Oliver, J.L., Meyers, R.W., Nimphius, S., & Jeffreys, I. (2013). Considerations for the development of agility during childhood and adolescence. *Strength and Conditioning Journal, 35*(3), 2-11.

Lockie, R.G., Murphy, A.J., & Spinks, C.D. (2003). Effects of resisted sled towing on sprint kinematics in field-sport athletes. *Journal of Strength and Conditioning Research, 17*(4), 760-767.

Lovell, R., Towlson, C., Parkin, G., Portas, M., Vaeyens, R., & Cobley, S. (2015). Soccer player characteristics in English lower-league development programmes: The relationships between relative age, maturation, anthropometry and physical fitness. *PLoS One, 10*(9), e0137238. doi:10.1371/journal.pone.0137238

Lubans, D.R., Morgan, P.J., Cliff, D.P., Barnett, L.M., & Okely, A.D. (2010). Fundamental movement skills in children and adolescents: Review of associated health benefits. *Sports Medicine, 40*(12), 1019-1035. doi:10.2165/11536850-000000000-00000

Malina, R.M., Bouchard, C., & Bar-Or, O. (2004). *Growth, maturation and physical activity.* Champaign, IL: Human Kinetics.

Mandelbaum, B.R., Silvers, H.J., Watanabe, D.S., Knarr, J.F., Thomas, S.D., Griffin, L.Y., . . . Garrett, W., Jr. (2005). Effectiveness of a neuromuscular and proprioceptive training program in preventing anterior cruciate ligament injuries in female athletes: 2-year follow-up. *The American Journal of Sports Medicine, 33*(7), 1003-1010. doi:10.1177/0363546504272261

Marques, M. C., A. Pereira, I. G. Reis, and R. van den Tillaar. 2013. Does an in-Season 6-Week Combined Sprint and Jump Training Program Improve Strength-Speed Abilities and Kicking Performance in Young Soccer Players? *Journal of Human Kinetics, 39*:157-66.

McNeal, J.R., & Sands, W.A. (2006). Stretching for performance enhancement. *Current Sports Medicine Reports, 5*(3), 141-146.

Mendez-Villanueva, A., Buchheit, M., Kuitunen, S., Douglas, A., Peltola, E., & Bourdon, P. (2011). Age-related differences in acceleration, maximum running speed, and repeated-sprint performance in young soccer players. *Journal of Sports Sciences, 29*(5), 477-484. doi:10.1080/02640414.2010.536248

Meyers, R.W., Moeskops, S., Oliver, J.L., Hughes, M.G., Cronin, J.B., & Lloyd, R.S. (in press). Lower limb stiffness and maximal running speed in 11-16-year-old-boys. *Journal of Strength and Conditioning Research.*

Meyers, R.W., Oliver, J., Hughes, M., Cronin, J.B., & Lloyd, R.S. (2015). Maximal sprint speed in boys of increasing maturity. *Pediatric Exercise Science, 27*, 85-94. doi:10.1123/pes.2013-0096

Meyers, R.W., Oliver, J.L., Hughes, M.G., Lloyd, R.S., & Cronin, J.B. (2015). The influence of age, maturity and body size on the spatiotemporal determinants of maximal sprint speed in boys. *Journal of Strength and Conditioning Research.* doi:10.1519/JSC.0000000000001310

Meyers, R.W., Oliver, J.L., Hughes, M.G., Lloyd, R.S., & Cronin, J.B. (2017). New insights into the development of maximal sprint speed in male youth. *Strength and Conditioning Journal, 39*(2), 2-10.

Meylan, C.M., Cronin, J., Oliver, J.L., Hopkins, W.G., & Pinder, S. (2014). Contribution of vertical strength and power to sprint performance in young male athletes. *International Journal of Sports Medicine, 35*(9), 749-754. doi:10.1055/s-0034-1377023

Meylan, C.M., Cronin, J.B., Oliver, J.L., Hopkins, W.G., & Contreras, B. (2014). The effect of maturation on adaptations to strength training and detraining in 11-15-year-olds. *Scandinavian Journal of Medicine & Science in Sports, 24*(3), e156-164. doi:10.1111/sms.12128

Meylan, C., & Malatesta, D. (2009). Effects of in-season plyometric training within soccer practice on explosive actions of young players. *Journal of Strength and Conditioning Research, 23*(9), 2605-2613. doi:10.1519/JSC.0b013e3181b1f330

Moran, J., Sandercock, G., Rumpf, M.C., & Parry, D.A. (2016). Variation in responses to sprint training in male youth athletes: A meta-analysis. *International Journal of Sports Medicine.* doi:10.1055/s-0042-111439

Morin, J.B., Bourdin, M., Edouard, P., Peyrot, N., Samozino, P., & Lacour, J.R. (2012). Mechanical determinants of 100-m sprint running performance. *European Journal of Applied Physiology, 112*(11), 3921-3930. doi:10.1007/s00421-012-2379-8

Morin, J.B., Edouard, P., & Samozino, P. (2011). Technical ability of force application as a determinant factor of sprint performance. *Medicine and Science in Sports and Exercise, 43*(9), 1680-1688. doi:10.1249/MSS.0b013e318216ea37

Morgan, D.W. (2008). Locomotor Economy. In N. Armstrong & W. van Mechelen (Eds.), *Paediatric exercise science and medicine* (pp. 283-296). Oxford, UK: Oxford University Press.

Myer, G.D., Faigenbaum, A.D., Chu, D.A., Falkel, J., Ford, K.R., Best, T.M., & Hewett, T.E. (2011). Integrative training for children and adolescents: Techniques and practices for reducing sports-related injuries and enhancing athletic performance. *The Physician and Sportsmedicine, 39*(1), 74-84. doi:10.3810/psm.2011.02.1864

Myer, G.D., Faigenbaum, A.D., Edwards, N.M., Clark, J.F., Best, T.M., & Sallis, R.E. (2015). Sixty minutes of what? A developing brain perspective for activating children with an integrative exercise approach. *British Journal of Sports Medicine.* doi:10.1136/bjsports-2014-093661

Myer, G.D., Ford, K.R., Brent, J.L., & Hewett, T.E. (2007). Differential neuromuscular training effects on ACL injury risk factors in"high-risk" versus "low-risk" athletes. *BMC Musculoskeletal Disorders, 8*, 39. doi:10.1186/1471-2474-8-39

Myer, G.D., Ford, K.R., Divine, J.G., Wall, E.J., Kahanov, L., & Hewett, T.E. (2009). Longitudinal assessment of noncontact anterior cruciate ligament injury risk factors during maturation in a female athlete: A case report. *Journal of Athletic Training, 44*(1), 101-109. doi:10.4085/1062-6050-44.1.101

Negra, Y., Chaabene, H., Hammami, M., Amara, S., Sammoud, S., Mkaouer, B., & Hachana, Y. (2017). Agility in young athletes: Is it a different ability from speed and power? *Journal of Strength and Conditioning Research, 31*(3), 727-735. doi:10.1519/JSC.0000000000001543

Nimphius, S. (2014). Increasing agility. In D. Joyce & D. Lewindon (Eds.), *High-performance training for sports* (pp. 185-197). Champaign: IL: Human Kinetics.

Nimphius, S., McGuigan, M.R., & Newton, R.U. (2010). Relationship between strength, power, speed, and change of direction performance of female softball players. *Journal of Strength and Conditioning Research, 24*(4), 885-895. doi:10.1519/JSC.0b013e3181d4d41d

Oliver, J.L., Lloyd, R.S., & Meyers, R.W. (2011). Training elite child athletes: Promoting welfare and well-being. *Strength and Conditioning Journal, 33*(4), 73-79.

Paul, D.J., Gabbett, T.J., & Nassis, G.P. (2016). Agility in team sports: Testing, training and factors affecting performance. *Sports Medicine, 46*(3), 421-442. doi:10.1007/s40279-015-0428-2

Paus, T., Zijdenbos, A., Worsley, K., Collins, D.L., Blumenthal, J., Giedd, J.N., . . . Evans, A.C. (1999). Structural maturation of neural pathways in children and adolescents: In vivo study. *Science, 283*(5409), 1908-1911.

Petrakos, G., Morin, J.B., & Egan, B. (2016). Resisted sled sprint training to improve sprint performance: A systematic review. *Sports Med, 46*(3), 381-400. doi:10.1007/s40279-015-0422-8

Philippaerts, R.M., Vaeyens, R., Janssens, M., Van Renterghem, B., Matthys, D., Craen, R., . . . Malina, R.M. (2006). The relationship between peak height velocity and physical performance in youth soccer players. *Journal of Sports Sciences, 24*(3), 221-230. doi:10.1080/02640410500189371

Rabinowickz, T. (1986). The differentiated maturation of the cerebral cortex. In F. Falkner & J. Tanner (Eds.), *Human growth: A comprehensive treatise—Postnatal growth, neurobiology* (Vol. 2, pp. 385-410). New York, NY: Plenum.

Radnor, J.M., Lloyd, R.S., & Oliver, J.L. (2017). Individual response to different forms of resistance training in school-aged boys. *Journal of Strength and Conditioning Research, 31*(3), 787-797. doi:10.1519/JSC.0000000000001527

Reilly, T., Williams, A.M., Nevill, A., & Franks, A. (2000). A multi-disciplinary approach to talent identification in soccer. *Journal of Sports Sciences, 18*(9), 695-702. doi:10.1080/02640410050120078

Richmond, S.A., Kang, J., Doyle-Baker, P.K., Nettel-Aguirre, A., & Emery, C.A. (2016). A school-based injury prevention program to reduce sport injury risk and improve healthy outcomes in youth: A pilot cluster-randomized controlled trial. *Clinical Journal of Sport Medicine, 26*(4), 291-298. doi:10.1097/JSM.0000000000000261

Roriz De Oliveira, M.S., Seabra, A., Freitas, D., Eisenmann, J.C., & Maia, J. (2014). Physical fitness percentile charts for children aged 6-10 from Portugal. *Journal of Sports Medicine and Physical Fitness, 54*(6), 780-792.

Rossler, R., Donath, L., Bizzini, M., & Faude, O. (2015). A new injury prevention programme for children's football—FIFA 11+ Kids—can improve motor performance: A cluster-randomised controlled trial. *Journal of Sports Sciences, 1-8.* doi:10.1080/02640414.2015.1099715

Rumpf, M.C., Cronin, J.B., Mohamad, I.N., Mohamad, S., Oliver, J., & Hughes, M. (2014). Acute effects of sled towing on sprint time in male youth of different maturity status. *Pediatric Exercise Science, 26*(1), 71-75. doi:10.1123/pes.2012-0185

Rumpf, M.C., Cronin, J.B., Mohamad, I.N., Mohamad, S., Oliver, J.L., & Hughes, M.G. (2015). The effect of resisted sprint training on maximum sprint kinetics and kinematics in youth. *European Journal of Sport Science, 15*(5), 374-381. doi:10.1080/17461391.2014.955125

Rumpf, M.C., Cronin, J.B., Oliver, J.L., & Hughes, M. (2011). Assessing youth sprint ability: Methodological issues, reliability and performance data. *Pediatric Exercise Science, 23*(4), 442-467.

Rumpf, M.C., Cronin, J.B., Oliver, J., & Hughes, M. (2015). Kinematics and kinetics of maximum running speed in youth across maturity. *Pediatric Exercise Science, 27*(2), 277-284. doi:10.1123/pes.2014-0064

Rumpf, M.C., Cronin, J.B., Pinder, S.D., Oliver, J., & Hughes, M. (2012). Effect of different training methods on running sprint times in male youth. *Pediatric Exercise Science, 24*(2), 170-186.

Rumpf, M.C., Lockie, R.G., Cronin, J.B., & Jalilvand, F. (2016). Effect of different sprint training methods on sprint performance over various distances: A brief review. *Journal of Strength and Conditioning Research, 30*(6), 1767-1785. doi:10.1519/JSC.0000000000001245

Salo, A.I., Bezodis, I.N., Batterham, A.M., & Kerwin, D.G. (2011). Elite sprinting: Are athletes individually step-frequency or step-length reliant? *Medicine and Science in Sports and Exercise, 43*(6), 1055-1062. doi:10.1249/MSS.0b013e318201f6f8

Sands, W.A., & McNeal, J. (2013). Mobility and flexibility development in youths. In R.S. Lloyd & J.L. Oliver (Eds.), *Strength and conditioning for young athletes: Science and application* (pp. 132-146). Oxon, UK: Routledge.

Serpell, B.G., Ford, M., & Young, W.B. (2010). The development of a new test of agility for rugby league. *Journal of Strength and Conditioning Research, 24*(12), 3270-3277. doi:10.1519/JSC.0b013e3181b60430

Serpell, B.G., Young, W.B., & Ford, M. (2011). Are the perceptual and decision-making components of agility trainable? A preliminary investigation. *Journal of Strength and Conditioning Research, 25*(5), 1240-1248. doi:10.1519/JSC.0b013e3181d682e6

Sheppard, J.M., & Young, W.B. (2006). Agility literature review: Classifications, training and testing. *Journal of Sports Sciences, 24*(9), 919-932. doi:10.1080/02640410500457109

Sohnlein, Q., Muller, E., & Stoggl, T.L. (2014). The effect of 16-week plyometric training on explosive actions in early to mid-puberty elite soccer players. *Journal of Strength and Conditioning Research, 28*(8), 2105-2114. doi:10.1519/JSC.0000000000000387

Spiteri, T., Newton, R.U., Binetti, M., Hart, N.H., Sheppard, J.M., & Nimphius, S. (2015). Mechanical determinants of faster change of direction and agility performance in female basketball athletes. *Journal of Strength and Conditioning Research, 29*(8), 2205-2214. doi:10.1519/JSC.0000000000000876

Spiteri, T., Nimphius, S., Hart, N.H., Specos, C., Sheppard, J.M., & Newton, R.U. (2014). Contribution of strength characteristics to change of direction and agility performance in female basketball athletes. *Journal of Strength and Conditioning Research, 28*(9), 2415-2423. doi:10.1519/JSC.0000000000000547

Stefanyshyn, D.J., & Nigg, B.M. (1998). Dynamic angular stiffness of the ankle joint during running and sprinting. *J Appl Biomech, 14,* 292-299.

Stojanovic, E., Aksovic, N., Stojilkovic, N., Stankovic, R., Scanlan, A.T., & Milanovic, Z. (in press). Reliability, usefulness, and factorial validity of change-of-direction speed tests in adolescent basketball players *Journal of Strength and Conditioning Research.*

Thomas, K., French, D., & Hayes, P.R. (2009). The effect of two plyometric training techniques on muscular power and agility in youth soccer players. *Journal of Strength and Conditioning Research, 23*(1), 332-335. doi:10.1519/JSC.0b013e318183a01a

Valente-dos-Santos, J., Coelho-e-Silva, M.J., Duarte, J., Pereira, J., Rebelo-Goncalves, R., Figueiredo, A., . . . Malina, R.M. (2014). Allometric multilevel modelling of agility and dribbling speed by skeletal age and playing position in youth soccer players. *International Journal of Sports Medicine, 35*(9), 762-771. doi:10.1055/s-0033-1358469

Vanderford, M.L., Meyers, M.C., Skelly, W.A., Stewart, C.C., & Hamilton, K.L. (2004). Physiological and sport-specific skill response of olympic youth soccer athletes. *Journal of Strength and Conditioning Research, 18*(2), 334-342. doi:10.1519/R-11922.1

Vanttinen, T., Blomqvist, M., Nyman, K., & Hakkinen, K. (2011). Changes in body composition, hormonal status, and physical fitness in 11-, 13-, and 15-year-old Finnish regional youth soccer players during a two-year follow-up. *Journal of Strength and Conditioning Research, 25*(12), 3342-3351. doi:10.1519/JSC.0b013e318236d0c2

Verschuren, O., Bloemen, M., Kruitwagen, C., & Takken, T. (2010). Reference values for anaerobic performance and agility in ambulatory children and adolescents with cerebral palsy. *Developmental Medicine and Child Neurology, 52*(10), e222-e228. doi:10.1111/j.1469-8749.2010.03747.x

Viru, A., Loko, J., Harro, M., Volver, A., Laaneot, L., & Viru, M. (1999). Critical periods in the development of performance capacity during childhood and adolescence. *European Journal of Physical Education, 4*, 75-119.

Weyand, P.G., Sandell, R.F., Prime, D.N., & Bundle, M.W. (2010). The biological limits to running speed are imposed from the ground up. *Journal of Applied Physiology, 108*(4), 950-961. doi:10.1152/japplphysiol.00947.2009

Weyand, P.G., Sternlight, D.B., Bellizzi, M.J., & Wright, S. (2000). Faster top running speeds are achieved with greater ground forces not more rapid leg movements. *Journal of Applied Physiology, 89*(5), 1991-1999.

Whitall, J. (2003). Development of locomotor co-ordination and control in children. In G.J.P. Savelsberg, K. Davids, & J. Van Der Kamp (Eds.), *Development of movement co-ordination in children* (pp. 251-270). London, UK: Routledge.

Wong, P.L., Chamari, K., & Wisloff, U. (2010). Effects of 12-week on-field combined strength and power training on physical performance among U-14 young soccer players. *Journal of Strength and Conditioning Research, 24*(3), 644-652. doi:10.1519/JSC.0b013e3181ad3349

Wrigley, R.D., Drust, B., Stratton, G., Atkinson, G., & Gregson, W. (2014). Long-term soccer-specific training enhances the rate of physical development of academy soccer players independent of maturation status. *International Journal of Sports Medicine, 35*(13), 1090-1094. doi:10.1055/s-0034-1375616

Yague, P.H., & De La Fuente, J.M. (1998). Changes in height and motor performance relative to peak height velocity: A mixed-longitudinal study of Spanish boys and girls. *American Journal of Human Biology, 10*, 647-660.

Young, W., & Rogers, N. (2014). Effects of small-sided game and change-of-direction training on reactive agility and change-of-direction speed. *Journal of Sports Sciences, 32*(4), 307-314. doi:10.1080/02640414.2013.823230

Chapter 11 Aerobic and Anaerobic Training

Abrantes, C., Macas, V., & Sampaio, J. (2004). Variation in football players' sprint test performance across different ages and levels of competition. *Journal of Sports Science & Medicine, 3*(YISI 1), 44-49.

Alexandre, D., da Silva, C.D., Hill-Haas, S., Wong del, P., Natali, A.J., De Lima, J.R., . . . Karim, C. (2012). Heart rate monitoring in soccer: interest and limits during competitive match play and training, practical application. *Journal of Strength and Conditioning Research, 26*(10), 2890-2906.

Ariens, G.A., van Mechelen, W., Kemper, H.C., & Twisk, J.W. (1997). The longitudinal development of running economy in males and females aged between 13 and 27 years: The Amsterdam Growth and Health Study. *European Journal of Applied Physiology and Occupational Physiology, 76*(3), 214-220.

Armstrong, N. (2016). Aerobic Fitness and Training in Children and Adolescents. *Pediatric Exercise Science, 28*(1), 7-10.

Armstrong, N., & Barker, A.R. (2011). Endurance training and elite young athletes. In N. Armstrong & A.M. McManus (Eds.), *The elite young athlete* (pp. 59-83). Basel: Karger.

Armstrong, N., Barker, A.R., & McManus, A.M. (2015). Muscle metabolism changes with age and maturation: How do they relate to youth sport performance? *British Journal of Sports Medicine, 49*(13), 860-864.

Armstrong, N., & Fawkner, S.G. (2008). Exercise metabolism. In N. Armstrong & W. van Mechelen (Eds.), *Paediatric exercise science and medicine* (pp. 213-226). Oxford, UK: Oxford University Press.

Armstrong, N., Kirby, B.J., McManus, A.M., & Welsman, J.R. (1995). Aerobic fitness of prepubescent children. *Annals of Human Biology, 22*(5), 427-441.

Armstrong, N., & Welsman, J.R. (2000). Development of aerobic fitness during childhood and adolescence. *Pediatric Exercise Science, 12*, 128-149.

Armstrong, N., & Welsman, J.R. (2008). Aerobic fitness. In N. Armstrong & W. van Mechelen (Eds.), *Paediatric exercise science and medicine* (pp. 97-108). Oxford, UK: Oxford University Press.

Bangsbo, J., Krustrup, P., Duda, J., Hillman, C., Andersen, L.B., Weiss, M., . . . Elbe, A.M. (2016). The Copenhagen Consensus Conference 2016: Children, youth, and physical activity in schools and during leisure time. *British Journal of Sports Medicine, 50*(19), 1177-1178.

Baquet, G., Berthoin, S., Dupont, G., Blondel, N., Fabre, C., & van Praagh, E. (2002). Effects of high intensity intermittent training on peak VO(2) in prepubertal children. *International Journal of Sports Medicine, 23*(6), 439-444.

Baquet, G., Gamelin, F.X., Mucci, P., Thevenet, D., Van Praagh, E., & Berthoin, S. (2010). Continuous vs. interval aerobic training in 8- to 11-year-old children. *Journal of Strength and Conditioning Research, 24*(5), 1381-1388.

Baquet, G., van Praagh, E., & Berthoin, S. (2003). Endurance training and aerobic fitness in young people. *Sports Medicine, 33*(15), 1127-1143.

Bar-Or, O., & Rowland, T.W. (2004). *Pediatric exercise medicine: From physiological principles to health care application.* Champaign, IL: Human Kinetics.

Baxter-Jones, A.D., & Maffulli, N. (2003). Endurance in young athletes: It can be trained. *British Journal of Sports Medicine, 37*(2), 96-97.

Bedoya, A.A., Miltenberger, M.R., & Lopez, R.M. (2015). Plyometric training effects on athletic performance in youth soccer athletes: A systematic review. *Journal of Strength and Conditioning Research, 29*(8), 2351-2360.

Behringer, M., Vom Heede, A., Matthews, M., & Mester, J. (2011). Effects of strength training on motor performance skills in children and adolescents: A meta-analysis. *Pediatric Exercise Science, 23*(2), 186-206.

Behringer, M., Vom Heede, A., Yue, Z., & Mester, J. (2010). Effects of resistance training in children and adolescents: A meta-analysis. *Pediatrics, 126*(5), e1199-1210.

Berg, A., Kim, S.S., & Keul, J. (1986). Skeletal muscle enzyme activities in healthy young subjects. *International Journal of Sports Medicine, 7*(4), 236-239.

Billows, D., Reilly, T., & George, K. (2005). Physiological demands of match play and training in elite adolescent footballers. In T. Reilly, J. Cabri, & D. Araujo (Eds.), *Science & Football V* (pp. 453-461). Oxford, UK: Routledge.

Boisseau, N., & Delamarche, P. (2000). Metabolic and hormonal responses to exercise in children and adolescents. *Sports Medicine, 30*(6), 405-422.

Buchan, D.S., Ollis, S., Young, J.D., Cooper, S.M., Shield, J.P., & Baker, J.S. (2013). High intensity interval running enhances measures of physical fitness but not metabolic measures of cardiovascular disease risk in healthy adolescents. *BMC Public Health, 13*, 498.

Buchheit, M., Laursen, P.B., Kuhnle, J., Ruch, D., Renaud, C., & Ahmaidi, S. (2009). Game-based training in young elite handball players. *International Journal of Sports Medicine, 30*(4), 251-258.

Buchheit, M., Mendez-Villanueva, A., Delhomel, G., Brughelli, M., & Ahmaidi, S. (2010). Improving repeated sprint ability in young elite soccer players: repeated shuttle sprints vs. explosive strength training. *Journal of Strength and Conditioning Research, 24*(10), 2715-2722.

Cadefau, J., Casademont, J., Grau, J.M., Fernandez, J., Balaguer, A., Vernet, M., . . . Urbano-Marquez, A. (1990). Biochemical and histochemical adaptation to sprint training in young athletes. *Acta Physiologica Scandinavica, 140*(3), 341-351.

Catley, M.J., & Tomkinson, G.R. (2013). Normative health-related fitness values for children: Analysis of 85347 test results on 9-17-year-old Australians since 1985. *British Journal of Sports Medicine, 47*(2), 98-108.

Costigan, S.A., Eather, N., Plotnikoff, R.C., Taaffe, D.R., & Lubans, D.R. (2015). High-intensity interval training for improving health-related fitness in adolescents: A systematic review and meta-analysis. *British Journal of Sports Medicine, 49*(19), 1253-1261.

Daniels, J., Oldridge, N., Nagle, F., & White, B. (1978). Differences and changes in VO2 among young runners 10 to 18 years of age. *Medicine and Science in Sports, 10*(3), 200-203.

Dipla, K., Tsirini, T., Zafeiridis, A., Manou, V., Dalamitros, A., Kellis, E., & Kellis, S. (2009). Fatigue resistance during high-intensity intermittent exercise from childhood to adulthood in males and females. *European Journal of Applied Physiology, 106*(5), 645-653.

Dorgo, S., King, G.A., Candelaria, N.G., Bader, J.O., Brickey, G.D., & Adams, C.E. (2009). Effects of manual resistance training on fitness in adolescents. *Journal of Strength and Conditioning Research, 23*(8), 2287-2294.

Eriksson, B.O., Gollnick, P.D., & Saltin, B. (1973). Muscle metabolism and enzyme activities after training in boys 11-13 years old. *Acta Physiologica Scandinavica, 87*(4), 485-497.

Faigenbaum, A.D., Bush, J.A., McLoone, R.P., Kreckel, M.C., Farrell, A., Ratamess, N.A., & Kang, J. (2015). Benefits of strength and skill-based training during primary school physical education. *Journal of Strength and Conditioning Research, 29*(5), 1255-1262.

Faigenbaum, A.D., Farrell, A., Fabiano, M., Radler, T., Naclerio, F., Ratamess, N.A., . . . Myer, G.D. (2011). Effects of integrative neuromuscular training on fitness performance in children. *Pediatric Exercise Science, 23*(4), 573-584.

Faigenbaum, A.D., & Mediate, P. (2008). Effects of medicine ball training on fitness performance of high-school physical education students. *The Physical Educator*, 160-167.

Fellmann, N., & Coudert, J. (1994). Physiology of muscular exercise in children. *Archives of Pediatrics, 1*(9), 827-840.

Ferrari Bravo, D., Impellizzeri, F.M., Rampinini, E., Castagna, C., Bishop, D., & Wisloff, U. (2008). Sprint vs. interval training in football. *International Journal of Sports Medicine, 29*(8), 668-674.

Foster, C.D., Twist, C., Lamb, K.L., & Nicholas, C.W. (2010). Heart rate responses to small-sided games among elite junior rugby league players. *Journal of Strength and Conditioning Research, 24*(4), 906-911.

Fournier, M., Ricci, J., Taylor, A.W., Ferguson, R.J., Montpetit, R.R., & Chaitman, B.R. (1982). Skeletal muscle adaptation in adolescent boys: Sprint and endurance training and detraining. *Medicine and Science in Sports and Exercise, 14*(6), 453-456.

Gamble, P. (2014). Metabolic conditioning development in youths. In R.L. Lloyd & J.L. Oliver (Eds.), *Strength and conditioning for young athletes: Science and application* (pp. 120-131). Abingdon, UK: Routledge.

Granacher, U., Muehlbauer, T., Doerflinger, B., Strohmeier, R., & Gollhofer, A. (2011). Promoting strength and balance in adolescents during physical education: Effects of a short-term resistance training. *Journal of Strength and Conditioning Research, 25*(4), 940-949.

Haralambie, G. (1982). Enzyme activities in skeletal muscle of 13-15 years old adolescents. *Bulletin Europeen de Physiopathologie Respiratoire, 18*(1), 65-74.

Harrison, C.B., Gill, N.D., Kinugasa, T., & Kilding, A.E. (2013). Quantification of physiological, movement, and technical outputs during a novel small-sided game in young team sport athletes. *Journal of Strength and Conditioning Research, 27*(10), 2861-2868.

Harrison, C.B., Gill, N.D., Kinugasa, T., & Kilding, A.E. (2015). Development of aerobic fitness in young team sport athletes. *Sports Medicine, 45*(7), 969-983.

Harrison, C.B., Kilding, A.E., Gill, N.D., & Kinugasa, T. (2014). Small-sided games for young athletes: Is game specificity influential? *Journal of Sports Sciences, 32*(4), 336-344.

Helgerud, J., Engen, L.C., Wisloff, U., & Hoff, J. (2001). Aerobic endurance training improves soccer performance. *Medicine and Science in Sports and Exercise, 33*(11), 1925-1931.

Hill-Haas, S.V., Coutts, A.J., Dawson, B.T., & Rowsell, G.J. (2010). Time-motion characteristics and physiological responses of small-sided games in elite youth players: The influence of player number and rule changes. *Journal of Strength and Conditioning Research, 24*(8), 2149-2156.

Hill-Haas, S.V., Coutts, A.J., Rowsell, G.J., & Dawson, B.T. (2009). Generic versus small-sided game training in soccer. *International Journal of Sports Medicine, 30*(9), 636-642.

Hill-Haas, S.V., Dawson, B.T., Coutts, A.J., & Rowsell, G.J. (2009). Physiological responses and time-motion characteristics of various small-sided soccer games in youth players. *Journal of Sports Sciences, 27*(1), 1-8.

Impellizzeri, F.M., Marcora, S.M., Castagna, C., Reilly, T., Sassi, A., Iaia, F.M., & Rampinini, E. (2006). Physiological and performance effects of generic versus specific aerobic training in soccer players. *International Journal of Sports Medicine, 27*(6), 483-492.

Jones, A. (2006). The physiology of the world record holder for the women's marathon. *International Journal of Sports Science & Coaching, 1*(2), 101-116.

Katch, V.L. (1983). Physical conditioning of children. *Journal of Adolescent Health Care, 3*(4), 241-246.

Katis, A., & Kellis, E. (2009). Effects of small-sided games on physical conditioning and performance in young soccer players. *Journal of Sports Science & Medicine, 8*(3), 374-380.

Kentta, G., Hassmen, P., & Raglin, J.S. (2001). Training practices and overtraining syndrome in Swedish age-group athletes. *International Journal of Sports Medicine, 22*(6), 460-465.

Krahenbuhl, G.S., & Williams, T.J. (1992). Running economy: changes with age during childhood and adolescence. *Medicine and Science in Sports and Exercise, 24*(4), 462-466.

Larsen, H.B., Nolan, T., Borch, C., & Sondergaard, H. (2005). Training response of adolescent Kenyan town and village boys to endurance running. *Scandinavian Journal of Medicine & Science in Sports, 15*(1), 48-57.

Lexell, J., Sjostrom, M., Nordlund, A.S., & Taylor, C.C. (1992). Growth and development of human muscle: A quantitative morphological study of whole vastus lateralis from childhood to adult age. *Muscle Nerve, 15*(3), 404-409.

Logan, G.R., Harris, N., Duncan, S., & Schofield, G. (2014). A review of adolescent high-intensity interval training. *Sports Medicine, 44*(8), 1071-1085.

Lussier, L., & Buskirk, E.R. (1977). Effects of an endurance training regimen on assessment of work capacity in prepubertal children. *Annals of the New York Academy of Sciences, 301*, 734-747.

Mahon, A.D. (2008). Aerobic training. In N. Armstrong & W. van Mechelen (Eds.), *Paediatric exercise science and medicine* (pp. 513-530). Oxford, UK: Oxford University Press.

Mahon, A.D., & Vaccaro, P. (1989). Ventilatory threshold and VO2max changes in children following endurance training. *Medicine and Science in Sports and Exercise, 21*(4), 425-431.

Malina, R.M., Bouchard, C., & Bar-Or, O. (2004). *Growth, maturation and physical activity* Champaign, IL: Human Kinetics.

Matos, N.F., Winsley, R.J., & Williams, C.A. (2011). Prevalence of nonfunctional overreaching/overtraining in young English athletes. *Medicine and Science in Sports and Exercise, 43*(7), 1287-1294.

Mayorga-Vega, D., Viciana, J., & Cocca, A. (2013). Effects of a circuit training program on muscular and cardiovascular endurance and their maintenance in schoolchildren. *Journal of Human Kinetics, 37*, 153-160.

McManus, A.M., Armstrong, N., & Williams, C.A. (1997). Effect of training on the aerobic power and anaerobic performance of prepubertal girls. *Acta Paediatrica, 86*(5), 456-459.

McManus, A.M., Cheng, C.H., Leung, M.P., Yung, T.C., & Macfarlane, D.J. (2005). Improving aerobic power in primary school boys: A comparison of continuous and interval training. *International Journal of Sports Medicine, 26*(9), 781-786.

McMillan, K., Helgerud, J., Macdonald, R., & Hoff, J. (2005). Physiological adaptations to soccer specific endurance training in professional youth soccer players. *British Journal of Sports Medicine, 39*(5), 273-277.

McNarry, M., Barker, A.R., Lloyd, R.S., Buchheit, M., Williams, C.A., & Oliver, J.L. (2014). The BASES expert statement on trainability during childhood and adolescence. *The Sport and Exercise Scientist*, 22-23.

Millet, G.P., Jaouen, B., Borrani, F., & Candau, R. (2002). Effects of concurrent endurance and strength training on running economy and $\dot{V}O_2$ kinetics. *Medicine and Science in Sports and Exercise, 34*(8), 1351-1359.

Morgan, D.W. (2008). Locomotor Economy. In N. Armstrong & W. van Mechelen (Eds.), *Paediatric exercise science and medicine* (pp. 283-296). Oxford, UK: Oxford University Press.

Naughton, G., Farpour-Lambert, N.J., Carlson, J., Bradney, M., & Van Praagh, E. (2000). Physiological issues surrounding the performance of adolescent athletes. *Sports Medicine, 30*(5), 309-325.

Obert, P., Courteix, D., Lecoq, A.M., & Guenon, P. (1996). Effect of long-term intense swimming training on the upper body peak oxygen uptake of prepubertal girls. *European Journal of Applied Physiology and Occupational Physiology, 73*(1-2), 136-143.

Oliver, J.L., Lloyd, R.S., & Meyers, R.W. (2011). Training elite child athletes: Welfare and well-being. *Strength and Conditioning Journal, 33*, 73-79.

Ortega, F.B., Ruiz, J.R., Castillo, M.J., & Sjostrom, M. (2008). Physical fitness in childhood and adolescence: A powerful marker of health. *International Journal of Obesity, 32*(1), 1-11.

Petray, C.K., & Krahenbuhl, G.S. (1985). Running training, instruction on running technique, and running economy in 10 y old males. *Research Quarterly for Exercise and Sport*, 251-255.

Philippaerts, R.M., Vaeyens, R., Janssens, M., Van Renterghem, B., Matthys, D., Craen, R., . . . Malina, R.M. (2006). The relationship between peak height velocity and physical performance in youth soccer players. *Journal of Sports Sciences, 24*(3), 221-230.

Racil, G., Ben Ounis, O., Hammouda, O., Kallel, A., Zouhal, H., Chamari, K., & Amri, M. (2013). Effects of high vs. moderate exercise intensity during interval training on lipids and adiponectin levels in obese young females. *European Journal of Applied Physiology, 113*(10), 2531-2540.

Raglin, J., Sawamura, S., Alexiou, S., Hassmén, P., & Kentta, G. (2000). Training practices and staleness in 13-18-year-old swimmers: A cross-cultural study. *Pediatric Exercise Science, 12*(1), 61-70.

Ratel, S., Duche, P., Hennegrave, A., Van Praagh, E., & Bedu, M. (2002). Acid-base balance during repeated cycling sprints in boys and men. *Journal of Applied Physiology, 92*(2), 479-485.

Ratel, S., Duche, P., & Williams, C.A. (2006). Muscle fatigue during high-intensity exercise in children. *Sports Medicine, 36*(12), 1031-1065.

Ratel, S., & Williams, C.A. (2008). Children's musculoskeletal system: New research perspectives. In N.P. Beaulieu (Ed.), *Physical activity and children: New research*. Hauppauge, NY: Nova Science.

Reilly, T., Williams, A.M., Nevill, A., & Franks, A. (2000). A multidisciplinary approach to talent identification in soccer. *Journal of Sports Sciences, 18*(9), 695-702.

Reybrouck, T., Weymans, M., Stijns, H., Knops, J., & van der Hauwaert, L. (1985). Ventilatory anaerobic threshold in healthy children. Age and sex differences. *European Journal of Applied Physiology and Occupational Physiology, 54*(3), 278-284.

Rotstein, A., Dotan, R., Bar-Or, O., & Tenenbaum, G. (1986). Effect of training on anaerobic threshold, maximal aerobic power and anaerobic performance of preadolescent boys. *International Journal of Sports Medicine, 7*(5), 281-286.

Rowland, T.W. (1993). Does peak VO2 reflect VO2max in children? Evidence from supramaximal testing. *Medicine and Science in Sports and Exercise, 25*(6), 689-693.

Rowland, T.W. (2005). *Children's exercise physiology*. Champaign; IL: Human Kinetics.

Ruiz, J.R., Cavero-Redondo, I., Ortega, F.B., Welk, G.J., Andersen, L.B., & Martinez-Vizcaino, V. (2016). Cardiorespiratory fitness cut points to avoid cardiovascular disease risk in children and adolescents; what level of fitness should raise a red flag? A systematic review and meta-analysis. *British Journal of Sports Medicine*.

Rumpf, M.C., Cronin, J.B., Pinder, S.D., Oliver, J., & Hughes, M. (2012). Effect of different training methods on running sprint times in male youth. *Pediatric Exercise Science, 24*(2), 170-186.

Sallis, J.F., Buono, M.J., & Freedson, P.S. (1991). Bias in estimating caloric expenditure from physical activity in children. Implications for epidemiological studies. *Sports Medicine, 11*(4), 203-209.

Sjodin, B., & Svedenhag, J. (1992). Oxygen uptake during running as related to body mass in circumpubertal boys: A longitudinal study. *European Journal of Applied Physiology and Occupational Physiology, 65*(2), 150-157.

Spencer, M., Lawrence, S., Rechichi, C., Bishop, D., Dawson, B., & Goodman, C. (2004). Time-motion analysis of elite field hockey, with special reference to repeated-sprint activity. *Journal of Sports Sciences, 22*(9), 843-850.

Sperlich, B., De Marees, M., Koehler, K., Linville, J., Holmberg, H.C., & Mester, J. (2011). Effects of 5 weeks of high-intensity interval training vs. volume training in 14-year-old soccer players. *Journal of Strength and Conditioning Research, 25*(5), 1271-1278.

Sperlich, B., Zinner, C., Heilemann, I., Kjendlie, P.L., Holmberg, H.C., & Mester, J. (2010). High-intensity interval training improves VO(2peak), maximal lactate accumulation, time trial and competition performance in 9-11-year-old swimmers. *European Journal of Applied Physiology, 110*(5), 1029-1036.

Spittle, M., Harrison, C.B., Lloyd, R.S., & Cronin, J.B. (2017). Modifying games for improved aerobic fitness and skill acquisition in youth. *Strength and Conditioning Journal, 39*(2), 82-88.

Spurrs, R.W., Murphy, A.J., & Watsford, M.L. (2003). The effect of plyometric training on distance running performance. *European Journal of Applied Physiology, 89*(1), 1-7.

Storen, O., Helgerud, J., Stoa, E.M., & Hoff, J. (2008). Maximal strength training improves running economy in distance runners. *Medicine and Science in Sports and Exercise, 40*(6), 1087-1092.

Tolfrey, K., & Armstrong, N. (1995). Child-adult differences in whole blood lactate responses to incremental treadmill exercise. *British Journal of Sports Medicine, 29*(3), 196-199.

Tomkinson, G.R., Annadale, M., & Ferrar, K. (2013). *Global changes in cardiovascular endurance of children and youth since 1964: Systematic analysis of 25 million fitness test results from 28 countries.* Paper presented at the American Heart Association Scientific Sessions, Dallas.

Tonnessen, E., Shalfawi, S.A., Haugen, T., & Enoksen, E. (2011). The effect of 40-m repeated sprint training on maximum sprinting speed, repeated sprint speed endurance, vertical jump, and aerobic capacity in young elite male soccer players. *Journal of Strength and Conditioning Research, 25*(9), 2364-2370.

Utter, A.C., Robertson, R.J., Nieman, D.C., & Kang, J. (2002). Children's OMNI Scale of Perceived Exertion: Walking/running evaluation. *Medicine and Science in Sports and Exercise, 34*(1), 139-144.

Verschuren, O., Ketelaar, M., Gorter, J.W., Helders, P.J., Uiterwaal, C.S., & Takken, T. (2007). Exercise training program in children and adolescents with cerebral palsy: A randomized controlled trial. *Archives of Pediatrics & Adolescent Medicine, 161*(11), 1075-1081.

Viru, A., Loko, J., Harrow, M., Volver, A., Laaneots, L., & M, V. (1999). Critical periods in the development of performance capacity during childhood and adolescence. *EuropeAmerican Journal ofournal of Physical Education, 4*, 75-119.

Wall, M., & Côt, J. (2007). Developmental activities that lead to dropout and investment in sport. *Physical Education and Sport*, 77-87.

Welsman, J.R., Armstrong, N., Nevill, A.M., Winter, E.M., & Kirby, B.J. (1996). Scaling peak VO2 for differences in body size. *Medicine and Science in Sports and Exercise, 28*(2), 259-265.

Williams, C.A. (2008). Maximal Intensity Exercise. In N. Armstrong & W. van Mechelen (Eds.), *Paediatric exercise science and medicine* (pp. 227-242). Oxford, UK: Oxford University Press.

Williams, C. A., Winsley, R. J., Pinho, G., De Ste Croix, M., Lloyd, R. S., & Oliver, J. L. (2017). Prevalence of non-functionall overreaching in elite male and female youth academy football players. *Science and Medicine in Football, 1*, 222-228.

Wong, P.C., Chia, M.Y., Tsou, I.Y., Wansaicheong, G.K., Tan, B., Wang, J.C., . . . Lim, D. (2008). Effects of a 12-week exercise training programme on aerobic fitness, body composition, blood lipids and C-reactive protein in adolescents with obesity. *Annals of the Academy of Medicine, Singapore, 37*(4), 286-293.

Wrigley, R.D., Drust, B., Stratton, G., Atkinson, G., & Gregson, W. (2014). Long-term soccer-specific training enhances the rate of physical development of academy soccer players independent of maturation status. *International Journal of Sports Medicine, 35*(13), 1090-1094.

Wrigley, R., Drust, B., Stratton, G., Scott, M., & Gregson, W. (2012). Quantification of the typical weekly in-season training load in elite junior soccer players. *Journal of Sports Sciences, 30*(15), 1573-1580.

Chapter 12 Integrative Program Design

Alves, A.R., Marta, C.C., Neiva, H.P., Izquierdo, M., & Marques, M.C. (2016). Concurrent training in prepubescent children: The effects of 8 weeks of strength and aerobic training on explosive strength and V̇O2max. *Journal of Strength and Conditioning Research, 30*(7), 2019-2032. doi:10.1519/JSC.0000000000001294

American College of Sports Medicine. (2009). American College of Sports Medicine position stand. Progression models in resistance training for healthy adults. *Medicine and Science in Sports and Exercise, 41*(3), 687-708. doi:10.1249/MSS.0b013e3181915670

Armstrong, N., & Barker, A.R. (2011). Endurance training and elite young athletes. *Medicine and Sport Science, 56*, 59-83.

Baar, K. (2014). Using molecular biology to maximize concurrent training. *Sports Med, 44*(Suppl 2), S117-S125. doi:10.1007/s40279-014-0252-0

Baker, D.G. (2013). 10-year changes in upper body strength and power in elite professional rugby league players—The effect of training age, stage, and content. *Journal of Strength and Conditioning Research, 27*(2), 285-292. doi:10.1519/JSC.0b013e318270fc6b

Balyi, I., & Hamilton, A. (2004). *Long-term athlete development: Trainability in childhood and adolescence. Windows of Opportunity. Optimal trainability.* Victoria, British Columbia, Canada:

National Coaching Institute & Advanced Training and Performance.

Banister, E.W., Calvert, I.W., Savage, M.V., & Bach, I.M. (1975). A system model of training for athletic performance. *Australian Journal of Sports Medicine, 7*(3), 57-61.

Baquet, G., van Praagh, E., & Berthoin, S. (2003). Endurance training and aerobic fitness in young people. *Sports Medicine, 33*(15), 1127-1143.

Barnett, L.M., Ridgers, N.D., Zask, A., & Salmon, J. (2015). Face validity and reliability of a pictorial instrument for assessing fundamental movement skill perceived competence in young children. *Journal of Science and Medicine in Sport, 18*(1), 98-102. doi:10.1016/j.jsams.2013.12.004

Behringer, M., Vom Heede, A., Yue, Z., & Mester, J. (2010). Effects of resistance training in children and adolescents: a meta-analysis. *Pediatrics, 126*(5), e1199-1210. doi:10.1542/peds.2010-0445

Bergeron, M.F., Laird, M.D., Marinik, E.L., Brenner, J.S., & Waller, J.L. (2009). Repeated-bout exercise in the heat in young athletes: Physiological strain and perceptual responses. *Journal of Applied Physiology, 106*(2), 476-485. doi:10.1152/japplphysiol.00122.2008

Bergeron, M.F., Mountjoy, M., Armstrong, N., Chia, M., Cote, J., Emery, C.A., . . . Engebretsen, L. (2015). International Olympic Committee consensus statement on youth athletic development. *British Journal of Sports Medicine, 49*(13), 843-851. doi:10.1136/bjsports-2015-094962

Bompa, T.O., & Haff, G.G. (2009). *Periodization: Theory and methodology of training.* Champaign, IL: Human Kinetics.

Borresen, J., & Lambert, M.I. (2009). The quantification of training load, the training response and the effect on performance. *Sports Medicine, 39*(9), 779-795. doi:10.2165/11317780-000000000-00000

Bosquet, L., Montpetit, J., Arvisais, D., & Mujika, I. (2007). Effects of tapering on performance: A meta-analysis. *Medicine and Science in Sports and Exercise, 39*(8), 1358-1365. doi:10.1249/mss.0b013e31806010e0

Bowen, L., Gross, A.S., Gimpel, M., & Li, F.X. (2016). Accumulated workloads and the acute:chronic workload ratio relate to injury risk in elite youth football players. *British Journal of Sports Medicine.* doi:10.1136/bjsports-2015-095820

Calvert, T.W., Banister, E.W., Savage, M.V., & Bach, T. (1976). A systems model of the effects of training on physical performance. *IEEE Transactions on Systems, Man, and Cybernetics, 6,* 94-102.

Chiu, L.Z.F., & Barnes, J.L. (2003). The fitness-fatigue model revisited: Implications for planning short- and long-term training. *Strength and Conditioning Journal, 25*(6), 42-51.

DeWeese, B., Hornsby, G., Stone, M.E., & Stone, M.H. (2015). The training process: Planning for strength-power training in track and field. Part 2: Practical and applied aspects. *Journal of Sport and Health Science, 4*(4), 318-324.

DiFiori, J.P., Benjamin, H.J., Brenner, J.S., Gregory, A., Jayanthi, N., Landry, G.L., & Luke, A. (2014). Overuse injuries and burnout in youth sports: A position statement from the American Medical Society for Sports Medicine. *British Journal of Sports Medicine, 48*(4), 287-288. doi:10.1136/bjsports-2013-093299

Eston, R.G., Lambrick, D.M., & Rowlands, A.V. (2009). The perceptual response to exercise of progressively increasing intensity in children aged 7-8 years: Validation of a pictorial curvilinear ratings of perceived exertion scale. *Psychophysiology, 46*(4), 843-851. doi:10.1111/j.1469-8986.2009.00826.x

Faigenbaum, A.D., Farrell, A.C., Fabiano, M., Radler, T.A., Naclerio, F., Ratamess, N.A., . . . Myer, G.D. (2013). Effects of detraining on fitness performance in 7-year-old children. *Journal of Strength and Conditioning Research, 27*(2), 323-330. doi:10.1519/JSC.0b013e31827e135b

Faigenbaum, A.D., & McFarland, J. (2006). Make time for less-intense training. *Strength and Conditioning Journal, 28*(5), 77-79.

Falk, B., & Dotan, R. (2006). Child-adult differences in the recovery from high-intensity exercise. *Exercise and Sport Sciences Reviews, 34*(3), 107-112.

Farrow, D., & Robertson, S. (2016). Development of a skill acquisition periodisation framework for high-performance sport. *Sports Medicine.* doi:10.1007/s40279-016-0646-2

Fernandez-Fernandez, J., Granacher, U., Sanz-Rivas, D., Marin, J.M.S., Hernandez-Davo, J.L., & Moya, M. (2018). Sequencing effects of neuromuscular training on physical fitness in youth elite tennis players. *Journal of Strength and Conditioning Research, 32*(3), 849-856.

Fleisig, G.S., Andrews, J.R., Cutter, G.R., Weber, A., Loftice, J., McMichael, C., . . . Lyman, S. (2011). Risk of serious injury for young baseball pitchers: A 10-year prospective study. *American Journal of Sports Medicine, 39*(2), 253-257. doi:10.1177/0363546510384224

Foster, C., Daines, E., Hector, L., Snyder, A.C., & Welsh, R. (1996). Athletic performance in relation to training load. *Wisconsin Medical Journal, 95*(6), 370-374.

Fyfe, J.J., Bishop, D.J., & Stepto, N.K. (2014). Interference between concurrent resistance and endurance exercise: Molecular bases and the role of individual training variables. *Sports Medicine, 44*(6), 743-762. doi:10.1007/s40279-014-0162-1

Garcia-Hermoso, A., Ramirez-Velez, R., Ramirez-Campillo, R., Peterson, M.D., & Martinez-Vizcaino, V. (2016). Concurrent aerobic plus resistance exercise versus aerobic exercise alone to improve health outcomes in paediatric obesity: A systematic review and meta-analysis. *British Journal of Sports Medicine.* doi:10.1136/bjsports-2016-096605

Granacher, U., Lesinski, M., Busch, D., Muehlbauer, T., Prieske, O., Puta, C., . . . Behm, D.G. (2016). Effects of resistance training in youth athletes on muscular fitness and athletic performance: A conceptual model for long-term athlete development. *Frontiers in Physiology, 7,* 164. doi:10.3389/fphys.2016.00164

Haff, G.G. (2013). Periodization strategies for youth development. In R.S. Lloyd & J.L. Oliver (Eds.), *Strength and conditioning for young athletes: Science and application* (pp. 149-168). Oxford, United Kingdom: Routledge.

Haff, G.G., & Haff, E.E. (2012). Training integration and periodization. In J.R. Hoffman (Ed.), *NSCA's Guide to Program Design* (pp. 213-258). Champaign, IL: Human Kinetics.

Haff, G.G., & Nimphius, S. (2012). Training principles for power. *Strength and Conditioning Journal, 34*(6), 2-12.

Harries, S.K., Lubans, D.R., & Callister, R. (2012). Resistance training to improve power and sports performance in adolescent athletes: A systematic review and meta-analysis. *Journal of Science and Medicine in Sport, 15*(6), 532-540. doi:10.1016/j.jsams.2012.02.005

Harrison, C.B., Gill, N.D., Kinugasa, T., & Kilding, A.E. (2015). Development of aerobic fitness in young team sport athletes. *Sports Medicine, 45*(7), 969-983. doi:10.1007/s40279-015-0330-y

Hawley, J.A. (2009). Molecular responses to strength and endurance training: Are they incompatible? *Applied Physiology, Nutrition, and Metabolism, 34*(3), 355-361. doi:10.1139/H09-023

Inoue, D.S., De Mello, M.T., Foschini, D., Lira, F.S., De Piano Ganen, A., Da Silveira Campos, R.M., . . . Damaso, A.R. (2015). Linear and undulating periodized strength plus aerobic training promote similar benefits and lead to improvement of insulin resistance on obese adolescents. *Journal of Diabetes and Its Complications, 29*(2), 258-264. doi:10.1016/j.jdiacomp.2014.11.002

Issurin, V. (2008a). Block periodization versus traditional training theory: A review. *Journal of Sports Medicine and Physical Fitness, 48*(1), 65-75.

Issurin, V. (2008b). *Principles and basics of advanced training of athletes.* Muskegon, MI: Ultimate Athletes Concepts.

Issurin, V.B. (2009). Generalized training effects induced by athletic preparation. A review. *Journal of Sports Medicine and Physical Fitness, 49*(4), 333-345.

Issurin, V.B. (2010). New horizons for the methodology and physiology of training periodization. *Sports Medicine, 40*(3), 189-206. doi:10.2165/11319770-000000000-00000

Jayanthi, N., Dechert, A., Durazo, R., Dugas, L., & Luke, A. (2011). Training and sport specialization risks in junior elite tennis. *Journal of Medicine and Science in Tennis, 16*, 14-20.

Jayanthi, N.A., LaBella, C.R., Fischer, D., Pasulka, J., & Dugas, L.R. (2015). Sports-specialized intensive training and the risk of injury in young athletes: A clinical case-control study. *American Journal of Sports Medicine, 43*(4), 794-801. doi:10.1177/0363546514567298

Keiner, M., Sander, A., Wirth, K., Caruso, O., Immesberger, P., & Zawieja, M. (2013). Strength performance in youth: Trainability of adolescents and children in the back and front squats. *Journal of Strength and Conditioning Research, 27*(2), 357-362. doi:10.1519/JSC.0b013e3182576fbf

Keiner, M., Sander, A., Wirth, K., & Schmidtbleicher, D. (2014). Long-term strength training effects on change-of-direction sprint performance. *Journal of Strength and Conditioning Research, 28*(1), 223-231. doi:10.1519/JSC.0b013e318295644b

Kiely, J. (2012). Periodization paradigms in the 21st century: Evidence-led or tradition-driven? *International Journal of Sports Physiology and Performance, 7*(3), 242-250.

Lesinski, M., Prieske, O., & Granacher, U. (2016). Effects and dose-response relationships of resistance training on physical performance in youth athletes: A systematic review and meta-analysis. *British Journal of Sports Medicine, 50*(13), 781-795. doi:10.1136/bjsports-2015-095497

*British Journal of Sports Medicine*Lloyd, R.S., Cronin, J.B., Faigenbaum, A.D., Haff, G.G., Howard, R., Kraemer, W.J., . . . Oliver, J.L. (2016). National Strength and Conditioning Association Position Statement on long-term athletic development. *Journal of Strength and Conditioning Research, 30*(6), 1491-1509. doi:10.1519/JSC.0000000000001387

Lloyd, R.S., Faigenbaum, A.D., Stone, M.H., Oliver, J.L., Jeffreys, I., Moody, J.A., . . . Myer, G.D. (2014). Position statement on youth resistance training: The 2014 international consensus. *British Journal of Sports Medicine, 48*(7), 498-505. doi:10.1136/bjsports-2013-092952

Lloyd, R.S., & Oliver, J.L. (2012). The youth physical development model: A new approach to long-term athletic development. *Strength and Conditioning Journal, 34*(3), 61-72.

Lloyd, R.S., Oliver, J.L., Faigenbaum, A.D., Howard, R., De Ste Croix, M.B., Williams, C.A., . . . Myer, G.D. (2015). Long-term athletic development, part 1: A pathway for all youth. *Journal of Strength and Conditioning Research, 29*(5), 1439-1450. doi:10.1519/JSC.0000000000000756

Lloyd, R.S., Oliver, J.L., Faigenbaum, A.D., Myer, G.D., & De Ste Croix, M.B. (2014). Chronological age vs. biological maturation: Implications for exercise programming in youth. *Journal of Strength and Conditioning Research, 28*(5), 1454-1464. doi:10.1519/JSC.0000000000000391

Lloyd, R.S., Radnor, J.M., De Ste Croix, M.B., Cronin, J.B., & Oliver, J.L. (2016). Changes in sprint and jump performances after traditional, plyometric, and combined resistance training in male youth pre- and post-peak height velocity. *Journal of Strength and Conditioning Research, 30*(5), 1239-1247. doi:10.1519/JSC.0000000000001216

Marta, C., Marinho, D.A., Barbosa, T.M., Izquierdo, M., & Marques, M.C. (2013). Effects of concurrent training on explosive strength and VO(2max) in prepubescent children. *International Journal of Sports Medicine, 34*(10), 888-896. doi:10.1055/s-0033-1333695

Matos, N., & Winsley, R.J. (2007). Trainability of young athletes and overtraining. *Journal of Sports Science & Medicine, 6*(3), 353-367.

Matveyev, L.P. (1965). *Periodization of sports.* Moscow, Russia: Fizkultura i Sport.

Matveyev, L.P., & Zdornyj, A.P. (1981). *Fundamentals of sports training.* Moscow, Russia: Progress Publishers.

McMaster, D.T., Gill, N., Cronin, J., & McGuigan, M. (2013). The development, retention and decay rates of strength and power in elite rugby union, rugby league and American football: A systematic review. *Sports Medicine, 43*(5), 367-384. doi:10.1007/s40279-013-0031-3

Meeusen, R., Duclos, M., Foster, C., Fry, A., Gleeson, M., Nieman, D., . . . American College of Sports Medicine. (2013). Prevention, diagnosis, and treatment of the overtraining syndrome:Joint consensus statement of the European College of Sport Science and the American College of Sports Medicine. *Medicine and Science in Sports and Exercise, 45*(1), 186-205. doi:10.1249/MSS.0b013e318279a10a

Meylan, C.M., Cronin, J.B., Oliver, J.L., Hopkins, W.G., & Contreras, B. (2014). The effect of maturation on adaptations to strength training and detraining in 11-15-year-olds. *Scandinavian Journal of Medicine & Science in Sports, 24*(3), e156-164. doi:10.1111/sms.12128

Meylan, C.M., Cronin, J.B., Oliver, J.L., Hughes, M.G., & Manson, S. (2014). An evidence-based model of power development in youth soccer. *International Journal of Sports Science & Coaching, 9*, 1241-1264.

Milewski, M.D., Skaggs, D.L., Bishop, G.A., Pace, J.L., Ibrahim, D.A., Wren, T.A., & Barzdukas, A. (2014). Chronic lack of sleep is associated with increased sports injuries in adolescent athletes. *Journal of Pediatric Orthopedics, 34*(2), 129-133. doi:10.1097/BPO.0000000000000151

Moliner-Urdiales, D., Ruiz, J.R., Ortega, F.B., Jimenez-Pavon, D., Vicente-Rodriguez, G., Rey-Lopez, J.P., . . . Groups, H.S. (2010). Secular trends in health-related physical fitness in Spanish adolescents: The AVENA and HELENA studies. *Journal of Science and Medicine in Sport, 13*(6), 584-588. doi:10.1016/j.jsams.2010.03.004

Moran, J., Sandercock, G., Rumpf, M.C., & Parry, D.A. (2016). Variation in responses to sprint training in male youth athletes: A meta-analysis. *International Journal of Sports Medicine.* doi:10.1055/s-0042-111439

Morris, R., Tod, D., & Eubank, M. (2016). From youth team to first team: An investigation into the transition experiences of young professional athletes in soccer. *International Journal of Sport and Exercise Psychology.* doi:10.1080/1612197X.2016.1152992

Myer, G.D., Faigenbaum, A.D., Edwards, N.M., Clark, J.F., Best, T.M., & Sallis, R.E. (2015). Sixty minutes of what? A developing brain perspective for activating children with an integrative exercise approach. *British Journal of Sports Medicine, 49*(23), 1510-1516. doi:10.1136/bjsports-2014-093661

Myer, G.D., Jayanthi, N., Difiori, J.P., Faigenbaum, A.D., Kiefer, A.W., Logerstedt, D., & Micheli, L.J. (2015). Sport specialization, part I: Does early sports specialization increase negative outcomes and reduce the opportunity for success in young athletes? *Sports Health, 7*(5), 437-442. doi:10.1177/1941738115598747

Nádori, L. (1962). *Training and competition.* Budapest: Sport.

Nikolic, Z., & Ilic, N. (1992). Maximal oxygen uptake in trained and untrained 15-year-old boys. *British Journal of Sports Medicine, 26*(1), 36-38.

Oliver, J.L., Lloyd, R.S., & Meyers, R.W. (2011). Training elite child athletes: Promoting welfare and well-being. *Strength and Conditioning Journal, 33*(4), 73-79.

Parsonage, J.R., Williams, R.S., Rainer, P., McKeown, I., & Williams, M.D. (2014). Assessment of conditioning-specific movement tasks and physical fitness measures in talent identified under 16-year-old rugby union players. *Journal of Strength and Conditioning Research, 28*(6), 1497-1506. doi:10.1519/JSC.0000000000000298

Pelletier, L.G., Rocchi, M.A., Vallerand, R.J., Deci, E.L., & Ryan, R.M. (2013). Validation of the revised sport motivation scale (SMS-II). *Psychology of Sport and Exercise, 14,* 329-341.

Pichardo, A.W., Oliver, J.L., Harrison, C.B., Maulder, P.S., & Lloyd, R.S. (2018). Integrating models of long-term athletic development to maximize the physical development of youth. *International Journal of Sports Science & Coaching, 13*(6), 1189-1199.

Radnor, J.M., Lloyd, R.S., & Oliver, J.L. (2017). Individual response to different forms of resistance training in school aged boys. *Journal of Strength and Conditioning Research, 31*(3), 787-797.

Rhea, M.R., & Alderman, B.L. (2004). A meta-analysis of periodized versus nonperiodized strength and power training programs. *Research Quarterly for Exercise and Sport, 75*(4), 413-422. doi:10.1080/02701367.2004.10609174

Rice, S.G., Congeni, J.A., & Council on Sports Medicine and Fitness. (2012). Baseball and softball. *Pediatrics, 129*(3), e842-e856. doi:10.1542/peds.2011-3593

Robertson, R.J., Goss, F.L., Aaron, D.J., Gairola, A., Kowallis, R.A., Liu, Y., . . . White, B. (2008). One repetition maximum prediction models for children using the OMNI RPE Scale. *Journal of Strength and Conditioning Research, 22*(1), 196-201. doi:10.1519/JSC.0b013e31815f6283

Robertson, R.J., Goss, F.L., Andreacci, J.L., Dube, J.J., Rutkowski, J.J., Frazee, K.M., . . . Snee, B.M. (2005). Validation of the children's OMNI-resistance exercise scale of perceived exertion. *Medicine and Science in Sports and Exercise, 37*(5), 819-826.

Robertson, R.J., Goss, F.L., Boer, N.F., Peoples, J.A., Foreman, A.J., Dabayebeh, I.M., . . . Thompkins, T. (2000). Children's OMNI scale of perceived exertion: Mixed gender and race validation. *Medicine and Science in Sports and Exercise, 32*(2), 452-458.

Robineau, J., Babault, N., Piscione, J., Lacome, M., & Bigard, A.X. (2016). Specific training effects of concurrent aerobic and strength exercises depend on recovery duration. *Journal of Strength and Conditioning Research, 30*(3), 672-683. doi:10.1519/JSC.0000000000000798

Rumpf, M.C., Cronin, J.B., Pinder, S.D., Oliver, J., & Hughes, M. (2012). Effect of different training methods on running sprint times in male youth. *Pediatric Exercise Science, 24*(2), 170-186.

Runhaar, J., Collard, D.C., Singh, A.S., Kemper, H.C., van Mechelen, W., & Chinapaw, M. (2010). Motor fitness in Dutch youth: Differences over a 26-year period (1980-2006). *Journal of Science and Medicine in Sport, 13*(3), 323-328. doi:10.1016/j.jsams.2009.04.006

Sander, A., Keiner, M., Wirth, K., & Schmidtbleicher, D. (2013). Influence of a 2-year strength training programme on power performance in elite youth soccer players. *European Journal of Sport Science, 13*(5), 445-451. doi:10.1080/17461391.2012.742572

Santos, A.P., Marinho, D.A., Costa, A.M., Izquierdo, M., & Marques, M.C. (2012). The effects of concurrent resistance and endurance training follow a detraining period in elementary school students. *Journal of Strength and Conditioning Research, 26*(6), 1708-1716. doi:10.1519/JSC.0b013e318234e872

Selye, H. (1956). *The stress of life.* New York, NY: McGraw-Hill.

Sharf, R.S. (2009). *Applying career development theory to counseling* (5th ed.). Pacific Grove, CA: Brooks/Cole.

Shea, C.H., & Wulf, G. (2005). Schema theory: A critical appraisal and reevaluation. *Journal of Motor Behavior, 37*(2), 85-101. doi:10.3200/JMBR.37.2.85-102

Sheppard, J.M., & Triplett, N.T. (2016). Program design for resistance training. In G.G. Haff & N.T. Triplett (Eds.), *Essentials of strength training and conditioning* (4th ed., pp. 439-469). Champaign, IL: Human Kinetics.

Stadulis, R.E., MacCracken, M.J., Eidson, T.A., & Sevrance, C. (2002). A children's form of the Competitive State Anxiety Inventory: The CSAI-2C. *Meas Phys Educ Exerc Sci, 6*(3), 147-165.

Stambulova, N., Alfermann, D., Statler, T., & Cote, J. (2009). ISSP position stand: Career development and transitions of athletes. *International Journal of Sport and Exercise Psychology, 7,* 395-412.

Terry, P.C., Lane, A.M., Lane, H.J., & Keohane, L. (1999). Development and validation of a mood measure for adolescents. *Journal of Sports Sciences, 17*(11), 861-872. doi:10.1080/026404199365425

Tofler, I.R., Knapp, P.K., & Larden, M. (2005). Achievement by proxy distortion in sports: a distorted mentoring of high-achieving youth: Historical perspectives and clinical intervention with children, adolescents, and their families. *Clinics in Sports Medicine, 24*(4), 805-828, viii. doi:10.1016/j.csm.2005.06.007

Tremblay, M.S., Barnes, J.D., Gonzalez, S.A., Katzmarzyk, P.T., Onywera, V.O., Reilly, J.J., . . . Global Matrix 2.0 Research, T. (2016). Global matrix 2.0: Report card grades on the physical activity of children and youth comparing 38 countries. *Journal of Physical Activity & Health, 13*(11 Suppl 2), S343-S366. doi:10.1123/jpah.2016-0594

Verkhoshansky, Y. (2009). *Supertraining* (6th ed.). Rome, Italy: Verkhoshansky.

Viru, A. (1988). Planning macrocycles. *Modern Athlete and Coach*, *26*, 7-10.

Viru, A. (1995). *Adaptation in sports training*. Boca Raton, FL: CRC Press.

Watson, A., Brickson, S., Brooks, A., & Dunn, W. (2016). Subjective well-being and training load predict in-season injury and illness risk in female youth soccer players. *British Journal of Sports Medicine*. doi:10.1136/bjsports-2016-096584

Williams, C.A., Winsley, R.J., Pinho, G., De Ste Croix, M., Lloyd, R.S., & Oliver, J.L. (2017). Prevalence of non-functional overreaching in elite male and female youth academy football players. *Science and Medicine in Football, 1*(3), 222-228.

Williams, T.D., Tolusso, D.V., Fedewa, M.V., & Esco, M.R. (2017). Comparison of periodized and non-periodized resistance training on maximal strength: A meta-analysis. *Sports Medicine*. doi:10.1007/s40279-017-0734-y

Wilson, J.M., Marin, P.J., Rhea, M.R., Wilson, S.M., Loenneke, J.P., & Anderson, J.C. (2012). Concurrent training: A meta-analysis examining interference of aerobic and resistance exercises. *Journal of Strength and Conditioning Research, 26*(8), 2293-2307. doi:10.1519/JSC.0b013e31823a3e2d

Woods, C.T., McKeown, I., Haff, G.G., & Robertson, S. (2016). Comparison of athletic movement between elite junior and senior Australian football players. *Journal of Sports Sciences, 34*(13), 1260-1265. doi:10.1080/02640414.2015.1107185

World Health Organization. (2010). *Global recommendations on physical activity for health*. Geneva, Switzerland: Author.

Zamparo, P., Minetti, A.E., & di Prampero, P.E. (2002). Interplay among the changes of muscle strength, cross-sectional area and maximal explosive power: Theory and facts. *European Journal of Applied Physiology, 88*(3), 193-202. doi:10.1007/s00421-002-0691-4

Zatsiorsky, V.M., & Kraemer, W.J. (2006). *Science and practice of strength training*. Champaign, IL: Human Kinetics.

Chapter 13 Young Athletes and Sport Participation

Akenhead, R., French, D., Thompson, K.G., & Hayes, P.R. (2014). The acceleration dependent validity and reliability of 10 Hz GPS. *Journal of Science and Medicine in Sport, 17*(5), 562-566. doi:10.1016/j.jsams.2013.08.005

Alentorn-Geli, E., Mendiguchia, J., Samuelsson, K., Musahl, V., Karlsson, J., Cugat, R., & Myer, G.D. (2014). Prevention of non-contact anterior cruciate ligament injuries in sports. Part II: Systematic review of the effectiveness of prevention programmes in male athletes. *Knee Surgery, Sports Traumatology, Arthroscopy, 22*(1), 16-25. doi:10.1007/s00167-013-2739-x

Alentorn-Geli, E., Myer, G.D., Silvers, H.J., Samitier, G., Romero, D., Lazaro-Haro, C., & Cugat, R. (2009). Prevention of non-contact anterior cruciate ligament injuries in soccer players. Part 1: Mechanisms of injury and underlying risk factors. *Knee Surgery, Sports Traumatology, Arthroscopy, 17*(7), 705-729. doi:10.1007/s00167-009-0813-1

Allender, S., Cowburn, G., & Foster, C. (2006). Understanding participation in sport and physical activity among children and adults: A review of qualitative studies. *Health Education Research, 21*(6), 826-835. doi:10.1093/her/cyl063

American Academy of Orthopaedic Surgeons. (2012). *A guide to safety for young athletes*. Retrieved from http://orthoinfo.aaos.org/topic.cfm?topic=A00307

Ara, I., Vicente-Rodriguez, G., Jimenez-Ramirez, J., Dorado, C., Serrano-Sanchez, J.A., & Calbet, J.A. (2004). Regular participation in sports is associated with enhanced physical fitness and lower fat mass in prepubertal boys. *International Journal of Obesity and Related Metabolic Disorders, 28*(12), 1585-1593. doi:10.1038/sj.ijo.0802754

Armstrong, N. (1998). Young people's physical activity patterns as assessed by heart rate monitoring. *Journal of Sports Sciences, 16*(Suppl), S9-S16. doi:10.1080/026404198366632

Armstrong, N., & Welsman, J. (2005). Essay: Physiology of the child athlete. *Lancet, 366*(Suppl 1), S44-S45. doi:10.1016/S0140-6736(05)67845-2

Armstrong, N., & Welsman, J.R. (2006). The physical activity patterns of European youth with reference to methods of assessment. *Sports Med, 36*(12), 1067-1086.

Ballester, R., Huertas, F., Yuste, F.J., Llorens, F., & Sanabria, D. (2015). The relationship between regular sports participation and vigilance in male and female adolescents. *PLoS One, 10*(4), e0123898. doi:10.1371/journal.pone.0123898

Baranto, A., Hellstrom, M., Nyman, R., Lundin, O., & Sward, L. (2006). Back pain and degenerative abnormalities in the spine of young elite divers: A 5-year follow-up magnetic resonance imaging study. *Knee Surgery, Sports Traumatology, Arthroscopy, 14*(9), 907-914. doi:10.1007/s00167-005-0032-3

Barron, D.J., Atkins, S., Edmundson, C., & Fewtrell, D. (2014). Accelerometer derived load according to playing position in competitive youth soccer. *International Journal of Performance Analysis in Sport, 14*, 734-743.

Bauer, R., & Steiner, M. (2009). *Injuries in the European Union statistics summary 2005-2007*. Retrieved from http://ec.europa.eu/health//sites/health/files/healthy_environments/docs/2009-idb-report_screen.pdf

Bell, D.R., Post, E.G., Trigsted, S.M., Hetzel, S., McGuine, T.A., & Brooks, M.A. (2016). Prevalence of sport specialization in high school athletics: A 1-year observational study. *The American Journal of Sports Medicine, 44*(6), 1469-1474. doi:10.1177/0363546516629943

Berz, K., Divine, J., Foss, K.B., Heyl, R., Ford, K.R., & Myer, G.D. (2013). Sex-specific differences in the severity of symptoms and recovery rate following sports-related concussion in young athletes. *The Physician and Sportsmedicine, 41*(2), 58-63. doi:10.3810/psm.2013.05.2015

Beunen, G.P., & Malina, R.M. (2008). Growth and biological maturation: Relevance to athletic performance. In H. Hebestreit & O. Bar-Or (Eds.), *The young athlete* (pp. 3-17). Oxford: Blackwell Publishing.

Birrer, D., Lienhard, D., Williams, C.A., Röthlin, P., & Morgan, G. (2013). Prevalence of non-functional overreaching and the overtraining syndrome in Swiss elite athletes. *Schweizerische Zeitschrift fur Medizin und Traumatologie, 61*(4), 23-29.

Boden, B.P., Dean, G.S., Feagin, J.A., Jr., & Garrett, W.E., Jr. (2000). Mechanisms of anterior cruciate ligament injury. *Orthopedics, 23*(6), 573-578.

Bourdon, P.C., Cardinale, M., Murray, A., Gastin, P., Kellmann, M., Varley, M.C., . . . Cable, N.T. (2017). Monitoring athlete training loads: Consensus statement. *International Journal of Sports Physiology and Performance, 12*(Suppl 2), S2161-S2170. doi:10.1123/IJSPP.2017-0208

Brazo-Sayavera, J., Martinez-Valencia, M.A., Muller, L., Andronikos, G., & Martindale, R.J. (2016). Identifying talented track and field athletes: The impact of relative age effect on selection to the Spanish National Athletics Federation training camps. *Journal of Sports Sciences*, 1-7. doi:10.1080/02640414.2016.1260151

Brenner, J.S., & Council on Sports Medicine & Fitness. (2016). Sports specialization and intensive training in young athletes. *Pediatrics, 138*(3). doi:10.1542/peds.2016-2148

Brink, M.S., Visscher, C., Coutts, A.J., & Lemmink, K.A. (2012). Changes in perceived stress and recovery in overreached young elite soccer players. *Scandinavian Journal of Medicine & Science in Sports, 22*(2), 285-292. doi:10.1111/j.1600-0838.2010.01237.x

Brooks, A., & Hammer, E. (2013). Acute upper extremity injuries in young athletes. *Clinical Pediatric Emergency Medicine, 14*(4), 289-303.

Buchheit, M., Rabbani, A., & Beigi, H.T. (2014). Predicting changes in high-intensity intermittent running performance with acute responses to short jump rope workouts in children. *Journal of Sports Science & Medicine, 13*(3), 476-482.

Caine, D., Caine, C., & Maffulli, N. (2006). Incidence and distribution of pediatric sport-related injuries. *Clinical Journal of Sport Medicine, 16*(6), 500-513. doi:10.1097/01.jsm.0000251181.36582.a0

Cassas, K.J., & Cassettari-Wayhs, A. (2006). Childhood and adolescent sports-related overuse injuries. *American Family Physician, 73*(6), 1014-1022.

Castagna, C., Manzi, V., Impellizzeri, F., Weston, M., & Barbero Alvarez, J.C. (2010). Relationship between endurance field tests and match performance in young soccer players. *Journal of Strength and Conditioning Research, 24*(12), 3227-3233. doi:10.1519/JSC.0b013e3181e72709

Chaouachi, A., Hammami, R., Kaabi, S., Chamari, K., Drinkwater, E.J., & Behm, D.G. (2014). Olympic weightlifting and plyometric training with children provides similar or greater performance improvements than traditional resistance training. *Journal of Strength and Conditioning Research, 28*(6), 1483-1496. doi:10.1519/JSC.0000000000000305

Chen, Y.L., Chiou, W.K., Tzeng, Y.T., Lu, C.Y., & Chen, S.C. (2017). A rating of perceived exertion scale using facial expressions for conveying exercise intensity for children and young adults. *Journal of Science and Medicine in Sport, 20*(1), 66-69. doi:10.1016/j.jsams.2016.05.009

Cobley, S., Baker, J., Wattie, N., & McKenna, J. (2009). Annual age-grouping and athlete development: A meta-analytical review of relative age effects in sport. *Sports Medicine, 39*(3), 235-256. doi:10.2165/00007256-200939030-00005

Covassin, T., & Elbin, R.J. (2011). The female athlete: The role of gender in the assessment and management of sport-related concussion. *Clinics in Sports Medicine, 30*(1), 125-131, x. doi:10.1016/j.csm.2010.08.001

Covassin, T., Elbin, R.J., 3rd, Stiller-Ostrowski, J.L., & Kontos, A.P. (2009). Immediate post-concussion assessment and cognitive testing (ImPACT) practices of sports medicine professionals. *Journal of Athletic Training, 44*(6), 639-644. doi:10.4085/1062-6050-44.6.639

Covassin, T., Savage, J.L., Bretzin, A.C., & Fox, M.E. (2017). Sex differences in sport-related concussion long-term outcomes. *International Journal of Psychophysiology.* doi:10.1016/j.ijpsycho.2017.09.010

Cumming, S.P., Brown, D.J., Mitchell, S., Bunce, J., Hunt, D., Hedges, C., . . . Malina, R.M. (2018). Premier League academy soccer players' experiences of competing in a tournament bio-banded for biological maturation. *Journal of Sports Sciences, 36*(7), 757-765. doi:10.1080/02640414.2017.1340656

Cumming, S.P., Lloyd, R.S., Oliver, J.L., Eisenmann, J.C., & Malina, R.M. (2017). Bio-banding in sport: Applications to competition, talent, identification, and strength and conditioning of youth athletes. *Strength and Conditioning Journal, 39*(2), 34-47.

Dayne, A.M., McBride, J.M., Nuzzo, J.L., Triplett, N.T., Skinner, J., & Burr, A. (2011). Power output in the jump squat in adolescent male athletes. *Journal of Strength and Conditioning Research, 25*(3), 585-589. doi:10.1519/JSC.0b013e3181c1fa83

d'Hemecourt, P.A., Gerbino, P.G., 2nd, & Micheli, L.J. (2000). Back injuries in the young athlete. *Clinics in Sports Medicine, 19*(4), 663-679.

Del Campo, D.G.D., Vicedo, J.C.P., Villora, S.G., & Jordan, O.R.C. (2010). The relative age effect in youth soccer players from Spain. *Journal of Sports Science & Medicine, 9*(2), 190-198.

de Loes, M., Dahlstedt, L.J., & Thomee, R. (2000). A 7-year study on risks and costs of knee injuries in male and female youth participants in 12 sports. *Scandinavian Journal of Medicine & Science in Sports, 10*(2), 90-97.

Delorme, N., Boiche, J., & Raspaud, M. (2010a). Relative age and dropout in French male soccer. *Journal of Sports Sciences, 28*(7), 717-722. doi:10.1080/02640411003663276

Delorme, N., Boiche, J., & Raspaud, M. (2010b). Relative age effect in female sport: A diachronic examination of soccer players. *Scandinavian Journal of Medicine & Science in Sports, 20*(3), 509-515. doi:10.1111/j.1600-0838.2009.00979.x

Dennis, R.J., Finch, C.F., & Farhart, P.J. (2005). Is bowling workload a risk factor for injury to Australian junior cricket fast bowlers? *British Journal of Sports Medicine, 39*(11), 843-846. doi:10.1136/bjsm.2005.018515

Dick, R.W. (2009). Is there a gender difference in concussion incidence and outcomes? *British Journal of Sports Medicine, 43*(Suppl 1), i46-i50. doi:10.1136/bjsm.2009.058172

DiFiori, J.P., Benjamin, H.J., Brenner, J., Gregory, A., Jayanthi, N., Landry, G.L., & Luke, A. (2014). Overuse injuries and burnout in youth sports: A position statement from the American Medical Society for Sports Medicine. *Clinical Journal of Sport Medicine, 24*(1), 3-20. doi:10.1097/JSM.0000000000000060

Dotan, R., Mitchell, C.J., Cohen, R., Gabriel, D., Klentrou, P., & Falk, B. (2013). Explosive sport training and torque kinetics in children. *Applied Physiology, Nutrition, and Metabolism, 38*(7), 740-745. doi:10.1139/apnm-2012-0330

Drew, M.K., & Finch, C.F. (2016). The relationship between training load and injury, illness and soreness: A systematic and literature review. *Sports Medicine, 46*(6), 861-883. doi:10.1007/s40279-015-0459-8

Ebben, W.P., Fauth, M.L., Garceau, L.R., & Petushek, E.J. (2011). Kinetic quantification of plyometric exercise intensity. *Journal of Strength and Conditioning Research, 25*(12), 3288-3298. doi:10.1519/JSC.0b013e31821656a3

Ebben, W.P., Simenz, C., & Jensen, R.L. (2008). Evaluation of plyometric intensity using electromyography. *Journal of Strength and Conditioning Research, 22*(3), 861-868. doi:10.1519/JSC.0b013e31816a834b

Ehrmann, F.E., Duncan, C.S., Sindhusake, D., Franzsen, W.N., & Greene, D.A. (2016). GPS and injury prevention in professional soccer. *Journal of Strength and Conditioning Research, 30*(2), 360-367. doi:10.1519/JSC.0000000000001093

Eime, R.M., Harvey, J.T., Charity, M.J., Casey, M.M., Westerbeek, H., & Payne, W.R. (2016). Age profiles of sport participants. *BMC Sports Science, Medicine & Rehabilitation, 8*, 6. doi:10.1186/s13102-016-0031-3

Eime, R.M., Young, J.A., Harvey, J.T., Charity, M.J., & Payne, W.R. (2013). A systematic review of the psychological and social benefits of participation in sport for children and adolescents: Informing development of a conceptual model of health through sport. *International Journal of Behavioral Nutrition and Physical Activity, 10*, 98. doi:10.1186/1479-5868-10-98

Elbin, R.J., Sufrinko, A., Schatz, P., French, J., Henry, L., Burkhart, S., . . . Kontos, A.P. (2016). Removal from play after concussion and recovery time. *Pediatrics, 138*(3). doi:10.1542/peds.2016-0910

Elliott, S.K., & Drummond, M.J.N. (2017). Parents in youth sport: What happens after the game? *Sport, Education and Society, 22*(3), 391-406.

Emery, C.A. (2010). Injury prevention in paediatric sport-related injuries: A scientific approach. *British Journal of Sports Medicine, 44*(1), 64-69. doi:10.1136/bjsm.2009.068353

Emery, C.A., & Meeuwisse, W.H. (2010). The effectiveness of a neuromuscular prevention strategy to reduce injuries in youth soccer: A cluster-randomised controlled trial. *British Journal of Sports Medicine, 44*(8), 555-562. doi:10.1136/bjsm.2010.074377

Emery, C.A., Meeuwisse, W.H., & McAllister, J.R. (2006). Survey of sport participation and sport injury in Calgary and area high schools. *Clinical Journal of Sport Medicine, 16*(1), 20-26.

Emery, C., & Tyreman, H. (2009). Sport participation, sport injury, risk factors and sport safety practices in Calgary and area junior high schools. *Paediatrics & Child Health, 14*(7), 439-444.

Faigenbaum, A.D., Milliken, L.A., Cloutier, G., & Westcott, W.L. (2004). Perceived exertion during resistance exercise by children. *Perceptual and Motor Skills, 98*(2), 627-637. doi:10.2466/pms.98.2.627-637

Fernhall, B., Kohrt, W., Burkett, L.N., & Walters, S. (1996). Relationship between the lactate threshold and cross-country run performance in high school male and female runners. *Pediatric Exercise Science, 8*, 37-47.

Field, M., Collins, M.W., Lovell, M.R., & Maroon, J. (2003). Does age play a role in recovery from sports-related concussion? A comparison of high school and collegiate athletes. *Journal of Pediatrics, 142*(5), 546-553. doi:10.1067/mpd.2003.190

Fleisig, G.S., Andrews, J.R., Cutter, G.R., Weber, A., Loftice, J., McMichael, C., . . . Lyman, S. (2011). Risk of serious injury for young baseball pitchers: A 10-year prospective study. *The American Journal of Sports Medicine, 39*(2), 253-257. doi:10.1177/0363546510384224

Ford, K.R., Myer, G.D., Brent, J.L., & Hewett, T.E. (2009). Hip and knee extensor moments predict vertical jump height in adolescent girls. *Journal of Strength and Conditioning Research, 23*(4), 1327-1331. doi:10.1519/JSC.0b013e31819bbea4

Fraser-Thomas, J., & Cote, J. (2009). Understanding adolescents' positive and negative developmental experiences in sport. *The Sport Psychologist, 23*(1), 3-23.

Fridman, L., Fraser-Thomas, J.L., McFaull, S.R., & Macpherson, A.K. (2013). Epidemiology of sports-related injuries in children and youth presenting to Canadian emergency departments from 2007-2010. *BMC Sports Science, Medicine & Rehabilitation, 5*(1), 30. doi:10.1186/2052-1847-5-30

Froberg, A., Alricsson, M., & Ahnesjo, J. (2014). Awareness of current recommendations and guidelines regarding strength training for youth. *International Journal of Adolescent Medicine and Health, 26*(4), 517-523. doi:10.1515/ijamh-2013-0329

Gabbett, T.J. (2016). The training-injury prevention paradox: Should athletes be training smarter and harder? *British Journal of Sports Medicine, 50*(5), 273-280. doi:10.1136/bjsports-2015-095788

Gessel, L.M., Fields, S.K., Collins, C.L., Dick, R.W., & Comstock, R.D. (2007). Concussions among United States high school and collegiate athletes. *Journal of Athletic Training, 42*(4), 495-503.

Gomez, J.E., & Hergenroeder, A.C. (2013). New guidelines for management of concussion in sport: Special concern for youth. *Journal of Adolescent Health, 53*(3), 311-313. doi:10.1016/j.jadohealth.2013.06.018

Goncalves, C.E., Rama, L.M., & Figueiredo, A.B. (2012). Talent identification and specialization in sport: An overview of some unanswered questions. *International Journal of Sports Physiology and Performance, 7*(4), 390-393.

Gonzalez-Badillo, J.J., & Sanchez-Medina, L. (2010). Movement velocity as a measure of loading intensity in resistance training. *International Journal of Sports Medicine, 31*(5), 347-352. doi:10.1055/s-0030-1248333

Goodwin, M.L., Harris, J.E., Hernandez, A., & Gladden, L.B. (2007). Blood lactate measurements and analysis during exercise: A guide for clinicians. *Journal of Diabetes Science and Technology, 1*(4), 558-569. doi:10.1177/193229680700100414

Gould, D., & Carson, S. (2008). Life skills development through sport: Current status and future directions. *International Review of Sport and Exercise Psychology, 1*(1), 58-78.

Gould, D., Eklund, R., Petlichkoff, L., Peterson, K., & Bump, L. (1991). Psychological predictors of state anxiety and performance in age-group wrestlers. *Pediatric Exercise Science, 3*, 198-208.

Grady, M.F. (2010). Concussion in the adolescent athlete. *Current Problems in Pediatric and Adolescent Health Care, 40*(7), 154-169. doi:10.1016/j.cppeds.2010.06.002

Granan, L.P., Forssblad, M., Lind, M., & Engebretsen, L. (2009). The Scandinavian ACL registries 2004-2007: Baseline epidemiology. *Acta Orthopaedica, 80*(5), 563-567. doi:10.3109/17453670903350107

Haddad, M., Chaouachi, A., Castagna, C., Wong del, P., Behm, D.G., & Chamari, K. (2011). The construct validity of session RPE during an intensive camp in young male Taekwondo athletes. *International Journal of Sports Physiology and Performance, 6*(2), 252-263.

Halin, R., Germain, P., Buttelli, O., & Kapitaniak, B. (2002). Differences in strength and surface electromyogram characteristics between pre-pubertal gymnasts and untrained boys during brief and maintained maximal isometric voluntary contractions. *European Journal of Applied Physiology, 87*(4-5), 409-415. doi:10.1007/s00421-002-0643-z

Hall, R., Barber Foss, K., Hewett, T.E., & Myer, G.D. (2015). Sport specialization's association with an increased risk of developing anterior knee pain in adolescent female athletes. *Journal of Sport Rehabilitation, 24*(1), 31-35. doi:10.1123/jsr.2013-0101

Halson, S.L. (2014). Monitoring training load to understand fatigue in athletes. *Sports Medicine, 44*(Suppl 2), S139-S147. doi:10.1007/s40279-014-0253-z

Hardie Murphy, M., Rowe, D.A., & Woods, C.B. (2017). Impact of physical activity domains on subsequent physical activity in youth: A 5-year longitudinal study. *Journal of Sports Sciences, 35*(3), 262-268. doi:10.1080/02640414.2016.1161219

Hartwig, T.B., Naughton, G., & Searl, J. (2011). Motion analyses of adolescent rugby union players: A comparison of training and game demands. *Journal of Strength and Conditioning Research, 25*(4), 966-972. doi:10.1519/JSC.0b013e3181d09e24

Harwood, C.G., & Knight, C.J. (2015). Parenting in youth sport: A position paper on parenting expertise. *Psychology of Sport and Exercise, 16*, 24-35.

Haugen, T., & Buchheit, M. (2016). Sprint running performance monitoring: Methodological and practical considerations. *Sports Medicine, 46*(5), 641-656. doi:10.1007/s40279-015-0446-0

Haus, B.M., & Micheli, L.J. (2012). Back pain in the pediatric and adolescent athlete. *Clinics in Sports Medicine, 31*(3), 423-440. doi:10.1016/j.csm.2012.03.011

Hecksteden, A., Kraushaar, J., Scharhag-Rosenberger, F., Theisen, D., Senn, S., & Meyer, T. (2015). Individual response to exercise training: A statistical perspective. *Journal of Applied Physiology, 118*(12), 1450-1459. doi:10.1152/japplphysiol.00714.2014

Helsen, W.F., Baker, J., Michiels, S., Schorer, J., Van Winckel, J., & Williams, A.M. (2012). The relative age effect in European professional soccer: Did ten years of research make any difference? *Journal of Sports Sciences, 30*(15), 1665-1671. doi:10.1080/02640414.2012.721929

Helsen, W.F., van Winckel, J., & Williams, A.M. (2005). The relative age effect in youth soccer across Europe. *Journal of Sports Sciences, 23*(6), 629-636. doi:10.1080/02640410400021310

Hendrix, C.L. (2005). Calcaneal apophysitis (Sever disease). *Clinics in Podiatric Medicine and Surgery, 22*(1), 55-62, vi. doi:10.1016/j.cpm.2004.08.011

Hennrikus, W.L. (2006). Elbow disorders in the young athlete. *Operative Techniques in Sports Medicine, 14*, 165-172.

Hewett, T.E., Di Stasi, S.L., & Myer, G.D. (2013). Current concepts for injury prevention in athletes after anterior cruciate ligament reconstruction. *The American Journal of Sports Medicine, 41*(1), 216-224. doi:10.1177/0363546512459638

Hewett, T.E., Ford, K.R., & Myer, G.D. (2006). Anterior cruciate ligament injuries in female athletes: Part 2, a meta-analysis of neuromuscular interventions aimed at injury prevention. *The American Journal of Sports Medicine, 34*(3), 490-498. doi:10.1177/0363546505282619

Hewett, T.E., Myer, G.D., & Ford, K.R. (2004). Decrease in neuromuscular control about the knee with maturation in female athletes. *Journal of Bone and Joint Surgery, 86*-A(8), 1601-1608.

Hewett, T.E., Myer, G.D., & Ford, K.R. (2006). Anterior cruciate ligament injuries in female athletes: Part 1, mechanisms and risk factors. *The American Journal of Sports Medicine, 34*(2), 299-311. doi:10.1177/0363546505284183

Hewett, T.E., Myer, G.D., Ford, K.R., Paterno, M.V., & Quatman, C.E. (2016). Mechanisms, prediction, and prevention of ACL injuries: Cut risk with three sharpened and validated tools. *Journal of Orthopaedic Research, 34*(11), 1843-1855. doi:10.1002/jor.23414

Hill-Haas, S., Coutts, A., Rowsell, G., & Dawson, B. (2008). Variability of acute physiological responses and performance profiles of youth soccer players in small-sided games. *Journal of Science and Medicine in Sport, 11*(5), 487-490. doi:10.1016/j.jsams.2007.07.006

Hislop, M.D., Stokes, K.A., Williams, S., McKay, C.D., England, M.E., Kemp, S.P.T., & Trewartha, G. (2017). Reducing musculoskeletal injury and concussion risk in schoolboy rugby players with a pre-activity movement control exercise programme: A cluster randomised controlled trial. *British Journal of Sports Medicine, 51*(15), 1140-1146. doi:10.1136/bjsports-2016-097434

Hoffman, A., Wulff, J., Busch, D., & Sandner, H. (2012, July). *Relative age effect in Olympic sports: A comparison of Beijing 2008 and Singapore 2010.* Paper presented at the European College of Sports Sciences Congress, Bruges.

Hoppe, M.W., Baumgart, C., Bornefeld, J., Sperlich, B., Freiwald, J., & Holmberg, H.C. (2014). Running activity profile of adolescent tennis players during match play. *Pediatric Exercise Science, 26*(3), 281-290. doi:10.1123/pes.2013-0195

Howell, D.R., Osternig, L.R., & Chou, L.S. (2015). Adolescents demonstrate greater gait balance control deficits after concussion than young adults. *The American Journal of Sports Medicine, 43*(3), 625-632. doi:10.1177/0363546514560994

Hui, S.S., & Chan, J.W. (2006). The relationship between heart rate reserve and oxygen uptake reserve in children and adolescents. *Research Quarterly for Exercise and Sport, 77*(1), 41-49. doi:10.1080/02701367.2006.10599330

Hulin, B.T., Gabbett, T.J., Blanch, P., Chapman, P., Bailey, D., & Orchard, J.W. (2014). Spikes in acute workload are associated with increased injury risk in elite cricket fast bowlers. *British Journal of Sports Medicine, 48*(8), 708-712. doi:10.1136/bjsports-2013-092524

Hulin, B.T., Gabbett, T.J., Lawson, D.W., Caputi, P., & Sampson, J.A. (2016). The acute:chronic workload ratio predicts injury: High chronic workload may decrease injury risk in elite rugby league players. *British Journal of Sports Medicine, 50*(4), 231-236. doi:10.1136/bjsports-2015-094817

Hulteen, R.M., Smith, J.J., Morgan, P.J., Barnett, L.M., Hallal, P.C., Colyvas, K., & Lubans, D.R. (2017). Global participation in sport and leisure-time physical activities: A systematic review and meta-analysis. *Preventive Medicine, 95*, 14-25. doi:10.1016/j.ypmed.2016.11.027

Hutchinson, M.R. (1999). Low back pain in elite rhythmic gymnasts. *Medicine and Science in Sports and Exercise, 31*(11), 1686-1688.

Huxley, D.J., O'Connor, D., & Healey, P.A. (2014). An examination of the training profiles and injuries in elite youth track and field athletes. *European Journal of Sport Science, 14*(2), 185-192. doi:10.1080/17461391.2013.809153

Jarvis, M.M., Graham-Smith, P., & Comfort, P. (2016). A methodological approach to quantifying plyometric intensity. *Journal of Strength and Conditioning Research, 30*(9), 2522-2532. doi:10.1519/JSC.0000000000000518

Jayanthi, N.A., LaBella, C.R., Fischer, D., Pasulka, J., & Dugas, L.R. (2015). Sports-specialized intensive training and the risk of injury in young athletes: A clinical case-control study. *The American Journal of Sports Medicine, 43*(4), 794-801. doi:10.1177/0363546514567298

Kennedy, J.G., Knowles, B., Dolan, M., & Bohne, W. (2005). Foot and ankle injuries in the adolescent runner. *Current Opinion in Pediatrics, 17*(1), 34-42.

Kentta, G., Hassmen, P., & Raglin, J.S. (2001). Training practices and overtraining syndrome in Swedish age-group athletes. *International Journal of Sports Medicine, 22*(6), 460-465. doi:10.1055/s-2001-16250

Kerssemakers, S.P., Fotiadou, A.N., de Jonge, M.C., Karantanas, A.H., & Maas, M. (2009). Sport injuries in the paediatric and adolescent patient: A growing problem. *Pediatric Radiology, 39*(5), 471-484. doi:10.1007/s00247-009-1191-z

Khamis, H.J., & Roche, A.F. (1994). Predicting adult stature without using skeletal age: The Khamis-Roche method. *Pediatrics, 94*(4 Pt 1), 504-507.

Knight, C.J., Berrow, S.R., & Harwood, C.G. (2017). Parenting in sport. *Current Opinion in Psychology, 16*, 93-97.

Koklu, Y., Alemdaroglu, U., Cihan, H., & Wong, D.P. (2017). Effects of bout duration on players' internal and external loads during small-sided games in young soccer players. *International Journal of Sports Physiology and Performance*, 1-23. doi:10.1123/ijspp.2016-0584

LaBella, C.R., Hennrikus, W., Hewett, T.E., Council on Sports Medicine and Fitness, & Section on Orthopaedics. (2014). Anterior cruciate ligament injuries: diagnosis, treatment, and prevention. *Pediatrics, 133*(5), e1437-1450. doi:10.1542/peds.2014-0623

LaBella, C.R., Huxford, M.R., Grissom, J., Kim, K.Y., Peng, J., & Christoffel, K.K. (2011). Effect of neuromuscular warm-up on injuries in female soccer and basketball athletes in urban public high schools: Cluster randomized controlled trial. *Archives of Pediatrics & Adolescent Medicine, 165*(11), 1033-1040. doi:10.1001/archpediatrics.2011.168

LaPrade, R.F., Agel, J., Baker, J., Brenner, J.S., Cordasco, F.A., Cote, J., . . . Provencher, M.T. (2016). AOSSM early sport specialization consensus statement. *Orthopaedic Journal of Sports Medicine, 4*(4), 2325967116644241. doi:10.1177/2325967116644241

Lauersen, J.B., Bertelsen, D.M., & Andersen, L.B. (2014). The effectiveness of exercise interventions to prevent sports injuries: A systematic review and meta-analysis of randomised controlled trials. *British Journal of Sports Medicine, 48*(11), 871-877. doi:10.1136/bjsports-2013-092538

Leard, J.S., Cirillo, M.A., Katsnelson, E., Kimiatek, D.A., Miller, T.W., Trebincevic, K., & Garbalosa, J.C. (2007). Validity of two alternative systems for measuring vertical jump height. *Journal of Strength and Conditioning Research, 21*(4), 1296-1299. doi:10.1519/R-21536.1

Leek, D., Carlson, J.A., Cain, K.L., Henrichon, S., Rosenberg, D., Patrick, K., & Sallis, J.F. (2011). Physical activity during youth sports practices. *Archives of Pediatrics & Adolescent Medicine, 165*(4), 294-299. doi:10.1001/archpediatrics.2010.252

Leonard, J., & Hutchinson, M.R. (2010). Shoulder injuries in skeletally immature throwers: Review and current thoughts. *British Journal of Sports Medicine, 44*(5), 306-310. doi:10.1136/bjsm.2009.062588

Lesinski, M., Prieske, O., & Granacher, U. (2016). Effects and dose-response relationships of resistance training on physical performance in youth athletes: A systematic review and meta-analysis. *British Journal of Sports Medicine.* doi:10.1136/bjsports-2015-095497

Lincoln, A.E., Caswell, S.V., Almquist, J.L., Dunn, R.E., Norris, J.B., & Hinton, R.Y. (2011). Trends in concussion incidence in high school sports: A prospective 11-year study. *The American Journal of Sports Medicine, 39*(5), 958-963. doi:10.1177/0363546510392326

Lloyd, R.S., Cronin, J.B., Faigenbaum, A.D., Haff, G.G., Howard, R., Kraemer, W.J., . . . Oliver, J.L. (2016). National Strength and Conditioning Association position statement on long-term athletic development. *Journal of Strength and Conditioning Research, 30*(6), 1491-1509. doi:10.1519/JSC.0000000000001387

Lloyd, R.S., Faigenbaum, A.D., Stone, M.H., Oliver, J.L., Jeffreys, I., Moody, J.A., . . . Myer, G.D. (2014). Position statement on youth resistance training: The 2014 international consensus. *British Journal of Sports Medicine, 48*(7), 498-505. doi:10.1136/bjsports-2013-092952

Lloyd, R.S., Oliver, J.L., Faigenbaum, A.D., Howard, R., De Ste Croix, M.B., Williams, C.A., . . . Myer, G.D. (2015). Long-term athletic development, part 1: A pathway for all youth. *Journal of Strength and Conditioning Research, 29*(5), 1439-1450. doi:10.1519/JSC.0000000000000756

Lloyd, R.S., Oliver, J.L., Faigenbaum, A.D., Myer, G.D., & De Ste Croix, M.B. (2014). Chronological age vs. biological maturation: Implications for exercise programming in youth. *Journal of Strength and Conditioning Research, 28*(5), 1454-1464. doi:10.1519/JSC.0000000000000391

Lloyd, R.S., Oliver, J.L., Hughes, M.G., & Williams, C.A. (2009). Reliability and validity of field-based measures of leg stiffness and reactive strength index in youths. *Journal of Sports Sciences, 27*(14), 1565-1573. doi:10.1080/02640410903311572

Lovell, G., Galloway, H., Hopkins, W., & Harvey, A. (2006). Osteitis pubis and assessment of bone marrow edema at the pubic symphysis with MRI in an elite junior male soccer squad. *Clinical Journal of Sport Medicine, 16*(2), 117-122.

Luke, A., Lazaro, R.M., Bergeron, M.F., Keyser, L., Benjamin, H., Brenner, J., . . . Smith, A. (2011). Sports-related injuries in youth athletes: Is overscheduling a risk factor? *Clinical Journal of Sport Medicine, 21*(4), 307-314. doi:10.1097/JSM.0b013e3182218f71

Lyman, S., Fleisig, G.S., Waterbor, J.W., Funkhouser, E.M., Pulley, L., Andrews, J.R., . . . Roseman, J.M. (2001). Longitudinal study of elbow and shoulder pain in youth baseball pitchers. *Medicine and Science in Sports and Exercise, 33*(11), 1803-1810.

Malina, R.M. (2009). Children and adolescents in the sport culture: The overwhelming majority to the select few. *Journal of Exercise Science & Fitness, 7*, S1-S10.

Malina, R.M., Bouchard, C., & Bar-Or, O. (2004). *Growth, maturation and physical activity*. Champaign, IL: Human Kinetics.

Malisoux, L., Frisch, A., Urhausen, A., Seil, R., & Theisen, D. (2013). Monitoring of sport participation and injury risk in young athletes. *Journal of Science and Medicine in Sport, 16*(6), 504-508. doi:10.1016/j.jsams.2013.01.008

Malone, J.J., Lovell, R., Varley, M.C., & Coutts, A.J. (2017). Unpacking the black box: Applications and considerations for using GPS devices in sport. *International Journal of Sports Physiology and Performance, 12*(Suppl 2), S218-S226. doi:10.1123/ijspp.2016-0236

Malone, S., Roe, M., Doran, D.A., Gabbett, T.J., & Collins, K.D. (2017). Protection against spikes in workload with aerobic fitness and playing experience: The role of the acute:chronic workload ratio on injury risk in elite Gaelic football. *International Journal of Sports Physiology and Performance, 12*(3), 393-401. doi:10.1123/ijspp.2016-0090

Mann, D.L., & van Ginneken, P.J. (2017). Age-ordered shirt numbering reduces the selection bias associated with the relative age effect. *Journal of Sports Sciences, 35*(8), 784-790. doi:10.1080/02640414.2016.1189588

Mann, T.N., Lamberts, R.P., & Lambert, M.I. (2014). High responders and low responders: factors associated with individual variation in response to standardized training. *Sports Medicine, 44*(8), 1113-1124. doi:10.1007/s40279-014-0197-3

Matos, N.F., Winsley, R.J., & Williams, C.A. (2011). Prevalence of nonfunctional overreaching/overtraining in young English athletes. *Medicine and Science in Sports and Exercise, 43*(7), 1287-1294. doi:10.1249/MSS.0b013e318207f87b

Matsuura, T., Suzue, N., Iwame, T., Arisawa, K., Fukuta, S., & Sairyo, K. (2016). Epidemiology of shoulder and elbow pain in youth baseball players. *The Physician and Sportsmedicine, 44*(2), 97-100. doi:10.1080/00913847.2016.1149422

Matsuura, T., Suzue, N., Kashiwaguchi, S., Arisawa, K., & Yasui, N. (2013). Elbow injuries in youth baseball players without prior elbow pain: A 1-year prospective study. *Orthopaedic Journal of Sports Medicine, 1*(5), 2325967113509948. doi:10.1177/2325967113509948

May, M.M., & Bishop, J.Y. (2013). Shoulder injuries in young athletes. *Pediatric Radiology, 43*(Suppl 1), S135-S140. doi:10.1007/s00247-012-2602-0

McBride, J.M., McCaulley, G.O., Cormie, P., Nuzzo, J.L., Cavill, M.J., & Triplett, N.T. (2009). Comparison of methods to quantify volume during resistance exercise. *Journal of Strength and Conditioning Research, 23*(1), 106-110.

McCarthy, P.J., & Jones, M.V. (2007). A qualitative study of sport enjoyment in the sampling years. *Sport Psychologist, 21*, 400-416.

McCrory, P., Meeuwisse, W., Dvorak, J., Aubry, M., Bailes, J., Broglio, S., ... Vos, P.E. (2017). Consensus statement on concussion in sport: The 5th international conference on concussion in sport held in Berlin, October 2016. *British Journal of Sports Medicine.* doi:10.1136/bjsports-2017-097699

McGladrey, B.W., Hannon, J.C., Faigenbaum, A.D., Shultz, B.B., & Shaw, J.M. (2014). High school physical educators' and sport coaches' knowledge of resistance training principles and methods. *Journal of Strength and Conditioning Research, 28*(5), 1433-1442. doi:10.1519/JSC.0000000000000265

McGuigan, M.R., Al Dayel, A., Tod, D., Foster, C., Newton, R.U., & Pettigrew, S. (2008). Use of session rating of perceived exertion for monitoring resistance exercise in children who are overweight or obese. *Pediatric Exercise Science, 20*(3), 333-341.

McGuine, T.A., Post, E.G., Hetzel, S.J., Brooks, M.A., Trigsted, S., & Bell, D.R. (2017). A prospective study on the effect of sport specialization on lower extremity injury rates in high school athletes. *The American Journal of Sports Medicine, 45*(12), 2706-2712. doi:10.1177/0363546517710213

McMaster, D.T., Gill, N., Cronin, J., & McGuigan, M. (2014). A brief review of strength and ballistic assessment methodologies in sport. *Sports Medicine, 44*(5), 603-623. doi:10.1007/s40279-014-0145-2

Meeusen, R., Duclos, M., Foster, C., Fry, A., Gleeson, M., Nieman, D., ... American College of Sports Medicine. (2013). Prevention, diagnosis, and treatment of the overtraining syndrome: Joint consensus statement of the European College of Sport Science and the American College of Sports Medicine. *Medicine and Science in Sports and Exercise, 45*(1), 186-205. doi:10.1249/MSS.0b013e318279a10a

Merkel, D.L. (2013). Youth sport: Positive and negative impact on young athletes. *Open Access Journal of Sports Medicine, 4*, 151-160. doi:10.2147/OAJSM.S33556

Micheli, L.J., & Ireland, M.L. (1987). Prevention and management of calcaneal apophysitis in children: An overuse syndrome. *Journal of Pediatric Orthopedics, 7*(1), 34-38.

Mirwald, R.L., Baxter-Jones, A.D., Bailey, D.A., & Beunen, G.P. (2002). An assessment of maturity from anthropometric measurements. *Medicine and Science in Sports and Exercise, 34*(4), 689-694.

Moran, J., Sandercock, G.R., Ramirez-Campillo, R., Meylan, C., Collison, J., & Parry, D.A. (2017). A meta-analysis of maturation-related variation in adolescent boy athletes' adaptations to short-term resistance training. *Journal of Sports Sciences, 35*(11), 1041-1051. doi:10.1080/02640414.2016.1209306

Mueller, S., Mueller, J., Stoll, J., Prieske, O., Cassel, M., & Mayer, F. (2016). Incidence of back pain in adolescent athletes: A prospective study. *BMC Sports Science, Medicine & Rehabilitation, 8*, 38. doi:10.1186/s13102-016-0064-7

Muller, L., Muller, E., Hildebrandt, C., & Raschner, C. (2016). Biological maturity status strongly intensifies the relative age effect in Alpine ski racing. *PLoS One, 11*(8), e0160969. doi:10.1371/journal.pone.0160969

Myer, G.D., Faigenbaum, A.D., Foss, K.B., Xu, Y., Khoury, J., Dolan, L.M., ... Hewett, T.E. (2014). Injury initiates unfavourable weight gain and obesity markers in youth. *British Journal of Sports Medicine, 48*(20), 1477-1481. doi:10.1136/bjsports-2012-091988

Myer, G.D., Ford, K.R., Divine, J.G., Wall, E.J., Kahanov, L., & Hewett, T.E. (2009). Longitudinal assessment of noncontact anterior cruciate ligament injury risk factors during maturation in a female athlete: A case report. *Journal of Athletic Training, 44*(1), 101-109. doi:10.4085/1062-6050-44.1.101

Myer, G.D., Sugimoto, D., Thomas, S., & Hewett, T.E. (2013). The influence of age on the effectiveness of neuromuscular training to reduce anterior cruciate ligament injury in female athletes: A meta-analysis. *The American Journal of Sports Medicine, 41*(1), 203-215. doi:10.1177/0363546512460637

Myer, G.D., Yuan, W., Barber Foss, K.D., Smith, D., Altaye, M., Reches, A., ... Krueger, D. (2016). The effects of external jugular compression applied during head impact exposure on longitudinal changes in brain neuroanatomical and neurophysiological biomarkers: A preliminary investigation. *Frontiers in Neurology, 7*, 74. doi:10.3389/fneur.2016.00074

Myer, G.D., Yuan, W., Barber Foss, K.D., Thomas, S., Smith, D., Leach, J., ... Altaye, M. (2016). Analysis of head impact exposure and brain microstructure response in a season-long application of a jugular vein compression collar: a prospective, neuroimaging investigation in American football. *British Journal of Sports Medicine, 50*(20), 1276-1285. doi:10.1136/bjsports-2016-096134

Nakata, H., & Sakamoto, K. (2012). Sex differences in relative age effects among Japanese athletes. *Perceptual and Motor Skills, 115*(1), 179-186. doi:10.2466/10.05.17.PMS.115.4.179-186

National Council of Youth Sports. (2008). *Report on trends and participation in organized youth sports 2008.* Retrieved from www.ncys.org/pdfs/2008/2008-ncys-market-research-report.pdf

Nimmerichter, A., & Williams, C.A. (2015). Comparison of power output during ergometer and track cycling in adolescent cyclists. *Journal of Strength and Conditioning Research, 29*(4), 1049-1056. doi:10.1519/JSC.0000000000000723

Noorbhai, M.H., Essack, F.M., Thwala, S.N., Ellapen, T.J., & van Heerden, J.H. (2012). Prevalence of cricket-related musculoskeletal pain among adolescent cricketers in KwaZulu-Natal. *South African Journal of Sports Medicine, 24*(1), 3-9.

Noyes, F.R., & Barber Westin, S.D. (2012). Anterior cruciate ligament injury prevention training in female athletes: A systematic review of injury reduction and results of athletic performance tests. *Sports Health, 4*(1), 36-46. doi:10.1177/1941738111430203

O'Neill, K.S., & Cotton, W.G. (2012, July). *Factors influencing the development of Australian Olympic athletes: The impact of relative age effect and early specialization*. Paper presented at the International Convention on Science, Education and Medicine in Sport, Glasgow.

Obert, P., Stecken, F., Courteix, D., Lecoq, A.M., & Guenon, P. (1998). Effect of long-term intensive endurance training on left ventricular structure and diastolic function in prepubertal children. *International Journal of Sports Medicine, 19*(2), 149-154. doi:10.1055/s-2007-971897

Oliver, J.L., Lloyd, R.S., & Meyers, R.W. (2011). Training elite child athletes: Promoting welfare and well-being. *Strength and Conditioning Journal, 33*(4), 73-79.

Oliver, J.L., Lloyd, R.S., & Whitney, A. (2015). Monitoring of in-season neuromuscular and perceptual fatigue in youth rugby players. *European Journal of Sport Science, 15*(6), 514-522.

Olsen, S.J., 2nd, Fleisig, G.S., Dun, S., Loftice, J., & Andrews, J.R. (2006). Risk factors for shoulder and elbow injuries in adolescent baseball pitchers. *The American Journal of Sports Medicine, 34*(6), 905-912. doi:10.1177/0363546505284188

Parkkari, J., Pasanen, K., Mattila, V.M., Kannus, P., & Rimpela, A. (2008). The risk for a cruciate ligament injury of the knee in adolescents and young adults: A population-based cohort study of 46 500 people with a 9 year follow-up. *British Journal of Sports Medicine, 42*(6), 422-426. doi:10.1136/bjsm.2008.046185

Pasulka, J., Jayanthi, N., McCann, A., Dugas, L.R., & LaBella, C. (2017). Specialization patterns across various youth sports and relationship to injury risk. *The Physician and Sportsmedicine*, 1-9. doi:10.1080/00913847.2017.1313077

Paterno, M.V., Rauh, M.J., Schmitt, L.C., Ford, K.R., & Hewett, T.E. (2012). Incidence of contralateral and ipsilateral anterior cruciate ligament (ACL) injury after primary ACL reconstruction and return to sport. *Clinical Journal of Sport Medicine, 22*(2), 116-121. doi:10.1097/JSM.0b013e318246ef9e

Paterno, M.V., Schmitt, L.C., Ford, K.R., Rauh, M.J., Myer, G.D., Huang, B., & Hewett, T.E. (2010). Biomechanical measures during landing and postural stability predict second anterior cruciate ligament injury after anterior cruciate ligament reconstruction and return to sport. *The American Journal of Sports Medicine, 38*(10), 1968-1978. doi:10.1177/0363546510376053

Pfister, T., Pfister, K., Hagel, B., Ghali, W.A., & Ronksley, P.E. (2016). The incidence of concussion in youth sports: A systematic review and meta-analysis. *British Journal of Sports Medicine, 50*(5), 292-297. doi:10.1136/bjsports-2015-094978

Pfitzinger, P., & Freedson, P. (1997). Blood lactate responses to exercise in children: Part 2. Lactate theshold. *Pediatric Exercise Science, 9*, 299-307.

Phibbs, P.J., Roe, G., Jones, B., Read, D.B., Weakley, J., Darrall-Jones, J., & Till, K. (2017). Validity of daily and weekly self-reported training load measures in adolescent athletes. *Journal of Strength and Conditioning Research, 31*(4), 1121-1126. doi:10.1519/JSC.0000000000001708

Potach, D.H., & Chu, D.A. (2016). Program design and technique for plyometric training. In G.G. Haff & N.T. Triplett (Eds.), *Essentials of strength training and conditioning* (4th ed., pp. 471-520). Champaign, IL: Human Kinetics.

Purcell, L. (2009). Causes and prevention of low back pain in young athletes. *Paediatrics & Child Health, 14*(8), 533-538.

Purcell, L., & Micheli, L. (2009). Low back pain in young athletes. *Sports Health, 1*(3), 212-222. doi:10.1177/1941738109334212

Raglin, J., Sawamura, S., Alexiou, S., Hassmen, P., & Kentta, G. (2000). Training practices and staleness in 13-18-year-old swimmers: A cross-cultural study. *Pediatric Exercise Science, 12*, 61-70.

Read, P.J., Oliver, J.L., Croix, M.B., Myer, G.D., & Lloyd, R.S. (2016). Consistency of field-based measures of neuromuscular control using force-plate diagnostics in elite male youth soccer players. *Journal of Strength and Conditioning Research, 30*(12), 3304-3311. doi:10.1519/JSC.0000000000001438

Renstrom, P., Ljungqvist, A., Arendt, E., Beynnon, B., Fukubayashi, T., Garrett, W., . . . Engebretsen, L. (2008). Non-contact ACL injuries in female athletes: An International Olympic Committee current concepts statement. *British Journal of Sports Medicine, 42*(6), 394-412. doi:10.1136/bjsm.2008.048934

Romann, M., & Fuchslocher, J. (2013). Relative age effects in Swiss junior soccer and their relationship with playing position. *European Journal of Sport Science, 13*(4), 356-363. doi:10.1080/17461391.2011.635699

Romero-Franco, N., Jimenez-Reyes, P., Castano-Zambudio, A., Capelo-Ramirez, F., Rodriguez-Juan, J.J., Gonzalez-Hernandez, J., . . . Balsalobre-Fernandez, C. (2017). Sprint performance and mechanical outputs computed with an iPhone app: Comparison with existing reference methods. *European Journal of Sport Science, 17*(4), 386-392. doi:10.1080/17461391.2016.1249031

Rowland, T. (2016). Morphologic features of the "athlete's heart" in children: A contemporary review. *Pediatric Exercise Science, 28*(3), 345-352. doi:10.1123/pes.2015-0239

Rowland, T., Unnithan, V., Fernhall, B., Baynard, T., & Lange, C. (2002). Left ventricular response to dynamic exercise in young cyclists. *Medicine and Science in Sports and Exercise, 34*(4), 637-642.

Rowland, T., Wehnert, M., & Miller, K. (2000). Cardiac responses to exercise in competitive child cyclists. *Medicine and Science in Sports and Exercise, 32*(4), 747-752.

Sanchez-Medina, L., & Gonzalez-Badillo, J.J. (2011). Velocity loss as an indicator of neuromuscular fatigue during resistance training. *Medicine and Science in Sports and Exercise, 43*(9), 1725-1734. doi:10.1249/MSS.0b013e318213f880

Saw, A.E., Main, L.C., & Gastin, P.B. (2015). Monitoring athletes through self-report: Factors influencing implementation. *Journal of Sports Science & Medicine, 14*(1), 137-146.

Schaefer, D.R., Simpkins, S.D., Vest, A.E., & Price, C.D. (2011). The contribution of extracurricular activities to adolescent friendships: New insights through social network analysis. *Developmental Psychology, 47*(4), 1141-1152. doi:10.1037/a0024091

Scharfbillig, R.W., Jones, S., & Scutter, S.D. (2008). Sever's disease: What does the literature really tell us? *Journal of the American Podiatric Medical Association, 98*(3), 212-223.

Schmikli, S.L., Brink, M.S., de Vries, W.R., & Backx, F.J. (2011). Can we detect non-functional overreaching in young elite soccer players and middle-long distance runners using field performance tests? *British Journal of Sports Medicine, 45*(8), 631-636. doi:10.1136/bjsm.2009.067462

Schorer, J., Cobley, S., Busch, D., Brautigam, H., & Baker, J. (2009). Influences of competition level, gender, player nationality, career stage and playing position on relative age effects. *Scandinavian Journal of Medicine & Science in Sports, 19*(5), 720-730. doi:10.1111/j.1600-0838.2008.00838.x

Schroeder, A.N., Comstock, R.D., Collins, C.L., Everhart, J., Flanigan, D., & Best, T.M. (2015). Epidemiology of overuse injuries among high-school athletes in the United States. *Journal of Pediatrics, 166*(3), 600-606. doi:10.1016/j.jpeds.2014.09.037

Scott, B.R., Duthie, G.M., Thornton, H.R., & Dascombe, B.J. (2016). Training monitoring for resistance exercise: Theory and applications. *Sports Medicine, 46*(5), 687-698. doi:10.1007/s40279-015-0454-0

Selye, H. (1956). *The stress of life.* New York, NY: McGraw-Hill.

Shanmugam, C., & Maffulli, N. (2008). Sports injuries in children. *British Medical Bulletin, 86,* 33-57. doi:10.1093/bmb/ldn001

Shea, K.G., Pfeiffer, R., Wang, J.H., Curtin, M., & Apel, P.J. (2004). Anterior cruciate ligament injury in pediatric and adolescent soccer players: An analysis of insurance data. *Journal of Pediatric Orthopedics, 24*(6), 623-628.

Shelbourne, K.D., Gray, T., & Haro, M. (2009). Incidence of subsequent injury to either knee within 5 years after anterior cruciate ligament reconstruction with patellar tendon autograft. *The American Journal of Sports Medicine, 37*(2), 246-251. doi:10.1177/0363546508325665

Sherar, L.B., Baxter-Jones, A.D., Faulkner, R.A., & Russell, K.W. (2007). Do physical maturity and birth date predict talent in male youth ice hockey players? *Journal of Sports Sciences, 25*(8), 879-886. doi:10.1080/02640410600908001

Sim, A., Terryberry-Spohr, L., & Wilson, K.R. (2008). Prolonged recovery of memory functioning after mild traumatic brain injury in adolescent athletes. *Journal of Neurosurgery, 108*(3), 511-516. doi:10.3171/JNS/2008/108/3/0511

Smoll, F.L. (1998). Improving the quality of coach-parent relationships in youth sports. In J.M. Williams (Ed.), *Applied sport psychology: Personal growth to peak performance* (3rd ed., pp. 63-73). Mountain View, CA: Mayfield.

Smoll, F.L., Cumming, S.P., & Smith, R.E. (2011). Enhancing coach-parent relationships in youth sports: Increasing harmony and minimzing hassle. *International Journal of Sports Science & Coaching, 6*(1), 13-26.

Soligard, T., Myklebust, G., Steffen, K., Holme, I., Silvers, H., Bizzini, M., . . . Andersen, T.E. (2008). Comprehensive warm-up programme to prevent injuries in young female footballers: Cluster randomised controlled trial. *BMJ, 337,* a2469. doi:10.1136/bmj.a2469

Sporting Goods Manufacturers Association. (2011). *U.S. trends in team sports report.* Retrieved from www.sfia.org/reports/280_2011-U.S-Trendsin-Team-Sports-Report

Steib, S., Rahlf, A.L., Pfeifer, K., & Zech, A. (2017). Dose-response relationship of neuromuscular training for injury prevention in youth athletes: A meta-analysis. *Front Physiol, 8,* 920. doi:10.3389/fphys.2017.00920

Stein, C.J., & Micheli, L.J. (2010). Overuse injuries in youth sports. *The Physician and Sportsmedicine, 38*(2), 102-108. doi:10.3810/psm.2010.06.1787

Steinberg, N., Siev-Ner, I., Peleg, S., Dar, G., Masharawi, Y., Zeev, A., & Hershkovitz, I. (2013). Injuries in female dancers aged 8 to 16 years. *Journal of Athletic Training, 48*(1), 118-123. doi:10.4085/1062-6050-48.1.06

Stracciolini, A., Casciano, R., Friedman, H.L., Meehan, W.P., 3rd, & Micheli, L.J. (2015). A closer look at overuse injuries in the pediatric athlete. *Clinical Journal of Sport Medicine, 25*(1), 30-35. doi:10.1097/JSM.0000000000000105

Stracciolini, A., Casciano, R., Levey Friedman, H., Meehan, W.P., 3rd, & Micheli, L.J. (2013). Pediatric sports injuries: An age comparison of children versus adolescents. *The American Journal of Sports Medicine, 41*(8), 1922-1929. doi:10.1177/0363546513490644

Stracciolini, A., Casciano, R., Levey Friedman, H., Stein, C.J., Meehan, W.P., 3rd, & Micheli, L.J. (2014). Pediatric sports injuries: A comparison of males versus females. *The American Journal of Sports Medicine, 42*(4), 965-972. doi:10.1177/0363546514522393

Stracciolini, A., Levey Friedman, H., Casciano, R., Howell, D., Sugimoto, D., & Micheli, L.J. (2016). The relative age effect on youth sports injuries. *Medicine and Science in Sports and Exercise, 48*(6), 1068-1074. doi:10.1249/MSS.0000000000000868

Sugimoto, D., Alentorn-Geli, E., Mendiguchia, J., Samuelsson, K., Karlsson, J., & Myer, G.D. (2015). Biomechanical and neuromuscular characteristics of male athletes: Implications for the development of anterior cruciate ligament injury prevention programs. *Sports Med, 45*(6), 809-822. doi:10.1007/s40279-015-0311-1

Sugimoto, D., Myer, G.D., Barber Foss, K.D., Pepin, M.J., Micheli, L.J., & Hewett, T.E. (2016). Critical components of neuromuscular training to reduce ACL injury risk in female athletes: Meta-regression analysis. *British Journal of Sports Medicine, 50*(20), 1259-1266. doi:10.1136/bjsports-2015-095596

Sugimoto, D., Myer, G.D., Foss, K.D., & Hewett, T.E. (2014). Dosage effects of neuromuscular training intervention to reduce anterior cruciate ligament injuries in female athletes: Meta- and sub-group analyses. *Sports Medicine, 44*(4), 551-562. doi:10.1007/s40279-013-0135-9

Sugimoto, D., Myer, G.D., McKeon, J.M., & Hewett, T.E. (2012). Evaluation of the effectiveness of neuromuscular training to reduce anterior cruciate ligament injury in female athletes: A critical review of relative risk reduction and numbers-needed-to-treat analyses. *British Journal of Sports Medicine, 46*(14), 979-988. doi:10.1136/bjsports-2011-090895

Sundberg, S., & Elovainio, R. (1982). Resting ECG in athletic and non-athletic adolescent boys: Correlations with heart volume and cardiorespiratory fitness. *Clinical Physiology, 2*(5), 419-426.

Sward, L. (1992). The thoracolumbar spine in young elite athletes: Current concepts on the effects of physical training. *Sports Medicine, 13*(5), 357-364.

Terry, P.C., Lane, A.M., Lane, H.J., & Keohane, L. (1999). Development and validation of a mood measure for adolescents. *Journal of Sports Sciences, 17*(11), 861-872. doi:10.1080/026404199365425

Thompson, A.H., Barnsley, R.H., & Stebelsky, G. (1991). "Born to play ball": The relative age effect and Major League Baseball. *Sociology of Sport Journal, 8*(2), 146-151.

Till, K., Cobley, S., Wattie, N., O'Hara, J., Cooke, C., & Chapman, C. (2010). The prevalence, influential factors and mechanisms of relative age effects in UK Rugby League. *Scandinavian Journal of Medicine & Science in Sports, 20*(2), 320-329. doi:10.1111/j.1600-0838.2009.00884.x

Tofler, I.R., Knapp, P.K., & Larden, M. (2005). Achievement by proxy distortion in sports: A distorted mentoring of high-achieving youth. Historical perspectives and clinical intervention with children, adolescents, and their families. *Clinics in Sports Medicine, 24*(4), 805-828, viii. doi:10.1016/j.csm.2005.06.007

Towlson, C., Cobley, S., Midgley, A.W., Garrett, A., Parkin, G., & Lovell, R. (2017). Relative age, maturation and physical biases on position allocation in elite-youth soccer. *International Journal of Sports Medicine, 38*(3), 201-209. doi:10.1055/s-0042-119029

Tremblay, M.S., Barnes, J.D., Gonzalez, S.A., Katzmarzyk, P.T., Onywera, V.O., Reilly, J.J., . . . Global Matrix 2.0 Research Team. (2016). Global Matrix 2.0: Report card grades on the physical activity of children and youth comparing 38 countries. *Journal of Physical Activity & Health, 13*(11 Suppl 2), S343-S366. doi:10.1123/jpah.2016-0594

Ulbricht, A., Fernandez-Fernandez, J., Mendez-Villanueva, A., & Ferrauti, A. (2015). The relative age effect and physical fitness characteristics in German male tennis players. *Journal of Sports Science & Medicine, 14*(3), 634-642.

Valovich McLeod, T.C., Decoster, L.C., Loud, K.J., Micheli, L.J., Parker, J.T., Sandrey, M.A., & White, C. (2011). National Athletic Trainers' Association position statement: Prevention of pediatric overuse injuries. *Journal of Athletic Training, 46*(2), 206-220. doi:10.4085/1062-6050-46.2.206

Vanrenterghem, J., Nedergaard, N.J., Robinson, M.A., & Drust, B. (2017). Training load monitoring in team sports: A novel framework separating physiological and biomechanical load-adaptation pathways. *Sports Medicine.* doi:10.1007/s40279-017-0714-2

Varley, M.C., Fairweather, I.H., & Aughey, R.J. (2012). Validity and reliability of GPS for measuring instantaneous velocity during acceleration, deceleration, and constant motion. *Journal of Sports Sciences, 30*(2), 121-127. doi:10.1080/02640414.2011.627941

Vella, S.A., Schranz, N.K., Davern, M., Hardy, L.L., Hills, A.P., Morgan, P.J., . . . Tomkinson, G. (2016). The contribution of organised sports to physical activity in Australia: Results and directions from the Active Healthy Kids Australia 2014 Report Card on physical activity for children and young people. *Journal of Science and Medicine in Sport, 19*(5), 407-412. doi:10.1016/j.jsams.2015.04.011

Vincent, J., & Glamser, F.D. (2006). Gender differences in the relative age effect among US Olympic development program youth soccer players. *Journal of Sports Sciences, 24*(4), 405-413. doi:10.1080/02640410500244655

Visek, A.J., Harris, B.S., & Blom, L.C. (2013). Mental training with youth sport teams: Developmental considerations and best-practice recommendations. *Journal of Sport Psychology in Action, 4*, 45-55.

Voskanian, N. (2013). ACL Injury prevention in female athletes: Review of the literature and practical considerations in implementing an ACL prevention program. *Current Reviews in Musculoskeletal Medicine, 6*(2), 158-163. doi:10.1007/s12178-013-9158-y

Weiss, M.R., & Smith, A.L. (2002). Friendship quality in youth sport: Relationship to age, gender, and motivation variables. *Journal of Sport & Exercise Psychology, 24*, 420-437.

Wiegerinck, J.I., Yntema, C., Brouwer, H.J., & Struijs, P.A. (2014). Incidence of calcaneal apophysitis in the general population. *European Journal of Pediatrics, 173*(5), 677-679. doi:10.1007/s00431-013-2219-9

Wiersma, L.D. (2000). Risks and benefits of youth sport specialization: Perspectives and recommendations. *Pediatric Exercise Science, 12*, 13-22.

Wiggins, A.J., Grandhi, R.K., Schneider, D.K., Stanfield, D., Webster, K.E., & Myer, G.D. (2016). Risk of secondary injury in younger athletes after anterior cruciate ligament reconstruction: A systematic review and meta-analysis. *The American Journal of Sports Medicine, 44*(7), 1861-1876. doi:10.1177/0363546515621554

Williams, A.M., & Reilly, T. (2000). Talent identification and development in soccer. *Journal of Sports Sciences, 18*(9), 657-667. doi:10.1080/02640410050120041

Williams, C.A., Winsley, R.J., Pinho, G., De Ste Croix, M., Lloyd, R.S., & Oliver, J.L. (2017). Prevalence of non-functional overreaching in elite male and female youth academy football players. *Science and Medicine in Football, 1*(3), 222-228.

Wright, A.D., & Cote, J. (2003). A retrospective analysis of leadership development through sport. *Sport Psychologist, 17,* 268-291.

Wrigley, R.D., Drust, B., Stratton, G., Atkinson, G., & Gregson, W. (2014). Long-term soccer-specific training enhances the rate of physical development of academy soccer players independent of maturation status. *International Journal of Sports Medicine, 35*(13), 1090-1094. doi:10.1055/s-0034-1375616

Young, W.K., & d'Hemecourt, P.A. (2011). Back pain in adolescent athletes. *The Physician and Sportsmedicine, 39*(4), 80-89. doi:10.3810/psm.2011.11.1942

Zimmermann-Sloutskis, D., Wanner, M., Zimmermann, E., & Martin, B.W. (2010). Physical activity levels and determinants of change in young adults: A longitudinal panel study. *International Journal of Behavioral Nutrition and Physical Activity, 7*, 2. doi:10.1186/1479-5868-7-2

Chapter 14 Exercise for Overweight and Obese Youth

Alberga, A., Prud'homme, D., Kenny, G., Goldfield, G., Hadjiyannakis, S., Gougeon, R., Sigal, R. (2015). Effects of aerobic and resistance training on abdominal fat, apolipoproteins and high-sensitivity C-reactive protein in adolescents with obesity: The HEARTY randomized clinical trial. *International Journal of Obesity (London), 39*(10), 1494-1500.

Alberti, K., Eckel, R., Grundy, S., Zimmet, P., Cleeman, J., Donato, K., Smith, S. (2009). Harmonizing the metabolic syndrome: A joint interim statement of the International Diabetes Federation Task Force on Epidemiology and Prevention; National Heart, Lung, and Blood Institute; American Heart Association; World Heart Federation; International Atherosclerosis Society; and International Association for the Study of Obesity. *Circulation, 120*(16), 1640-1645.

American Academy of Pediatrics Council on Communications and Media. (2016). Media use by school-age children and adolescents. *Pediatrics, 138*(5), e 20162592.

Anderson, E., Howe, L., Jones, H., Higgins, J., Lawlor, D., & Fraser, A. (2015). The prevalence of non-alcoholic fatty liver disease in children and adolescents: A systematic review and meta-analysis. *PLoS ONE, 10*(10), e0140908.

Aversano, M., Moazzaz, P., Scaduto, A., & Otsuka, N. (2016). Association between body mass index-for-age and slipped capital femoral epiphysis: The long-term risk for subsequent slip in patients followed until physeal closure. *Journal of Child Orthopedics, 10*(3), 209-213.

Barlow, S. (2007). Expert committee recommendations regarding the prevention, assessment, and treatment of child and adolescent overweight and obesity: Summary report. *Pediatrics, 120*(Suppl 4), S164-S192.

Bea, J., Blew, R., Howe, C., Hetherington-Rauth, M., & Going, S. (2017). Resistance training effects on metabolic function among youth: A systematic review. *Pediatric Exercise Science, 29*(3), 297-315.

Behringer, M., Vom Heede, A., Matthews, M., & Mester, J. (2011). Effects of strength training on motor performance skills in children and adolescents: A meta-analysis. *Pediatric Exercise Science, 23*(2), 186-206.

Bharath, L., Choi, W., Cho, J., Skobodzinski, A., Wong, A., Sweeney, T., & Park, S. (2018). Combined resistance and aerobic exercise training reduces insulin resistance and central adiposity in adolescent girls who are obese: Randomized clinical trial. *European Journal of Applied Physiology.* 118(8): 1653-1660 doi: 10.1007/s00421-018-3898-8.

Bhushan, B., Ayub, B., Thompson, D., Abdullah, F., & Billings, K. (2017). Impact of short sleep on metabolic variables in obese children with obstructive sleep apnea. *Laryngoscope, 127*(9), 2176-2181.

Bond, B., Weston, K., Williams, C., & Barker, A. (2017). Perspectives on high-intensity interval exercise for health promotion in children and adolescents. *Open Access Journal of Sports Medicine, 8,* 243-265.

Buchan, D., Ollis, S., Young, J., Thomas, N., Cooper, S., Tong, T., . . . Baker, J. (2011). The effects of time and intensity of exercise on novel and established markers of CVD in adolescent youth. *American Journal of Human Biology, 23*(4), 517-526.

Bugge, A., El-Naaman, B., McMurray, R., Froberg, K., & Andersen, L. (2013). Tracking of clustered cardiovascular disease risk factors from childhood to adolescence. *Pediatric Research, 73*(2), 245-249.

Buscot, M., Thomson, R., Juonala, M., Sabin, M., Burgner, D., Lehtimäki, T., . . . Magnussen, C.G. (2018). BMI trajectories associated with resolution of elevated youth BMI and incident adult obesity. *Pediatrics, 141*(1), e20172003.

Cesario, S., & Hughes, L. (2007). Precocious puberty: A comprehensive review of literature. *Journal of Obstetric, Gynecologic, and Neonatal Nursing, 36*(3), 263-274.

Ciocca, M., Ramonet, M., & Álvarez, F. (2016). Non-alcoholic fatty liver disease: A new epidemic in children. *Archivos Argentinos de Pediatría, 114*(6), 563-569.

Corte de Araujo, A., Roschel, H., Picanço, A., do Prado, D., Villares, S., de Sá Pinto, A., & Gualano, B. (2012). Similar health benefits of endurance and high-intensity interval training in obese children. *PLoS ONE, 7*(8), e42747.

Costigan, S., Eather, N., Plotnikoff, R., Taaffe, D., & Lubans, D. (2015). High-intensity interval training for improving health-related fitness in adolescents: A systematic review and meta-analysis. *British Journal of Sports Medicine, 49*(19), 1253-1261.

Crisp, N., Fournier, P., Licari, M., , , Braham, R., & Guelfi, K. (2012). Optimising sprint interval exercise to maximise energy expenditure and enjoyment in overweight boys. *Applied Physiology Nutrition and Metabolism, 37*(6), 1222-1231.

Cvetković, N, Stojanović,E, Stojiljković, N, Nikolić, D, Scanlan, A, Milanović, Z. (2018). Exercise training in overweight and obese children: Recreational football and high-intensity interval training provide similar benefits to physical fitness. *Scandinavian Journal of Medicine and Science in Sports.* 28(suppl 1): 18-32.

D'Hondt, E., Deforche, B., Gentier, I., De Bourdeaudhuij, I., Vaeyens, R., Philippaerts, R., & Lenoir, M. (2013). A longitudinal analysis of gross motor coordination in overweight and obese children versus normal-weight peers. *International Journal of Obesity (London), 37*(1), 61-67.

Dâmaso, A., da Silveira Campos, R., Caranti, D., de Piano, A., Fisberg, M., Foschini, D., . . . de Mello, M. (2014). Aerobic plus resistance training was more effective in improving the visceral adiposity, metabolic profile and inflammatory markers than aerobic training in obese adolescents. *Journal of Sports Science, 32*(15), 1435-1445.

Daniels, S. (2009). Complications of obesity in children and adolescents. *International Journal of Obesity (London), 33*(Suppl 1), S60-S65.

Danielsson, P., Bohlin A., Bendito, A., Svensson, A., & Klaesson, S. (2016). Five-year outpatient programme that provided children with continuous behavioural obesity treatment enjoyed high success rate. *Acta Paediatrica, 105*(10), 1181-1190.

Danielsson, P., Kowalski, J., Ekblom, Ö., & Marcus, C. (2012). Response of severely obese children and adolescents to behavioral treatment. *Archives of Pediatric and Adolescent Medicine, 166*(12), 1103-1108.

das Virgens Chagas, D., Carvalho, J., & Batista, L. (2016). Do girls with excess adiposity perform poorer motor skills than leaner peers? *International Journal of Exercise Science, 9*(3), 318-326.

Davis, C., Tomporowski, P., McDowell, J., Austin, B., Miller, P., Yanasak, N., . . . Naglieri, J. (2011). Exercise improves executive function and achievement and alters brain activation in overweight children: A randomized, controlled trial. *Health Psychology, 30*(1), 91-98.

De Leonibus, C., Marcovecchio, M., Chiavaroli, V., de Giorgis, T., Chiarelli, F., & Mohn, A. (2014). Timing of puberty and physical growth in obese children: A longitudinal study in boys and girls. *Pediatric Obesity, 9*(4), 292-299.

De Miguel-Etayo, P., Bueno, G., Garagorri, J., & Moreno, L. (2013). Interventions for treating obesity in children. *World Review of Nutrition and Dietetics, 108,* 98-106.

Dias, I., Farinatti, P., de Souza, M., Manhanini, D., Balthazar, E., Dantas, D., . . . Kraemer-Aguiar, L. (2015). Effects of resistance training on obese adolescents. *Medicine and Science in Sports and Exercise, 47*(12), 2636-2644.

Dias, K., Green, D., Ingul, C., Pavey, T., & Coombes, J. (2015). Exercise and vascular function in child obesity: A meta-analysis. *Pediatrics, 136*(3), e648-659.

Dietz, P., Hoffmann, S., Lachtermann, E., & Simon, P. (2012). Influence of exclusive resistance training on body composition and cardiovascular risk factors in overweight or obese children: A systematic review. *Obesity Facts, 5*(4), 546-560.

Dowda, M., Taverno Ross, S., McIver, K., Dishman, R., & Pate, R. (2017). Physical activity and changes in adiposity in the transition from elementary to middle school. *Childhood Obesity, 13*(1), 53-62.

Dumuid, D., Olds, T., Lewis, L., Martin-Fernández, J., Barreira, T., Broyles, S., . . . ISCOLE Research Group. (2018). The adiposity of children is associated with their lifestyle behaviours: A cluster analysis of school-aged children from 12 nations. *Pediatric Obesity, 13*(2), 111-119.

Dunford, E., & Popkin, B. (2018). 37 year snacking trends for US children 1977-2014. *Pediatric Obesity, 13*(4), 247-255.

Ebbeling, C.B., Pawlak, D.B., & Ludwig, D.S. (2002). Childhood obesity: Public-health crisis, common sense cure. *Lancet, 360*(9331), 473-482.

Eime, R., Young, J., Harvey, J., Charity, M., & Payne, W. (2013). A systematic review of the psychological and social benefits of participation in sport for children and adolescents: Informing development of a conceptual model of health through sport. *International Journal of Behavioral Nutrition and Physical Activity, 10*(98). doi:10.1186/1479-5868-10-98.

Eisenberg, M., Neumark-Sztainer, D., & Story, M. (2003). Associations of weight-based teasing and emotional well-being among adolescents. *Archives of Pediatric and Adolescent Medicine, 157*(8), 733-738.

Evensen, E., Wilsgaard, T., Furberg, A., & Skeie, G. (2016). Tracking of overweight and obesity from early childhood to adolescence in a population-based cohort: The Tromsø Study, Fit Futures. *BMC Pediatrics, 16*(64).

Faigenbaum, A. (2009). Resistance training for overweight and obese youth: Beyond sets and reps. *Obesity Management, 5*(6), 282-285.

Fairchild, T., Klakk, H., Heidemann, M., Andersen, L., & Wedderkopp, N. (2016). Exploring the relationship between adiposity and fitness in young children. *Medicine and Science in Sports and Exercise, 48*(9), 1708-1714.

Faith, M., Butryn, M., Wadden. T., Fabricatore, A., Nguyen, A., & Heymsfield, S. (2011). Evidence for prospective associations among depression and obesity in population-based studies. *Obesity Review, 12*(5), e438-453.

Falaschetti, E., Hingorani, A., Jones, A., Charakida, M., Finer, N., Whincup, P., . . . Deanfield, J. (2010). Adiposity and cardiovascular risk factors in a large contemporary population of pre-pubertal children. *European Heart Journal, 31*(24), 3063-3072.

Finkelstein, E., Graham, W., & Malhotra, R. (2014). Lifetime direct medical costs of childhood obesity. *Pediatrics, 133*(5), 854-862.

Fiorilli, G., Iuliano, E., Aquino, G., Campanella, E., Tsopani, D., Di Costanzo, A., . . . di Cagno, A. (2017). Different consecutive training protocols to design an intervention program for overweight youth: A controlled study. *Diabetes Metabolic Syndrome and Obesity, 10*, 37-45.

Fisberg, M., Maximino, P., Kain, J., & Kovalskys, I. (2016). Obesogenic environment: Intervention opportunities. *Journal of Pediatrics (Rio J), 92*(3 Suppl 1), S30-S39.

Fraser, B., Huynh, Q., Schmidt, M., Dwyer, T., Venn, A., & Magnussen, C. (2016). Childhood muscular fitness phenotypes and adult metabolic syndrome. *Medicine and Science in Sports and Exercise, 48*(9), 1715-1722.

Fraser, B., Schmidt, M., Huynh, Q., Dwyer, T., Venn, A., & Magnussen, C. (2017). Tracking of muscular strength and power from youth to young adulthood: Longitudinal findings from the Childhood Determinants of Adult Health Study. *Journal of Science and Medicine in Sport, 20*(10), 927-931.

Freedman, D, & Berenson, G. (2017). Tracking of BMI *z* scores for severe obesity. *Pediatrics, 140*(3): e20171072

Freedman, D., Ogden, C., Blanck, H., Borrud, L., & Dietz, W. (2013). The abilities of body mass index and skinfold thicknesses to identify children with low or elevated levels of dual-energy X-ray absorptiometry-determined body fatness. *Journal of Pediatrics, 163*(1), 160-166.

García-Hermoso, A., Cerrillo-Urbina, A., Herrera-Valenzuela, T., Cristi-Montero, C., Saavedra, J., & Martínez-Vizcaíno, V. (2016). Is high-intensity interval training more effective on improving cardiometabolic risk and aerobic capacity than other forms of exercise in overweight and obese youth? A meta-analysis. *Obesity Review, 17*(6), 531-540.

García-Hermoso, A., González-Ruiz, K., Triana-Reina, H., Olloquequi, J., & Ramírez-Vélez, R. (2017). Effects of exercise on carotid arterial wall thickness in obese pediatric populations: A meta-analysis of randomized controlled trials. *Childhood Obesity, 13*(2), 138-145.

García-Hermoso, A., Ramírez-Vélez, R., Ramírez-Campillo, R., Peterson, M., & Martínez-Vizcaíno, V. (2018). Concurrent aerobic plus resistance exercise versus aerobic exercise alone to improve health outcomes in paediatric obesity: A systematic review and meta-analysis. *British Journal of Sports Medicine.* 52(3): 161-166

García-Hermoso, A, Ramírez-Vélez, R, Saavedra J (2019). Exercise, health outcomes, and paediatric obesity: A systematic review of meta-analyses. *Journal of Science and Medicine in Sport.* 22(1): 76-84.

Gillis, L., Kennedy, L., & Bar-Or, O. (2006). Overweight children reduce their activity levels earlier in life than healthy weight children. *Clinical Journal of Sports Medicine, 16*(1), 51-55.

Gishti, O., Gaillard, R., Durmus, B., Abrahamse, M., van der Beek, E., Hofman, A., . . . Jaddoe, V. (2015). BMI, total and abdominal fat distribution, and cardiovascular risk factors in school-age children. *Pediatric Research, 77*(5), 710-718.

Golden, N., Schneider, M., Wood, C., & AAP Committee on Nutrition. (2016). Preventing obesity and eating disorders in adolescents. *Pediatrics, 138*(3), e20161649.

Goldfield, G., Kenny, G., Alberga, A., Prud'homme, D., Hadjiyannakis, S., Gougeon, R., . . . Sigal, R. (2015). Effects of aerobic training, resistance training, or both on psychological health in adolescents with obesity: The HEARTY randomized controlled trial. *Journal of Consulting and Clinical Psychology, 83*(6), 1123-1135.

Goldfield, G., Kenny, G., Alberga, A., Tulloch, H., Doucette, S., Cameron, J., & Sigal, R. (2017). Effects of aerobic or resistance training or both on health related quality of life in youth with obesity: The HEARTY trial. *Applied Physiology Nutrition and Metabolism.* 42(4): 361-370. doi: 10.1139/apnm-2016-0386

Gomes, T., Dos Santos, F., Katzmarzyk, P., & Maia, J. (2017). Active and strong: physical activity, muscular strength, and metabolic risk in children. *American Journal of Human Biology, 29*(1).

Grant-Guimaraes, J., Feinstein, R., Laber, E., & Kosoy, J. (2016). Childhood overweight and obesity. *Gastroenterology Clinics of North America, 45*(4), 715-728.

Greco, M., Sood, A., Kwon, S., & Ariza, A. (2016). Cardiovascular risk factor screening and management of obese patients at an outpatient pediatric cardiology center. *Springerplus, 5*(1), 1868.

Griffiths, L., Sera, F., Cortina-Borja, M., Law, C., Ness, A., & Dezateux, C. (2016). Objectively measured physical activity and sedentary time: Cross-sectional and prospective associations with adiposity in the Millennium Cohort Study. *BMJ Open, 6*(4), e010366.

Hales, C., Fryar, C, Carroll, M, Freedman, D, Ogden, C (2018). Trends in obesity and severe obesity prevalence in US youth and adults by sex and age, 2007-2008 to 2015-2016. *Journal of the American Medical Association.* 319(16) 1723-1725..

Han, A., Fu, A., Cobley, S., & Sanders, R. (2017). Effectiveness of exercise intervention on improving fundamental movement skills and motor coordination in overweight/obese children and adolescents: A systematic review. *Journal of Science and Medicine in Sport, 21*(1), 89-102.

Hayden-Wade, H., Stein, R., Ghaderi, A., Saelens, B., Zabinski, M., & Wilfley, D. (2005). Prevalence, characteristics, and correlates of teasing experiences among overweight children vs. non-overweight peers. *Obesity Research, 13*(8), 1381-1392.

He, J., Cai, Z., & Fan, X. (2017). Prevalence of binge and loss of control eating among children and adolescents with overweight and obesity: An exploratory meta-analysis. *International Journal of Eating Disorders, 50*(2), 91-103.

Henrique, R., Bustamante, A., Freitas, D., Tani, G., Katzmarzyk, P., & Maia, J. (2018). Tracking of gross motor coordination in Portuguese children. *Journal of Sports Science, 36*(2), 220-228.

Heymsfield, S., & Wadden, T. (2017). Mechanisms, pathophysiology, and management of obesity. *New England Journal of Medicine, 376*(3), 254-266.

Hills, A., Andersen, L., & Byrne, N. (2011). Physical activity and obesity in children. *British Journal of Sports Medicine, 45*(11), 866-870.

Hirschfeld-Dicker, L, Samuel, R, Tiram Vakrat, E, Dubnov-Raz, G, (2019). Preferred weight-related terminology by parents of children with obesity. *Acta Paediatrica,* 108(4): 712-717

Ho, N., Olds, T., Schranz, N., & Maher, C. (2017). Secular trends in the prevalence of childhood overweight and obesity across Australian states: A meta-analysis. *Journal of Sports Science, 20*(5), 480-488.

Hochdorn, A., Faleiros, V., Camargo, B., Bousfield, A., Wachelke, J., Quintão, I., . . . Gregori, D. (2018). Obese children are thin in parents' eyes: A psychologically, socially, or culturally driven bias? *Journal of Health Psychology, 23*(1), 114-126.

Hruby, A., Manson, J., Qi, L., Malik, V., Rimm, E., Sun, Q., . . . Hu, F. (2016). Determinants and consequences of obesity. *American Journal of Public Health, 106*(9), 1656-1662.

Hudson, L., Rapala, A., Khan, T., Williams, B., & Viner, R. (2015). Evidence for contemporary arterial stiffening in obese children and adolescents using pulse wave velocity: A systematic review and meta-analysis. *Atherosclerosis, 241*(2), 376-386.

Institute of Medicine. (2015). *Physical activity: Moving toward obesity solutions.* Washington, DC: National Academies Press.

Juonala, M., Magnussen, C., Berenson, G., Venn, A., Burns, T., Sabin, M., . . . Raitakari, O. (2011). Childhood adiposity, adult adiposity, and cardiovascular risk factors. *New England Journal of Medicine, 365*(20), 1876-1885.

Juonala, M., Magnussen, C., Venn, A., Dwyer, T., Burns, T., Davis, P., . . . Raitakari, O. (2010). Influence of age on associations between childhood risk factors and carotid intima-media thickness in adulthood: The Cardiovascular Risk in Young Finns Study, the Childhood Determinants of Adult Health Study, the Bogalusa Heart Study, and the Muscatine Study for the International Childhood Cardiovascular Cohort (i3C) Consortium. *Circulation, 122*(24), 2514-2520.

Jung, H, Jeon, S, Lee, N, Kim, K, Kang, M, Lee, S (2018). Effects of exercise intervention on visceral fat in obese children and adolescents: meta-analysis. *Journal of Sports Medicine and Physical Fitness.* doi: 10.23736/S0022-4707.18.08935-1

Kaplowitz, P. (2008). Link between body fat and the timing of puberty. *Pediatrics, 121*(Suppl 3), S208-S217.

Kelleher, E., Davoren, M., Harrington, J., Shiely, F., Perry, I., & McHugh, S. (2017). Barriers and facilitators to initial and continued attendance at community-based lifestyle programmes among families of overweight and obese children: A systematic review. *Obesity Review, 18*(2), 183-194.

Kelley, G., Kelley, K., & Pate, R. (2017). Exercise and BMI z-score in overweight and obese children and adolescents: A systematic review and network meta-analysis of randomized trials. *Journal of Evidence-based Medicine, 10*(2), 108-128.

Kelly, A., Barlow, S., Rao, G., Inge, T., Hayman, L., Steinberger, J., . . . Daniels, S. (2013). Severe obesity in children and adolescents: Identification, associated health risks, and treatment approaches: A scientific statement from the American Heart Association. *Circulation, 128*(15), 1689-1712.

Khalsa, A., Kharofa, R., Ollberding, N., Bishop, L., & Copeland, K. (2017). Attainment of "5-2-1-0" obesity recommendations in preschool-aged children. *Preventive Medicine Reports, 8,* 79-87.

Koebnick, C., Smith, N., Black, M., Porter, A., Richie, B., Hudson, S., . . . Longstreth, G. (2012). Pediatric obesity and gallstone disease: Results from a cross-sectional study of over 510,000 youth. *Journal of Pediatric Gastroenterology and Nutrition, 55*(3), 328-333.

Koh, Y., Lee, J., Kim, E., & Moon, K. (2016). Acanthosis nigricans as a clinical predictor of insulin resistance in obese children. *Pediatric Gastroenterology, Hepatology & Nutrition, 19*(4), 251-258.

Krul, M., van der Wouden, J., Schellevis, F., van Suijlekom-Smit, L., & Koes, B. (2009). Musculoskeletal problems in overweight and obese children. *Annals of Family Medicine, 7*(4), 352-356.

Kuczmarski, R., Ogden, C., Grummer-Strawn, L., Flegal, K., Guo, S., Wei, R., . . . Johnson, C. (2000). CDC growth charts: United States. *Advance Data, 314,* 1-27.

Kumar, S., & Kelly, A. (2017). Review of childhood obesity: From epidemiology, etiology, and comorbidities to clinical assessment and treatment. *Mayo Clinic Proceedings, 92*(2), 251-265.

Kurpad, A., Varadharajan, K., & Aeberli, I. (2011). The thin-fat phenotype and global metabolic disease risk. *Current Opinion in Clinical Nutrition and Metabolic Care, 14*(6), 542-547.

Lang, J., Belanger, K., Poitras, V., Janssen, I., Tomkinson, G., & Tremblay, M. (2018). Systematic review of the relationship between 20m shuttle run performance and health indicators among children and youth. *Journal of Science and Medicine in Sport, 21*(4), 83-397.

Le, J., Zhang, D., Menees, S., Chen, J., & Raghuveer, G. (2010). "Vascular age" is advanced in children with atherosclerosis-promoting risk factors. *Circulation Cardiovascular Imaging, 3,* 8-11.

Lee, A., Fermin, C., Filipp, S., Gurka, M., & DeBoer, M. (2017). Examining trends in prediabetes and its relationship with the metabolic syndrome in US adolescents, 1999-2014. *Acta Diabetologica, 54*(4), 373-381.

Lee, B., Adam, A., Zenkov, E., Hertenstein, D., Ferguson, M., Wang, P., . . . Brown, S. (2017). Modeling the economic and health impact of increasing children's physical activity in the United States. *Health Affairs (Millford), 36*(5), 902-908.

Leinaar, E., Alamian, A., & Wang, L. (2016). A systematic review of the relationship between asthma, overweight, and the effects of physical activity in youth. *Annals of Epidemiology, 26*(7), 504-510.

Levitt Katz, L., Bacha, F., Gidding, S., Weinstock, R., El Ghormli, L., Libman, I., . . . TODAY Study Group. (2018). Lipid profiles, inflammatory markers, and insulin therapy in youth with type 2 diabetes. *Journal of Pediatrics, 196,* 208-216.

Li, L., Zhang, S., Huang, Y., & Chen, K. (2017). Sleep duration and obesity in children: A systematic review and meta-analysis of prospective cohort studies. *Journal of Paediatric Child Health, 53*(4), 378-385.

Lima, R., Bugge, A., Pfeiffer, K., & Andersen, L. (2017). Tracking of gross motor coordination from childhood into adolescence. *Research Quarterly in Exercise and Sport, 88*(1), 52-59.

Lloyd, R., Oliver, J., Faigenbaum, A., Howard, R., De Ste Croix, M., Williams, C., . . . Myer, G. (2015). Long-term physical development: Barriers to success and potential solutions—Part 2. *Journal of Strength and Conditioning Research, 29*(5), 1451-1464.

Lo, J., Maring, B., Chandra, M., Daniels, S., Sinaiko, A., Daley, M., . . . Greenspan, L. (2014). Prevalence of obesity and extreme obesity in children aged 3-5 years. *Pediatric Obesity, 9*(3), 167-175.

Lobstein, T., & Jackson-Leach, R. (2016). Planning for the worst: Estimates of obesity and comorbidities in school-age children in 2025. *Pediatric Obesity, 11*(5), 321-325.

Lopes, V., Malina R.M., Gomez-Campos, R., Cossio-Bolaños, M., Arruda, M., & Hobold, E. (2018). Body mass index and physical fitness in Brazilian adolescents. *Journal of Pediatrics (Rio J)*. doi: 10.1016/j.jped.2018.04.003.

Lu, H., Tarasenko, Y., Asgari-Majd, F., Cottrell-Daniels, C., Yan, F., & Zhang, J. (2015). More overweight adolescents think they are just fine: Generational shift in body weight perceptions among adolescents in the U.S. *American Journal of Preventative Medicine, 49*(5), 670-677.

Lu, K., Manoukian, K., Radom-Aizik, S., Cooper, D., & Galant, S. (2016). Obesity, asthma, and exercise in child and adolescent health. *Pediatric Exercise Science, 28*(2), 264-274.

Luger, M., Lafontan, M., Bes-Rastrollo, M., Winzer, E., Yumuk, V., & Farpour-Lambert, N. (2017). Sugar-sweetened beverages and weight gain in children and adults: A systematic review from 2013 to 2015 and a comparison with previous studies. *Obesity Facts, 10*(6), 674-693.

Lustig, R., Mulligan, K., Noworolski, S., Tai, V., Wen, M., Erkin-Cakmak, A., . . . Schwarz, J. (2016). Isocaloric fructose restriction and metabolic improvement in children with obesity and metabolic syndrome. *Obesity (Silver Springs), 24*(2), 453-460.

Malik, A., Williams, C., Bond, B., Weston, K., & Barker, A. (2017). Acute cardiorespiratory, perceptual and enjoyment responses to high-intensity interval exercise in adolescents. *European Journal of Sport Science, 17*(10), 1335-1342.

Malik, A., Williams, C., Weston, K., & Barker, A. (2018). Perceptual responses to high- and moderate-intensity interval exercise in adolescents. *Medicine and Science in Sports and Exercise, 50*(5), 1021-1030.

Manios, Y., Moschonis, G., Karatzi, K., Androutsos, O., Chinapaw, M., Moreno, L., . . . ENERGY Consortium. (2015). Large proportions of overweight and obese children, as well as their parents, underestimate children's weight status across Europe. The ENERGY (EuropeaN Energy balance Research to prevent excessive weight Gain among Youth) project. *Public Health Nutrition, 18*(12), 2183-2190.

Marmeleira, J., Veiga, G., Cansado, H., & Raimundo, A. (2017). Relationship between motor proficiency and body composition in 6- to 10-year-old children. *Journal of Paediatric Child Health, 53*(4), 348-353.

Marson, E., Delevatti, R., Prado, A., Netto, N., & Kruel, L. (2016). Effects of aerobic, resistance, and combined exercise training on insulin resistance markers in overweight or obese children and adolescents: A systematic review and meta-analysis. *Preventive Medicine, 93*, 211-218.

Martin-Calvo, N., Moreno-Galarraga, L., & Martinez-Gonzalez, M. (2016). Association between body mass index, waist-to-height ratio and adiposity in children: A systematic review and meta-analysis. *Nutrients, 8*(8), E512.

McCrindle, B. (2015). Cardiovascular consequences of childhood obesity. *Canadian Journal of Cardiology, 31*(2), 124-130.

McGuigan, M.R., Tatasciore, M., Newton, R.U., & Pettigrew, S. (2009). Eight weeks of resistance training can significantly alter body composition in children who are overweight or obese. *Journal of Strength and Conditioning Research, 23*(1), 80-85.

McHugh, M. (2010). Oversized young athletes: A weighty concern. *British Journal of Sports Medicine, 44*(1), 45-49.

McMurray, R., & Ondrak, K. (2013). Cardiometabolic risk factors in children: The importance of physical activity. *American Journal of Lifestyle Medicine, 7*(5), 292-303.

Mebrahtu, T., Feltbower, R., Greenwood, D., & Parslow, R. (2015). Childhood body mass index and wheezing disorders: A systematic review and meta-analysis. *Pediatric Allergy and Immunology, 26*(1), 62-72.

Melnyk, B., Jacobson, D., Kelly, S., Belyea, M., Shaibi, G., Small, L., . . . Marsiglia, F. (2015). Twelve-month effects of the COPE healthy lifestyles TEEN program on overweight and depressive symptoms in high school adolescents. *Journal of School Health, 85*(12), 861-870.

Meredith-Jones, K., Haszard, J., Moir, C., Heath, A., Lawrence, J., Galland, B., . . . Taylor, R. (2018). Physical activity and inactivity trajectories associated with body composition in pre-schoolers. *International Journal of Obesity (London)*. 42(9): 1621-1630. doi: 10.1038/s41366-018-0058-5

Meyer, A., Kundt, G., Steiner, M., Schuff-Werner, P., & Kienast, W. (2006). Impaired flow-mediated vasodilation, carotid artery intima-media thickening, and elevated endothelial plasma markers in obese children: The impact of cardiovascular risk factors. *Pediatrics, 117*(5), 1560-1567.

Michalsky, M., Inge, T., Simmons, M., Jenkins, T., Buncher, R., Helmrath, M., . . . Teen-LABS Consortium. (2015). Cardiovascular risk factors in severely obese adolescents: The Teen Longitudinal Assessment of Bariatric Surgery (Teen-LABS) study. *Journal of the American Medical Association Pediatrics, 169*(5), 438-444.

Mitchell, J., Pate, R., España-Romero, V., O'Neill, J., Dowda, M., & Nader, P. (2013). Moderate-to-vigorous physical activity is associated with decreases in body mass index from ages 9 to 15 years. *Obesity (Silver Spring), 21*(3), E280-E293.

Mogri, M., Dhindsa, S., Quattrin, T., Ghanim, H., & Dandona, P. (2013). Testosterone concentrations in young pubertal and post-pubertal obese males. *Clinical Endocrinology, 78*(4), 593-599.

Myer, G., Faigenbaum, A., Ford, K., Best, T., Bergeron, M., & Hewett, T. (2011). When to initiate integrative neuromuscular training to reduce sports-related injuries and enhance health in youth? *Current Sports Medicine Reports, 10*(3), 155-166.

Nadeau, K., Anderson, B., Berg, E., Chiang, J., Chou, H., Copeland, K., . . . Zeitler, P. (2016). Youth-onset type 2 diabetes consensus report: Current status, challenges, and priorities. *Diabetes Care, 39*(9), 1635-1642.

Nader, P., O'Brien, M., Houts, R., Bradley, R., Belsky, J., Crosnoe, R., . . . Susman, E. (2006). Identifying risk for obesity in early childhood. *Pediatrics, 118*, e594-e601.

Næss, M., Holmen, T., Langaas, M., Bjørngaard, J., & Kvaløy, K. (2016). Intergenerational transmission of overweight and obesity from parents to their adolescent offspring: The HUNT study. *PLoS ONE, 11*(11), e0166585.

National Academies of the Sciences, E.a.M. (2016). *Obesity in th early childhood years:State of the science and implementation of promising solutions: Workshop summary.* Washington, DC: National Academies Press.

NCD Risk Factor Collaboration. (2017). Worldwide trends in body-mass index, underweight, overweight, and obesity from 1975 to 2016: A pooled analysis of 2416 population-based measurement studies in 128·9 million children, adolescents, and adults. *Lancet Medical Journal, 390*(10113), 2627-2642.

Ng, M., Fleming, T., Robinson, M., Thomson, B., Graetz, N., Margono, C., . . . Gakidou, E. (2014). Global, regional, and national prevalence of overweight and obesity in children and adults during 1980-2013: A systematic analysis for the Global Burden of Disease Study 2013. *Lancet, 384*(9945), 766-781.

Ortega, F., Labayen, I., Ruiz, J., Kurvinen, E., Loit, H., Harro, J., . . . Sjöström, M. (2011). Improvements in fitness reduce the risk of becoming overweight across puberty. *Medicine and Science in Sports and Exercise, 43*(10), 1891-1897.

Oude Luttikhuis, H., Baur, L., Jansen. H., Shrewsbury, V., O'Malley, C., Stolk, R., & Summerbell, C. (2009). Interventions for treating obesity in children. *Cochrane Database of Systematic Reviews,* CD001872.

Paruthi, S., Brooks, L., D'Ambrosio, C., Hall, W., Kotagal, S., Lloyd, R., . . . Wise, M. (2016). Consensus Statement of the American Academy of Sleep Medicine on the recommended amount of sleep for healthy children: Methodology and discussion. *Clinical Journal of Sleep Medicine, 12*(11), 1549-1561.

Patinkin, Z., Feinn, R., & Santos, M. (2017). Metabolic consequences of obstructive sleep apnea in adolescents with obesity: A systematic literature review and meta-analysis. *Childhood Obesity, 13*(2), 102-110.

Paulis, W., Silva, S., Koes, B., & van Middelkoop, M. (2014). Overweight and obesity are associated with musculoskeletal complaints as early as childhood: A systematic review. *Obesity Review, 15*(1), 52-67.

Pereira, H., Bobbio, T., Antonio, M., & Barros Filho Ade, A. (2013). Childhood and adolescent obesity: How many extra calories are responsible for excess of weight? *Revista Paulista de Pediatria, 31*(2), 252-257.

Pescud, M., Pettigrew, S., McGuigan, M., & Newton, R. (2010). Factors influencing overweight children's commencement of and continuation in a resistance training program. *BMC Public Health, 10,* 709.

Poitras, V., Gray, C., Borghese, M., Carson, V., Chaput, J., Janssen, I., . . . Tremblay, M. (2016). Systematic review of the relationships between objectively measured physical activity and health indicators in school-aged children and youth. *Applied Physiology Nutrition and Metabolism, 41,* S197-S239.

Pont, S., Puhl, R., Cook, S., & Slusser, W. (2017). Stigma experienced by children and adolescents with obesity. *Pediatrics, 140*(6), e20173034.

Prentice, P., & Viner, R. (2013). Pubertal timing and adult obesity and cardiometabolic risk in women and men: A systematic review and meta-analysis. *International Journal of Obesity, 37*(8), 1036-1043.

Rääsk, T., Konstabel, K., Mäestu, J., Lätt, E., Jürimäe, T., & Jürimäe, J. (2015). Tracking of physical activity in pubertal boys with different BMI over two-year period. *Journal of Sport Sciences, 33*(16), 1649-1657.

Racil, G., Ben Ounis, O., Hammouda, O., Kallel, A., Zouhal, H., Chamari, K., & Amri, M. (2013). Effects of high vs. moderate exercise intensity during interval training on lipids and adiponectin levels in obese young females. *European Journal of Applied Physiology, 113*(10), 2531-2540.

Racil, G., Zouhal, H., Elmontassar, W., Ben Abderrahmane, A., De Sousa, M., Chamari, K., . . . Coquart, J. (2016). Plyometric exercise combined with high-intensity interval training improves metabolic abnormalities in young obese females more so than interval training alone. *Applied Physiology Nutrition and Metabolism, 41*(1), 103-109.

Rankin, J., Matthews, L., Cobley, S., Han, A., Sanders, R., Wiltshire, H., & Baker, J. (2016). Psychological consequences of childhood obesity: Psychiatric comorbidity and prevention. *Adolescent Health, Medicine and Therapeutics, 7,* 125-146.

Rao, D., Kropac, E., Do, M., Roberts, K., & Jayaraman, G. (2016). Childhood overweight and obesity trends in Canada. *Health Promotion and Chronic Disease Prevention in Canada, 36*(9), 194-198.

Resnicow, K., Harris, D., Wasserman, R., Schwartz, R., Perez-Rosas, V., Mihalcea, R., & Snetselaar, L. (2016). Advances in motivational interviewing for pediatric obesity: Results of the brief motivational interviewing to reduce body mass index trial and future directions. *Pediatric Clinics of North America, 63*(3), 539-562.

Robinson, E., & Sutin, A. (2016). Parental perception of weight status and weight gain across childhood. *Pediatrics, 137*(5), e20153957.

Rodrigues, L., Stodden, D., & Lopes, V. (2016). Developmental pathways of change in fitness and motor competence are related to overweight and obesity status at the end of primary school. *Journal of Science and Medicine in Sport, 19*(1), 87-92.

Roman-Viñas, B., Chaput, J., Katzmarzyk, P., Fogelholm, M., Lambert, E., Maher, C., . . . ISCOLE Research Group. (2016). Proportion of children meeting recommendations for 24-hour movement guidelines and associations with adiposity in a 12-country study. *International Journal of Behavior, Nutrition and Physical Activity, 13*(1), 123.

Rosenfield, R. (2015). The diagnosis of polycystic ovary syndrome in adolescents. *Pediatrics, 136*(6), 1154-1165.

Roura, E., Milà-Villarroel, R., Lucía Pareja, S., & Adot Caballero, A. (2016). Assessment of eating habits and physical activity among Spanish adolescents. The "Cooking and Active Leisure" TAS Program. *PLoS ONE, 11*(7), e0159962.

Roy, S., Spivack, J., Faith, M., Chesi, A., Mitchell, J., Kelly, A., . . . Zemel, B. (2016). Infant BMI or weight-for-length and obesity risk in early childhood. *Pediatrics, 137*(5), e20153492.

Rukavina, P., & Doolittle, S. (2016). Fostering inclusion and positive physical education experiences. *Journal of Physical Education Recreation and Dance, 87*(4), 36-45.

Ryder, J., Edwards, N., Gupta, R., Khoury, J., Jenkins, T., Bout-Tabaku, S., . . . Kelly, A. (2016). Changes in functional mobility and musculoskeletal pain after bariatric surgery in teens with severe obesity: Teen-Longitudinal Assessment of Bariatric Surgery (LABS) study. *JAMA Pediatrics, 170*(9), 871-977.

Saavedra, J., Escalante, Y., & Garcia-Hermoso, A. (2011). Improvement of aerobic fitness in obese children: A meta-analysis. *International Journal of Pediatric Obesity, 6*(3-4), 169-177.

Salvy, S., Bowker, J., Germeroth, L., & Barkley, J. (2012). Influence of peers and friends on overweight/obese youths' physical activity. *Exercise and Sport Science Reviews, 40,* 127-132.

Sampasa-Kanyinga, H., Hamilton, H., Willmore, J., & Chaput, J. (2017). Perceptions and attitudes about body weight and adherence to the physical activity recommendation among adolescents: The moderating role of body mass index. *Public Health, 146,* 75-83.

Schranz, N., Tomkinson, G., & Olds, T. (2013). What is the effect of resistance training on the strength, body composition and psychosocial status of overweight and obese children and adolescents? A systematic review and meta-analysis. *Sports Medicine, 43*(9), 893-907.

Schwarzfischer, P., Gruszfeld, D., Socha, P., Luque, V, Closa-Monasterolo, R, Rousseaux, D, Moretti M, Mariani B, Verduci E, Koletzko B, Grote V. (2018). Longitudinal analysis of physical activity, sedentary behaviour and anthropometric measures from ages 6 to 11 years. *International Journal of Behavioral Nutrition and Physical Activity.* 15(1): 126

Schwimmer, J., Burwinkle, T., & Varni, J. (2003). Health-related quality of life of severely obese children and adolescents. *Journal of the American Medical Association, 289*(14), 1813 1819.

Shaibi, G., Cruz, M., Ball, G.D., Weigensberg, M., Salem, G., Crespo, N., & Goran, M. (2006). Effects of resistance training on insulin sensitivity in overweight Latino adolescent males. *Medicine and Science in Sports and Exercise, 38*(7), 1208-1215.

Shaibi, G., Ryder, J., Kim, J., & Barraza, E. (2015). Exercise for obese youth: Refocusing attention from weight loss to health gains. *Exercise and Sport Science Reviews, 43*(1), 41-47.

Shalitin, S., & Kiess, W. (2017). Putative effects of obesity on linear growth and puberty. *Hormonal Research in Paediatrics, 88*(1), 101-110.

Sigal, R., Alberga, A., Goldfield, G., Prud'homme, D., Hadjiyannakis, S., Gougeon, R., . . . Kenny, G. (2014). Effects of aerobic training, resistance training, or both on percentage body fat and cardiometabolic risk markers in obese adolescents: The healthy eating aerobic and resistance training in youth randomized clinical trial. *Journal of the American Medical Association Pediatrics, 168*(11), 1006-1014.

Silva-Santos, S., Santos, A., Vale, S., & Mota, J. (2017). Motor fitness and preschooler children obesity status. *Journal of Sports Science.* 35(17): 1704-1708. doi: 10.1080/02640414.2016

Skinner, A, Perrin, E, Moss, L, Skelton, J. (2015). Cardiometabolic risks and severity of obesity in children and young adults. *New England Journal of Medicine.* 373(14):1307–1317.

Skinner, A., Ravanbakht, S., Skeleton, J., Perrin, E., & Armstrong. (2018). Prevalence of obesity and severe obesity in US children, 1999-2016. *Pediatrics,* 141(3):e20173459.

Slining, M., Adair, L., Goldman, B., Borja, J., & Bentley, M. (2010). Infant overweight is associated with delayed motor development. *Journal of Pediatrics, 157*(1), 20-25.

Slyper, A., Rosenberg, H., Kabra, A., Weiss, M., Blech, B., Gensler, S., & Matsumura, M. (2014). Early atherogenesis and visceral fat in obese adolescents. *International Journal of Obesity (London), 38*(7), 954-958.

Smith, J., Eather, N., Morgan, P., Plotnikoff, R., Faigenbaum, A., & Lubans, D. (2014). The health benefits of muscular fitness for children and adolescents: A systematic review and meta-analysis. *Sports Medicine, 44*(9), 1209-1223.

Sonntag, D., Ali, S., & De Bock, F. (2016). Lifetime indirect cost of childhood overweight and obesity: A decision analytic model. *Obesity (Silver Spring), 24*(1), 200-206.

Sothern, M.S., Loftin, J.M., Udall, J.N., Suskind, R.M., Ewing, T.L., Tang, S.C., & Blecker, U. (2000). Safety, feasibility, and efficacy of a resistance training program in preadolescent obese children. *American Journal of the Medical Sciences, 319*(6), 370-375.

Spilsbury, J., Storfer-Isser, A., Rosen, C., & Redline, S. (2015). Remission and incidence of obstructive sleep apnea from middle childhood to late adolescence. *Sleep, 38*(1), 23-29.

Spinelli A, Buoncristiano M, Kovacs V et al. (2019). Prevalence of severe obesity among primary school children in 21 European countries. *Obesity Facts.* 12(2): 244-258.

Steene-Johannessen, J., Anderssen, S., & Kolle, E. (2009). Low muscle fitness is associated with metabolic risk in youth. *Medicine and Science in Sports and Exercise, 41,* 1361-1367.

Steinberger, J., Daniels, S., Hagberg, N., Isasi, C., Kelly, A., Lloyd-Jones, D., . . . Stroke Council. (2016). Cardiovascular health promotion in children: Challenges and opportunities for 2020 and beyond. *Circulation, 134*(12), e236-e255.

Stoner, L., Rowlands, D., Morrison, A., Credeur, D., Hamlin, M., Gaffney, K., . . . Matheson, A. (2016). Efficacy of exercise intervention for weight loss in overweight and obese adolescents: Meta-analysis and implications. *Sports Medicine, 46*(11), 1737-1751.

Stoner, L., Weatherall, M., Skidmore, P., Castro, N., Lark, S., Faulkner, J., & Williams, M. (2017). Cardiometabolic risk variables in preadolescent children: A factor analysis. *Journal of the American Heart Association, 6* (10), e007071.

Sutaria, S., Devakumar, D., Yasuda, S., Das, S., & Saxena, S. (2019). Is obesity associated with depression in children? Systematic review and meta-analysis. *Archives of Disease in Childhood.* 104(1): 64-74 doi: 10.1136/archdischild-2017-314608.

Tan, S., Chen, C., Sui, M., Xue, L., & Wang, J. (2017). Exercise training improved body composition, cardiovascular function, and physical fitness of 5-year-old children with obesity or normal body mass. *Pediatric Exercise Science, 29*(2), 245-253.

Tanrikulu, M., Agirbasli, M., & Berenson, G. (2017). Primordial prevention of cardiometabolic risk in childhood. *Advances in Experimental Medicine and Biology.* 956: 489-496. doi: 10.1007/5584_2016_172.

Telama, R., Yang, X., Leskinen, E., Kankaanpää, A., Hirvensalo, M., Tammelin, T., . . . Raitakari, O. (2014). Tracking of physical activity from early childhood through youth into adulthood. *Medicine and Science in Sports and Exercise, 46*(5), 955-962.

Theim, K., Sinton, M., Goldschmidt, A., Van Buren, D., Doyle, A., Saelens, B., . . . Wilfley, D. (2013). Adherence to behavioral targets and treatment attendance during a pediatric weight control trial. *Obesity (Silver Springs), 21*(2), 394-397.

Thivel, D., Masurier, J., Baquet, G., Timmons, B., Pereira, B., Berthoin, S., . . . Aucouturier, J. (2019). High-intensity interval training in overweight and obese children and adolescents: Systematic review and meta-analysis. *Journal of Sports Medicine and Physical Fitness.* 59(2): 310-324. doi: 10.23736/S0022-4707.18.08075-1

Thivel, D., Ring-Dimitriou, S., Weghuber, D., Frelut, M., & O'Malley, G. (2016). Muscle strength and fitness in pediatric obesity: A systematic review from the European Childhood Obesity Group. *Obesity Facts, 9*(1), 52-63.

Thota, P., Perez-Lopez, F., Benites-Zapata, V., Pasupuleti, V., & Hernandez, A. (2017). Obesity-related insulin resistance in adolescents: A systematic review and meta-analysis of observational studies. *Gynecological Endocrinology, 33*(3), 179-184.

Toomey, C., Whittaker, J., Nettel-Aguirre, A., Reimer, R., Woodhouse, L., Ghali, B., . . . Emery, C. (2017). Higher fat mass is associated with a history of knee injury in youth sport. *Journal of Orthopaedic and Sports Physical Therapy, 47*(2), 80-87.

Tsiros, M., Buckley, J., Olds, T., Howe, P., Hills, A., Walkley, J., . . . Coates, A. (2016). Impaired physical function associated with childhood obesity: How should we Intervene? *Childhood Obesity, 12*(2), 126-134.

Twig, G., Yaniv, G., Levine, H., Leiba, A., Goldberger, N., Derazne, E., . . . Kark, J. (2016). Body-mass index in 2.3 million adolescents and cardiovascular death in adulthood. *New England Journal of Medicine, 374*(25), 2430-2440.

U.S. Preventive Services Task Force, Grossman, D., Bibbins-Domingo, K., Curry, S., Barry, M., Davidson, K., . . . Tseng, C. (2017). Screening for obesity in children and adolescents: US Preventive Services Task Force recommendation statement. *Journal of the American Medical Association, 317*(23), 2417-2426.

Utz-Melere, M., Targa-Ferreira, C., Lessa-Horta, B., Epifanio, M., Mouzaki, M., & Mattos, A. (2018). Non-alcoholic fatty liver disease in children and adolescents: Lifestyle change: A systematic review and meta-analysis. *Annals of Hepatology, 17*(3), 34-354.

Valaiyapathi, B., Gower, B., & Ashraf, A. (2018). Pathophysiology of type 2 diabetes in children and adolescents. *Current Diabetes Reviews*.doi: 10.2174/1573399814666180608074510

van Leeuwen, J., Hoogstrate, M., Duiverman, E., & Thio, B. (2014). Effects of dietary induced weight loss on exercise-induced bronchoconstriction in overweight and obese children. *Pediatrics Pulmonology, 49*(12), 1155-1161.

Vasconcellos, F., Seabra, A., Cunha, F., Montenegro, R., Penha, J., Bouskela, E., . . . Farinatti, P. (2016). Health markers in obese adolescents improved by a 12-week recreational soccer program: A randomised controlled trial. *Journal of Sport Sciences, 34* (6), 564-575.

Viswanathan, V., & Eugster, E. (2014). Etiology and treatment of hypogonadism in adolescents. *Pediatric Clinics of North America, 58*(5), 1181.

Ward, Z., Long, M., Resch, S., Giles, C., Cradock, A., & Gortmaker, S. (2017). Simulation of growth trajectories of childhood obesity into adulthood. *New England Journal of Medicine, 377*(22), 2145-2153.

White, D., Place, R., Michael, T., Hoffman, E., Gordon, P., & Visich, P. (2017). The relationship between coronary artery disease risk factors and carotid intima-media thickness in children. *Journal of Pediatrics, 190*, 38-42.

Wijnhoven, T., van Raaij, J., Spinelli, A., Rito, A., Hovengen, R., Kunesova, M., . . . Breda, J. (2013). WHO European Childhood Obesity Surveillance Initiative 2008: Weight, height and body mass index in 6-9-year-old children. *Pediatric Obesity, 8*(2), 79-97.

Witbreuk, M., van Kemenade, F., van der Sluijs, J., Jansma, E., Rotteveel, J., & van Royen, B. (2013). Slipped capital femoral epiphysis and its association with endocrine, metabolic and chronic diseases: A systematic review of the literature. *Journal of Child Orthopedics, 7*(3), 213-223.

Wong, E., & Cheng, M. (2013). Effects of motivational interviewing to promote weight loss in obese children. *Journal of Clinical Nursing, 22*(17-18), 2519-2530.

Yu, C., Sung, R., So, R., Lui, K., Lau, W., Lam, P., & Lau, E. (2005). Effects of strength training on body composition and bone mineral content in children who are obese. *Journal of Strength and Conditioning Research, 19*, 667-672.

Zhao, C., Ma, Y., Pan, C., Chen, X., & Sun, H. (2016). Prevalence and trends of obesity among Chinese Korean nationality children and adolescents, 1991-2010. *Iran Journal of Public Health, 45*(6), 721-728.

Zhu, K., Allen, K., Mountain, J., Lye, S., Pennell, C., & Walsh, J. (2017). Depressive symptoms, body composition and bone mass in young adults: A prospective cohort study. *International Journal of Obesity, 41* (4), 576-581.

Zwolski, C., Quatman-Yates, C., & Paterno, M. (2017). Resistance training in youth: Laying the foundation for injury prevention and physical literacy. *Sports Health, 9*(5), 436-443.

Chapter 15 Exercise for Youth With Selected Clinical Conditions

Akinbami, L., Simon, A., & Rossen, L. (2016). Changing trends in asthma prevalence among children. *Pediatrics, 137*(1), e20152354.

Aljebab, F., Choonara, I., & Conroy, S. (2017). Systematic review of the toxicity of long-course oral corticosteroids in children. *PLoS ONE, 12*(1), e0170259.

American College of Sports Medicine. (2018). *ACSM's guidelines for exercise testing and prescription* (10th ed.). Baltimore, MD: Lippincott, Williams and Wilkins.

American Diabetes Association. (2015). Section 2: Classification and diagnosis of diabetes. *Diabetes Care, 38*(1 Suppl), S8-S16.

Amutha, A., Anjana, R., Venkatesan, U., Ranjani, H., Unnikrishnan, R., Venkat Narayan, K., Ali, M. (2017). Incidence of complications in young-onset diabetes: Comparing type 2 with type 1 (the young diab study). *Diabetes Research in Clinical Practice, 123*, 1-8.

Anderson, S., & Kippelen, P. (2008). Airway injury as a mechanism for exercise-induced bronchoconstriction in elite athletes. *Journal of Allergy and Clinical Immunology, 122*(2), 225-235.

Andersson, M., Hedman, L., Nordberg, G., Forsberg, B., Eriksson, K., & Rönmark, E. (2015). Swimming pool attendance is related to asthma among atopic school children: A population-based study. *Environmental Research, 14*(37).

Andrade, L., Britto, M., Lucena-Silva, N., Gomes, R., & Figueroa, J. (2014). The efficacy of aerobic training in improving the inflammatory component of asthmatic children. Randomized trial. *Respiratory Medicine, 108*(10), 1438-1445.

Ash, T., Bowling, A., Davison, K., & Garcia, J. (2017). Physical activity interventions for children with social, emotional, and behavioral disabilities: A systematic review. *Journal of Developmental and Behavioral Pediatrics, 38*(6), 431-445.

Bailey, A., Hetrick, S., Rosenbaum, S., Purcell, R., & Parker, A. (2018). Treating depression with physical activity in adolescents and young adults: A systematic review and meta-analysis of randomised controlled trials. *Psychological Medicine, 48*(7), 1068-1083.

Baksjøberget, P.E., Nyquist, A., Moser, T., & Jahnsen, R. (2017). Having fun and staying active! children with disabilities and participation in physical activity: A follow-up study. *Physical & Occupational Therapy In Pediatrics, 37*(4), 347-358. doi:10.1080/01942638.2017.1281369

Baran, F., Aktop, A., Özer, D., Nalbant, S., A⊠lam⊠, E., Barak, S., & Hutzler, Y. (2013). The effects of a Special Olympics Unified Sports Soccer training program on anthropometry, physical fitness and skilled performance in Special Olympics soccer athletes and non-disabled partners. *Research in Developmental Disabilities, 34*(1), 695-709.

Bar-Or, O., & Rowland, T. (2004). *Pediatric exercise medicine.* Champaign, IL: Human Kinetics.

Basaran, S., Guler-Uysal, F., Ergen, N., Seydaoglu, G., Bingol-Karakoc, G., & Ufuk Altintas, D. (2006). Effects of physical exercise on quality of life, exercise capacity and pulmonary function in children with asthma. *Journal of Rehabilitation Medicine, 38*(2), 130-135.

Bax, M., Flodmark, O., & Tydeman, C. (2007). Definition and classification of cerebral palsy. From syndrome toward disease. *Developmental Medicine & Child Neurology, 109* (Suppl), 39-41.

Bea, J., Blew, R., Howe, C., Hetherington-Rauth, M., & Going, S. (2017). Resistance training effects on metabolic function among youth: A systematic review. *Pediatric Exercise Science, 29*(3), 297-315.

Beggs, S., Foong, Y., Le, H., Noor, D., Wood-Baker, R., & Walters, J. (2013). Swimming training for asthma in children and adolescents aged 18 years and under. *Cochrane Database of Systematic Reviews, 30*(4), CD009607.

Bernard, A., Nickmilder, M., & Dumont, X. (2015). Chlorinated pool attendance, airway epithelium defects and the risks of allergic diseases in adolescents: Interrelationships revealed by circulating biomarkers. *Environmental Research, 140,* 119-126.

Bertapelli, F., Pitetti, K., Agiovlasitis, S., & Guerra-Junior, G. (2016). Overweight and obesity in children and adolescents with Down syndrome—Prevalence, determinants, consequences, and interventions: A literature review. *Research in Developmental Disabilities, 57,* 181-192.

Bloemen, M., Backx, F., Takken, T., Wittink, H., Benner, J., Mollema, J., & de Groot, J. (2015). Factors associated with physical activity in children and adolescents with a physical disability: A systematic review. *Developmental Medicine & Child Neurology, 57*(2), 137-148.

Bond, B., Weston, K., Williams, C., & Barker, A. (2017). Perspectives on high-intensity interval exercise for health promotion in children and adolescents. *Open Access Journal of Sports Medicine, 8,* 243-265.

Brackney, D., & Cutshall, M. (2015). Prevention of type 2 diabetes among youth: A systematic review, implications for the school nurse. *Journal of School Nursing, 31,* 6-21.

Bull, M., & Committee on Genetics. (2011). Health supervision for children with Down syndrome. *Pediatrics, 128*(2), 393-406.

Caggiano, S., Cutrera, R., Di Marco, A., & Turchetta, A. (2017). Exercise-induced bronchospasm and allergy. *Frontiers in Pediatrics, 5,* 131.

Cairney, J., Veldhuizen, S., King-Dowling, S., Faught, B., & Hay, J. (2017). Tracking cardiorespiratory fitness and physical activity in children with and without motor coordination problems. *Journal of Science and Medicine in Sport, 20*(4), 380-385.

Carlsen, K., Anderson, S., & Bjermer, L. (2008). Exercise-induced asthma, respiratory and allergic disorders in elite athletes: epidemiology, mechanisms and diagnosis: Part I of the report from the Joint Task Force of the European Respiratory Society

(ERS) and the European Academy of Allergy and Clinical Immunology (EAACI) in cooperation with GA2LEN. *Allergy, 63,* 387-403.

Carroll, D., Courtney-Long, E., Stevens, A., Sloan, M., Lullo, C., Visser, S., . . . Centers for Disease Control and Prevention. (2014). Vital signs: Disability and physical activity—United States, 2009-2012. *Morbidity and Mortality Weekly Report, 63*(18), 407-413.

Carson, V., Barnes, J., LeBlanc, C., Moreau, E., & Tremblay, M. (2017). Increasing Canadian paediatricians' awareness and use of the new Canadian Physical Activity and Sedentary Behaviour Guidelines for ages 0 to 17 years. *Paediatrics & Child Health, 22*(1), 17-22.

Cockcroft, E., Williams, C., Tomlinson, O., Vlachopoulos, D., Jackman, S., Armstrong, N., & Barker, A. (2015). High intensity interval exercise is an effective alternative to moderate intensity exercise for improving glucose tolerance and insulin sensitivity in adolescent boys. *Journal of Science and Medicine in Sport, 18*(6), 720-724.

Colberg, S., Sigal, R., Yardley, J., Riddell, M., Dunstan, D., Dempsey, P., . . . Tate, D. (2016). Physical activity/exercise and diabetes: A position statement of the American Diabetes Association. *Diabetes Care, 39*(11), 2065-2079.

Couto, M., Kurowski, M., Moreira, A., Bullens, D., Carlsen, K., Delgado, L., . . . Seys, S. (2018). Mechanisms of exercise-induced bronchoconstriction in athletes: Current perspectives and future challenges. *Allergy.* 73(1): 8-16. doi: 10.1111/all.13224

Crawford, C., Burns, J., & Fernie, B. (2015). Psychosocial impact of involvement in the Special Olympics. *Research in Developmental Disabilities, 45-46,* 93-102.

Crosbie, A. (2012). The effect of physical training in children with asthma on pulmonary function, aerobic capacity and health-related quality of life: A systematic review of randomized control trials. *Pediatric Exercise Science, 24*(3), 472-489.

Dabelea, D., Stafford, J.M., Mayer-Davis, EJ, D'Agostino, R., Dolan, L., Imperatore, G., . . . SEARCH for Diabetes in Youth Research Group. (2017). Association of type 1 diabetes vs type 2 diabetes diagnosed during childhood and adolescence with complications during teenage years and young adulthood. *Journal of the American Medical Association, 317*(8), 825-835.

Dart, A., Martens, P., Rigatto, C., Brownell, M., Dean, H., & Sellers, E. (2014). Earlier onset of complications in youth with type 2 diabetes. *Diabetes Care, 37*(2), 436-443.

de Aguiar, K., Anzolin, M., & Zhang, L. (2018). Global prevalence of exercise-induced bronchoconstriction in childhood: A meta-analysis. *Pediatric Pulmonology, 53*(4), 412-425.

de Greeff, J., Bosker, R., Oosterlaan, J., Visscher, C., & Hartman, E. (2018). Effects of physical activity on executive functions, attention and academic performance in preadolescent children: A meta-analysis. *Journal of Science and Medicine in Sport, 21*(5), 501-507.

de Lima, V., Mascarenhas, L., Decimo, J., de Souza, W., Monteiro, A., Lahart, I., . . . Leite, N. (2017). Physical activity levels of adolescents with type 1 diabetes physical activity in T1D. *Pediatric Exercise Science, 29*(2), 213-219.

Donnelly, J., Hillman, C., Castelli, D., Etnier, J., Lee, S., Tomporowski, P., . . . Szabo-Reed, A. (2016). Physical activity, fitness, cognitive function, and academic achievement in children: A systematic review. *Medicine and Science in Sports and Exercise, 48*(6), 1197-1222.

Eichenberger, P., Diener, S., Kofmehl, R., & Spengler, C. (2013). Effects of exercise training on airway hyperreactivity in asthma: A systematic review and meta-analysis. *Sports Medicine, 43*(11), 1157-1170.

Einarsson, I., Jóhannsson, E., Daly, D., & Arngrímsson, S. (2016). Physical activity during school and after school among youth with and without intellectual disability. *Research in Developmental Disabilities, 56*, 60-70.

Fanelli, A., Cabral, A., Neder, J., Martins, M., & Carvalho, C. (2007). Exercise training on disease control and quality of life in asthmatic children. *Medicine and Science in Sports and Exercise, 39*(9), 1474-1480.

Fragala-Pinkham, M., Haley, S., & O'Neil, M. (2008). Group aquatic aerobic exercise for children with disabilities. *Developmental Medicine & Child Neurology, 50*(11), 822-827.

Glazebrook, C., McPherson, A., Macdonald, I., Swift, J., Ramsay, C., Newbould, R., & Smyth, A. (2006). Asthma as a barrier to children's physical activity: Implications for body mass index and mental health. *Pediatrics, 118*(6), 2443-2449.

Gómez-Bruton, A., Matute-Llorente, Á., González-Agüero, A., Casajús, J., & Vicente-Rodríguez, G. (2017). Plyometric exercise and bone health in children and adolescents: A systematic review. *World Journal of Pediatrics, 13*(2), 112-121.

Gordon, J., Dolinsky, V., Mughal, W., Gordon, G., & McGavock, J. (2015). Targeting skeletal muscle mitochondria to prevent type 2 diabetes in youth. *Biochemistry and Cell Biology, 93*(5), 452-465.

Grover, S., Aubert-Broche B1, Fetco, D., Collins, D., Arnold, D., Finlayson, M., . . . Yeh, E. (2015). Lower physical activity is associated with higher disease burden in pediatric multiple sclerosis. *Neurology, 85*(19), 1663-1669.

Guarnaccia, S., Holliday, C., D'Agata, E., Pluda, A., Pecorelli, G., Gretter, V., . . . Ricci, E. (2016). Clinical and health promotion asthma management: An intervention for children and adolescents. *Allergy and Asthma Proceedings, 37*(4), 70-76.

Guarnaccia, S., Pecorelli, G., Bianchi, M., Cartabia, M., Casadei, G., Pluda, A., . . . Bonati, M. (2017). IOEASMA: An integrated clinical and educational pathway for managing asthma in children and adolescents. *Italian Journal of Pediatrics, 43*(1), 58.

Gullach, A., Risgaard, B., Lynge, T., Jabbari, R., Glinge, C., Haunsø, S., . . . Tfelt-Hansen, J. (2015). Sudden death in young persons with uncontrolled asthma: A nationwide cohort study in Denmark. *BMC Pulmonary Medicine, 15*, 35.

Gupta, S., Rao, B., & Kumaran, S. (2011). Effect of strength and balance training in children with Down's syndrome: A randomized controlled trial. *Clinical Rehabilitation, 25*(5), 425-432.

Hands, B. (2008). Changes in motor skill and fitness measures among children with high an low motor competence: A five year longitudinal study. *Journal of Science and Medicine in Sport, 11*, 155-162.

Hankinson, T., & Anderson, R. (2010). Craniovertebral junction abnormalities in Down syndrome. *Neurosurgery, 66*(3 Suppl), 32-38.

Hannon, T., & Arslanian, S. (2015). The changing face of diabetes in youth: Lessons learned from studies of type 2 diabetes. *Annals of the New York Academy of Science, 1353*(1), 113-137.

Hannon, T., Janosky, J., & Arslanian, S. (2006). Longitudinal study of physiologic insulin resistance and metabolic changes of puberty. *Pediatric Research, 60*(6), 759-763.

Hartman, E., Smith, J., Houwen, S., & Visscher, C. (2017). Skill-related physical fitness versus aerobic fitness as a predictor of executive functioning in children with intellectual disabilities or borderline intellectual functioning. *Research in Developmental Disabilities, 64*, 1-11.

Hartman, E., Smith, J., Westendorp, M., & Visscher, C. (2015). Development of physical fitness in children with intellectual disabilities. *Journal of Intellectual Disability Research, 59*(5), 439-449.

Hastie, P., & Martin, E. (2006). *Teaching elementary physical education.* San Francisco, CA: Benjamin Cummings.

Hinckson, E., & Curtis, A. (2013). Measuring physical activity in children and youth living with intellectual disabilities: A systematic review. *Research in Developmental Disabilities, 34* (1), 72-86.

Ho, M., Garnett, S., Baur, L., Burrows, T., Stewart, L., Neve, M., & Collins, C. (2013). Impact of dietary and exercise interventions on weight change and metabolic outcomes in obese children and adolescents: A systematic review and meta-analysis of randomized trials. *Journal of the American Medical Association, 167*(8), 759-768.

Holderness, H., Chin, N., Ossip, D., Fagnano, M., Reznik, M., & Halterman, J. (2017). Physical activity, restrictions in activity, and body mass index among urban children with persistent asthma. *Annals of Allergy Asthma & Immunology, 118*(4), 433-438.

Hsu, J., Qin, X., Beavers, S., & Mirabelli, M. (2016). Asthma-related school absenteeism, morbidity, and modifiable factors. *American Journal of Preventative Medicine, 51*(1), 23-32.

Ishiguro, H., Kodama, S., Horikawa, C., Fujihara, K., Hirose A., Hirasawa, R., . . . Sone, H. (2016). In search of the ideal resistance training program to improve glycemic control and its indication for patients with type 2 diabetes mellitus: A systematic review and meta-analysis. *Sports Medicine, 46*(1), 67-77.

Jaarsma, E., Dijkstra, P., Geertzen, J., & Dekker, R. (2014). Barriers to and facilitators of sports participation for people with physical disabilities: a systematic review. *Scandinavian Journal of Medicine and Science in Sport, 24*(6), 871-881.

Jago R., Searle, A., Henderson, A., & Turner, K. (2017). Designing a physical activity intervention for children with asthma: A qualitative study of the views of healthcare professionals, parents and children with asthma. *BMJ Open, 7*(3), e014020.

Jemtå, L., Fugl-Meyer, K., Oberg, K., & Dahl, M. (2009). Self-esteem in children and adolescents with mobility impairment: Impact on well-being and coping strategies. *Acta Paediatrica, 98*(3), 567-572.

Johnson, C. (2009). The benefits of physical activity for youth with developmental disabilities: A systematic review. *American Journal of Health Promotion, 23*(3), 157-167.

Kachouri, H., Borji, R., Baccouch, R., Laatar, R., Rebai, H., & Sahli, S. (2016). The effect of a combined strength and proprioceptive training on muscle strength and postural balance in boys with intellectual disability: An exploratory study. *Research in Developmental Disabilities, 53-54*, 367-376.

Kanikowska, A, Napiórkowska-Baran, K, Graczyk, M, Kucharski, M. (2018). Influence of chlorinated water on the development of allergic diseases - An overview. *Annals of Agriculture and Environmental Medicine.* 25(4): 651-655.

Karges, B., Schwandt, A., Heidtmann, B., Kordonouri, O., Binder, E., Schierloh, U., . . . Holl, R. (2017). Association of insulin pump therapy vs insulin injection therapy with severe hypoglycemia, ketoacidosis, and glycemic control among children, adolescents, and young adults with type 1 diabetes. *Journal of the American Medical Association, 318*(14), 1358-1366.

Kelsey, M., & Zeitler, P. (2016). Insulin resistance of puberty. *Current Diabetes Reports, 16*(7), 64.

Kim, S., Kim, S., Yang, Y., Lee, I., & Koh, S. (2017). Effect of weight bearing exercise to improve bone mineral density in children with cerebral palsy: A meta-analysis. *Journal of Musculoskeletal and Neuronal Interactions, 17*(4), 334-340.

Korczak, D., Madigan, S., & Colasanto, M. (2017). Children's physical activity and depression: A meta-analysis. *Pediatrics, 139*(4), e20162266.

Kriska, A., El Ghormli, L., Copeland, K., Higgins, J., Ievers-Landis, C., Levitt Katz, L., . . . TODAY Study Group. (2018). Impact of lifestyle behavior change on glycemic control in youth with type 2 diabetes. *Pediatric Diabetes, 19*(1), 36-44.

Lahart, I., & Metsios, G. (2018). Chronic physiological effects of swim training interventions in non-elite swimmers: A systematic review and meta-analysis. *Sports Medicine, 48*(2), 337-359.

Larsen, M., Nielsen, C., Helge, E., Madsen, M., Manniche, V., Hansen, L., . . . Krustrup, P. (2018). Positive effects on bone mineralisation and muscular fitness after 10 months of intense school-based physical training for children aged 8-10 years: The FIT FIRST randomised controlled trial. *British Journal of Sports Medicine, 52*, 254-260.

Lee, A., Fermin, C., Filipp, S., Gurka, M., & DeBoer, M. (2017). Examining trends in prediabetes and its relationship with the metabolic syndrome in US adolescents, 1999-2014. *Acta Diabetologica, 54*(4), 373-381.

Lee, B., Adam, A., Zenkov, E., Hertenstein, D., Ferguson, M., Wang, P., . . . Brown, S. (2017). Modeling the economic and health impact of increasing children's physical activity in the United States. *Health Affairs (Millford), 36*(5), 902-908.

Leser, K., Pirie, P., Ferketich, A., Havercamp, S., & Wewers, M. (2017). Dietary and physical activity behaviors of adults with developmental disabilities and their direct support professional providers. *Disability and Health Journal, 10*(4), 532-541.

Lin, H., Lin, H., Yu, H., Wang, L., Lee, J., Lin, Y., . . . Chiang, B. (2017). Tai-Chi-Chuan exercise improves pulmonary function and decreases exhaled nitric oxide level in both asthmatic and nonasthmatic children and improves quality of life in children with asthma. *Evidence Based Complementary Alternative Medicine, 2017*, 6287642.

Lochte, L., Nielsen, K., Petersen, P., & Platts-Mills, T. (2016). Childhood asthma and physical activity: A systematic review with meta-analysis and graphic appraisal tool for epidemiology assessment. *BMC Pediatrics, 16*(50).

Lu, K, Cooper, D, Haddad, F, Radom-Aizik, S. (2018). Four months of a school-based exercise program improved aerobic fitness and clinical outcomes in a low-SES population of normal weight and overweight/obese children with asthma. *Frontiers in Pediatrics, 6*: 380. doi: 10.3389/fped.2018.00380

Macêdo, T., Freitas, D., Chaves, G., Holloway, E., & Mendonça, K. (2016). Breathing exercises for children with asthma. *Cochrane Database of Systematic Reviews, 4*, CD011017.

MacMillan, F., Kirk, A., Mutrie, N., Matthews, L., Robertson, K., & Saunders, D. (2014). A systematic review of physical activity and sedentary behavior intervention studies in youth with type 1 diabetes: Study characteristics, intervention design, and efficacy. *Pediatric Diabetes, 15*(3), 175-189.

Magnussen, C., Koskinen, J., Juonala, M., Chen, W., Srinivasan, S., Sabin, M., . . . Raitakari, O. (2012). A diagnosis of the metabolic syndrome in youth that resolves by adult life is associated with a normalization of high carotid intima-media thickness and type 2 diabetes mellitus risk: The Bogalusa heart and cardiovascular risk in young Finns studies. *Journal of the American College of Cardiology, 60*(17), 1631-1639.

Maher, C., Crettenden, A., Evans, K., Thiessen, M., Toohey, M., Watson, A., & Dollman, J. (2015). Fatigue is a major issue for children and adolescents with physical disabilities. *Developmental Medicine & Child Neurology, 57*(8), 742-747.

Marson, E., Delevatti, R., Prado, A., Netto, N., & Kruel, L. (2016). Effects of aerobic, resistance, and combined exercise training on insulin resistance markers in overweight or obese children and adolescents: A systematic review and meta-analysis. *Preventive Medicine, 93*, 211-218.

Mayer-Davis, E., Lawrence, J., Dabelea, D., Divers, J., Isom, S., Dolan, L., . . . SEARCH for Diabetes in Youth Study. (2017). Incidence trends of type 1 and type 2 diabetes among youths, 2002-2012. *New England Journal of Medicine, 376*(15), 1419-1429.

McMahon, S., Ferreira, L., Ratnam, N., Davey, R., Youngs, L., Davis, E., . . . Jones, T. (2007). Glucose requirements to maintain euglycemia after moderate-intensity afternoon exercise in adolescents with type 1 diabetes are increased in a biphasic manner. *Journal of Clinical Endocrinology and Metabolism, 92*(3), 963-968.

McMurray, R.G., Harrell, J.S., Creighton, D., Wang, Z., & Bangdiwala, S.I. (2008). Influence of physical activity on change in weight status as children become adolescents. *International Journal of Pediatric Obesity, 3*(2), 69-77.

Michaud, I., Henderson, M., Legault, L., & Mathieu, M. (2017). Physical activity and sedentary behavior levels in children and adolescents with type 1 diabetes using insulin pump or injection therapy: The importance of parental activity profile. *Journal of Diabetes and Its Complications, 31*(2), 381-386.

Molis, M., & Molis, W. (2010). Exercise-induced bronchospasm. *Sports Health, 2*(4), 311-317.

Moore, G., Durstein, J., & Painter, P. (2016). *ACSM's exercise management for persons with chronic diseases and disabilities* (4th ed.). Champaign, IL: Human Kinetics.

Mtshali, B., Mokwena, K., & Oguntibeju, O. (2015). Effect of submaximal warm-up exercise on exercise-induced asthma in African school children. *West Indian Medical Journal, 64*(2), 117-125.

Murphy, N., Carbone, P., & American Academy of Pediatrics Council on Children With Disabilities. (2008). Promoting the participation of children with disabilities in sports, recreation, and physical activities. *Pediatrics, 121*(5), 1057-1061.

Myśliwiec, A., & Damentko, M. (2015). Global initiative of the Special Olympics movement for people with intellectual disabilities. *Journal of Human Kinetics, 45*(7), 253-259.

Nadeau, K., Anderson, B., Berg, E., Chiang, J., Chou, H., Copeland, K., . . . Zeitler, P. (2016). Youth-onset type 2 diabetes consensus report: Current status, challenges, and priorities. *Diabetes Care, 39*(9), 1635-1642.

Narasimhan, S., & Weinstock, R. (2014). Youth-onset type 2 diabetes mellitus: Lessons learned from the TODAY study. *Mayo Clinic Proceedings, 89*(6), 806-816. doi:10.1016/j.mayocp.2014.01.009

National Association for Sport and Physical Education. (2011). *Physical education for lifelong fitness* (3rd ed.). Champaign, IL: Human Kinetics.

National Heart, Lung, and Blood Institute & National Asthma Education and Prevention Program. (2007). *Expert panel report 3: Guidelines for the diagnosis and management of asthma.* Bethesda, MD: U.S. Department of Health and Human Services, National Institutes of Health, National Heart, Lung, and Blood Institute.

National Institute for Health and Clinical Excellence. (2013). *NCE Quality Standards [QS25]: Asthma.* Manchester, UK: National Institute for Health and Clinical Excellence.

Nievas, I., & Anand, K. (2013). Severe acute asthma exacerbation in children: A stepwise approach for escalating therapy in a pediatric intensive care unit. *Journal of Pediatric Pharmacology Therapy, 18*(2), 88-104.

O'Brien, T., Noyes, J., Spencer, L., Kubis, H., Hastings, R., & Whitaker, R. (2016). Systematic review of physical activity and exercise interventions to improve health, fitness and well-being of children and young people who use wheelchairs. *BMJ Open Sport & Exercise Medicine, 2*(1), e000109.

Oppewal, A., Hilgenkamp, T., van Wijck, R., & Evenhuis, H. (2013). Cardiorespiratory fitness in individuals with intellectual disabilities—A review. *Research in Developmental Disabilities, 34*(10), 3301-3316.

Papas, M., Trabulsi, J., Axe, M., & Rimmer, J. (2016). Predictors of obesity in a US sample of high school adolescents with and without disabilities. *Journal of School Health, 86*(11), 803-812.

Philpott, J., Houghton, K., & Luke, A. (2010). Physical activity recommendations for children with specific chronic health conditions: Juvenile idiopathic arthritis, hemophilia, asthma and cystic fibrosis. *Paediatric Child Health, 15*(4), 213-225.

Pivovarov, J., Taplin, C., & Riddell, M. (2015). Current perspectives on physical activity and exercise for youth with diabetes. *Pediatric Diabetes, 16*(4), 242-255.

Poitras, V., Gray, C., Borghese, M., Carson, V., Chaput, J., Janssen, I., . . . Tremblay, M. (2016). Systematic review of the relationships between objectively measured physical activity and health indicators in school-aged children and youth. *Applied Physiology Nutrition and Metabolism, 41*, S197-S239.

Pulcini, C., Zima, B., Kelleher, K., & Houtrow, A. (2017). Poverty and trends in three common chronic disorders. *Pediatrics, 139*(3), e20162539.

Quirk, H., Blake, H., Tennyson, R., Randell, T., & Glazebrook, C. (2014). Physical activity interventions in children and young people with type 1 diabetes mellitus: A systematic review with meta-analysis. *Diabetic Medicine, 31*(10), 1163-1173.

Riddell, M., Gallen, I., Smart, C., Taplin, C., Adolfsson, P., Lumb, A., . . . Laffel, L. (2017). Exercise management in type 1 diabetes: A consensus statement. *Lancet Diabetes Endocrinology, 5*(5), 377-390.

Rimmer, J., & Marques, A. (2012). Physical activity for people with disabilities. *Lancet, 380*(9838), 193-195.

Riner, W., & Hunt Sellhorst, S. (2017). Physical activity and exercise in children with chronic health conditions. *Journal of Sport and Health Science, 2*, 12-20.

Roberts, A., & Taplin, C. (2015). Exercise in youth with type 1 diabetes. *Current Pediatric Reviews, 11*(2), 120-125.

Rustler, V., Hagerty, M., Daeggelmann, J., Marjerrison, S., Bloch, W., & Baumann, F. (2017). Exercise interventions for patients with pediatric cancer during inpatient acute care: A systematic review of literature. *Pediatric Blood and Cancer, 64*(11).

San Juan, A., Wolin, K., & Lucía, A. (2011). Physical activity and pediatric cancer survivorship. *Recent Results in Cancer Research, 186*, 319-347.

Savoye, M., Caprio, S., Dziura, J., Anne Camp, A., Greg Germain, G., Craig Summers, C., . . . Tamborlane, W. (2014). Reversal of early abnormalities in glucose metabolism in obese youth: Results of an intensive lifestyle randomized controlled trial. *Diabetes Care, 37*, 317–324.

Schalock, R., Borthwick-Duffy, S., Bradley, V., Buntix, W., Coulter, D., & Craig, E. (2010). *Intellectual disability: Definition, classification and systems of support* (11th ed.). Washington, DC: American Association on Intellectual and Developmental Disability.

Segal, M., Eliasziw, M., Phillips, S., Bandini, L., Curtin, C., Kral, T., . . . Must, A. (2016). Intellectual disability is associated with increased risk for obesity in a nationally representative sample of U.S. children. *Disability and Health Journal, 9*(3), 392-398.

Shields, N., & Synnot, A. (2016). Perceived barriers and facilitators to participation in physical activity for children with disability: A qualitative study. *BMC Pediatrics, 16*(9).

Shields, N., Synnot, A., & Kearns, C. (2015). The extent, context and experience of participation in out-of-school activities among children with disability. *Research in Developmental Disabilities, 47*, 165-174.

Sit, C., McKenzie, T., Cerin, E., Chow, B., Huang, W., & Yu, J. (2017). Physical activity and sedentary time among children with disabilities at school. *Medicine and Science in Sports and Exercise, 49*(2), 292-297.

Skoner, D. (2016). Inhaled corticosteroids: Effects on growth and bone health. *Annals of Allergy Asthma & Immunology, 117*(6), 595-600.

Special Olympics. (2019).Retrieved from www.specialolympics. org. accessed April 30, 2019.

Spruit, A., Assink, M., van Vugt, E., van der Put, C., & Stams, G. (2016). The effects of physical activity interventions on psychosocial outcomes in adolescents: A meta-analytic review. *Clinical Psychological Review, 45*(56-71).

Stickland, M., Rowe, B., Spooner, C., Vandermeer, B., & Dryden, D. (2013). Effect of warm-up exercise on exercise-induced bronchoconstriction. *Medicine and Science in Sports and Exercise, 44*(3), 383-391.

Stoner, L., Rowlands, D., Morrison, A., Credeur, D., Hamlin, M., Gaffney, K., . . . Matheson, A. (2016). Efficacy of exercise intervention for weight loss in overweight and obese adolescents: Meta-analysis and implications. *Sports Medicine, 46*(11), 1737-1751.

Sugimoto, D., Bowen, S., Meehan, W., & Stracciolini, A. (2016). Effects of neuromuscular training on children and young adults with Down Syndrome: Systematic review and meta-analysis. *Research in Developmental Disabilities*, 197-206.

Tremblay, M., Barnes, J., González, S., Katzmarzyk, P., Onywera, V., Reilly, J., . . . Global Matrix 2.0 Research Team. (2016). Global Matrix 2.0: Report card grades on the physical activity of children and youth comparing 38 countries. *Journal of Physical Activity and Health, 13*(Suppl 2), S343-S366.

Umpierre, D., Ribeiro, P., Kramer, C., Leitão, C., Zucatti, A., Azevedo, M., . . . Schaan, B. (2011). Physical activity advice only or structured exercise training and association with HbA1c levels in type 2 diabetes: A systematic review and meta-analysis. *Journal of the American Medical Association, 305*(17), 1709-1799.

U.S. Department of Health and Human Services. (2016). *Healthy people 2020. Physical activity objectives.* Retrieved from www.healthypeople.gov/2020/topics-objectives

Uzark, K., King, E., Cripe, L., Spicer R, Sage, J., Kinnett, K., . . . Varni, J. (2012). Health-related quality of life in children and adolescents with Duchenne muscular dystrophy. *Pediatrics, 130*(6), e1559-1566.

Van Cleave, J., Gortmaker, S., & Perrin, J. (2010). Dynamics of obesity and chronic health conditions among children and youth. *Journal of the American Medical Association, 303*(7), 623-630.

van den Driessen Mareeuw, F., Hollegien, M., Coppus, A., Delnoij, D., & de Vries, E. (2017). In search of quality indicators for Down syndrome healthcare: A scoping review. *BMC Health Services Research, 17*(1), 284.

Vanlancker, T., Schaubroeck, E., Vyncke, K., Cadenas-Sanchez, C., Breidenassel, C., González-Gross, M., . . . HELENA project group. (2017). Comparison of definitions for the metabolic syndrome in adolescents. The HELENA study. *European Journal of Pediatrics, 176*(2), 241-252.

Verschuren, O., Peterson, M., Balemans, A., & Hurvitz, E. (2016). Exercise and physical activity recommendations for people with cerebral palsy. *Developmental Medicine & Child Neurology, 58*(8), 798-808.

Viner, R., White, B., & Christie, D. (2017). Type 2 diabetes in adolescents: A severe phenotype posing major clinical challenges and public health burden. *Lancet, 389*(10085), 2252-2260.

Wanrooij, V., Willeboordse, M., Dompeling, E., & van de Kant, K. (2014). Exercise training in children with asthma: A systematic review. *British Journal of Sports Medicine, 48*(13), 1024-1031.

Westergren, T., Fegran, L., Nilsen, T., Haraldstad, K., Kittang, O., & Berntsen, S. (2016). Active play exercise intervention in children with asthma: A pilot study. *BMJ Open, 6*(1), e009721.

Wiart, L., Darrah, J., Kelly, M., & Legg, D. (2015). Community fitness programs: What is available for children and youth with motor disabilities and what do parents want? *Physical and Occupational Therapy in Pediatrics, 35*(1), 73-87.

Willeboordse, M., van de Kant, K., van der Velden, C., van Schayck, C., & Dompeling, E. (2016). Associations between asthma, overweight and physical activity in children: A cross-sectional study. *BMC Public Health, 16*, 919.

Winn, C., Mackintosh, K., Eddolls, W., Stratton, G., Wilson, A., Rance, J., . . . Davies, G. (2018). Perceptions of asthma and exercise in adolescents with and without asthma. *Journal of Asthma.* 55(8): 868-876 doi: 10.1080/02770903.2017.1369992

Wouters, M, Evenhuis, H, Hilgenkamp, T. (2019). Physical fitness of children and adolescents with moderate to severe intellectual disabilities. *Disability and Rehabilitation.* doi: 10.1080/09638288.2019.1573932

World Health Organization. (2001). *The international classification of functioning, disability and health.* Geneva, Switzerland: Author.

World Health Organization. (2018). *Global action plan on physical activity 2018-2030: More active people for a healthier world.* Geneva, Switzerland: Author.

Wright A, Roberts R, Bowman G, A. (2018). Barriers and facilitators to physical activity participation for children with physical disability: comparing and contrasting the views of children, young people, and their clinicians. *Disability and Rehabilitation.* doi: 10.1080/09638288.2018.1432702

Wu, W., Yang, Y., Chu, I., Hsu, H., Tsai, F., & Liang, J. (2017). Effectiveness of a cross-circuit exercise training program in improving the fitness of overweight or obese adolescents with intellectual disability enrolled in special education schools. *Research in Developmental Disabilities, 60*, 83-95.

Yang, Z., Scott, C., Mao, C., Tang, J., & Farmer, A. (2014). Resistance exercise versus aerobic exercise for type 2 diabetes: A systematic review and meta-analysis. *Sports Medicine, 44*(4), 487-499.

Yawn, B., Rank, M., Cabana, M., Wollan, P., & Juhn, Y. (2016). Adherence to asthma guidelines in children, tweens, and adults in primary care settings: A practice-based network assessment. *Mayo Clinical Proceedings, 91*(4), 411-421.

Zeitler, P., Hirst, K., Pyle, L., Linder, B., Copeland, K., Arslanian, S., . . . Kaufman, F. (2012). A clinical trial to maintain glycemic control in youth with type 2 diabetes. *New England Journal of Medicine, 366*(24), 2247-2256.

Zwinkels, M., Verschuren, O., Balemans, A., Lankhorst, K., Te Velde, S., van Gaalen, L., . . . Takken, T. (2018). Effects of a school-based sports program on physical fitness, physical activity, and cardiometabolic health in youth with physical disabilities: Data from the Sport-2-Stay-Fit Study. *Frontiers in Pediatrics, 6*, 75.

Zwinkels, M, Verschuren, O, de Groot, J, Backx, F, Wittink, H, Visser-Meily, A, Takken, T. Sport-2-Stay-Fit study group. (2019). Effects of high-intensity interval training on fitness and health in youth with physical disabilities. *Pediatric Physical Therapy.* 31(1): 84-93

Chapter 16 Nutrition for Youth

Adolphus, K., Lawton, C.L., & Dye, L. (2013). The effects of breakfast on behavior and academic performance in children and adolescents. *Frontiers in Human Neuroscience, 7*, 425.

Alaimo, K., Olson, C.M., & Frongillo, E.A., Jr. (2001). Food insufficiency and American school-aged children's cognitive, academic, and psychosocial development. *Pediatrics, 108*(1), 44-53.

Alves, C., & Lima, R.V. (2009). Dietary supplement use by adolescents. *Journal of Pediatrics (Rio J), 85*(4), 287-294.

American Academy of Pediatrics. (2011). Clinical report: Sports drinks and energy drinks for children and adolescents: are they appropriate? *Pediatrics, 127*(6), 1182-1189.

American Diabetes Association. (2000). Type 2 diabetes in children and adolescents. *Pediatrics, 105*(3 Pt 1), 671-680.

Amiel, S.A., Sherwin, R.S., Simonson, D.C., Lauritano, A.A., & Tamborlane, W.V. (1986). Impaired insulin action in puberty. A contributing factor to poor glycemic control in adolescents with diabetes. *New England Journal of Medicine, 315*(4), 215-219.

Arnaoutis, G., Kavouras, S.A., Angelopoulou, A., Skoulariki, C., Bismpikou, S., Mourtakos, S., & Sidossis, L.S. (2015). Fluid balance during training in elite young athletes of different sports. *Journal of Strength and Conditioning Research, 29*(12), 3447-3452.

Astrup, A., Dyerberg, J., Elwood, P., Hermansen, K., Hu, F.B., Jakobsen, M.U., . . . Willett, W.C. (2011). The role of reducing intakes of saturated fat in the prevention of cardiovascular disease: Where does the evidence stand in 2010? *American Journal of Clinical Nutrition, 93*(4), 684-688.

Atkinson, F.S., Foster-Powell, K., & Brand-Miller, J.C. (2008). International tables of glycemic index and glycemic load values: 2008. *Diabetes Care, 31*(12), 2281-2283.

Bachrach, L.K. (2001). Acquisition of optimal bone mass in childhood and adolescence. *Trends in endocrinology and metabolism, 12*(1), 22-28.

Backhouse, S.H., Whitaker, L., & Petroczi, A. (2013). Gateway to doping? Supplement use in the context of preferred competitive situations, doping attitude, beliefs, and norms. *Scandinavian Journal of Medicine & Science in Sports, 23*(2), 244-252.

Bailey, D.A., Faulkner, R.A., & McKay, H.A. (1996). Growth, physical activity, and bone mineral acquisition. *Exercise and Sport Sciences Reviews, 24*, 233-266.

Bailey, R.L., Gahche, J.J., Thomas, P.R., & Dwyer, J.T. (2013). Why US children use dietary supplements. *Pediatric Research, 74*(6), 737-741.

Baker, S.S., Cochran, W.J., Flores, C.A., Georgieff, M.K., Jacobson, M.S., Jaksic, T., & Krebs, N.F. (1999). Calcium requirements of infants, children, and adolescents. *Pediatrics, 104*(5 Pt 1), 1152-1157.

Barclay, A.W., Petocz, P., McMillan-Price, J., Flood, V.M., Prvan, T., Mitchell, P., & Brand-Miller, J.C. (2008). Glycemic index, glycemic load, and chronic disease risk-—Meta-analysis of observational studies. *American Journal of Clinical Nutrition, 87*(3), 627-637.

Bell, A., Dorsch, K.D., McCreary, D.R., & Hovey, R. (2004). A look at nutritional supplement use in adolescents. *Journal of Adolescent Health, 34*(6), 508-516.

Bernadot, D., Schwarz, M., & Heller, D.W. (1989). Nutrient intake in young, highly competitive gymnasts. *Journal of American Dietetic Association, 3*, 401.

Birch, L.L., Johnson, S.L., Andresen, G., Peters, J.C., & Schulte, M.C. (1991). The variability of young children's energy intake. *New England Journal of Medicine, 324*(4), 232-235.

Bourre, J.M. (2006a). Effects of nutrients (in food) on the structure and function of the nervous system: Update on dietary requirements for brain. Part 1: Micronutrients. *Journal of Nutrition, Health & Aging, 10*(5), 377-385.

Bourre, J.M. (2006b). Effects of nutrients (in food) on the structure and function of the nervous system: update on dietary requirements for brain. Part 2: Macronutrients. *Journal of Nutrition, Health & Aging, 10*(5), 386-399.

Brandao-Neto, J., Stefan, V., Mendonca, B.B., Bloise, W., Ana Valeria, B., & Castro, M.D. (1995). The essential role of zinc in growth. *Nutrition Research, 15*(3), 335-358.

Branum, A.M., & Rossen, L.M. (2014). The contribution of mixed dishes to vegetable intake among US children and adolescents. *Public Health Nutrition, 17*(9), 2053-2060.

Briefel, R.R., Bialostosky, K., Kennedy-Stephenson, J., McDowell, M.A., Ervin, R.B., & Wright, J.D. (2000). Zinc intake of the U.S. population: Findings from the third National Health and Nutrition Examination Survey, 1988-1994. *Journal of Nutrition, 130*(5S Suppl), 1367S-1373S.

Caballero, B. (2007). The global epidemic of obesity: An overview. *Epidemiologic Reviews, 29*, 1-5.

Canadian Paediatric Society. (2004). Dieting in adolescence. *Paediatrics & Child Health, 9*(7), 487-503.

Centers for Disease Control and Prevention. (2011). School health guidelines to promote healthy eating and physical activity. *Morbidity and Mortality Weekly Report, 60*(5), 1-75.

Centers for Disease Control and Prevention. (2016). *High sodium intake in children and adolescents: Cause for concern*: Retrieved from www.cdc.gov/salt/pdfs/children_sodium.pdf

Cohen, J.F., Gorski, M.T., Gruber, S.A., Kurdziel, L.B., & Rimm, E.B. (2016). The effect of healthy dietary consumption on executive cognitive functioning in children and adolescents: A systematic review. *British Journal of Nutrition, 116*(6), 989-1000.

Constantini, N.W., Arieli, R., Chodick, G., & Dubnov-Raz, G. (2010). High prevalence of vitamin D insufficiency in athletes and dancers. *Clinical Journal of Sport Medicine, 20*(5), 368-371.

Croll, J.K., Neumark-Sztainer, D., Story, M., Wall, M., Perry, C., & Harnack, L. (2006). Adolescents involved in weight-related and power team sports have better eating patterns and nutrient intakes than non-sport-involved adolescents. *Journal of the American Dietetic Association, 106*(5), 709-717.

Cupisti, A., D'Alessandro, C., Castrogiovanni, S., Barale, A., & Morelli, E. (2002). Nutrition knowledge and dietary composition in Italian adolescent female athletes and non-athletes. *International Journal of Sport Nutrition and Exercise Metabolism, 12*(2), 207-219.

Dabelea, D., Lawrence, J.M., Pihoker, C., Dolan, L., D'Agostino, R.B., Jr., Marcovina, S., . . . SEARCH for Diabetes in Youth Study. (2014). Re: "Prevalence of diagnosed and undiagnosed type 2 diabetes mellitus among US adolescents: Results from the continuous NHANES, 1999-2010." *American Journal of Epidemiology, 179*(3), 396-397.

Dehghan, M., Mente, A., Zhang, X., Swaminathan, S., Li, W., Mohan, V., . . . Prospective Urban Rural Epidemiology Study Investigators. (2017). Associations of fats and carbohydrate intake with cardiovascular disease and mortality in 18 countries from five continents (PURE): A prospective cohort study. *Lancet, 390*(10107), 2050-2062.

Desbrow, B., McCormack, J., Burke, L.M., Cox, G.R., Fallon, K., Hislop, M., . . . Leveritt, M. (2014). Sports Dietitians Australia position statement: Sports nutrition for the adolescent athlete. *International Journal of Sport Nutrition and Exercise Metabolism, 24*(5), 570-584.

Escobar, K.A., McLain, T.A., & Kerksick, C.M. (2016). Protein needs of young athletes. In C.M. Kerksick & E. Fox (Eds.), *Sports nutrition needs for child and adolescent athletes* (pp. 59-76). Washington, DC: CRC Press.

Evans, M.W., Jr., Ndetan, H., Perko, M., Williams, R., & Walker, C. (2012). Dietary supplement use by children and adolescents in the United States to enhance sport performance: Results of the National Health Interview Survey. *Journal of Primary Prevention, 33*(1), 3-12.

Fajcsak, Z., Gabor, A., Kovacs, V., & Martos, E. (2008). The effects of 6-week low glycemic load diet based on low glycemic index foods in overweight/obese children—Pilot study *Journal of the American College of Nutrition, 27*(1), 12-21.

Fink, H.F., Mikesky, A.E., & Burgoon, L.A. (2012). *Practical applications in sports nutrition.* Burlington, MA: Jones & Bartlett Learning.

Florence, M.D., Asbridge, M., & Veugelers, P.J. (2008). Diet quality and academic performance. *Journal of School Health, 78*(4), 209-215.

Fogelholm, M. (2013). New Nordic nutrition recommendations are here. *Food & Nutrition Research, 57*.

Foster-Powell, K., Holt, S.H., & Brand-Miller, J.C. (2002). International table of glycemic index and glycemic load values: 2002. *American Journal of Clinical Nutrition, 76*(1), 5-56.

Fox, E., & Kerksick, C.M. (2016). Sport nutrition and youth. In C.M. Kerksick & E. Fox (Eds.), *Sports nutrition needs for child and adolescent athletes* (pp. 3-16). Boca Raton, FL: CRC Press.

Fox, E.A., McDaniel, J.L., Breitbach, A.P., & Weiss, E.P. (2011). Perceived protein needs and measured protein intake in collegiate male athletes: An observational study. *Journal of the International Society of Sports Nutrition, 8,* 9.

Fung, T.T., Hu, F.B., Pereira, M.A., Liu, S., Stampfer, M.J., Colditz, G.A., & Willett, W.C. (2002). Whole-grain intake and the risk of type 2 diabetes: A prospective study in men. *American Journal of Clinical Nutrition, 76*(3), 535-540.

Galemore, C.A. (2011). Sports drinks and energy drinks for children and adolescents—Are they appropriate? A summary of the clinical report. *NASN School Nurse, 26*(5), 320-321.

Geiker, N.R.W., Hansen, M., Jakobsen, J., Kristensen, M., Larsen, R., Jorgensen, N.R., . . . Bugel, S. (2017). Vitamin D status and muscle function among adolescent and young swimmers. *International Journal of Sport Nutrition and Exercise Metabolism, 27*(5), 399-407.

Gibson, J.C., Stuart-Hill, L., Martin, S., & Gaul, C. (2011). Nutrition status of junior elite Canadian female soccer athletes. *International Journal of Sport Nutrition and Exercise Metabolism, 21*(6), 507-514.

Gidding, S.S., Dennison, B.A., Birch, L.L., Daniels, S.R., Gillman, M.W., Lichtenstein, A.H., . . . American Academy of Pediatrics. (2005). Dietary recommendations for children and adolescents: A guide for practitioners: Consensus statement from the American Heart Association. *Circulation, 112*(13), 2061-2075.

Goran, M.I., & Gower, B.A. (2001). Longitudinal study on pubertal insulin resistance. *Diabetes, 50*(11), 2444-2450.

Grantham-McGregor, S., & Ani, C. (2001). A review of studies on the effect of iron deficiency on cognitive development in children. *Journal of Nutrition, 131*(2S-2), 649S-666S.

Greer, F.R., Krebs, N.F., & American Academy of Pediatrics Committee on Nutrition. (2006). Optimizing bone health and calcium intakes of infants, children, and adolescents. *Pediatrics, 117*(2), 578-585.

Grimes, C.A., Riddell, L.J., Campbell, K.J., Beckford, K., Baxter, J.R., He, F.J., & Nowson, C.A. (2017). Dietary intake and sources of sodium and potassium among Australian schoolchildren: Results from the cross-sectional Salt and Other Nutrients in Children (SONIC) study. *BMJ Open, 7*(10), e016639.

He, F.J., & MacGregor, G.A. (2006). Importance of salt in determining blood pressure in children: Meta-analysis of controlled trials. *Hypertension, 48*(5), 861-869.

Herriman, M., Fletcher, L., Tchaconas, A., Adesman, A., & Milanaik, R. (2017). Dietary supplements and young teens: Misinformation and access provided by retailers. *Pediatrics, 139*(2).

Hess, J., & Slavin, J. (2014). Snacking for a cause: Nutritional insufficiencies and excesses of U.S. children, a critical review of food consumption patterns and macronutrient and micronutrient intake of U.S. children. *Nutrients, 6*(11), 4750-4759.

Heyman, M.B., Abrams, S.A., Section on Gastroenterology, Hepatology, and Nutrition, & Committee on Nutrition. (2017). Fruit juice in infants, children, and adolescents: Current recommendations. *Pediatrics, 139*(6).

Hildebrandt, T., Harty, S., & Langenbucher, J.W. (2012). Fitness supplements as a gateway substance for anabolic-androgenic steroid use. *Psychology of Addictive Behaviors, 26*(4), 955-962.

Hill, J.O., Wyatt, H.R., & Peters, J.C. (2012). Energy balance and obesity. *Circulation, 126*(1), 126-132.

Hoch, A.Z., Goossen, K., & Kretschmer, T. (2008). Nutritional requirements of the child and teenage athlete. *Physical Medicine and Rehabilitation Clinics of North America, 19*(2), 373-398.

Holick, M.F., Binkley, N.C., Bischoff-Ferrari, H.A., Gordon, C.M., Hanley, D.A., Heaney, R.P., . . . Endocrine Society. (2011). Evaluation, treatment, and prevention of vitamin D deficiency: An Endocrine Society clinical practice guideline. *Journal of Clinical Endocrinology and Metabolism, 96*(7), 1911-1930.

Imamura, F., O'Connor, L., Ye, Z., Mursu, J., Hayashino, Y., Bhupathiraju, S.N., & Forouhi, N.G. (2016). Consumption of sugar sweetened beverages, artificially sweetened beverages, and fruit juice and incidence of type 2 diabetes: Systematic review, meta-analysis, and estimation of population attributable fraction. *British Journal of Sports Medicine, 50*(8), 496-504.

Institute of Medicine. (2001). *Dietary reference intakes for vitamin A, vitamin K, arsenic, boron, chromium, copper, iodine, iron, manganese, molybdenum, nike, silicon, vanadium, and zinc.* Washington, DC: National Academies Press.

Institute of Medicine. (2004). *Dietary reference intakes for water, potassium, sodium, chloride, and sulfate.* Washington, DC: National Academies Press.

Institute of Medicine. (2005). *Dietary reference intakes for energy, carbohydrate, fiber, fat, fatty acids, cholesterol, protein, and amino acids.* Washington, DC: National Academies Press.

Institute of Medicine. (2010). *Report brief: Dietary reference intakes or calcium and vitamin D.* Washington, DC: National Academy of Sciences.

International Zinc Nutrition Consultative Group. (2004). International Zinc Nutrition Consultative Group (IZiNCG) technical document #1. Assessment of the risk of zinc deficiency in populations and options for its control. *Food and Nutrition Bulletin, 25*(1 Suppl 2), S99-S203.

Jager, R., Kerksick, C.M., Campbell, B.I., Cribb, P.J., Wells, S.D., Skwiat, T.M., . . . Antonio, J. (2017). International Society of Sports Nutrition position stand: Protein and exercise. *Journal of the International Society of Sports Nutrition, 14,* 20.

Kaganov, B., Caroli, M., Mazur, A., Singhal, A., & Vania, A. (2015). Suboptimal micronutrient intake among children in Europe. *Nutrients, 7*(5), 3524-3535.

Kalkwarf, H.J., Khoury, J.C., & Lanphear, B.P. (2003). Milk intake during childhood and adolescence, adult bone density, and osteoporotic fractures in US women. *American Journal of Clinical Nutrition, 77*(1), 257-265.

Keast, R.S.J., & Breslin, P.A.S. (2003). An overview of binary taste-taste interactions. *Food Quality and Preference, 14*(2), 111-124.

Kenney, E.L., Long, M.W., Cradock, A.L., & Gortmaker, S.L. (2015). Prevalence of inadequate hydration among US children and disparities by gender and race/ethnicity: National health and nutrition examination survey, 2009-2012. *American Journal of Public Health, 105*(8), e113-118.

Kenney, W.L., & Chiu, P. (2001). Influence of age on thirst and fluid intake. *Medicine and Science in Sports and Exercise, 33*(9), 1524-1532.

Keskin, M., Kurtoglu, S., Kendirci, M., Atabek, M.E., & Yazici, C. (2005). Homeostasis model assessment is more reliable than the fasting glucose/insulin ratio and quantitative insulin sensitivity check index for assessing insulin resistance among obese children and adolescents. *Pediatrics, 115*(4), e500-503.

Kit, B.K., Carroll, M.D., & Ogden, C.L. (2011). Low-fat milk consumption among children and adolescents in the United States, 2007-2008. *NCHS Data Brief*(75), 1-8.

Koehler, K., Braun, H., Achtzehn, S., Hildebrand, U., Predel, H.G., Mester, J., & Schanzer, W. (2012). Iron status in elite young athletes: Gender-dependent influences of diet and exercise. *European Journal of Applied Physiology, 112*(2), 513-523.

Kurpad, A.V., Muthayya, S., & Vaz, M. (2005). Consequences of inadequate food energy and negative energy balance in humans. *Public Health Nutrition, 8*(7A), 1053-1076.

LaBotz, M., Griesemer, B.A., & Council on Sports Medicine and Fitness. (2016). Use of performance-enhancing substances. *Pediatrics, 138*(1).

Larson, N., Dewolfe, J., Story, M., & Neumark-Sztainer, D. (2014). Adolescent consumption of sports and energy drinks: Linkages to higher physical activity, unhealthy beverage patterns, cigarette smoking, and screen media use. *Journal of Nutrition Education and Behavior, 46*(3), 181-187.

Leites, G.T., & Meyer, F. (2016). The importance of proper fluid and hydration. In C.M. Kerksick & E. Fox (Eds.), *Sports nutrition for child and adolescent athletes* (pp. 113-133). Washington, DC: CRC Press.

Lipek, T., Igel, U., Gausche, R., Kiess, W., & Grande, G. (2015). Obesogenic environments: Environmental approaches to obesity prevention. *Journal of Pediatric Endocrinology & Metabolism, 28*(5-6), 485-495.

Lozoff, B., Beard, J., Connor, J., Barbara, F., Georgieff, M., & Schallert, T. (2006). Long-lasting neural and behavioral effects of iron deficiency in infancy. *Nutrition Reviews, 64*(5 Pt 2), S34-S43.

Luger, M., Lafontan, M., Bes-Rastrollo, M., Winzer, E., Yumuk, V., & Farpour-Lambert, N. (2017). Sugar-sweetened beverages and weight gain in children and adults: A systematic review from 2013 to 2015 and a comparison with previous studies. *Obesity Facts, 10*(6), 674-693.

Lustig, R.H., Mulligan, K., Noworolski, S.M., Tai, V.W., Wen, M.J., Erkin-Cakmak, A., . . . Schwarz, J.M. (2016). Isocaloric fructose restriction and metabolic improvement in children with obesity and metabolic syndrome. *Obesity (Silver Spring), 24*(2), 453-460.

Malina, R.M., Bouchard, C., & Bar-Or, O. (2004). *Growth, maturation and physical activity* Champaign, IL: Human Kinetics.

Mangieri, H. (2017). *Fueling young athletes.* Champaign, IL: Human Kinetics.

McDaniel, J., & Fox, E. (2016). How to fuel your day. In C.M. Kerksick & E. Fox (Eds.), *Sports nutrition for child and adolescent athletes.* Washington, DC: CRC Press.

McGill, C.R., Fulgoni, V.L., 3rd, & Devareddy, L. (2015). Ten-year trends in fiber and whole grain intakes and food sources for the United States population: National Health and Nutrition Examination Survey 2001-2010. *Nutrients, 7*(2), 1119-1130.

McLain, T.A., & Conn, C.A. (2016). Fat needs. In C.M. Kerksick & E. Fox (Eds.), *Sports nutrition needs for child and adolescent athletes* (pp. 77-98). Washington, DC: CRC Press.

Mensink, R.P., Zock, P.L., Kester, A.D., & Katan, M.B. (2003). Effects of dietary fatty acids and carbohydrates on the ratio of serum total to HDL cholesterol and on serum lipids and apolipoproteins: A meta-analysis of 60 controlled trials. *American Journal of Clinical Nutrition, 77*(5), 1146-1155.

Mesias, M., Seiquer, I., & Navarro, M.P. (2011). Calcium nutrition in adolescence. *Critical Reviews in Food Science and Nutrition, 51*(3), 195-209.

Morgan, D. (2017). Children and adolescents: Birth to 17 years old. In B. Bushman (Ed.), *American College of Sports Medicine Complete Guide to Fitness and Health* (pp. 207-227). Champaign, IL: Human Kinetics

Movassagh, E.Z., Baxter-Jones, A.D.G., Kontulainen, S., Whiting, S.J., & Vatanparast, H. (2017). Tracking dietary patterns over 20 Years from childhood through adolescence into young adulthood: The Saskatchewan pediatric bone mineral accrual study. *Nutrients, 9*(9).

Mozaffarian, D., Katan, M.B., Ascherio, A., Stampfer, M.J., & Willett, W.C. (2006). Trans fatty acids and cardiovascular disease. *New England Journal of Medicine, 354*(15), 1601-1613.

Mozaffarian, D., Micha, R., & Wallace, S. (2010). Effects on coronary heart disease of increasing polyunsaturated fat in place of saturated fat: A systematic review and meta-analysis of randomized controlled trials. *PLoS Medicine, 7*(3), e1000252.

Murphy, M.M., Douglass, J.S., Johnson, R.K., & Spence, L.A. (2008). Drinking flavored or plain milk is positively associated with nutrient intake and is not associated with adverse effects on weight status in US children and adolescents. *Journal of the American Dietetic Association, 108*(4), 631-639.

Nawrot, P., Jordan, S., Eastwood, J., Rotstein, J., Hugenholtz, A., & Feeley, M. (2003). Effects of caffeine on human health. *Food Additives and Contaminants, 20*(1), 1-30.

Nead, K.G., Halterman, J.S., Kaczorowski, J.M., Auinger, P., & Weitzman, M. (2004). Overweight children and adolescents: A risk group for iron deficiency. *Pediatrics, 114*(1), 104-108.

Nordic Council of Ministers. (2014). *Nordic nutritional recommendations 2012, integrating nutrition and physical activity.* Copenhagen: Nordic Council of Ministers.

Norton, L.E., Wilson, G.J., Layman, D.K., Moulton, C.J., & Garlick, P.J. (2012). Leucine content of dietary proteins is a determinant of postprandial skeletal muscle protein synthesis in adult rats. *Nutrition & Metabolism, 9*(1), 67.

Ogden, C.L., Carroll, M.D., Lawman, H.G., Fryar, C.D., Kruszon-Moran, D., Kit, B.K., & Flegal, K.M. (2016). Trends in obesity prevalence among children and adolescents in the United States, 1988-1994 through 2013-2014. *Journal of the American Medical Association, 315*(21), 2292-2299.

Papadopoulou, S.K., Papadopoulou, S.D., & Gallos, G.K. (2002). Macro- and micro-nutrient intake of adolescent Greek female volleyball players. *International Journal of Sport Nutrition and Exercise Metabolism, 12*(1), 73-80.

Parnell, J.A., Wiens, K.P., & Erdman, K.A. (2016). Dietary intakes and supplement use in pre-adolescent and adolescent Canadian athletes. *Nutrients, 8*(9).

Pekkinen, M., Viljakainen, H., Saarnio, E., Lamberg-Allardt, C., & Makitie, O. (2012). Vitamin D is a major determinant of bone mineral density at school age. *PLoS One, 7*(7), e40090.

Pereira, M.A., O'Reilly, E., Augustsson, K., Fraser, G.E., Goldbourt, U., Heitmann, B.L., . . . Ascherio, A. (2004). Dietary fiber and risk of coronary heart disease: A pooled analysis of cohort studies. *Archives of Internal Medicine, 164*(4), 370-376.

Petrie, H.J., Stover, E.A., & Horswill, C.A. (2004). Nutritional concerns for the child and adolescent competitor. *Nutrition, 20*(7-8), 620-631.

Petroczi, A., Naughton, D.P., Pearce, G., Bailey, R., Bloodworth, A., & McNamee, M. (2008). Nutritional supplement use by elite young UK athletes: Fallacies of advice regarding efficacy. *Journal of the International Society of Sports Nutrition, 5,* 22.

Picciano, M.F., Dwyer, J.T., Radimer, K.L., Wilson, D.H., Fisher, K.D., Thomas, P.R., . . . Marriott, B.M. (2007). Dietary supplement use among infants, children, and adolescents in the United States, 1999-2002. *Archives of Pediatrics & Adolescent Medicine, 161*(10), 978-985.

Pinhas-Hamiel, O., & Zeitler, P. (2007). Acute and chronic complications of type 2 diabetes mellitus in children and adolescents. *Lancet, 369*(9575), 1823-1831.

Poti, J.M., Slining, M.M., & Popkin, B.M. (2014). Where are kids getting their empty calories? Stores, schools, and fast-food restaurants each played an important role in empty calorie intake among US children during 2009-2010. *Journal of the Academy of Nutrition and Dietetics, 114*(6), 908-917.

Pritchett, K., Bishop, P., Pritchett, R., Green, M., & Katica, C. (2009). Acute effects of chocolate milk and a commercial recovery beverage on postexercise recovery indices and endurance cycling performance. *Applied Physiology, Nutrition, and Metabolism, 34*(6), 1017-1022.

Public Health England. (2016). *Government recommednations for energy and nutrients for males and females aged 1-18 yars and 19+ years*. London, UK: PHE Publications.

Purcell, L.K., & Canadian Paediatric Society Paediatric Sports and Exercise Medicine Section. (2013). Sport nutrition for young athletes. *Paediatrics & Child Health, 18*(4), 200-205.

Reinehr, T. (2013). Type 2 diabetes mellitus in children and adolescents. *World Journal of Diabetes, 4*(6), 270-281.

Rockett, H.R., Berkey, C.S., & Colditz, G.A. (2007). Comparison of a short food frequency questionnaire with the youth/adolescent questionnaire in the Growing Up Today Study. *International Journal of Pediatric Obesity, 2*(1), 31-39.

Rodriguez, N.R., DiMarco, N.M., Langley, S., American Dietetic, A., Dietitians of, C., American College of Sports Medicine, N., & Athletic, P. (2009). Position of the American Dietetic Association, Dietitians of Canada, and the American College of Sports Medicine: Nutrition and athletic performance. *Journal of the American Dietetic Association, 109*(3), 509-527.

Roemmich, J.N., & Sinning, W.E. (1997). Weight loss and wrestling training: Effects on nutrition, growth, maturation, body composition, and strength. *Journal of Applied Physiology, 82*(6), 1751-1759.

Rogol, A.D., Clark, P.A., & Roemmich, J.N. (2000). Growth and pubertal development in children and adolescents: Effects of diet and physical activity. *American Journal of Clinical Nutrition, 72*(2 Suppl), 521S-528S.

Ross, A.C., Manson, J.E., Abrams, S.A., Aloia, J.F., Brannon, P.M., Clinton, S.K., . . . Shapses, S.A. (2011). The 2011 report on dietary reference intakes for calcium and vitamin D from the Institute of Medicine: What clinicians need to know. *Journal of Clinical Endocrinology and Metabolism, 96*(1), 53-58.

Rouhani, M.H., Kelishadi, R., Hashemipour, M., Esmaillzadeh, A., & Azadbakht, L. (2013). The effect of an energy restricted low glycemic index diet on blood lipids, apolipoproteins and lipoprotein (a) among adolescent girls with excess weight: A randomized clinical trial. *Lipids, 48*(12), 1197-1205.

Sacks, F.M., Lichtenstein, A.H., Wu, J.H.Y., Appel, L.J., Creager, M.A., Kris-Etherton, P.M., . . . American Heart Association. (2017). Dietary fats and cardiovascular disease: A presidential advisory from the American Heart Association. *Circulation, 136*(3), e1-e23.

Savage, J.S., Peterson, J., Marini, M., Bordi, P.L., Jr., & Birch, L.L. (2013). The addition of a plain or herb-flavored reduced-fat dip is associated with improved preschoolers' intake of vegetables. *Journal of the Academy of Nutrition and Dietetics, 113*(8), 1090-1095.

Schoenfeld, B., & Aragon, A. (2016). Vitamin and mineral needs. In C.M. Kerksick & E. Fox (Eds.), *Sports nutrition needs for child and adolescent athletes* (pp. 99-112). Washington, DC: CRC Press.

Schulze, M.B., Liu, S., Rimm, E.B., Manson, J.E., Willett, W.C., & Hu, F.B. (2004). Glycemic index, glycemic load, and dietary fiber intake and incidence of type 2 diabetes in younger and middle-aged women. *American Journal of Clinical Nutrition, 80*(2), 348-356.

Seifert, S.M., Schaechter, J.L., Hershorin, E.R., & Lipshultz, S.E. (2011). Health effects of energy drinks on children, adolescents, and young adults. *Pediatrics, 127*(3), 511-528.

Semba, R.D., Shardell, M., Sakr Ashour, F.A., Moaddel, R., Trehan, I., Maleta, K.M., . . . Manary, M.J. (2016). Child stunting is associated with low circulating essential amino acids. *EBioMedicine, 6*, 246-252.

Serairi Beji, R., Megdiche Ksouri, W., Ben Ali, R., Saidi, O., Ksouri, R., & Jameleddine, S. (2016). Evaluation of nutritional status and body composition of young Tunisian weightlifters. *La Tunisie Medicale, 94*(2), 112-117.

Shaikh, U., Byrd, R.S., & Auinger, P. (2009). Vitamin and mineral supplement use by children and adolescents in the 1999-2004 National Health and Nutrition Examination Survey: Relationship with nutrition, food security, physical activity, and health care access. *Archives of Pediatrics & Adolescent Medicine, 163*(2), 150-157.

Shenkin, A. (2006). Micronutrients in health and disease. *Postgraduate Medical Journal, 82*(971), 559-567.

Simopoulos, A.P. (2002). The importance of the ratio of omega-6/omega-3 essential fatty acids. *Biomedicine & Pharmacotherapy, 56*(8), 365-379.

Spodaryk, K. (2002). Iron metabolism in boys involved in intensive physical training. *Physiology and Behavior, 75*(1-2), 201-206.

Sports Dietitians Australia. (2015). *Fuelling active kids: Junior swimmer, a guide for parents, coaches and team managers*: Retrieved from www.sportsdietitians.com.au/wp-content/uploads/2015/04/SDA_Junior-Swimmer_Web.pdf

St-Onge, M.P., Keller, K.L., & Heymsfield, S.B. (2003). Changes in childhood food consumption patterns: A cause for concern in light of increasing body weights. *American Journal of Clinical Nutrition, 78*(6), 1068-1073.

Story, M., & Stang, J. (2005). Nutrition needs of adolescents. In J. Stang & M. Story (Eds.), *Guidelines for adolescent nutrition services*. Minneapolis, MN: University of Minnesota, Centre for Leadership, Education and Training in Maternal and Child Nutrition, Division of Epidemiology and Community Health, School of Public Health.

Swinburn, B.A., Sacks, G., Hall, K.D., McPherson, K., Finegood, D.T., Moodie, M.L., & Gortmaker, S.L. (2011). The global obesity pandemic: Shaped by global drivers and local environments. *Lancet, 378*(9793), 804-814.

Te Morenga, L., & Montez, J.M. (2017). Health effects of saturated and trans-fatty acid intake in children and adolescents: Systematic review and meta-analysis. *PLoS One, 12*(11), e0186672.

Tipton, C.M., & Tcheng, T.K. (1970). Iowa wrestling study. Weight loss in high school students. *Journal of the American Medical Association, 214*(7), 1269-1274.

Trommelen, J., & van Loon, L.J. (2016). Pre-sleep protein ingestion to improve the skeletal muscle adaptive response to exercise training. *Nutrients, 8*(12).

U.S. Department of Agriculture. (2015). *2015-2020 Dietary Guidelines for Americans: 8th Edition.* Retrieved from http://health.gov/dietaryguidelines/2015/guidelines

van Vught, A.J., Heitmann, B.L., Nieuwenhuizen, A.G., Veldhorst, M.A., Brummer, R.J., & Westerterp-Plantenga, M.S. (2009). Association between dietary protein and change in body composition among children (EYHS). *Clinical Nutrition, 28*(6), 684-688.

Viner, R., White, B., & Christie, D. (2017). Type 2 diabetes in adolescents: A severe phenotype posing major clinical challenges and public health burden. *Lancet, 389*(10085), 2252-2260.

Visram, S., Cheetham, M., Riby, D.M., Crossley, S.J., & Lake, A.A. (2016). Consumption of energy drinks by children and young people: A rapid review examining evidence of physical effects and consumer attitudes. *BMJ Open, 6*(10), e010380.

Vos, M.B., Kaar, J.L., Welsh, J.A., Van Horn, L.V., Feig, D.I., Anderson, C.A.M., . . . Council on Hypertension. (2017). Added sugars and cardiovascular disease risk in children: A scientific statement from the American Heart Association. *Circulation, 135*(19), e1017-e1034.

Walsh, M., Cartwright, L., Corish, C., Sugrue, S., & Wood-Martin, R. (2011). The body composition, nutritional knowledge, attitudes, behaviors, and future education needs of senior schoolboy rugby players in Ireland. *International Journal of Sport Nutrition and Exercise Metabolism, 21*(5), 365-376.

Welsh, J.A., Sharma, A., Cunningham, S.A., & Vos, M.B. (2011). Consumption of added sugars and indicators of cardiovascular disease risk among US adolescents. *Circulation, 123*(3), 249-257.

Whitton, C., Nicholson, S.K., Roberts, C., Prynne, C.J., Pot, G.K., Olson, A., . . . Stephen, A.M. (2011). National Diet and Nutrition Survey: UK food consumption and nutrient intakes from the first year of the rolling programme and comparisons with previous surveys. *British Journal of Nutrition, 106*(12), 1899-1914.

World Health Organization. (2011). *Prevention of iron deficiency anaemia in adolescents.* New Delhi, India: Author.

World Health Organization. (2015). *Guideline: Sugars intake for adults and children.* Geneva, Switzerland: Author.

Yang, Q., Zhang, Z., Kuklina, E.V., Fang, J., Ayala, C., Hong, Y., . . . Merritt, R. (2012). Sodium intake and blood pressure among US children and adolescents. *Pediatrics, 130*(4), 611-619.

Zakrewski, J.K., & Tolfrey, K. (2016). Carbohyhdrate needs of the yound athlete. In C.M. Kerksick & E. Fox (Eds.), *Sports nutrition needs for child and adolescent athletes.* Washington, DC: CRC Press.

Ziegler, P.J., Khoo, C.S., Kris-Etherton, P.M., Jonnalagadda, S.S., Sherr, B., & Nelson, J.A. (1998). Nutritional status of nationally ranked junior US figure skaters. *Journal of the American Dietetic Association, 98*(7), 809-811.

INDEX

Note: The italicized *f* and *t* following page numbers refer to figures and tables, respectively.

Avery D. Faigenbaum, EdD, is a full professor in the department of health and exercise science at The College of New Jersey. His research interests focus on pediatric exercise science, resistance exercise, and preventive medicine, and he is devoted to bridging the gap between the laboratory and the playing field. As an active researcher and practitioner, Faigenbaum has coauthored over 250 peer-reviewed publications, 50 book chapters, and 10 books, including *Youth Strength Training, Strength and Power for Young Athletes,* and *Progressive Plyometrics for Kids.* He has been an invited speaker at more than 300 conferences throughout the world. Faigenbaum is a fellow of the American College of Sports Medicine (ACSM) and the National Strength and Conditioning Association (NSCA), and

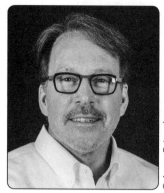

© Avery Faigenbaum

he serves as associate editor of *Pediatric Exercise Science* and the *Journal of Strength and Conditioning Research.* He was elected vice president of the NSCA in 2005 and served on the Massachusetts Governor's Committee on Physical Fitness and Sports from 1998 to 2004. Faigenbaum was awarded the Boyd Epley Award for Lifetime Achievement from the NSCA in 2017.

Rhodri S. Lloyd, PhD, is a reader in pediatric strength and conditioning and chair and co-founder of the Youth Physical Development Centre at Cardiff Metropolitan University. He also holds a research associate position with Auckland University of Technology. Lloyd's research interests surround the impact of growth and maturation on long-term athletic development and the neuromuscular mechanisms underpinning training adaptations in youth. To date he has published in excess of 100 peer-reviewed publications and more than 20 book chapters on the topics of youth fitness and pediatric strength and conditioning. He is a senior associate editor for the *Journal of Strength and Conditioning Research* and an associate editor for the *Strength and Conditioning Journal.* In 2016, he received the Strength

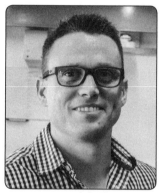

© Rhodri Lloyd

and Conditioning Coach of the Year award for research and education from the UK Strength and Conditioning Association, and in 2017 he was awarded the Terry J. Housh Outstanding Young Investigator Award from the National Strength and Conditioning Association (NSCA). In 2019, he was again recognized by the NSCA, receiving both the *Journal of Strength and Conditioning Research* Editorial Excellence Award and the Educator of the Year Award.

Jon L. Oliver, PhD, is a professor of applied pediatric exercise science at Cardiff Metropolitan University, where he cofounded the Youth Physical Development Centre. He is also an adjunct professor at the Sport Performance Research Institute New Zealand (SPRINZ). His research focuses on youth physical development across performance, injury, and health perspectives, with an emphasis on the role of strength and conditioning to promote athletic development at all levels. He has published over 100 international peer-reviewed articles, contributed to international position and consensus statements, and authored numerous book chapters. Oliver's research has been influential in informing both academics and practitioners on factors related to the development of physical fitness in youth. This

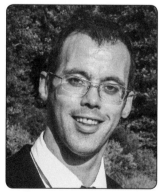

© Jon Oliver

has included developing coach education materials for professional sports organizations and national governing bodies. His research is supported by a network of research students and is built on collaborations with professional sports organizations and pediatric exercise scientists, both in the United Kingdom and in other countries.

ABOUT THE ACSM

The **American College of Sports Medicine (ACSM)**, founded in 1954, is the largest sports medicine and exercise science organization in the world. With more than 50,000 members and certified professionals worldwide, ACSM is dedicated to improving health through science, education, and medicine. ACSM members work in a wide range of medical specialties, allied health professions, and scientific disciplines.

Members are committed to the diagnosis, treatment, and prevention of sport-related injuries and the advancement of the science of exercise. The ACSM promotes and integrates scientific research, education, and practical applications of sports medicine and exercise science to maintain and enhance physical performance, fitness, health, and quality of life.

You read the book—now complete the companion CE exam to earn continuing education credit!

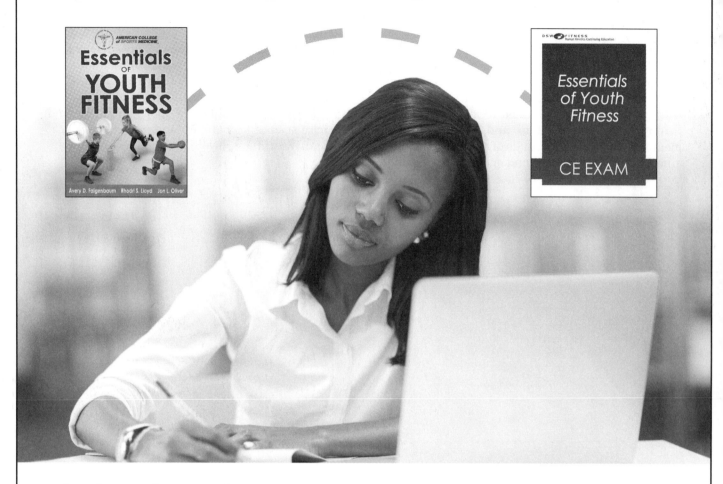

Find and purchase the companion CE exam here:
US.HumanKinetics.com/collections/CE-Exam
Canada.HumanKinetics.com/collections/CE-Exam
UK.HumanKinetics.com/collections/CE-Exam

50% off the companion CE exam with this code

EYF2020

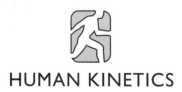

HUMAN KINETICS